An Introduction to
Clinical Neurology

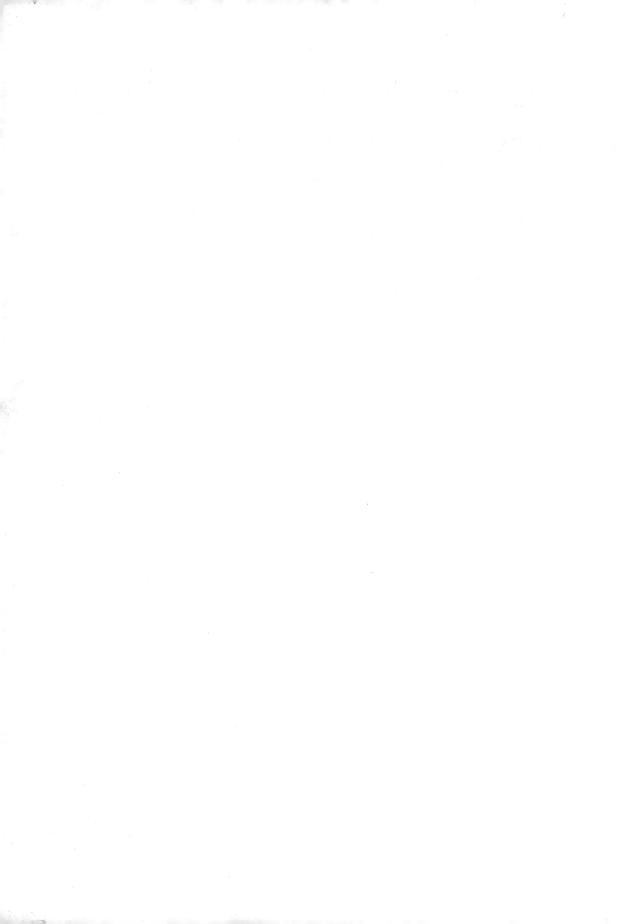

An Introduction to Clinical Neurology

Pathophysiology, Diagnosis, and Treatment

Alan Guberman, M.D., C.M., F.R.C.P.(C)
Associate Professor of Medicine (Neurology),
University of Ottawa Faculty of Medicine;
Staff Neurologist, Division of Neurology,
Ottawa General Hospital, Ottawa

Little, Brown and Company
Boston/New York/Toronto/London

Library of Congress Cataloging-in-Publication Data

Guberman, Alan.
    An introduction to clinical neurology : pathophysiology, diagnosis, and treatment / Alan Guberman.
        p.   cm.
    Includes bibliographical references and index.
    ISBN 0-316-33073-6
    1. Neurology.   2. Nervous system—Diseases.   I. Title.
    [DNLM: 1. Nervous System Diseases—physiopathology.
    2. Nervous System Diseases—diagnosis.   3. Nervous System
    Diseases—therapy.
    WL 100 G921i   1993]
    RC346.G83   1993
    616.8—dc20
    DNLM/DLC
    for Library of Congress   93-20527
                                                            CIP

Printed in the United States of America

MV-NY

Third Printing

Sponsoring Editor: Nancy Megley
Production Editor: Anne Holm
Copyeditor: Betty Notzon
Indexer: Alexandra Nickerson
Production Supervisors: F. David Bell and Louis C. Bruno, Jr.
Designer: F. David Bell
Cover Designers: Miriam Recio and Louis C. Bruno, Jr.

To my devoted wife, Solange, whose energy, inspiration, and constant support appear on every page, and to our children, Daniel and Liana, who give us untold happiness

Contents

Contributing Authors

Peter Humphreys, M.D., C.M., F.R.C.P.(C)
Associate Professor of Pediatrics,
University of Ottawa Faculty of Medicine;
Head, Division of Neurology,
Children's Hospital of Eastern Ontario, Ottawa
27. Inherited Metabolic and Developmental Disorders

Alex MacKenzie, M.D., Ph.D., F.R.C.P.(C)
Assistant Professor of Pediatrics,
University of Ottawa Faculty of Medicine;
Pediatric Molecular Geneticist,
Children's Hospital of Eastern Ontario, Ottawa
26. Molecular Genetic Aspects of Neurological Disease

Brian G. Weinshenker, M.D., F.R.C.P.(C)
Assistant Professor of Neurology,
Mayo Medical School;
Consultant in Neurology,
Mayo Clinic, Rochester, Minnesota
25. Multiple Sclerosis

Preface

My purpose in setting out to write *An Introduction to Clinical Neurology* was to offer a synthesis of the essentials of clinical neurology. In this day and age, with the enormous explosion of knowledge in basic and clinical neurological sciences, one person alone cannot possibly cover such a vast subject. Three of my expert colleagues have therefore kindly dealt with the areas of inherited metabolic and developmental disorders of childhood, molecular genetics, and neuroimmunology. The text is certainly stronger for their contributions.

I have endeavored throughout to provide a balanced account of neurology, combining a traditional clinical approach with an emphasis on pathophysiology and applied neurosciences. It is only through an increasing awareness of both types of knowledge at the bedside that we can provide optimal care for our patients. Therapeutics, which is becoming ever more important in neurology, has been attributed ample space in the book.

This work is intended for students of neurology at all levels: medical students, postgraduate trainees (particularly in areas other than neurology), non-neurologist practicing physicians, paramedical personnel, and basic neuroscientists who wish to have an overview of clinical neurology. Hopefully, the depth of coverage will permit undergraduate students to use the text as a reference source in their postgraduate years as well. The abundant references have been carefully selected and can serve to direct those so inclined toward further exploration.

Since this is primarily a textbook of adult neurology, except for the chapter on inherited metabolic and developmental disorders encountered both in adults and children, pediatric topics have been sparsely covered. In addition, the areas of neuroendocrinology and neuropsychiatry have not been dealt with separately.

I have attempted to impart the enthusiasm that those working in the clinical and basic neurosciences feel in this, the "Decade of the Brain." This sense of excitement is based on the realization that we are currently unravelling many mysteries of the human nervous system and the illnesses to which it is prone. Progress has been based on the application of powerful new molecular genetic and immunological techniques that have helped unearth the etiology of heretofore obscure conditions. Other innovations include the development of diagnostic tools such as positron emission tomography and magnetic resonance imaging, which have shed light on the structure and function of the living brain, and the utilization of pharmacological discoveries to devise effective new therapies for previously untreatable disorders.

An Introduction to Clinical Neurology is a book written for learners of neurology; it also reflects the challenges and insights that students have offered me, as a teacher, over the last two decades. I have been molded as a neurologist by dedicated, knowledgeable, and insightful masters. I hope this work passes on the torch, guiding each reader to new thresholds and levels of professional growth.

A.G.

Acknowledgments

I would like to express my heartfelt gratitude to the following colleagues for their invaluable advice and critical reading of various chapters: Dr. G. Garber, Dr. M. Hassan, Dr. J. Henderson, Dr. R. Hughes, Dr. J. Marsan, Dr. R. F. Nelson, and Dr. D. Zackon. I would also like to thank the following colleagues and co-workers who kindly contributed material for the figures: Dr. O. Benavente, Dr. R. Broughton, Dr. S. Grahovac, Dr. B. Lach, Dr. V. Montpetit, Dr. T. Picton, Dr. D. Ramsay, Dr. R. Wee, David Barker, and Jagdish Maru. I wish to express my appreciation to Emil Purgina for his excellent work in preparing original illustrations and to Zuzanna Purgina for her photographic assistance. My appreciation to Anne Holm, production editor at Little, Brown, for lending her linguistic expertise to the final text as well as Nancy Megley and the other editors at Little, Brown who have supported this project. I also wish to express a special thank you to my secretary, Claire Loyer, whose expert typing skills, patience, and diligence were called upon throughout the preparation of the manuscript.

An Introduction to
Clinical Neurology

Notice

The indications and dosages of all drugs in this book have been recommended in the medical literature and conform to the practices of the general medical community. The medications described do not necessarily have specific approval by the Food and Drug Administration for use in the diseases and dosages for which they are recommended. The package insert for each drug should be consulted for use and dosage as approved by the FDA. Because standards for usage change, it is advisable to keep abreast of revised recommendations, particularly those concerning new drugs.

Diagnosis and Decision-Making

UNIQUENESS OF NEUROLOGY

In neurology, the ability to elicit data directly from the patient through the process of history-taking and physical examination assumes particular importance. No matter how sophisticated laboratory tests become, careful bedside observation will remain the special tool of neurologists by which they gain firsthand information about the workings of the patient's nervous system and gather the basic data needed for the purposes of diagnostic, prognostic, and therapeutic decision-making. Carefully elicited and recorded signs and symptoms and the subsequent formulation of diagnostic possibilities allow the rational selection of appropriate tests from among an array of special tests now available—some costly and uncomfortable, and not without risk to the patient. Interpretation of laboratory and radiological results frequently depends on a detailed knowledge of the patient's clinical state. The decision to order urgent diagnostic tests or therapeutic measures in an acutely ill patient is often based on signs of neurological deterioration gleaned from serial bedside observations. The decision whether to continue a particular therapy often depends on changes revealed by the neurological examination. For these reasons, the neurological history and examination reign supreme in the practice of clinical neurology, and are likely to continue to do so.

Another distinctive feature of neurology is the close link between basic and clinical neurosciences. Neuroanatomical, neurophysiological, neuropharmacological, and neuropathological principles are considered in a clinical framework on a daily basis by the neurologist. It is only through a thorough understanding of pathophysiological principles that the complexities of a disordered nervous system and its symptomatic expressions can be unraveled. Although there are recurrent themes and patterns in neurological illness, the unexpected and unfamiliar are frequently encountered, even by experienced neurologists, and this requires ongoing consideration of basic pathophysiological principles.

THE NEUROLOGICAL DIAGNOSTIC PROCESS

Diagnosis in neurology is a two-part process: first localization and then establishment of the cause (etiology). In **localizing** a lesion, the topography of the lesion, or lesions, in the nervous system is determined in terms of the **level** of involvement and the **systems** affected. **Type localization** involves identifying whether the lesion is unifocal, multifocal, diffuse, or confined to a system, or a combination of these. Determining whether the lesion involves the neuraxis, and its coverings and vasculature directly, or whether it lies primarily outside the nervous system in neighboring structures (e.g., sinuses, pituitary gland, or vertebral bodies) is also part of the process. Attempting to localize the lesion or delineate the process involved also helps determine whether the patient's problem is psychogenic rather than primarily neurological, as many "functional" disorders have inconsistent or "nonanatomical" features. Data for localization are derived mainly from the neurological examination, and to a lesser extent from the patient's history.

Once localization has been tentatively accomplished, the second part of the neurological diagnostic process, establishment of **etiology,** can be attempted. The reason for localizing first is that once the location of the lesion in the nervous system is known, it is much easier to determine its nature. Localization helps limit the etiological possibilities. Historical details such as the patient's age, acuteness of onset of the disease, family history, and so on, provide further important clues to the etiology. Confirmation of both the location and the cause of the lesion frequently depends on radiological, electrophysiological, and other special laboratory tests. The main levels and types of localization, manifestations pointing to involvement of specific systems, and general etiological categories are listed in Tables 1-1 to 1-4.

The step from clinical examination to neuroanatomical localization requires a knowledge of (1) tools that reliably elicit signs and symptoms from the patient (i.e., the neurological history and examination) and (2) the typical signs and

Table 1-1. Topographical Localization (Level)

Supratentorial
    Cranial nerves I and II
    Cerebral hemispheres
Posterior fossa (infratentorial)
    Brainstem
    Cranial nerves III–XII
    Cerebellum
Spinal cord
Peripheral
    Anterior horn cells
    Spinal nerve roots and ganglia
    Plexuses
    Nerves
    Neuromuscular junction
    Muscle

Table 1-2. Type Localization

Focal (right, left, midline)
Multifocal
Diffuse
Confined to a system
Combination of the above

Table 1-3. Systems in Neurological Diagnosis

Cerebrospinal fluid and brain coverings
Consciousness system
Sensory system
Motor system
Autonomic system
Vascular system

Table 1-4. Etiological Categories in Neurological Diagnosis

Genetic
Congenital–developmental
Metabolic
Degenerative
Toxic–nutritional
Infectious
Immunological–demyelinating
Vascular
Neoplastic
Traumatic
Psychogenic

symptoms of lesions of the nervous system involving various levels and systems (i.e., functional neuroanatomy and neurophysiology). These signs and symptoms, along with their most important localizing significance, are listed in Tables 1-5 and 1-6. The next step— the transition from neuroanatomical localization to diagnosis of the cause—is based on (1) a knowledge of which causes are most likely to give rise to lesions at a given location; (2) historical data; and (3) confirmation by appropriate laboratory and special tests.

MANAGEMENT VERSUS TREATMENT

The goal of the physician must be to help ease the physical, psychological, and socioeconomic burden of illness whenever possible. In illnesses for which there is no specific therapy, as in many neurological disorders, the skills of the physician in **managing** the patient's overall condition are put to the test. In certain cases, this may consist only of offering a precise diagnosis

and prognosis, thereby alleviating the patient's anxiety stemming from his or her perception that the physician will not be able to "find out what's wrong." A definite diagnosis may also spare the patient further discomfort, expense, and even danger as he or she consults one physician after another in an effort to seek a diagnosis or perhaps recklessly pursues "experimental" treatments. With many of the degenerative diseases, multiple sclerosis, stroke, and brain tumor, the role of the physician and health-care team is often limited to providing emotional support; prescribing symptomatic treatment for complaints such as pain, urinary incontinence, or spasticity; or recommending appropriate physiotherapy and rehabilitation facilities. Although these measures cannot cure and may not halt the underlying disease process, the patient's quality of life may benefit immeasurably from their use. It is by understanding the importance of proper management in these cases that the health-care worker can maintain a positive attitude when faced with chronically debilitating, incurable, and at times fatal neurological illness.

Table 1-5. Main Signs and Symptoms Attributable to Disease at Various Levels of the Nervous System

Supratentorial	Posterior fossa	Spinal	Peripheral
Delirium	Loss of consciousness	Low back or neck pain	Distal symmetrical sensory loss and/or weakness
Dementia	Vertigo	Radicular pain	
Mental retardation	Diplopia	Weakness (upper motor neuron or lower motor neuron segmental)	Sensory loss or weakness conforming to a root or peripheral nerve distribution
Memory loss	Facial numbness		
Language disorders (aphasia)	Gaze disturbances	Changes in deep tendon reflexes	
	Facial weakness		Muscle atrophy
Agnosia	Hearing loss	Sensory level	Fasciculations
Apraxia	Dysarthria	Segmental sensory loss	Reduced deep tendon reflexes
Seizures	Dysphagia	Dissociated sensory loss	
Gaze disturbances	Ataxia	Bladder symptoms	
Hemianopsia	Nystagmus	Scoliosis	
Hemiplegia (especially affecting mainly arm and face)	Palatal myoclonus		
	Bilateral motor or sensory findings		
Monocular blindness	Hemiplegia		
Hemisensory loss	Hemisensory loss		
Cortical sensory loss			
Loss of smell (anosmia)			

Table 1-6. Main Signs and Symptoms Attributable to Disease of Various Systems of the Nervous System

CSF	Consciousness	Sensory	Motor	Autonomic	Vascular
Headache	Stupor	Pain	Upper motor neuron	Sleep and temperature regulation disturbances	Neurological signs conform to vascular distribution
Neck stiffness	Coma	Paresthesias	Pseudobulbar syndrome	Orthostatic hypotension	Bruit over neck or head
Kernig's sign	Syncope	Sensory loss (cortical or primary) in extremities	Weakness	Pupillary abnormalities	Headache
Papilledema	Seizures	Ataxia	Spasticity	Bladder and bowel disturbances	Alterations in pulses about head and neck
Hydrocephalus	Delerium–confusion	Diminished deep tendon reflexes	Increased deep tendon reflexes	Cardiac arrhythmias	
	Narcolepsy	Vertigo	Reduced superficial reflexes	Sweating disturbances	
		Loss of vision	Babinski's sign	Impotence	
		Loss of hearing	Flexor spasms		
			Lower motor neuron		
			Weakness		
			Atrophy		
			Hypotonia		
			Fasciculations		
			Reduced deep tendon reflexes		
			Cramps		
			Myotonia		
			Other		
			Involuntary movement (choreoathetosis, dystonias, myoclonus)		
			Rigidity		
			Tremor		
			Ataxia		

DECISION-MAKING ANALYSIS

In neurology, as in all of medicine, complex diagnostic and therapeutic decisions are often reached on the basis of incomplete data and are accompanied by a relative degree of uncertainty. Medical decision analysis utilizes quantitative and objectively based methods in place of the intuitive clinical reasoning usually employed to solve clinical problems. Neurology is an area that lends itself to decision analysis, as there are numerous areas of controversy in which decision-making can be facilitated by a more quantitative approach. In this section two aspects of decision analysis will be briefly discussed: calculation of post-test probability and use of decision trees to select appropriate therapy.

Probability

To determine probability, a 2 × 2 table can be constructed that characterizes the performance of a particular test in a specific disease state (Table 1-7). In this table, *TP* represents the number of **true positives**, or those patients who have the disease and a positive test result. *FN* represents the number of **false negatives**, or those patients with the disease but a negative test result. *FP* stands for **false positives**, patients who do not have the disease in question but have a positive test result. *TN* stands for **true negatives**, patients who do not have the disease in question and show a negative test result.

Specificity and Sensitivity

The most important measures of the usefulness of a particular test (or clinical sign) are its speci-

Table 1-7. A 2 × 2 Table Relating Test Results to Disease Status in a Population

Test results	Disease status	
	D+	D−
T+	TP	FP
T−	FN	TN

T = test; D = disease; TP, FP = true positive, false positive; TN, FN = true negative, false negative.

ficity and **sensitivity**. The sensitivity of a test is defined as the proportion of patients with the disease who show a positive test result or: $\frac{TP}{TP + FN}$. Specificity is defined as the proportion of patients without the disease who show a negative test result or $\frac{TN}{FP + TN}$. Another useful measure is the **false-positive rate**, which is equal to 1 − specificity. Specificities and sensitivities have been studied for various tests used in neurology. For example, the presence of oligoclonal bands in patients with active multiple sclerosis has a sensitivity of 90 percent, which is relatively high, but a specificity of approximately 80 percent because oligoclonal bands are also encountered in a number of other conditions such as central nervous system sarcoidosis, lupus, and syphilis.

When evaluating the published sensitivities and specificities for various tests, it is important to take note of certain biases introduced because the values are based on specific characteristics of the particular patient population in which the test parameters were determined. For example, the derived sensitivities and specificities are markedly influenced by whether a basically healthy or diseased population was studied. In addition, the characteristics of the practitioner's own particular patient population and the experience of local laboratories must be taken into consideration when using published test parameters.

Another factor that influences sensitivity and specificity is the cutoff point chosen for a particular test result. For most tests (except "gold standard" tests that are used to define a disease state), there is a numerical value or range of values that defines normality and abnormality for that particular test. If the continuum of test result values is plotted for those patients with and without the disease in question, the two curves will usually overlap. Selection of a high cutoff point to exclude virtually all patients who do not have the disease and have low test values will translate into few false positives and therefore a high specificity. Conversely, a greater number of patients with the disease will be deemed normal, thereby increasing the number of false negatives and reducing the sensitivity of the test. A highly sensitive test is most useful in screening large populations for the disease, but a highly specific, and oftentimes more expensive, test is most useful to confirm a diagnosis. In this situation, it is important to keep the false-positive rate low.

Two other useful measures of test performance are the positive and negative predictive values. PV(+), or the **positive predictive value**, equals $\dfrac{TP}{TP + FP}$, that proportion of all patients with a positive test result who actually have the disease. PV(−), or the **negative predictive value**, equals $\dfrac{TN}{TN + FN}$, the proportion of all patients with a negative test result who actually do not have the disease.

Using the defined test parameters and estimates of the *a priori* probability of a particular disease in a given patient, it is possible to calculate whether a positive or negative test result will change the likelihood of a particular diagnosis. Such calculations will help the clinician decide if a particular test is worth doing, both in terms of whether it will significantly alter the likelihood of a particular diagnosis and how a positive or negative result should change the clinical diagnostic impression.

Bayes' Theorem

Bayes' theorem is used in the following manner to calculate post-test probabilities *(p)*, with *D* referring to the disease and *T* to the test result:

$$p\,(D+/T+) = \frac{p\,(T+/D+) \times p\,(D+)}{\begin{array}{c}p\,(T+/D+) \times p\,(D+) \,+\\ p\,(T+/D-) \times p\,(D-)\end{array}}$$

$p\,(D+/T+)$ = Probability of the disease being present, given a positive test result

$p\,(D+)$ = The *a priori* probability of disease in the patient, which is usually equal to the estimated prevalence of the disease in the practitioner's particular patient population

$p\,(D-)$ = *A priori* probability of non-disease in the population = $1 - p\,(D+)$

$p\,(T+/D+)$ = The sensitivity of the test (i.e., proportion of patients with the disease who test positive)

$p\,(T+/D-)$ = The false-positive rate (i.e., probability of a positive test result in patients without the disease)

Nomograms or computer programs permit much quicker calculation of post-test probabilities using pre-test probabilities and likelihood ratios for a particular test. The **positive likelihood ratio** is defined as the sensitivity (i.e., true-positive rate) divided by the false-positive rate.

Bayes' theorem can also be used to calculate the probability of disease if a test result is negative, as follows:

$$p\,(D+/T-) = \frac{p\,(T-/D+) \times p\,(D+)}{\begin{array}{c}p\,(T-/D+) \times p\,(D+) \,+\\ p\,(T-/D-) \times p\,(D-)\end{array}}$$

where

$p\,(T-/D+)$ = The false-negative rate = $1 -$ sensitivity, and

$p\,(T-/D-)$ = The true-negative rate = specificity

The following will illustrate the application of Bayes' theorem. A patient is seen who has spells that resemble complex partial seizures, and the likelihood of epilepsy, based on a 1 percent overall prevalence and only mildly suggestive clinical description of the spells, is judged to be 20 percent. Standard electroencephalography (EEG), which has a sensitivity of 80 percent and specificity of 95 percent, is performed to look for interictal epileptiform features. Utilizing Bayes' theorem, the post-test probabilities can be calculated for positive and negative test results, as follows:

$$p\,(D+/T+) = \frac{(0.8)(0.2)}{(0.8)(0.2) + (0.05)(0.8)} = 0.80$$

$$p\,(D+/T-) = \frac{(0.2)(0.2)}{(0.2)(0.2) + (0.95)(0.8)} = 0.05$$

In other words, a positive EEG increases the probability of epilepsy to 80 percent in this patient and will likely surpass the **treatment threshold**, leading to a recommendation for therapy. A negative EEG will very likely be the deciding factor in a decision not to treat.

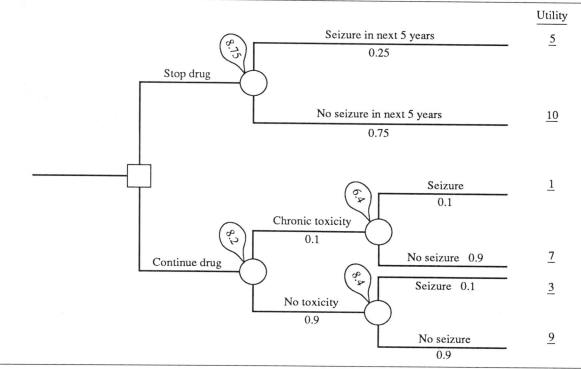

Utility

Seizure in next 5 years — 5
0.25

Stop drug — 8.75

No seizure in next 5 years — 10
0.75

Continue drug — 8.2

Chronic toxicity 0.1 — 6.4
Seizure 0.1 — 1
No seizure 0.9 — 7

No toxicity 0.9 — 8.4
Seizure 0.1 — 3
No seizure 0.9 — 9

Fig. 1-1. *Decision tree applied in determining whether to continue or stop anticonvulsant drugs. Adjustments to the utility values in the outcomes for the bottom four terminal branches were made to take into account a reduction in the quality of life resulting from chronic drug toxicity plus the inconvenience and expense of taking long-term medication. In assigning a utility value of 5 to seizure recurrence, this took into account the fact that the patient was a policeman and would likely lose his job if he had any further seizures.*

One of the most important conclusions made apparent by this method is that the post-test probability depends on the pre-test probability; the diagnostic usefulness of a particular test cannot be considered separately from the estimated prevalence of the disease in the particular population involved. Many tests are most useful when the *a priori* probability of disease falls in the intermediate range, neither too low nor too high. For example, if clinically it is 98 percent certain that a patient has polymyositis, performance of a muscle biopsy, which has a relatively low sensitivity (i.e., fairly high chance of missing the lesions), will not significantly alter the likelihood of the diagnosis or the decision to treat. There may, however, be reasons to perform the test in a particular case, other than to guide the decision to treat.

Decision Trees

Decision trees are a means of representing schematically the step-by-step sequential thinking and choices involved in reaching a particular decision. This technique clarifies the various assumptions and uncertainties attending each step of the decision-making process, compares the various choices in quantitative terms, and assesses the impact on the decision-making process when one or more of the assigned variables in the equation (sensitivity analysis) are altered. The decision tree consists of a series of **chance nodes** (circles), leading to branches where probabilities are assigned, and **choice nodes** (squares), representing the possible decisions. The probabilities assigned to the branches to the right of a chance node must add up to 1, since they represent all the possible outcomes and are mutually exclusive.

A **relative utility value** that corresponds to the various outcomes is assigned at the end of each branch of the decision tree. Assigning utilities is a somewhat arbitrary and difficult part of the analysis. It must take into account the particular preferences and characteristics of the patient. Utilities may be specified in terms of quality-adjusted years of survival, or arbitrary utility units may be assigned in which 0 stands for the worse possible outcome (often death) and 1, the best possible outcome. When the decision analysis is used to examine cost effectiveness, utilities may also be expressed in terms of the dollars spent per additional year of life saved. Once utilities are assigned for the various outcomes, the **expected values** of each of the alternatives are calculated using the process of **averaging out and folding back**, working from the right side to the left side of the tree.

Following is an example of the use of a deci-sion tree. A policeman who has had a single seizure has been on drug treatment for a year. His physician must now decide whether to dis-continue the anticonvulsant medications. A simple decision tree can be constructed, as fol-lows (Fig. 1-1). If the assumptions about seizure recurrence are correct, the analysis indicates a slight advantage to stopping treatment (8.75 versus 8.2). However, if the probability of sei-zure recurrence while off treatment is 0.4 in-stead of 0.25, the conclusion of the analysis favors continuance of therapy (8.2 versus 8).

BIBLIOGRAPHY

Sox, H.C., Jr., et al. *Medical Decision Making.* Boston: Butterworths, 1988.

Koprowski, C.D., Longstreth, W.T., Jr., and Cebul, R.D. Clinical neuroepidemiology. III: Decisions. *Arch. Neurol.* 46:223–229, 1989.

Examination and History-Taking

HISTORY-TAKING

In no area of medicine are the principles of good history-taking more important than in neurology. A carefully obtained initial history, supplemented, if necessary, by information acquired at later sessions, will frequently direct the appropriate selection of special tests and the formulation of a definite diagnosis. This is all the more true in the practice of neurology because, in most cases, the patient with neurological symptoms has normal examination findings. The history-taking also yields valuable clues about the etiology and, to a lesser extent, the localization of the process.

The neurological patient with impaired brain function who is perhaps suffering from dementia, anosognosia, aphasia, or periodic loss of consciousness may not be able to provide a reliable or comprehensible history. It is then necessary to interview the patient's family or contacts. Even when a patient seems lucid and reliable, family members may frequently provide new insights into the patient's condition.

Avoiding Suggestion

The principles of good history-taking also apply to the neurological interview. One begins by listening to the patient tell his or her story, interrupting only for the purposes of clarification or amplification. The importance of not leading the patient cannot be overemphasized. For example, an examiner who is considering a diagnosis of classic migraine in a patient whose complaint is headaches may be tempted to ask: "Do you ever see little flashing lights or zigzag lines off to one side which last for about 15 minutes prior to your headache?" After some reflection, the patient may answer: "Yes, I've had that." However, the significance of this information is dubious because it may be based more on the patient's desire to come up with the "right answers" than on the actual features of the illness. It would have been much better not to directly suggest these symptoms to the patient but to have approached the subject indirectly, as follows:

Interviewer: "Do you have any other symptoms around the time of your headaches?"

Patient:	"I usually get irritable."
Interviewer:	"What about your eyes?"
Patient:	"They burn and sometimes the light bothers me."
Interviewer:	"Do you ever see anything unusual or does your vision change?"
Patient:	"That reminds me—sometimes I see bright spots in my right eye before the headache starts."

This information, spontaneously offered by the patient, can be given credence in making a diagnosis. However, no matter how objective and nondirective an interviewer may be, because neurological patients have frequently seen several physicians, they may describe symptoms that have been previously suggested to them. This must be kept in mind when questioning such patients.

Testing Hypotheses

Besides listening to the reason for consultation or admission to hospital (chief complaint) and hearing the patient's story from beginning to end, a good interviewer must select and weigh the importance of the data, focusing on significant features and ignoring irrelevant details. As the history unfolds and new information revealed, the interviewer should be constantly formulating possible diagnoses and composing critical questions to elicit further relevant information. For example, when confronted with a patient who has experienced the subacute onset of weakness in the hands and feet, it would be important to ask whether the patient makes lead glass as a hobby or whether he or she has ever had wine-colored urine. This would not be an obvious line of questioning unless one recognizes the possibility of an acute motor neuropathy and knows its causes (e.g., lead poisoning and porphyria). At the completion of the history-taking, one or more diagnostic possibilities should be under consideration, to be later verified during the physical examination. These clinical skills require the knowledge and judgment which can be acquired only through experience.

The Interview as an Examination

Because history-taking is an opportunity to observe the patient's nervous system in action, the interview is also the initial step in the neurological examination. By noting the patient's general appearance, his or her gait when walking into the room, the speech, gestures, eye movements, facial expression, and movements, as well as the workings of memory, attention, and intellect, valuable data are obtained under spontaneous and informal conditions that may be more revealing than the information gained during the formal neurological examination. The interviewer should also keep in mind from the outset that patients form their initial impression of the physician during the history-taking. Ultimate rapport with the patient will depend on how successfully the physician demonstrates a concerned, caring attitude and competence in dealing with the patient's problems. Gaining the patient's confidence and establishing rapport may determine whether the patient will later agree, for example, to undergo an uncomfortable test such as angiography or take anticonvulsant medication four times a day for several years.

Recording Data in Concrete Terms

Neurological complaints should be quantified or translated into specific terms whenever possible. For example, if a patient complains of weakness in the upper extremities, it is useful to determine its proximal or distal distribution by finding out if the patient has difficulty turning a key in a lock, opening a jar, holding heavy pots, lifting heavy objects onto a high shelf, or holding the arms elevated to do up the hair or shave. If the patient complains of diplopia, it is important to know whether the two images are side-by-side or vertically separated, whether they are farther apart with any particular direction or gaze, whether the diplopia is relieved by covering one eye, whether the complaint is constant or occurs sporadically in attacks of a specific duration, and whether the symptom tends to appear as the day advances or with fatigue. It is important to know if a patient with gait difficulty can walk up only one flight of stairs before having to pause due to leg weakness. Vague terms such as *numbness* and *dizziness* must be explained in the recorded history.

Details regarding the patient's ability to perform specific tasks at work or to engage in previously enjoyed leisure activities and sports are often revealing. Old photographs may reveal that a problem such as ptosis, muscle atrophy, or facial asymmetry is long-standing. When information is recorded in a precise and concrete manner, this allows subsequent assessment of the progression of the illness.

Recurrent Episodes

A situation requiring special history-taking techniques, frequently encountered in neurology, is recurrent attacks of one sort or another. Headaches, dizzy spells, epileptic seizures, speech difficulty, visual loss, diplopia, hemiparesis, and hemisensory loss are merely some of the symptoms that can occur as discrete attacks. The following line of questioning should be pursued in each instance:

1. Detailed description and circumstances of the first attack
2. Description of the typical attack and variations; are they stereotyped?
3. Duration
4. Frequency and temporal profile (e.g., daily? weekly? monthly? occurring in clusters? most recent?)
5. Evolution (e.g., are they increasing or decreasing in frequency or severity?)
6. Specific circumstances of their occurrence or precipitating factors (e.g., related to emotional upset? menstrual cycle? meals? exercise? specific movements?)
7. Relieving factors (e.g., cold cloth on the forehead, aspirin, lying down and resting)
8. Accompanying symptoms

The responses to this questioning frequently point toward a definitive diagnosis and they assume special importance when there are no physical findings and test results are negative. When a patient has more than one episodic complaint, such as dizziness, headaches, and loss of consciousness, it is also necessary to determine how often various permutations and combinations of the complaints occur. Although this is often a time-consuming task, there is no substitute for it and both the patient and physician may be spared much frustration through its rigorous application.

Some Areas of Emphasis

The family history is important, particularly in the practice of pediatric neurology, because of the many hereditary neurological conditions. It is not sufficient to ask merely: "Is there any problem like this in your family?" The patient's memory may need to be jogged by direct inquiry about each family member. The parent of a patient with migraine or epilepsy may have had similar complaints earlier in his or her life of which the patient is unaware. The patient and other family members may not report a particular neurological deficit, such as the gait ataxia seen in spinocerebellar degeneration, because it is so commonplace in family members that it ceases to be considered abnormal. Families may also conceal a neurological illness because it is perceived as a stigma. When the interviewer suspects a hereditary illness, it is therefore mandatory to examine family members personally. Family photographs may also provide useful data in the context of conditions such as muscular dystrophy or certain movement disorders.

The patient should always be asked about a history of hypertension, heart disease, diabetes mellitus, head trauma, alcohol or drug abuse, and exposure to toxins. In addition, a patient's sexual history must be discreetly elicited when the myriad neurological complications of AIDS are under consideration. All of these conditions are frequently associated with neurological disease. A detailed history of medication use, including oral contraceptives and over-the-counter preparations, should also be obtained in view of the high incidence of iatrogenic neurological symptoms or illness.

Certain features of history-taking should be stressed depending on the age of the patient. In children or adolescents, gestational and developmental history as well as infectious illness or reactions to immunizations early in life may be important. Questions bearing on generalized vascular and cardiac disease are often appropriate in elderly patients.

The Neurological Functional Inquiry

If not already covered, every patient with neurological complaints should be directly asked about each of the following symptoms:

1. Loss of intellectual abilities, memory problems, concentration difficulties, change in personality, depression, and loss of drive
2. Headache
3. Convulsive seizures, loss of consciousness
4. Dizziness or vertigo
5. Loss or blurring of vision (monocular or other), diplopia
6. Loss of hearing, tinnitus
7. Incoordination or gait difficulty
8. Speech difficulties
9. Dysphagia
10. Weakness, involuntary movements
11. Paresthesias, sensory loss, pain
12. Urinary difficulties, impotence
13. Sleep difficulties (insomnia, hypersomnia)

THE PHYSICAL AND NEUROLOGICAL EXAMINATION

Further history-taking may become necessary as findings are unearthed during the formal neurological examination. There are various schemes for the neurological examination, but, more important than the approach itself, is its consistent and fixed use, so that the examiner becomes familiar and comfortable with it. It is not necessary to follow a strict neuroanatomically based order and shortcuts can be taken for the sake of efficiency. For example, once the flashlight is taken out, pupillary responses and palatal elevation can be examined sequentially. In the same way, sensation can be tested over the body and face together. However, irrespective of the order of the examination, findings should always be recorded in a formal and consistent fashion. Most of the examination can be done with the patient sitting, but the recumbent position is used for testing the plantar re-

sponses, abdominal reflexes, and muscle tone in the lower extremities. The six-part scheme outlined later in this chapter starts with the head region and moves down, and includes many traditional elements.

The interpretation of signs in neurology depends on the examiner's having a definite concept of what is normal, including both the normal range of responses and age-related variations in the results of various neurological tests. This knowledge can be gained only through application of the same techniques to a large number of patients. Heavy reliance is also placed on differences between sides (assuming one side is normal) or comparison with the examiner's ability (e.g., for strength or visual field testing).

A complete examination may take a few hours in difficult cases but only about 10 minutes in a neurologically healthy and cooperative patient. The depth of the examination and use of more specialized bedside procedures (e.g., complete aphasia testing) must be governed by the nature of the problem at hand. If either the examiner or patient is fatigued, this may influence the findings. Therefore, rather than unduly prolonging a difficult examination, it should either be completed in a reasonable time or equivocal findings checked at a later session.

The patient's comfort must be taken into account at all times. A room that is too cold or a manner that is too stern and mechanical may make the patient uncooperative and destroy rapport. The patient should be forewarned about the discomfort from testing the corneal, gag, and plantar reflexes as well as pinprick sensation.

Instrumentation

The following instruments should be readily accessible for a full neurological examination:

1. Ophthalmoscope for funduscopy and an otoscope for examining the ear canal and eardrum
2. Stethoscope for auscultating the heart, neck vessels, and cranium
3. Flashlight for testing pupillary responses and examining the palate

4. Substances such as coffee, soap, tobacco, or peppermint for testing smell
5. Tape measure for measuring head and muscle circumference
6. Reflex hammer (preferably with a long handle and heavy head)
7. Cotton or tissue to test the corneal reflex and touch perception
8. Tongue depressor for testing the gag reflex
9. 128-Hz tuning fork for testing vibratory sensation
10. Safety pin for testing pain sensation and the abdominal reflexes
11. Several small objects such as a key, bolt, paper clip, and coin for testing stereognosis
12. Glass tubes to fill with hot and cold water for testing temperature sensation

Optional equipment includes calipers and a ruler for testing two-point discrimination, a pinwheel for pain testing, a red glass for the cover test, a 256-Hz tuning fork for more sensitive vibration testing (e.g., the Weber and Rinne tests), and small sticks or blocks for testing constructional ability.

The General Physical Examination

Before undertaking the formal neurological examination, a general physical examination should be done with particular attention to areas frequently showing abnormalities associated with neurological disease.

Skull

An abnormally sized skull often indicates an underlying developmental brain abnormality. The skull circumference should be measured in its largest frontooccipital dimension. In adults, the frontooccipital circumference (FOC) normally ranges from 53 to 59 cm in males and 51 to 58 cm in females. In children, the FOC should be plotted on the standard graphs relating FOC to age that can be found in most pediatrics textbooks. A small head (<50 cm in adults) occurs with microcephaly. A large head in adults (>62 cm) is seen in patients with hydrocephalus, Paget's disease, or megalencephaly (a congenitally large brain). Additional causes in children

consist of subdural hematomas or effusions, various childhood metabolic (e.g., Tay-Sachs) and degenerative (e.g., Alexander's and Canavan's) diseases that cause the brain to enlarge, subgaleal effusions following trauma, and diseases such as osteopetrosis, which cause increased thickness of the cranial vault.

The **shape of the skull** should be examined as well. Premature fusion of the sutures (craniosynostosis) brings about an abnormally shaped skull that may be elongated when the sagittal suture is involved (dolichocephaly) or broadened and foreshortened with a high forehead when the coronal suture is affected (brachycephaly). Plagiocephaly consists of asymmetry of the skull with flattening on one side. Localized bulges arise as the result of early life lesions such as subarachnoid or porencephalic cysts and may also be seen in patients with large superficial tumors such as meningiomas or osteomas of the cranial vault.

The **cranium** should also be examined for the presence of visible and palpable defects that may sometimes by hidden by scalp hair. This may reveal sinuses connecting to the subarachnoid space, encephaloceles, burrholes or scars indicating previous head trauma or intracranial surgery, skull metastases, a large meningioma eroding the skull or producing hyperostosis, and multiple myeloma involving the calvaria. Palpation of the frontal and maxillary sinuses, to detect tenderness, is carried out in patients with headache or facial pain who may have sinusitis.

Auscultation should be done with the stethoscope over the mastoids, temporal bones, and the orbits. In the last instance, this can best be accomplished by placing a pediatric bell on the stethoscope and asking the patient first to close the eyes and then to try and hold them open to silence the sound produced by blinking. Intracranial bruits stemming from arteriovenous malformations, large aneurysms, or very vascular tumors can be detected in this manner. Benign intracranial bruits may be found in the presence of fever or anemia and are not uncommon in children.

Neck

The neck is examined with regard to its appearance and mobility. An abnormally short neck may be seen in patients with certain anomalies at the base of the skull, such as basilar impression. It is also common in patients with syringomyelia. Neck flexion is limited and painful due to irritation of the meninges in meningitis and subarachnoid hemorrhage. Neck stiffness is also seen with lesions of the posterior fossa that cause tonsillar herniation through the foramen magnum and in children with meningismus produced by conditions such as retropharyngeal abscess, viral myositis, and migraine. Limitation of neck movements in several directions is found with spondylotic, arthritic, and degenerative disc disease affecting the cervical spine. Lhermitte's sign, which is a sudden shocklike sensation or tingling traveling down the spine when the neck is flexed, is most commonly associated with multiple sclerosis but can also be seen in the presence of cervical spondylosis and cervical spine tumors.

The **common carotid pulses** should be gently palpated in the neck using the three middle fingers and then the two sides compared. An increased pulse may be seen in the following conditions: tortuosity of the common carotid, increased flow due to hyperdynamic circulation (e.g., anemia, fever, or hyperthyroidism), occlusion of the opposite internal carotid artery requiring contralateral collateral circulation, and an intracranial arteriovenous malformation that is supplied by the carotid circulation. A decreased pulse may be due to overlying muscle and soft tissue but may also indicate reduced flow through a stenotic common or internal carotid artery. However, it is usually the internal carotid artery that is of greatest interest to the examiner and its pulsations cannot be reliably felt in the neck. Theoretically it can be detected in the tonsillar fossa, but this is usually impractical. The rest of the neurovascular examination can be carried out at this point.

The **facial pulses** comprising the facial artery as it crosses the angle of the jaw, the angular artery at the junction of the nasal bridge and supraorbital ridge, and the supraorbital artery, can be palpated and both sides compared. The superficial temporal arteries should also be felt to look for the irregularity, induration, tortuosity, and tenderness which are found in elderly patients with temporal arteritis. These arteries

are branches of the external carotid and may exhibit increased pulses on the side of an internal carotid artery occlusion when there is significant extracranial-intracranial collateral flow.

A bruit may be heard over the carotid artery in the neck, but it is often necessary to have the patient hold his or her breath while listening for this. It may be due to turbulence in either the internal, external, or rarely common carotid artery stemming from stenosis or increased flow. Bruits of vertebral artery origin are best heard in the supraclavicular fossa or more posteriorly at the base of the neck. Subclavian artery stenosis also produces bruits in this location. A venous bruit can be distinguished from an arterial bruit because it is obliterated when gentle pressure is exerted over the internal jugular vein above the site of the sound. Heart murmurs radiating to the carotid arteries are usually heard bilaterally, possess a different quality from carotid bruits, and are loudest over the base of the neck, gradually fading as the stethoscope is moved upward. The thyroid can also be inspected and palpated as part of the neck examination.

Spine

The spine or vertebral column should first be inspected and examined for mobility. An abnormally straight spine with loss of the usual lumbar lordosis may indicate paravertebral muscle spasm due to lumbosacral disc disease. An exaggerated lumbar lordosis, often seen with obesity, may indicate a predisposition to lumbosacral strain and is also common in the presence of muscle weakness due to muscular dystrophy or other myopathic illnesses. Scoliosis is associated with a number of neurological conditions. It can either arise as the result of progressive paravertebral muscle weakness, such as in the muscular dystrophies, or as an associated developmental anomaly, such as in syringomyelia and spinocerebellar degeneration. Sinuses and patches of hair in the lumbosacral region can be associated with occult spina bifida, which may also indicate an Arnold-Chiari malformation. The vertebral spines should also be firmly palpated to detect tenderness arising from a metastatic tumor or infectious process.

Heart

The heart is carefully auscultated to detect any murmurs arising from valvular disease such as mitral stenosis or from subacute bacterial endocarditis or to identify a midsystolic click associated with mitral valve leaflet prolapse. Any arrhythmias such as atrial fibrillation should be noted. These and other cardiac findings can suggest a source of emboli to the brain or retina or a cause for syncopal attacks. Signs of generalized atherosclerosis such as diminished peripheral pulses, hardened arteries, a femoral bruit, xanthelasma, and tendinous xanthoma suggest concomitant extracranial or intracranial atherosclerotic disease.

Skin

Because of its common ectodermal origin with the nervous system, the skin can exhibit visible evidence pointing to possible underlying nervous system involvement in a group of neurocutaneous developmental disorders called the *phakomatoses*. These disorders include neurofibromatosis, (von Recklinghausen's disease), tuberous sclerosis, Sturge-Weber syndrome, von Hippel–Lindau disease, and ataxia telangiectasia, and are further discussed in Chapter 27. Skin ulcers and trophic changes may also be seen in sensory neuropathies, syringomyelia, and conditions in which pain is absent because of a congenital cause. There are a variety of other skin manifestations in, for example, systemic vasculitis, dermatomyositis, meningococcal meningitis, subacute bacterial meningitis, and Osler-Weber-Rendu disease (hereditary hemorrhagic telangiectasia), and these serve as clues to the etiology of a neurological illness.

The Neurological Examination

As mentioned earlier, the neurological examination consists of six parts and usually starts with an assessment of higher functions.

Higher Functions (Mental Status)

With the recent increased interest in neuropsychology, more emphasis has been placed on the evaluation of higher functions as part of the neurological examination. Because it is time-consuming and requires special techniques, it is often the most poorly done aspect of the examination. Unlike the psychiatric mental status examination, attention focuses mainly on those aspects of higher brain function that are most commonly disturbed in the context of organic cerebral disease. In no other area of the neurological examination is it more important for the examiner to have a set technique with a definite series of questions which he or she can use repeatedly in order to judge the range of normal responses. Beginners often tend to give the patient the benefit of the doubt when encountering mildly deviant responses that the more experienced tester would deem abnormal.

Orientation is tested with regard to person (name? age? occupation?), place (current location? city? building? street? floor? room number?), and time (day? date? time of day? season?). Orientation to time is usually the earliest affected with that to person the best preserved.

Memory is tested in recent (learning) and remote (recall) spheres. The three-object test (e.g., "number 237," "color blue," and "apple") or reading a short story is commonly used to test recent memory. The three objects are named and patients are asked to repeat them immediately to be sure they were paying attention. Patients are told that they will be tested again in 5 minutes, and are then distracted so that they cannot rehearse in the interval. Anything but 100 percent recall is abnormal. Long-term memory is tested by having patients recount details from their past such as the names of schoolteachers, former jobs, military service, and important dates or places. It may be necessary to verify this information with an outside source.

Attention mechanisms are examined by tests of immediate recall. The patient is asked to repeat a series of digits forward and backward. The normal digit span is 5 or more forward and 3 or more backward. Having patients subtract serial 7s as quickly as possible starting from 100 or, for someone less apt at calculation, serial 3s starting from 20 tests both calculation and attention mechanisms. The time taken and the number of errors are recorded.

Calculation can be tested by having the patient perform mental arithmetic (e.g., 3×17)

as well as written calculations, when necessary. The patient's facility at these tests must be viewed in the context of his or her education, previous mathematical ability, and current use of figures.

Judgment may be examined by asking the traditional: "What would you do if you found a sealed, addressed, stamped letter lying in the street?" or "What would you do if you were in a theater and you smelled smoke?" Other more challenging questions can be used such as: "What would you do if you were in a restaurant and, when it came time to pay the bill, you found you'd left your wallet at home?" or "What would you do if you were driving down the street and another car struck you, denting your fender?" **Insight** and the patient's awareness of his or her neurological problems should also be assessed by asking patients to explain why they are in the hospital or why they were sent to see you, or what is wrong with them.

The patient's prevailing affect (e.g., depression or euphoria), appropriateness of emotional responses, and any excessive lability of emotion should be noted.

The patient's fund of information is also assessed to gain a general idea of his or her intellectual level and everyday contact with the environment. Questions designed to test information should be selected with the patient's educational and occupational background in mind. Traditional questions are to name five large cities in the patient's country, the last several government leaders, and details of salient current events.

In special circumstances, supplementary tests can be administered, such as having patients explain proverbs and identify similarities (e.g., ball, an orange, and the moon) and differences (e.g., king and president, or reputation and character).

Visuospatial Abilities. Visuospatial functions and constructional abilities, which may be abnormal especially with right, but also with left or bilateral parietooccipital lesions, are examined by having the patient copy drawings such as a simple house, three-dimensional cube, or a more complex standardized figure such as

the Rey-Osterreith figure. The patient's strategy or approach to copying the figure and his or her speed, accuracy, and ability in reproducing the figure later from memory (nonverbal learning) should also be noted. The patient should also be asked to produce drawings spontaneously, such as a clock with the numbers on it or a daisy with the petals equally arranged around the center. This may reveal the hemispatial neglect that occurs with nondominant parietal lesions (Fig. 2-1). Constructional ability can be tested further by having the patient use small sticks, wooden matches, or blocks to create various designs and structures.

Early in the examination, the **handedness** of the patient should be determined. It is not sufficient to ask the patient which hand he or she writes with, since many lefthanders have been taught to write with their right hand. Foot preference in kicking a ball, eye preference in sighting a gun, hand preference in sports such as baseball, golf, and hockey, and a family history of left-handedness are also determined.

Language and Speech. There are several tests that evaluate language and speech function when aphasia (see Chapter 6) is suspected. For screening purposes, it is sufficient to listen to the fluency and other aspects of the patient's spontaneous speech and to note his or her ability to comprehend questions and commands during the regular neurological history and examination and to name several objects. For more comprehensive aphasia testing, the following should be specifically examined:

1. Fluency during spontaneous speech. The patient's ability to produce sentences of three words or more and a flowing speech output (60 words per minute) are noted. The prosody, volume, grammar, word choice, and the use of any paraphasias or neologisms in spontaneous speech should also be noted.

2. Comprehension. This can be tested in three increasingly difficult ways. First, by having patients answer questions such as: "Are you Mr. Johnston?" "Does a board float on water?" "What do I use to cut wood with?" or "The lion was killed by the tiger. Who is dead?" Second, by testing their ability to follow one-,

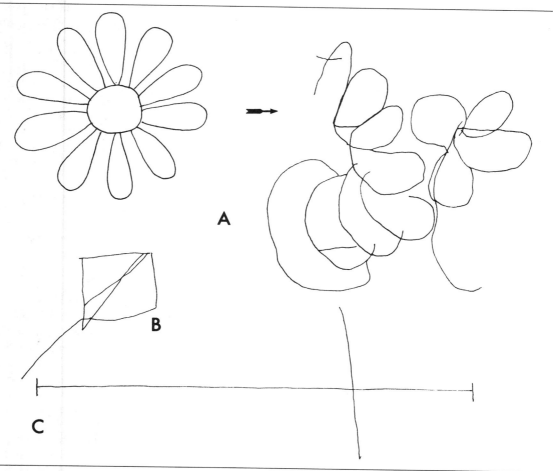

Fig. 2-1. *Visuospatial dysfunction and hemispatial neglect in a 69-year-old woman with a right parietotemporal glioma. The patient had a left homonymous hemianopia, mild left hemiparesis, left-sided astereognosis, dressing apraxia, and mild left apractagnosia. (A) Attempt to copy a daisy and (B) a three-dimensional box and (C) to bisect a line.*

two-, and three-step commands, such as "Point to the window, then the door, and then clap your hands." In the third approach, a pen, coin, and rubber band are placed in front of the patients and they are asked to perform several tasks in response to commands, such as: "Put the pen between the coin and rubber band," "Pick the pen up, turn it around, and put it on top of the coin," or "Flip the metal object over and put it inside the rubber band."

3. Repetition. Start with letters and simple words like "cat" and "table," then proceed to more difficult words and phrases like "basketball," "here she comes," and "today is a nice day," and finally pose a more challenging phrase such as "no if's, and's, or but's."

4. Naming. At least ten objects should be shown to the patient in turn. If patients cannot think of the word, they can be prompted by giving them the first letter or phoneme in the word. If they still cannot name the object, they can be given a list of three or four possibilities and asked to pick the correct name. If this is not helpful, patients should be asked to show whether they recognize the object, thus ruling out a visual agnosia, by showing how it is used or by describing its function. If comprehension is intact, naming should also be tested in re-

sponse to verbal description. For example, "I use it to cut wood with, it's a _____" or "This animal can go in the desert for a long time without water, it's a _____." The use of paraphasias and neologisms should be noted. There are two types of paraphasias: verbal (words that resemble the correct word in meaning but are not exact) and literal, or phonemic, (words that resemble the correct word in sound but are not exact). Neologisms are nonsense terms that have no resemblance to the correct word.

5. Writing. Patients should be asked to write their name, a sentence or two to dictation, and then a spontaneous description of how they came to the office or the hospital. If the right hand is plegic, writing can be done with the left hand. In an acutely aphasic patient who is alert with good comprehension but mute, writing may be the only way to demonstrate the presence of an aphasia.

6. Reading. Single letters, progressively more difficult words, and then sentences are read aloud by the patient. The patient's ability to carry out written commands and understand material from newspapers or magazines can be used to evaluate reading comprehension. Standardized tests such as the Boston Diagnostic Aphasia Evaluation or the Western Aphasia Battery are also available.

Apraxia and Agnosia. Apraxia is the inability to perform a learned skilled motor act (usually in response to verbal command) in the absence of a comprehension deficit, paralysis, uncooperation, or other obvious reason. Oral-buccal-lingual-facial apraxia can be tested for by asking the patient to pretend to drink from a straw, lick crumbs from the lips, pucker the lips as for a kiss, blow out an imaginary match, sniff a flower, pretend to chew gum, and express surprise. Apraxia is looked for in each arm by asking patients to pretend to brush their teeth, comb their hair, salute, strike a match, or hammer a nail. The ability to pantomime whole-body activities such as dancing or swimming and to carry out an imaginary series of actions, such as folding a letter, placing it in an envelope, sealing it, and stamping it, is also tested. In severe cases, patients will not even be able to

attempt the action. Patients with milder apraxia can often approximate the correct gesture but in a somewhat hesitant or clumsy fashion and may use part of their hand as the imaginary object (e.g., the fist to drive in an imaginary nail). Often giving them the actual object will serve as a visual and tactile cue and allow them to perform the task smoothly and accurately.

Agnosia, which is an inability to recognize or grasp the significance of a sensory stimulus (visual, auditory, or tactile) in the absence of a primary sensory deficit (see Chapter 6), is much less frequently encountered than apraxia. Testing for agnosia may be difficult when aphasic deficits exist, and the intactness of the sensory modality concerned must always be demonstrated as well.

Cranial Nerves

The twelve paired cranial nerves all leave or enter the brainstem, except for the first two which are supratentorial. A great deal of attention is paid to cranial nerve testing during the neurological examination because these nerves or the muscles that they supply are frequently compromised in lesions of both the central and peripheral nervous system as well as in myopathic disorders. Moreover, specific cranial nerve deficits are often valuable objective signs of a true lesion of the nervous system and are very helpful for purposes of localization.

Olfactory Nerve (Cranial nerve I). The olfactory nerve has its primary receptor in the nasal mucosa and is formed on each side from the olfactory bulbs and tracts that course across the floor of the anterior cranial fossa beneath the frontal lobes. Because of its location, the first cranial nerve is subject to pressure from subfrontal tumors such as meningiomas arising from the olfactory groove, and may also sustain damage as the result of fractures of the floor of the anterior cranial fossa. Before anosmia (loss of smell) can be attributed to an olfactory nerve lesion, an intranasal disorder, which is much more common, such as allergic rhinitis, benign growths, and upper respiratory infections, has to be excluded. Although smell is not examined routinely by most neurologists, when testing is indicated, each nostril can be assessed separately using nonirritating substances such as tobacco, coffee, or a bar of soap.

Optic Nerve (Cranial Nerve II). The optic nerve is embryologically an extension of the brain. It is therefore the only part of the central nervous system that can be directly visualized.

Funduscopy. The optic nerve head (disc) and the retina, macula, and retinal vessels are all observed through the ophthalmoscope (funduscopy). The patient is asked to fixate on a distant object, gazing slightly toward the side where the examiner is standing. A darkened room facilitates the task by allowing maximal pupillary dilatation; however, it is important to learn to perform funduscopy without mydriatic drops because, in many acute neurological conditions, a dilated pupil is an important sign of imminent transtentorial herniation, thus contraindicating their use.

The main findings of interest are optic pallor, indicative of optic atrophy, and papilledema (Fig. 2-2), usually arising from elevated intra-cranial pressure. In **optic atrophy,** the disc is grayish-white and there is a reduced number of capillaries crossing the disc margins. Temporal pallor of the disc due to previous demyelination of the maculopapular bundle (part of the optic nerve transmitting macular or central vision) is a common sequela of retrobulbar neuritis in patients with multiple sclerosis. Segmental areas of pallor may be seen in vascular lesions of the disc. The earliest funduscopic sign of raised intracranial pressure is loss of venous pulsations. These pulsations can be seen as the veins emerge from the optic disc and are elicited by gentle lateral pressure over the eyeball. They are not always present in normal subjects or easily seen, but, when viewed, are reliable evidence against a significant elevation of intra-cranial pressure.

Dilatation and tortuosity of the veins with loss of the optic cup and a congested appearance of the disc with slightly indistinct disc margins are early signs of **papilledema**. In more advanced cases, there are definite elevation and blurring of the disc margins, with tortuosity and

Fig. 2-2. *Funduscopic study showing papilledema in a 28-year-old woman with pseudotumor cerebri. Note hemorrhages around the optic disc.*

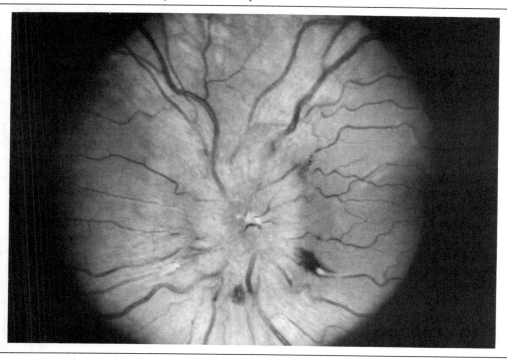

dilatation of the retinal vessels, a reddened appearance of the disc, linear hemorrhages over the disc and retina, and retinal edema. Conditions such as optic drusen, congenital abnormalities of the disc (some of which are familial), and medullated nerve fibers may be mistaken for papilledema.

Papillitis, which is a swollen optic nerve head with vascular, toxic, demyelinating, or inflammatory optic neuritis, can resemble early papilledema. The distinction is best made on the basis of central vision and visual acuity, which are affected early in papillitis but only late in papilledema. Vitreous floaters may also be seen in papillitis. In late papilledema, before vision is permanently lost, attacks of transient blindness lasting a few seconds, known as visual obscurations, may occur. Rarely papilledema may occur in the presence of normal intracranial pressure due to a retroorbital lesion causing venous congestion or in reduced intraocular pressure. Unilateral papilledema is not always found on the side of the intracranial lesion causing the elevated pressure, however.

Visual Acuity. Visual acuity is measured in each eye using either a standard wall-mounted chart or a special card for use at a distance of 14 inches (35 cm). Visual acuity should be tested with the patient wearing glasses because the state of the optic nerve is of greater interest than refractive errors in this setting. A useful and very sensitive test for determining impaired afferent visual input from one eye, usually due to a previous optic nerve lesion, is the swinging flashlight test. The light is swung from one pupil to the other and, when the light is flashed at the abnormal eye, the pupil will transiently dilate rather than constrict. The term *Gunn pupil* is used to describe this phenomenon which, when present, strongly suggests the existence of an optic nerve lesion even when visual acuity is normal. The ability to perceive a red object normally is another sensitive test of optic nerve function. The patient with retrobulbar neuritis, for example, may report that red objects appear less bright or brownish to the involved eye.

Visual Fields. The third step in optic nerve evaluation is testing the visual fields by confrontation. To do this, the examiner stands facing the patient about 3 feet (1 meter) away. The patient is told to fixate on the examiner's eyes and then the patient's ability to pick up slight finger movement or count fingers at the extremes of the four quadrants of the visual fields is gauged. The examiner compares the patient's fields to his or her own. Each eye need not be tested individually except in unusual circumstances. It is sometimes useful after examining each quadrant individually to present bilateral simultaneous stimuli so that unilateral visual neglect or extinction can be detected. In an uncooperative or aphasic patient, screening for gross visual field defects such as a hemianopia can be done by visual threat. To do this, a stimulus such as the examiner's finger is presented suddenly from the side and moved rapidly toward the eye. If this maneuver elicits a blink or startle response, then a hemianopia is excluded.

The **blind spot**, which lies about 15 degrees temporally from the point of fixation, can also be assessed and compared to the examiner's by using a small white or red object (such as the tip of a cotton swab). The points where it disappears and reemerges are carefully plotted. More complete evaluation of the central visual fields requires use of a tangent screen. A rapid screening test for scotomata, which are discrete areas of visual loss within the visual fields, is to have the patient fixate with one eye on a dot placed at the center of an ordinary piece of graph paper and outline any areas where the lines appear distorted or unclear. Prepared sheets with a pattern printed on them, known as the Amsler grid, can also be used for this purpose.

Oculomotor, Trochlear, and Abducens Nerves (Cranial Nerves III, IV, and VI). The oculomotor nerve operates in conjunction with the fourth and sixth nerves to control extraocular movements but has certain additional functions. Its nuclear complex lies in the midbrain and the nerve courses forward through the substance of the brainstem to emerge in the interpeduncular space before traversing the cavernous sinus and supraorbital fissure. Pupillary constrictor function, which is involved in the **light and accommodation reflexes**, is mediated by parasympathetic fibers carried in the third nerve. The light reflex afferents arise from optic nerve fibers before they synapse in the lateral geniculate nucleus of the thalamus. These fibers reach the pretectal area of the dorsal midbrain and are distributed bilaterally before synapsing more ventrally in the Edinger-Westphal nucleus. The pupilloconstrictor muscle is ultimately supplied by fibers arising from the ciliary ganglion behind the eyeball.

When the light is shined into one pupil, this elicits a direct response as well as constriction of the opposite pupil (a consensual response). The consensual response may be used to test the pupillary response in a blind eye. During testing of the light reflexes, the size, symmetry, regularity, shape, and any eccentricity of the pupils are noted. Pupillary constriction with accommodation is tested by having patients rapidly shift their fixation from a distant to a near object. To observe this response in patients with dark eyes, it is sometimes necessary to shine a light onto the cornea from the side. The abbreviation PERRLA (pupils equal, round, regular, and react to light and accommodation) is commonly used to denote normal findings. Abnormalities of pupillary function are further discussed in Chapter 11. Ptosis is also looked for at this point because the nerve supply to the levator palpebrae muscle arises partially from the third nerve. There can be a fairly complete ptosis with interruption of the third nerve. Ptosis is bilateral if a lesion involves the third nerve nuclear complex in the midbrain. Other causes of ptosis include Horner's syndrome, myasthenia gravis, various myopathic disorders, congenital familial ptosis, and lax eyelids with old age.

Extraocular Movements. The extraocular movements are controlled by the third nerve, which supplies the muscles for adduction (medial rectus), depression (inferior rectus), and elevation (superior rectus and inferior oblique), as well as by the fourth and sixth nerves. In the presence of a third nerve lesion, the involved eye does not fully adduct or elevate but tends to lie in a down-and-out position.

The **trochlear nerve** emerges dorsally from the midbrain and traverses the cavernous sinus and superior orbital fissure to supply the superior oblique muscle. This muscle is responsible for depressing the adducted eye and internally rotating the abducted eye. An isolated fourth nerve lesion tends to cause vertical diplopia with a compensatory head tilt away from the side of the lesion. To test the nerve, the patient is asked to look downward and inward. In the presence of a third nerve palsy with the eye abducted, evaluation of the fourth nerve is most easily carried out. If the fourth nerve is intact, asking the patient to look downward and inward will produce an observable internal rotation (intortion) of the eye that is obvious from the movement of the capillaries on the surface of the sclera.

The **abducens** nucleus lies in the pons and the nerve sweeps dorsally around the seventh nerve nucleus before exiting ventrally, passing over the apex of the petrous bone, then through the cavernous sinus and the superior orbital fissure. Only abduction (the lateral rectus muscle) is supplied by the sixth nerve, and a severe lesion affecting it will leave the eye in an adducted position at rest.

To test the function of the sixth nerve, the patient is asked to look to the side being tested. When a patient is complaining of diplopia and there is no obvious ocular deviation to indicate a particular nerve or muscle involvement, either the **red glass test** may be used at the bedside or more sophisticated ophthalmological techniques performed to identify the particular nerve involved. To perform the red glass test, the patient's right eye is covered with a red glass and the patient is told to gaze in the direction of maximum diplopia, while looking at a yellow light. In a paretic eye, the image seen will fall outside the image seen by the intact eye. This can identify which muscle is involved.

Gaze Mechanisms. The third, fourth, and sixth cranial nerves can be assessed in conjunction with gaze mechanisms. The anatomical pathways for gaze begin in the frontal and occipital areas, descend in the internal capsule to the prerubral and pretectal areas, where the centers for contralateral up-gaze and down-gaze lie slightly separated, and cross to make contact with the pontine center for horizontal gaze (parapontine reticular formation). The patient is asked to look vertically and horizontally and the parallelism of the eyes is observed. To detect slight ocular deviations, it is useful to hold a light in front of the eyes and observe any discrepancies in the position of the light reflection in the pupils as the patient gazes in various directions. When the two eyes do not move in parallel (dysconjugate gaze), a lesion of cranial nerves III, IV, or VI; a lesion of one or more of the extraocular muscles; myasthenia gravis; or a congenital strabismus should be suspected. In **strabismus**, testing of the eyes individually will reveal a full range of motion.

Because the anatomical pathways for pursuit and saccadic gaze differ, the two functions should be tested separately. In testing **pursuit gaze**, the patient is asked to follow a slowly moving object in various directions. **Saccadic gaze** is examined by having the patient rapidly refixate from one object (e.g., a pencil) to another (e.g., the examiner's finger) held about 18 inches (46 cm) away and 6 inches (15 cm) apart. To fully evaluate extraocular movements, it is necessary to assess **fixation** on an object. To do this, the patient maintains the eyes in the primary position (i.e., gazing straight ahead) while the examiner looks for any extraneous oscillations or drifting of the eyes. **Convergence**, which is the ability to adduct both eyes in order to follow an object or the patient's thumb as it is moved toward the nose, is also assessed.

Nystagmus.   When gaze is examined, it is also convenient to look for any spontaneous or gaze-evoked nystagmus. **Nystagmus** is a rhythmic oscillation, usually of both eyes, that is most frequently elicited at the extremes of gaze and commonly has a rapid component in one direction and slow component in the other (jerk nystagmus). In some forms of congenital nystagmus, the movements are equal in both directions and there is no fast and slow phase (pendular nystagmus). Nystagmus may be seen in a variety of congenital and acquired lesions affecting the vestibular pathways and their cerebellar connections as well as in toxic-metabolic disorders, weakness of gaze (gaze-paretic nystagmus), and blindness. One should also note whether the nystagmus occurs in the primary position or with gaze in a particular direction; whether it is vertical, horizontal, oblique, or rotatory; its direction (named according to the fast phase); whether it is coarse or fine; and whether it is different in the two eyes (dissociated). Nystagmus may be detected during the funduscopic examination when fine oscillations of the retina become apparent and visual fixation is removed. When nystagmus is present, the patient may complain of oscillopsia, or a visual sensation of the environment moving to-and-fro. During testing for nystagmus, patients should hold their gaze about 20 degrees short of the limit, as physiological end-gaze nystagmus is seen in many normal subjects.

Optokinetic nystagmus (OKN) is a physiological nystagmus seen in normal subjects when following a series of moving visual stimuli such as a train or a rotating striped drum. The slow phase is mediated by pursuit mechanisms, and fast-phase or corrective movements are controlled by saccadic mechanisms as the limit of gaze is reached and the eyes flick back. This reflex can be elicited at the bedside using an alternately colored striped band (or striped necktie) moved horizontally or vertically in front of the patient's eyes. Horizontal OKN impairment is typically seen in patients with deep parietal lesions, in which case the fast phase is irregular or absent as the tape is moved toward the side of the lesion. A homonymous hemianopia does not impair the OKN unless the lesion causing it extends into the parietal area, in which case tumor rather than a vascular cause is more probable (Cogan's rule).

Trigeminal Nerve (Cranial Nerve V).
The trigeminal nerve supplies sensation over the face (except for the angle of the jaw), the anterior half of the scalp, and the mucosa of the mouth and nose (Fig. 2-3). The three sensory divisions (ophthalmic, maxillary, and mandibular) enter the skull through separate foramina and form the trigeminal ganglion (gasserian), which lies on the sphenoid wing not far from the internal carotid artery as it enters the skull. The roots from the ganglion enter the

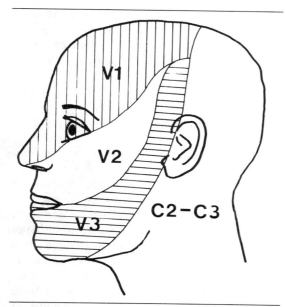

Fig. 2-3. *Sensory distribution of the three branches of the trigeminal nerve over the face. (V1 = ophthalmic; V2 = maxillary; V3 = mandibular.)*

ventrolateral pons and split to enter the main and descending (spinal) sensory nuclei. The spinal nucleus mainly mediates pain and temperature sensation, and thus there may be a dissociated sensory loss over the face (i.e., loss of pain and temperature with preservation of touch) in the event of a brainstem lesion. This sensory loss extends as far down as the medulla, and lesions in its inferior portion mainly affect upper face sensation because of a somatotopic arrangement.

Touch sensation (lightly touching the patient with a cotton or tissue) and pinprick sensation are evaluated in all three divisions, always comparing the two sides. If there is a complete lesion of the fifth nerve on one side, sensation is lost over the whole hemiface, sparing an area over the angle of the jaw and to a variable extent in front of the ear. Sensation is also preserved over the scalp posterior to a line joining the ears and passing through the vertex. Because the sensory fields from the two sides overlap, the sensory loss usually extends almost, but not quite, to the midline. The patient's unawareness of the anatomical borders between the fifth nerve and C2–C3 sensory supply is often useful for distinguishing functional complaints of facial numbness from true fifth nerve lesions.

The **corneal reflex** is assessed by lightly touching a twisted cotton or tissue to the edge of the patient's cornea, then observing the speed of the direct (eye-stimulated) and consensual (opposite eye) blink responses. It is important to touch the cornea and not the relatively insensitive sclera. Patients should be asked whether the stimulus feels the same on both sides. A blink response may be reduced with a seventh nerve lesion that impairs the efferent side of the reflex arc, but, in this case, the preservation of corneal sensation is confirmed by the presence of a normally brisk consensual blink response and equal subjective sensation on the two sides. When reporting a reduced corneal reflex, by convention this is described as an interruption in the afferent (fifth nerve) component of the reflex arc. Contact lenses, a false eye, and anesthetic drops will all obviously cause a reduced corneal reflex.

Somewhat less consistent and reliable, but at times useful as a partially objective assessment of the second division of the fifth nerve, is the sternutatory or *nose-tickle reflex*. Lightly tickling the nasal hairs and mucosa produces wrinkling of the nose and a withdrawal response that should be similar on both sides. The motor components of the fifth nerve are anatomically associated with the third division and supply the muscles of mastication (masseter and temporalis) as well as the pterygoids, the anterior belly of the digastric muscles, and the mylohyoid muscles. This division is tested by palpating and observing the masseters and temporalis muscles as the patient bites down, holds the jaw open against resistance, and moves it from side to side against resistance. In fifth motor lesions, masseter or temporalis wasting may cause a hollowing of the cheek or temple area. Jaw deviation toward the side of the lesion may also occur when the patient opens his or her mouth.

Facial Nerve (Cranial Nerve VII). The facial nerve innervates the muscles that control facial expression, mediates taste over the anterior two thirds of the tongue, and supplies the tensor tympani muscle, which is responsible for reflexly dampening loud sounds (the stapedius reflex). The facial nucleus in the pons sends its fibers along with the nervus intermedius and eighth nerve through the internal auditory meatus. The fibers pass through the facial canal, traverse the geniculate ganglion lying near the middle ear, and emerge at the styloid foramen at the angle of the jaw behind the ear. The nerve branches out at this point to supply its various muscles.

The **facial movements** involved in smiling (orbicularis oris), eye closure (orbicularis oculi), turning down the corners of the mouth (platysma), puffing out the cheeks, and wrinkling of the forehead are compared between sides. Eye closure strength can be assessed by comparing the patient's ability to bury the eyelashes on both sides and to resist attempts by the examiner to open the eyes. At rest, flattening of the nasolabial fold on one side is an early sensitive sign of facial weakness. Other signs consist of drooping of the corner of the mouth, decreased blinking, widening of the palpebral fissure (distance between the eyelids), and smoothing-out of forehead wrinkles and wrinkles at the corner of the eye.

Comparisons between sides are important in evaluating facial function, but minor degrees of bilateral facial weakness can easily pass unnoticed. For example, the patient's mouth and facial movements observed during spontaneous talking and smiling may at times be a better way to detect minimal degrees of facial weakness than asking the patient to smile. Dissociations between voluntary and spontaneous smiling may occur.

A lower motor neuron facial weakness (from the nucleus to the periphery) is characterized by equal involvement of the upper and lower facial muscles (unless there is selective branch involvement after the nerve emerges from the styloid foramen, as can happen with a parotid tumor or trauma). In an upper motor neuron facial weakness, as occurs with lesions of the cortex or the corticobulbar projections (e.g., cerebral infarction), the lower facial muscles are usually selectively involved contralateral to the lesion but eye closure and forehead wrinkling are relatively well preserved. The weak-

ness is distributed in this way because in most people, those neurons in the facial nucleus supplying the muscles of the lower face receive a strictly contralateral supranuclear input, whereas those supplying muscles of the upper face have a bilateral supranuclear supply. Because of anatomical variations, the upper face may also rarely be significantly weak in the presence of upper motor neuron lesions.

Taste testing is carried out only when there is obvious evidence of a facial nerve lesion, such as in Bell's palsy. To perform this, the patient's tongue is pulled out and held with a piece of gauze wrapped around it. The words *sweet, salt, sour*, and *bitter* are written on a piece of paper and the patient is asked to point to the corresponding taste each time a substance in solution is applied to the tongue. The test substances are sugar, salt, lemon juice, and quinine or tonic water, although the first two are adequate for screening purposes. The mouth is rinsed between each application of a different substance and the findings for the two sides of the tongue are compared.

Auditory-Vestibular Nerve (Cranial Nerve VIII). The auditory-vestibular nerve has two divisions, as its name implies. It is formed by cochlear and vestibular afferent fibers, passes through the internal auditory canal and the internal auditory meatus, crosses the cerebellar pontine angle, and joins its nuclei in the lower brainstem. Once the external ears have been examined, hearing is tested on both sides by assessing the patient's ability to hear a ticking watch, whispered numbers, or fingers rubbed gently together. If this shows reduced hearing, the Rinne and Weber tests are used to help distinguish neurosensory from conductive (middle ear disease) hearing loss. In the **Rinne test**, a vibrating 256-Hz tuning fork is placed on the mastoid (bone conduction) and the patient is asked to indicate when the sound stops. The tuning fork is then immediately held close to the ear (air conduction) and the additional time the patient hears the sound is noted. In normal subjects, the air conduction time is about double the bone conduction time, but, in patients with conductive deafness, the bone conduction time will be longer than the air conduction time. To perform the **Weber test**, the tuning fork is placed firmly over the vertex. In normal subjects, the sound will be heard equally in both ears, but, in patients with a conductive hearing loss, the sound will be referred to the involved ear because of less competition from external noise. These tests have been largely supplanted by modern audiometric methods using special equipment operated by trained personnel.

The **vestibular component** of the eighth nerve is partially evaluated by looking for nystagmus, gait ataxia, and performing the **Romberg test**. Past-pointing can also be easily looked for. Patients with a suspected vestibular nerve or end-organ lesion are asked to close their eyes and hold the arms extended out in front with their fingertips opposite the examiner's. They are then asked to raise their arms above their head one or more times and to return them to the same place. Deviation of the arms, known as past-pointing, may occur toward the side of a vestibular lesion. More direct examination requires specialized procedures such as caloric testing or electronystagmography (see Chapter 10).

Glossopharyngeal and Vagus Nerves (Cranial Nerves IX and X).

The glossopharyngeal and vagus nerves are generally evaluated together because their functions partially overlap. Sensation over the posterior tongue and oropharynx, which are supplied by the ninth nerve, can be tested by touching these areas with a cotton swab. The gag reflex can be tested by touching the posterior pharynx with a tongue blade or cotton swab. The unilateral absence or reduction of gag is a significant finding, but a bilateral reduction may be seen in normal subjects as well as in pathological states. The symmetry of the palatal elevation is also examined, and this includes looking at the midline white raphe of the soft palate, both during gag reflex testing or when the patient opens the mouth and says "aaah . . ." In the event of unilateral palatal weakness, the palate will be pulled up and deviate toward the normal side. Uvular deviation is a less reliable sign. Having the patient say "ga-ga-ga-ga . . ." as rapidly

as possible is also useful for testing palatal function.

The vagus nerve supplies the vocal cords via recurrent laryngeal branches, and lesions (usually originating from carcinoma of the lung) cause hoarseness and a weak cough due to unilateral vocal cord paralysis, which can be confirmed by direct laryngoscopy. More extensive testing of vagus nerve function can be done as part of a complete evaluation of the autonomic nervous system (see Chapter 21).

Spinal Accessory Nerve (Cranial Nerve XI).

The spinal accessory nerve is formed principally by roots from the upper cervical segments that enter the intracranial cavity through the foramen magnum and exit through the jugular foramen to supply the sternocleidomastoid and upper trapezius muscles. This nerve is not uncommonly injured in the neck during radical neck surgery, and this may lead to significant disability of the upper extremity due to poor scapular stabilization. The trapezius and sternocleidomastoid are inspected and palpated for signs of wasting. The sternocleidomastoid is a strong muscle, and the examiner should not be able to overcome head-turning to one side by pressing on the patient's chin and jaw. Both sternocleidomastoids are involved in flexing the neck against resistance or lifting the head from the supine position. Most patients do not realize that the sternocleidomastoid turns the head to the opposite side, and this can be used to detect a hemiparesis stemming from hysteria or malingering. Trapezius function is tested by having the patient shrug the shoulders against resistance.

Hypoglossal Nerve (Cranial Nerve XII).

The hypoglossal nerve emerges from the medulla and leaves the base of the skull through the hypoglossal foramen to supply the muscles of the tongue. This nerve may be damaged by trauma, vascular lesions, or infiltrative processes along the base of the skull, or its motor neurons may be affected in amyotrophic lateral sclerosis. Twelfth nerve dysfunction, especially when bilateral, produces dysarthria and dysphagia. Wasting of the tongue may be observable as a deep furrowing, especially along the edges of the tongue. Twelfth nerve or nuclear lesions involving lower motor neurons may also produce fasciculations of the tongue which consist of spontaneous brief contractions of individual motor units. Fine individual muscle fiber contractions, termed *fibrillations*, may be observed with denervation of the tongue. These movements are best seen with the tongue at rest on the floor of the mouth and may be difficult to distinguish from normal spontaneous tongue muscle movements. The patient is also asked to protrude the tongue to see if it remains in the midline. In the event of unilateral tongue weakness, the tongue will deviate toward the weak side as the unopposed intact muscles pull it over (Fig. 2-4). In some cases, analogous to the situation with upper motor neuron facial weakness, tongue deviation can be caused by a contralateral supranuclear lesion such as a cerebral infarction. The strength of the tongue can also be assessed by comparing

Fig. 2-4. *Right-sided tongue atrophy and deviation in a 68-year-old woman with a glomus jugulare tumor invading the base of the skull. The patient also had involvement of cranial nerves VIII to XI.*

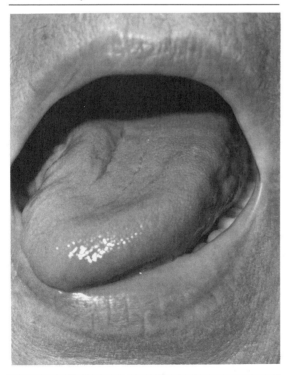

the patient's ability to press his or her tongue to either side against a tongue blade or into the cheek against the examiner's hand. Tongue agility should also be tested by having the patient move the tongue rapidly from side to side while protruded and to repeat sounds such as "ta-ta-ta-ta."

Motor System

Much of the nervous system is geared toward movement, and therefore evaluation of the motor system is a central part of the neurological examination. Establishing the level of the lesion as well as diagnosing specific system degenerations frequently depend on accurate motor assessment. The extent of individual muscle testing depends on the particular problem.

Muscle Bulk. Muscle bulk is evaluated with the patient's body well exposed. The contours of certain muscles such as the deltoids, supraspinatus, palmar eminences, first dorsal interosseous, quadriceps, gastrocnemius, and extensor digitorum brevis (the round bulge over the lateral dorsum of the foot when the toes are extended) are easily noted and compared between sides (Fig. 2-5). The muscle circumference can be measured at a standard location on the two sides (e.g., 6 cm above the patella for the quadriceps or 6 cm below the patella for the gastrocnemius).

Muscle hypertrophy produces increased bulk and may be due to physiological hypertrophy, such as that seen in weight lifters and athletes; pseudohypertrophy, such as occurs in the calf muscles in Duchenne's and other forms of muscular dystrophy as well as in myotonia congenita; or infiltrative processes, such as certain lipidoses (Kufs' disease), glycogenoses (Pompe's disease), or forms of hypothyroidism. There may be decreased muscle bulk in patients with hypotrophy, which is the failure of muscle to develop due to congenital or early life lesions such as polio, but is more commonly seen with **atrophy**. Atrophy is mostly characteristic of processes that affect the lower motor neuron or the muscle itself, but can also occur with disuse following upper motor neuron paralysis or immobilization of a limb.

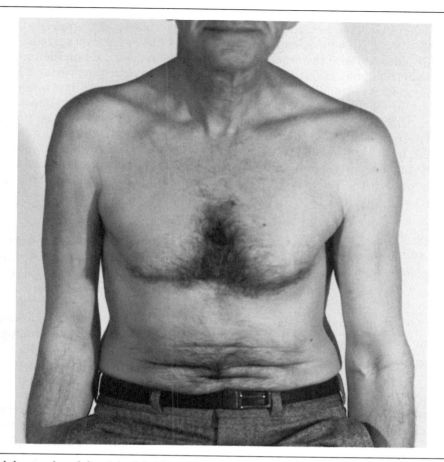

Fig. 2-5. *Subtle atrophy of the right deltoid muscle in a patient with a localized inflammatory myopathy.*

Nonneurological conditions such as cachexia or rheumatoid arthritis can also produce generalized or localized muscle wasting. Following denervation, atrophy may be apparent within as early as 3 to 4 weeks in muscles such as the quadriceps.

Fasciculations. With denervation, atrophy may be accompanied by fasciculations. These muscle twitches are detected by having the patient completely relax the muscle, making sure that the patient is not too cold, and looking tangentially across the muscle under good lighting. Their presence, especially when there is no atrophy, is not necessarily pathological because many normal subjects experience fasciculations during fatigue or stress, or after excessive coffee drinking or exercise. However, fasciculations are commonly found in the context of motor neuron disease, irritative spinal root lesions such as disc compression and spondylosis, and other neuropathic disorders. These movements may be difficult to distinguish from other involuntary muscle movements such as myokymia.

Muscle Strength. To test for **drift**, the patient is asked to extend both arms out in front while in a hypersupinated position with the eyes closed (Barré maneuver) for about 30 seconds. If there is a mild degree of hemiparesis, the hand will pronate slowly and the arm will drift downward. It may also drift upward or outward with sensory abnormalities and cerebellar lesions. This is a convenient time to inspect the musculature of the hands and arms and to look for tremor or other involuntary movements.

The patient's muscle strength is compared between the two sides and with the examiner's power. Specific detailed muscle testing is well outlined in other sources (see bibliography) and is not dealt with at length here. For reliable assessment, the patient must be fully cooperative. Functional, hysterical, or feigned weakness will often have a "sudden-give" and variable quality, and pain may significantly impair the accuracy of testing. Strength is graded on a scale of 0 to 5, as follows:

0   No trace of movement
1   A flicker of muscle contraction
2   Able to produce some movement around
    a joint but not against gravity
3   Able to move against gravity
4   Able to move against some resistance
4½ Able to move against moderate resistance
5   Full strength

Use of the 4½ grade is not standard, but is recommended because of the large gap between 4 and 5. More objective quantitative testing can be done utilizing specialized equipment such as hand dynamometers, which are available in most physiotherapy departments. At the bedside, having the patient squeeze a blood pressure cuff to assess grip pressure is sometimes a convenient quantitative test. In most instances, however, assessment of proximal and distal strength in the upper and lower extremities is adequate. This can be done using the following maneuvers: attempting to overcome the patient's arms as they are held in abduction with the elbows flexed (deltoids), having the patient squeeze two of the examiner's fingers in each hand (grip strength), attempting to overcome the patient's extended wrists, examining the patient's ability to flex the thigh while sitting as the examiner exerts downward pressure on the knee, and asking the patient to walk on his heels with the feet dorsiflexed (tibialis anterior).

Certain strong muscles such as the quadriceps and gastrocnemius are best tested against the patient's own weight. The quadriceps can be tested by having the patient step onto a low stool or a chair several times and the gastrocnemius, by having the patient stand, balancing on one foot and rising up on the toes repeatedly.

Muscle strength testing in large groups of normal subjects has shown that a woman lying supine should be able to hold one leg elevated at 45 degrees for a minimum of 30 seconds and her head elevated off the couch for a minimum of 30 seconds as well. The corresponding figures for males are 60 seconds and 90 seconds. The nervous supply and function of the various muscles are shown in Table 2-1.

Muscle Tone. Muscle tone is defined as the resistance of a relaxed muscle to passive movement. Tone may be decreased in conditions affecting the lower motor neuron, the muscle itself, tendons or ligaments, or the cerebellum. In newborns and infants, a wide variety of diffuse cerebral and systemic conditions also produce hypotonia. Hypertonia is a more important finding and such patients may complain of stiffness, cramps, and slowness of movement.

Rigidity is a form of hypertonia that is best seen in parkinsonism and other extrapyramidal diseases. It is present even when the muscle is at rest. Increased resistance to passive movements is fairly even in the "lead pipe" variety, which gives the impression of bending a metal pipe, or the "cogwheel" variety, which exhibits a ratchety effect produced by the tremor. Slow passive rotation of the wrist is the best maneuver for demonstrating rigidity in the parkinsonian patient.

Spasticity is a special type of increased tone that always indicates an abnormality in the corticospinal tracts. Its main characteristic is a velocity-dependent increase in tone accompanied by a "clasp-knife" reflex, or a sudden give or release of tone at a certain point following a gradual increase in tone starting from the onset of the movement. Spasticity is best felt in the upper extremity by grasping the patient's hand in a "hand-shake" position and quickly supinating the forearm, whereupon the catch-and-give phenomenon can be detected. To test spasticity in the lower extremities, the patient is placed supine and the examiner clasps his or her hands

Table 2-1. Nerve Supply and Functions of Principal Muscles

Nerve	Nerve roots	Muscle	Function
Phrenic	C3, C4, C5	Diaphragm	Inspiration
BRACHIAL PLEXUS			
Medial and lateral pectoral	C5, C6	Pectoralis major: Clavicular part	Adduction of elevated arm
	C7, C8, T1	Sternocostal part	Adduction and forward depression of arm
Long thoracic	C5, C6, C7	Anterior serratus	Fixation of the scapula during forward thrusting of the arm
Dorsal scapular	C4, C5	Rhomboids	Elevation and fixation of scapula
Suprascapular	C4, C5, C6	Supraspinatus	Initiation of abduction of arm
Suprascapular	(C4), C5, C6	Infraspinatus	External rotation of arm
Thoracodorsal	C6, C7, C8	Latissimus dorsi	Adduction of horizontal, externally rotated arm; coughing
Lower subscapular	C5, C6	Teres major	Adduction and medial rotation of arm
	C5	Teres minor	Lateral rotation of arm
Axillary	C5, C6	Deltoid	Lateral and forward elevation of arm to horizontal
Musculocutaneous	C5, C6	Biceps, brachial	Flexion of supinated forearm
	C6, C7, C8	Triceps	Extension of forearm
Radial (from posterior cord of plexus)	C5, C6	Brachioradialis	Flexion of semipronated forearm
	C6, C7, C8	Extensor carpi radialis	Extension of wrist to radial side
Posterior interosseous (from radial)	C5, C6	Supinator	Supination of extended forearm
	C7, C8	Extensor digitorum	Extension of proximal phalanges
	C7, C8	Extensor carpi ulnaris	Extension of wrist to ulnar side
	C7, C8	Extensor indicis	Extension of proximal phalanx of index finger
	C7, C8	Abductor pollicis longus	Abduction of first metacarpal in plane at right angle to palm
	C7, C8	Extensor pollicis longus	Extension at first interphalangeal joint
	C7, C8	Extensor pollicis brevis	Extension at first metacarpophalangeal joint
Median (C6–C7 from lateral cord of plexus, C8–T1 from medial cord)	C6, C7	Pronator teres	Pronation of extended forearm
	C6, C7	Flexor carpi radialis	Flexion of wrist to radial side
	C7, C8, T1	Flexor digitorum superficialis	Flexion of middle phalanges
	C8–T1	Flexor digitorum profundus (lateral part)	Flexion of terminal phalanges, index, and middle fingers
	C8, T1	Flexor pollicis longus (anterior interosseous nerve)	Flexion of distal phalanx, thumb
	C8, T1	Abductor pollicis brevis (ulnar nerve rarely)	Abduction of first metacarpal in plane at right angle to palm

Table 2-1 (Continued).

Nerve	Nerve roots	Muscle	Function
	C8, T1	Flexor pollicis brevis (sometimes ulnar nerve)	Flexion of proximal phalanx, thumb
	C8, T1	Opponens pollicis (sometimes ulnar nerve)	Opposition of thumb against 5th finger
	C8, T1	1st and 2nd lumbricals	Extension of middle phalanges while proximal phalanges are fixed in extension
Ulnar (from medial cord of plexus)	C7, C8	Flexor carpi ulnaris	Observe tendon while testing abductor digiti minimi
	C8, T1	Flexor digitorum profundus (medial part)	Flexion of distal phalanges of ring and little fingers
	C8, T1	Hypothenar	Abduction and opposition of little finger
	C8, T1	3rd and 4th lumbricals	Extension of middle phalanges while proximal phalanges are fixed in extension
	C8, T1	Adductor pollicis	Adduction of thumb against palmar surface of index finger
	C8, T1	Flexor pollicis brevis (sometimes median nerve)	Flexion of proximal phalanx, thumb
	C8, T1	Interosseous	Abduction and adduction of fingers
LUMBOSACRAL PLEXUS			
Twigs from lumbar plexus	L1, L2, L3	Iliopsoas	Hip flexion from semiflexed position
Femoral	L2, L3	Sartorius	Hip flexion from externally rotated position
	L2, L3, L4	Quadriceps	Extension at knee
Obturator	L2, L3, L4	Adductor longus, adductor magnus, adductor brevis	Adduction of thigh
	L2, L3, L4	Gracilis	
Superior gluteal	L4, L5, S1	Gluteus medius	Adduction, internal rotation of thigh
	L4, L5, S1	Tensor fasciae latae	
Inferior gluteal	L5, S1, S2	Gluteus maximus	Extension of thigh
Sciatic	L5, S1, S3	Biceps femoris	Flexion at knee, assist in extension of thigh
	L5, S1, S3	Semitendinosus	
	L5, S1, S2	Semimembranosus	
Peroneal (deep)	L4, L5	Anterior tibial	Dorsiflexion of foot
	L5, S1	Extensor digitorum longus	Dorsiflexion of toes
	L5, (S1)	Extensor hallucis longus	Dorsiflexion of great toe
	L5, S1	Extensor digitorum brevis	Dorsiflexion of toes

Table 2-1 (Continued).

Nerve	Nerve roots	Muscle	Function
Peroneal (superficial)	L5, S1	Peroneus longus	Eversion of foot
		Peroneus brevis	
Tibial	S1, S2	Gastrocnemius	Plantar flexion of foot
	S1, S2	Soleus	Plantar flexion of foot
	L4, L5, S1	Posterior tibial	Inversion of plantar-flexed foot
	L5, S1, S2	Flexor digitorum longus	Flexion of toes (distal phalanges)
	L5, S1, S2	Flexor hallucis longus	Flexion of great toe (distal phalanx)
	L5, S1	Flexor digitorum brevis	Flexion of toes (middle phalanges)
	L5, S1	Flexor hallucis brevis	Flexion of great toe (proximal phalanx)
Pudendal	S2, S3, S4	Perineal and sphincters	Voluntary control of pelvic floor

behind the patient's knee and quickly lifts the leg to produce hip and knee flexion. In a relaxed patient with spasticity, the knee will remain extended, the heel will come off the bed, and the knee will flex only gradually as the clasp-knife reflex comes into play. Spasticity is also found in association with other evidence of an upper motor neuron lesion, such as hyperreflexia, clonus, and a Babinski sign.

Clonus is the repetitive, rhythmic contraction of a muscle produced by a sudden stretch. When well developed, it is sustained for as long as the muscle is kept in the stretched state and its amplitude parallels the force of stretch. Clonus is most easily elicited at the ankle, patella, wrist, and jaw.

Another form of increased muscle tone that is often exhibited by demented patients with diffuse cerebral disease is **paratonia** or gegenhalten. The characteristics of this form of rigidity are fairly nondescript, but it is variable from moment to moment and appears as if the patient is voluntarily failing to relax.

As part of the motor examination, any tremor, dystonia, and involuntary movements such as choreoathetosis or myoclonus should be noted (see Chapter 13).

Reflexes

Reflex testing has an important place in the neurological examination because of the relative objectivity of the information provided and

the conclusions that can be drawn about both segmental and suprasegmental function. The **deep tendon reflexes** are elicited by a sudden stretch when a tendon is tapped; this triggers the transmission of afferent impulses from muscle stretch receptors to the spinal segments involved. The anterior horn cells thus contacted then send an efferent discharge to the muscles to contract. These reflexes are elicited with the patient in a relaxed, symmetrical position. It is important to strike the tendon rather than the muscle because even a denervated muscle will contract when directly percussed, sometimes more briskly than normal. The most important deep tendon reflexes to test, together with their corresponding segmental and nerve supplies, are shown in Table 2-2. There is no reflex test for the L5 segment, although the posterior tibial reflex and hamstring reflex have sometimes been used even though the responses are inconsistent. Sides are compared and the reflexes are graded on a five-point scale, as follows:

0 Absent, even with reinforcement
1 Present, but reduced
2 Normal
3 Increased
4 Increased and pathological, often with clonus

An absent reflex is always pathological, but, before a reflex is judged absent, every effort

Table 2-2. Deep Tendon Reflexes

Reflex	Segments	Nerve
Biceps	C5–C6	Musculocutaneous
Brachioradialis (supinator)	C5–C6	Radial
Triceps	C6–C7–C8	Radial
Finger flexion	C8–T1	Median, ulnar
Patellar or knee jerk (quadriceps)	L2–L3–L4	Femoral
Ankle or Achilles (gastrocnemius)	S1–S2	Sciatic (posterior tibial branch)

must be made to obtain it. The patient must be relaxed and positioned properly, and a large hammer should be used. Reinforcement should be carried out, which is a way of facilitating the reflex by having the patient hook his or her hands together and pull outward, or bite down or squeeze his or her fist when the tendon is struck. A difficult ankle jerk can best be obtained by having patients kneel on the bench with their back facing the examiner and feet hanging over the edge while hooking their hands together and pulling. If a reflex can be obtained at least once, this confirms its presence. It is sometimes easier to detect a reflex by feeling the tendon contract (as in the biceps reflex) or the foot flex (as in the Achilles reflex) than by trying to visualize it.

With lesions of the upper motor neuron, dysinhibition may result in excessive spread of the afferent reflex signal to adjacent or contralateral spinal segments. This may produce such phenomena as the simultaneous contraction of the biceps when the brachioradialis reflex is elicited or a crossed adductor reflex whereby the legs "scissor" when the knee adductor tendons are tapped on one side. Reflexes are reduced or absent in disorders of the lower motor neurons that interrupt the reflex arc either peripherally or within the spinal cord, in myopathies, and in hypothyroidism as well as other metabolic disorders. Ankle jerks are frequently difficult to elicit in elderly patients. Hyperreflexia occurs in very tense individuals as well as in those with upper motor neuron disorders or hyperthyroidism.

The **jaw jerk** is a useful deep tendon reflex because it is mediated by afferent and efferent fibers that travel via the fifth cranial nerve. To perform it, the patient is asked to hold the jaw partially open and slack; the examiner places a finger over the chin and strikes it with a moderate downward, glancing blow. The resultant jaw closure can be seen and felt. The reflex is variable in normal subjects. An abnormally brisk jaw jerk implies a bilateral lesion of the corticobulbar pathways above the fifth nerve nuclei in the pons. In a patient with spastic quadriparesis or paraparesis, a hyperactive jaw jerk suggests that the level of the lesion is at least above the pons.

The **Hoffman reflex** is another deep tendon reflex, related to hyperactive finger flexor jerks; its presence suggests hyperreflexia but is not necessarily a pathological sign. If it is only obtained unilaterally, it is a significant finding. To best elicit it, the examiner places his or her middle finger under the patient's middle finger while the patient's wrist is extended and the other fingers are lightly flexed. The examiner then quickly flicks the terminal phalanx of the patient's middle finger with the other hand, which produces flexion of all the terminal phalanges including the thumb.

Superficial Reflexes. The superficial reflexes may be reduced in the presence of upper motor neuron lesions, but this finding is less reliable than other signs of corticospinal tract involvement. These reflexes are also impaired with segmental lesions interrupting the reflex arc.

The **abdominal reflexes** are tested by lightly scratching on the surface of skin away from the umbilicus in all four quadrants. The response is a slight movement of the umbilicus in the direction of the stimulus. The upper abdominal reflexes depend on segments T8–T10 and the lower ones on segments T10–T12. Abdominal reflexes are commonly missing in obese individuals, multiparous women, and patients who have undergone extensive abdominal surgery.

The **cremasteric reflex** is a retraction of the scrotum following a light scratch on the upper inner thigh, and relies on segments L1–L2. The **bulbocavernous reflex** consists of a contraction of the anus when the head of the penis is squeezed and may be useful for evaluating the intactness of the lower sacral segments. These segments may also be assessed by observing for contraction of the anus in response to a light scratch over the perianal skin.

Pathological Reflexes. There are several pathological reflexes that are sought, some of which normally exist in infants and are therefore considered to represent release phenomena stemming from dysinhibition. The most useful of these is the **Babinski response** (Fig. 2-6). Normally, when a noxious stimulus is applied to the sole of the foot, there is plantar flexion of the toes and triple flexion of the

ankle, knee, and hip provoking a withdrawal response. To elicit a possible Babinski response, a sharp instrument such as a key or applicator stick is used to scratch from the lateral sole of the foot to the medial aspect under the ball of the first toe. The Babinski response, or extensor plantar response, consists of extension (upward movement) of the first toe often accompanied by fanning of the other toes.

Even more sensitive than the Babinski response is the **Chaddock response**, which is an upgoing toe elicited by scratching along the lateral border of the foot near the sole. The Babinski response is important because its presence is excellent evidence of a lesion in the corticospinal tract above L5 or its cells of origin in the motor cortex. It is also an early and sensitive sign of such a lesion. Rarely there is a false extensor response when plantar flexion is limited due to selective paralysis of the toe flexors or to arthritic disease. Attention should also be paid to any right-left asymmetry of the plantar responses, even if a full-blown Babinski response is not obtained.

Sucking, snout, rooting, and **grasping reflexes**

Fig. 2-6. *Babinski response in a patient with multiple sclerosis.*

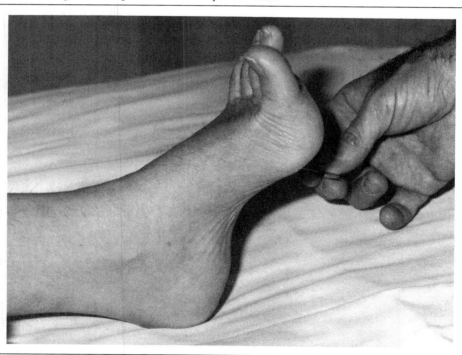

are primitive phenomena seen most commonly in patients with dementia and diffuse or bifrontal brain impairment. In testing for a grasp reflex, the patient should be clearly told not to squeeze the examiner's hand as it is moved lightly across the patient's open palm, and then distracted as further attempts are made. The **glabellar reflex** (Myerson's sign) consists of obligatory blinking each time the glabellar area between the eyes is tapped. This sign is most frequently encountered in parkinsonian patients. A **palmomental reflex** involves a twitch of the mentalis muscle (at the chin) when the thenar eminence on the same side is scratched with a pin. Although this reflex may be found in normal subjects, it is prominent in demented patients and, on rare occasions, may be one of the only signs of a contralateral frontal lesion.

The **corneomandibular reflex** is a lateral deviation of the jaw toward the side opposite a brisk corneal stimulus. This reflex, mediated by the fifth nerve, is most commonly encountered in comatose patients and implies interruption of the corticobulbar fibers, usually at the midbrain level, as occurs in transtentorial herniation.

Gait and Coordination

Gait requires the coordinated functioning of many neuroanatomical systems, including the motor cortex and corticospinal tracts, peripheral neurons and muscles, the basal ganglia, the cerebellum, the vestibular system, and visual and proprioceptive sensory afferents. Therefore, gait may be disturbed in the context of a wide variety of neurological disorders and gait testing is a good overall screening device. Every attempt should be made to have patients walk, even if some effort and support are needed to prevent their falling. Conditions such as arthritis and back pain may interfere with evaluation of the neurological aspects of gait. While engaged in **natural gait**, the patient's overall posture, arm-swing, width of stance, springiness, length of stride, and balance are observed. Some abnormal gaits are listed in Table 2-3.

Hopping or standing on one leg may provide further useful information. The patient should walk on his or her toes and heels so that distal lower extremity muscle strength can be assessed. **Tandem gait**, or walking heel-to-toe

along a straight line, may be done forward and backward principally to test midline cerebellar function. The **Romberg test** is fairly sensitive for determining the status of the patient's proprioceptive pathways from the lower extremities. Results may also be positive with vestibular impairment. The patient is asked first to stand with his or her feet together and the arms extended out in front and the eyes open. If imbalance is increased when the eyes are closed, this is a positive result. Caution must be exercised to prevent the patient from falling.

Coordination of the individual limbs may be affected by lesions of the cerebellum and its connections, weakness, alterations of sensory input with certain neuropathies, and rarely cortical lesions in the absence of weakness. Limb **ataxia** and **dysmetria**, which is a difficulty in achieving a precise movement toward a specific target with a tendency to overshoot, should be sought in the upper extremities using the **finger-nose-finger test**, in which the patient is asked to alternately touch the examiner's finger while in motion, then his or her nose, and back to the examiner's finger, and so on.

An analogous test for the lower extremities is the **heel-knee-shin** test, in which the patient slides his or her heel, with the toes pointing upward, smoothly up and down the front of the shin between the knee and ankle.

Intention tremor, which is usually a sign of a cerebellar efferent lesion, is also looked for during these tests. It consists of an oscillating movement perpendicular to the line of motion that increases in amplitude as the goal is approached. **Distal fine movements** are influenced not only by cerebellar function but also by strength, muscle tone, and, to a certain degree, by sensory input. Useful tests to assess this are to have the patient tap the index finger on the most distal thumb crease as rapidly as possible, describe small circles continuously on the back of the hand with the second and third fingers, rapidly alternate touching of the thumb to each of the other fingers, and tap a foot on the floor with the heel planted against the examiner's hand while the patient is supine. When interpreting the results of these tests, normal right-left differences must be taken into account. When the ability to perform rapid alter-

Table 2-3. Some Types of Gait Disturbance

Gait	Description	Cause or main example
Hemiparetic	Arm held adducted, flexed at elbow and wrist; leg dragged and circumducted with poor hip flexion and foot extension	Spastic hemiparesis (e.g., cerebral infarct)
Parkinsonian	Stooped posture, reduced arm swing, small steps, shuffling, hesitation, propulsion (festination) or retropulsion, poor balance, turns en bloc	Parkinsonism
Cerebellar	Wide-based, ataxic	Midline (vermis) cerebellar lesions (e.g., alcoholic degeneration)
Steppage	Marching appearance, lifting knees high and slapping feet on ground	Peripheral neuropathy (e.g., tabes, dorsalis, bilateral foot drop)
Waddling	Excessive dropping of the pelvis toward non-weightbearing side with each step	Hip-girdle weakness (e.g., muscular dystrophy)
Spastic	Stiff-legged, scissoring, may walk on toes	Paraparesis due to upper motor neuron lesions
Sensory ataxic	Ataxic, patient may keep eyes fixed on floor	Peripheral sensory neuropathy
Frontal lobe	Slow, ataxic, short steps, trouble initiating gait ("stuck to floor")	e.g., normal pressure hydrocephalus
Hysterical	Bizarre, nondescript, may be wildly ataxic, astasia-abasia	Psychogenic

nating movements is impaired, this is referred to as dysdiadochokinesia.

Sensory System

The sensory examination is the least reliable part of the neurological examination (Fig. 2-7). Great care must be taken to apply stimuli in a consistent fashion. Differences between sides are less likely suggested to patients if they are asked "Does this feel the same on both sides?" To get an idea of the degree of sensory loss, the patient is asked to quantitatively compare areas of reduced sensation with normal areas, which are given a grade of 10 out of 10. It is best to move the test stimulus toward the normal areas from an area of sensory loss to define its borders. Marking the boundaries of sensory loss with a pen on the skin and then later retesting the patient with his or her eyes closed may help distinguish real from functional sensory loss and better define affected areas.

Other clues to hysterically related sensory loss or malingering are: noncorrespondence of the apparent dermatomal distribution over the front and back of the body, stocking-and-glove sensory loss with very sharp borders,

unilateral sensory loss below a certain level equal to all modalities, and large discrepancies in vibration sensation over the two sides when the tuning fork is applied to each side of the forehead and sternum. Any areas of sensory loss are best recorded on a diagram for future reference.

Primary Modalities. The primary modalities are assessed first, taking into account that there are two main sensory pathways: the **posterior columns**, which carry vibratory sensation and synapse ipsilaterally in the nuclei gracilis and cuneatus of the medulla, and the **spinothalamic tracts**, which carry pain and temperature and are formed by neurons crossing and synapsing as they enter the spinal cord before ascending to the thalamus. Touch is mediated by both sensory pathways, and therefore, for screening purposes, testing of vibration and pain is adequate.

Vibratory sensation is tested using a 128-Hz tuning fork that is applied to bony prominences such as the toes, medial malleolus, patella, iliac crest, fingers, wrist, and elbow, and may be timed or compared with the examiner's sensa-

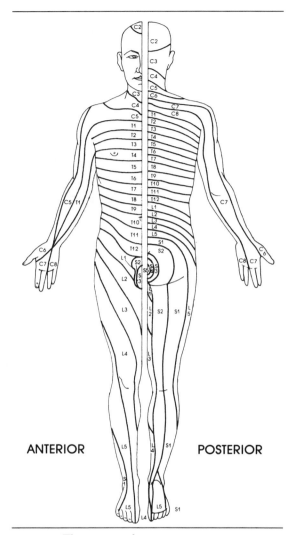

ANTERIOR   **POSTERIOR**

Fig. 2-7. *The sensory dermatomes.*

tion. In the elderly, vibratory sensation is commonly absent or reduced in the feet.

Pain is tested using a sharp safety pin, taking care not to draw blood, and applying one or two stimuli each time. The patient is asked to report differences between sides or any areas where the pinprick feels dull. Patients with irritative root lesions, painful neuropathies, and spinothalamic tract or thalamic lesions may exhibit **hyperalgesia**, or an exaggerated response to pinprick.

Temperature may also be tested when there is loss of pain sensation by asking patients to report whether they feel heat or cold as test

tubes filled with hot or cold water are applied to the skin. Touch can be examined by lightly touching the skin with a cotton or tissue while the patient's eyes are closed and having them say "touch" each time.

Joint position sense, or proprioception, which is mediated by fibers ascending in the posterior columns but also involves cortical integrative functions, is tested by grasping the sides of a distal phalanx of a finger or toe (or more proximal part of the limb when the loss is substantial) and having the patient, with the eyes covered, report small (about 5–10 degrees) random displacements in the upward or downward direction.

Cortical Sensory Modalities. Cortical sensory modalities depend on the contralateral parietal lobe. They can be meaningfully tested only after it has been shown that primary modalities are relatively well preserved. Traditionally only the hands are examined, but other parts of the body can be tested when indicated. There are a large number of tests available for this purpose, but only two or three are necessary in most instances. **Stereognosis** (the ability to identify objects by feel), **graphesthesia** (the ability to recognize numbers or letters written on the skin with a pointed object), and **two-point discrimination** (the ability to distinguish the sites of placement when two pins or pointed objects, held at various distances apart, are applied simultaneously to the skin in a nonpainful manner) are the most widely tested. For adequate interpretation of the findings from the latter two tests, the normal limits of discrimination over various bodily areas must be known. For example, on the tips of the index finger, a normal individual can distinguish two points as little as 2 mm apart and correctly identify a number that is 5-mm high. Other tests for assessing cortical modalities include touch localization (the ability to localize a touch stimulus on the skin without seeing it), sense of texture, weight perception, and wet-dry perception.

Double simultaneous stimulation is tested by touching a part of the body bilaterally after first touching each part individually. Each time, the patient reports "right," "left," or "both." **Extinction**, or failure to acknowledge the stimulus on one side may occur initially or with subsequent double stimuli and this may result from a contralateral parietal lesion that is producing a degree of sensory neglect.

Other Considerations in the Neurological Examination

The Screening Examination

A rapid screening of nervous system function can be carried out in a cooperative patient when no major neurological findings are expected. Following is an outline of the basic screening examination and how it can be recorded in concise form:

Neck: supple
Carotid pulses: 2/2, no bruits
Skull: normal in size and shape, no bruits
Spine: no tenderness or deformity
    Higher functions: alert
        Oriented × 3
        Memory: 3 objects after 5 minutes
        Speech and naming: normal
    Cranial nerves
          II—Normal discs
          —Visual fields intact
          —Visual acuity grossly normal
      III, IV, VI—PERRLA
          —extraocular movements: full and conjugate
          —No nystagmus
        V—Pinprick: normal over face
          —Corneals: normal bilaterally
      VII—Face (smile and eye closure): strong and symmetrical
     VIII—Hears fingers rubbed together
    IX, X—Palate elevates well symmetrically
      XI—Symmetrical shoulder shrug
          —Sternocleidomastoids: normal
     XII—Tongue protrudes in midline, no atrophy

Motor
    Normal strength, bulk, and tone bilaterally proximally and distally
    No drift of outstretched arms
Reflexes (Fig. 2-8)
Gait and coordination
    Natural gait, heel walking, toe walking, tandem: all normal
    Romberg test: negative
    Finger-nose-finger: normal
    Heel-knee-shin: normal
    Fine motor and rapid alternating movements in hands and feet: normal

Fig. 2-8. *Method for recording deep tendon and abdominal reflexes. (Downgoing arrows indicate flexor plantar responses.)*

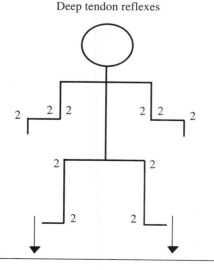

Deep tendon reflexes

Abdominal reflexes

Sensory
  Pinprick and vibration: normal and equal
    bilaterally in hands and feet
  Stereognosis in hands: normal

Examination of the Pediatric Patient

Specialized techniques are used in a neonate, infant, or young child, and one relies heavily on observation of the child during spontaneous play and reflex testing. The child's motor, language, and social behavior are compared to established norms, such as those contained in the Denver Developmental Schedule. In the infant, various reflexes such as the suck, dazzle, fixing and following, Moro, tonic neck, parachute, and Landau are examined. More attention is paid to the skull and sutures than in an adult, and the skull may be transilluminated using a strong flashlight in a dark room.

The Comatose Patient

In a comatose patient, the neurological examination has to be adapted to the patient's inability to cooperate. Heavy reliance is placed on brainstem and other reflexes. Further discussion of the topic is presented in Chapter 5.

BIBLIOGRAPHY

Brazis, P.W., Masdeu, J.C., and Biller, J. *Localization in Clinical Neurology*, 2nd ed. Boston: Little, Brown, 1990.

DeJong, R.N., and Heaver, A.F. Case-taking and the neurological examination. In R.J. Joynt (editor). *Clinical Neurology*, Vol. 1. Philadelphia: Lippincott, 1989, Pp. 1–89.

Guarantors of *Brain. Aids to the Examination of the Peripheral Nervous System.* London: Baillière Tindall, 1986.

Nakano, K.K. *Neurology of Musculoskeletal and Rheumatic Disorders.* Boston: Houghton Mifflin, 1979.

Rodnitsky, R.L. *Van Allen's Pictorial Manual of Neurologic Tests*, 3rd ed. Chicago: Year Book, 1987.

Ross, R.T. *How to Examine the Nervous System*, 2nd Ed. New York: Medical Examination, 1985.

Wilson-Pauwels, L., Akesson, E.J., and Stewart, P.A. *Cranial Nerves: Anatomy and Clinical Comments.* Toronto: Decker, 1988.

Laboratory, Bedside, and Neuroradiological Test Procedures

Because of the proliferation of special tests, it has become more important than ever to use good judgment when ordering these procedures. For the most part, special tests and neuroradiological procedures are used to confirm the clinical localization of lesions within the nervous system, to provide data pertaining to the etiology of the process, and to help gauge the progression of a disease or the patient's response to therapy. When considering which tests to order in a particular patient, the following must be considered: the probability of the test contributing useful information concerning the patient's problem and its treatment, the potential discomfort or serious complications from the test, and the cost of the test. The expertise of the neurologist is at times best put to use in sparing the patient exposure to unnecessary investigations. A clinical maxim worth remembering is: "The second examination is the most helpful diagnostic test in a difficult neurological case."

SPECIAL BEDSIDE TESTS

Lumbar Puncture

There are several indications for performing a lumbar puncture (LP):

1. To obtain cerebrospinal fluid (CSF) for analysis to aid in the diagnosis of conditions such as meningitis, encephalitis, subarachnoid hemorrhage, multiple sclerosis, central nervous system (CNS) and meningeal neoplasms, and Guillain-Barré syndrome
2. To measure intracranial pressure in conditions such as pseudotumor cerebri
3. To perform myelography, radionuclide cisternography, a CSF infusion test, computed tomography (CT) with metrizamide enhancement, and other related diagnostic studies
4. To instill drugs such as antibiotics or chemotherapeutic agents

5. To determine the presence of a spinal block using Queckenstedt's test

The following are contraindications to performing LP:

1. Absolute: infection in the path of the needle (e.g., skin or epidural abscess)
2. Relative:
   Raised intracranial pressure, especially due to lateralized supratentorial expanding lesions or posterior fossa lesions
   Suspected incomplete spinal block
   Bleeding disorders
   Developmental abnormalities in which the spinal cord may be tethered to the sacrum and has a low termination
   The intention of performing an LP in the near future for a radiological or radionuclide diagnostic study

Although LP can sometimes be done safely in a patient with raised intracranial pressure, suspicion or signs of intracranial hypertension such as papilledema mandate that CT or magnetic resonance imaging be done first. In the setting of pseudotumor cerebri or subarachnoid hemorrhage, the danger of herniation following an LP is minimal, despite elevated intracranial pressure. Although the risk is greater in meningitis, early LP is vital for diagnosis and treatment and the elevated pressure can be managed simultaneously.

Because an incomplete spinal block can become a complete block with consequential severe spinal cord compression if pressure is reduced below the site of the block, ideally an MRI or CT scan should be obtained first to search for a compressive lesion in suspected cases of spinal block (e.g., following spinal trauma with paraparesis). LP using a small needle can be done to instill a few milliliters of myelographic dye to delineate the level of the block and determine whether neurosurgical decompression is indicated. Queckenstedt's test (discussed later) has been used in the past for identifying spinal block and may still be useful on occasion.

In patients with bleeding disorders (e.g., hemophilia or thrombocytopenia, or those on an-

ticoagulant therapy), LP can be performed cautiously but the patient's coagulation status should be improved as much as possible before the procedure. Neurological function in the lower extremities should also be carefully monitored following the test. Massive hematomas causing cauda equina compression have occasionally occurred in such patients.

Caution should also be exercised in patients with Arnold-Chiari malformation or anomalies at the base of the spine, because an LP needle may pierce a low-lying spinal cord. When a neuroradiological procedure requiring LP is contemplated, a CSF sample should be obtained at that time as subsequent CSF leakage may cause the lumbar thecal sac to collapse and make a later LP difficult to perform for several days or even a few weeks. This can lead to a subdural injection of contrast medium, which can delay the radiological procedure for days.

Technique

The LP procedure and its purpose are first explained to the patient, who is then made to relax and positioned at the edge of the bed or table lying on the side in extreme flexion. Having an aid hold the patient's neck and legs in flexion and pillows placed between the knees and supporting the head can improve positioning, especially in an uncooperative patient. Because the spinal cord ends at L1–L2 in adults, the needle is inserted at the L3–L4 vertebral spinal interspace, opposite the top of the iliac crests (Fig. 3-1). The desired interspinous space is marked in the midline by making a fingernail impression on the skin. The area is then sterilized, surgical gloves are donned (and rinsed with alcohol to remove powder granules), and the LP tray prepared. The manometer and valve, test tubes for fluid collection, and a No. 20 LP needle with stylet are all prepared.

One or 2 ml of xylocaine is injected intradermally at the site of entry; freezing of subcutaneous areas is unnecessary. The LP needle is then advanced in the midline about 3 to 4 cm, and kept parallel to the bed and pointing toward the umbilicus. As the needle is further advanced a few millimeters at a time, the stylet is withdrawn each time to verify whether CSF is returning.

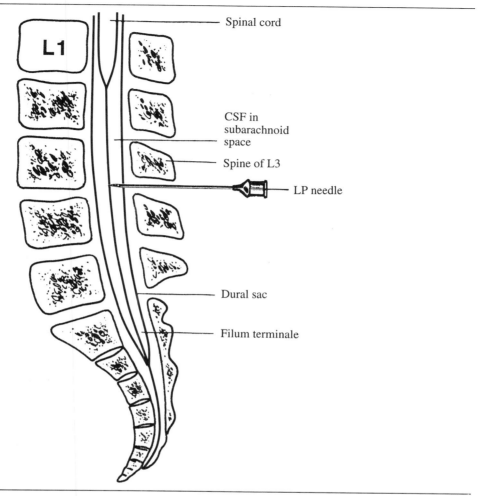

Fig. 3-1. *Position of lumbar puncture* (LP) *needle passing between the spines of the L3 and L4 vertebrae and entering the subarachnoid space. (CSF = cerebrospinal fluid.)*

When the subarachnoid space is entered, the manometer should be attached immediately and the pressure measured before any fluid is allowed to escape. The legs of the patient must be extended when the pressure reading is taken. Fluctuation of the fluid column with respirations indicates that the needle is lying well within the subarachnoid space. A low CSF pressure with very slowly flowing fluid may occur with spinal block, severe dehydration, and partial obstruction of the LP needle. It may also occur after earlier attempts at LP that have punctured the thecal sac. Fluid is then collected for the determination of protein or glucose con-

tent, cell count, and any other indicated tests. The needle is withdrawn, a Band-Aid placed over the site, and the patient kept horizontal, preferably prone, for 12 to 24 hours.

If it proves difficult to enter the subarachnoid space and bone is struck repeatedly, the needle must be withdrawn to below the skin surface so that its course can be redirected. A cooperative patient may be able to tell whether the needle is to the right or left of the midline.

If LP cannot be accomplished after trying two or three interspaces, the procedure should be undertaken by someone else. If still unsuccessful, the LP can be attempted with the patient in the sitting position and leaning forward over a bedside table. A neurosurgeon can also be requested to perform a cisternal puncture when CSF sampling is mandatory.

In cases of severe scoliosis, ankylosing spondylitis, or previous low back surgery with fusion, LP is best performed in the fluoroscopy suite under radiological guidance.

Post LP Headache

Because fluid may continue to leak out of the hole left in the lumbar thecal sac, especially if the patient is in the upright position, traction may be exerted on pain-sensitive structures at the base of the skull as the brain settles downward with standing, producing a post-LP headache. The chances of this happening are lessened by using a relatively small needle with a clean initial entry into the subarachnoid space and also having the patient remain horizontal for awhile after the LP. If a post-LP headache occurs, the patient should be kept strictly horizontal for at least 12 hours after the headache has disappeared and fluids forced. In intractable cases, in which the headache persists for weeks, an anesthesiologist may be called upon to inject 10 ml of the patient's venous blood, collected under sterile conditions, into the epidural space around the site of the LP (epidural blood patch).

Queckenstedt's Test

Queckenstedt's test is used mainly in cases of suspected spinal block, to aid in the decision whether to perform emergency myelography or obtain urgent neurosurgical consultation. The test can determine whether there is free communication between lumbar and intracranial subarachnoid spaces. To perform the test, once the LP needle is well in place, the examiner exerts gentle pressure by placing his or her hands around the patient's neck and occluding jugular venous flow. The resulting rise in intracranial pressure will then be transmitted to the lumbar CSF, provided there is no blockage in the spinal canal above the LP site, and will be reflected by a prompt rise in the CSF column within the manometer. Once the examiner's hands are released, the CSF column will fall equally promptly. This test is contraindicated in

cases of known or suspected raised intracranial pressure.

CSF Findings

The normal CSF values are shown in Table 3-1. Various tests may be ordered on the CSF specimen, depending on the problem at hand. A VDRL test is requested when CNS syphilis is suspected. Gram's staining, culture, India ink preparations, cryptococcal antigen and antibody measurement, and special viral studies can be done when meningitis or encephalitis are possibilities. Testing for oligoclonal bands is particularly useful when multiple sclerosis is a consideration. Cytological studies, utilizing a Millipore filter and ultracentrifugation, can help in the diagnosis of carcinomatous meningitis and certain CNS tumors.

The routine tests are the cell count and determining the protein and glucose content. Neurologists should learn to do their own cell counts rather than relying on laboratory personnel. Cells must be examined within about an hour following the LP before lysis occurs.

Cell count is done using a microscope and an ordinary hematological counting chamber. The white cells can be differentiated by staining the CSF with methylene blue, coating the sides of a capillary tube, or lysing the red cells with a dilute acetic acid solution. Wright's stain is used for obtaining a differential white blood cell count. Although a few mononuclear cells may be found in the CSF of normal subjects, even one polymorphonuclear cell suggests active inflammation or infection. Occasional contami-

Table 3-1. Normal Cerebrospinal Fluid Values

Measurement	Value
Opening pressure	<200 mm H_2O (CSF)
Fluid appearance	Clear, colorless
Cells	≤3 mononuclear white blood cells per mm^3
Glucose	> one half blood glucose level drawn at time of lumbar puncture
Protein	<45 mg/dl (lumbar), <15 mg/dl (ventricular)
Protein electrophoresis	gamma globulin, <14%

nation by vertebral bone marrow cells, particularly in elderly osteoporotic patients and in patients who had difficult LPs, may result in misleading cell counts. Red cells may be seen in the CSF after hemorrhage into the subarachnoid space or a traumatic tap. However, not just difficult LPs can cause a traumatic tap, as epidural veins may be punctured even during an "easy" tap. A traumatic tap can be usually distinguished from a subarachnoid hemorrhage due to ruptured aneurysm using the criteria listed in Table 3-2.

Xanthochromia in a spundown specimen of CSF presents a yellow-golden appearance imparted mainly by the presence of bilirubin. Faint degrees of xanthochromia are best detected by holding the CSF specimen and a test tube of water against a white background. When blood is released into the CSF, the red cells lyse and produce free hemoglobin that breaks down to methemoglobin. This makes the fluid pinkish. Xanthochromia occurs after about 12 hours as the bilirubin forms. There is normally a minute quantity of bilirubin, bound to albumin, in the CSF in equilibrium with the plasma bilirubin and albumin levels. Xanthochromia may also occur when the CSF protein or the serum bilirubin concentration is markedly raised (approximately >10 mg/dl).

The CSF protein content, largely albumin, may reach very high levels in the presence of a spinal block, tuberculous meningitis, or the Guillain-Barré syndrome. The upper limits of the protein level also tend to increase slightly with each decade in older individuals. When blood is found in the CSF, the protein and red cell count should be determined in the same tube because a correction factor of 1.5 mg/dl of protein for every 1,000 red cells should be added to the normal upper limit. A raised gamma globulin level in the CSF is found in patients with multiple sclerosis, subacute sclerosing panencephalitis, CNS syphilis, collagen diseases involving the CNS, CNS sarcoidosis, and in other conditions that cause an increase in the serum gamma globulin level, such as multiple myeloma. Oligoclonal bands detected by agar gel electrophoresis are frequently found in multiple sclerosis and subacute sclerosing panencephalitis but can also be seen in other conditions.

The glucose level in CSF is normally one half to two thirds that in a specimen of blood drawn at the time of LP. In meningitis, the glucose level may be near zero. Conditions causing a low CSF glucose content include infectious meningitis (bacterial, tuberculous, syphilitic, sarcoid, fungal, and occasionally viral, e.g., herpes, mumps), carcinomatous meningitis, subarachnoid hemorrhage (occasionally), and systemic hypoglycemia.

Ophthalmodynamometry

Ophthalmodynamometry is a bedside method for measuring intraocular blood pressure. To perform it, pressure is applied to the eyeball with an ophthalmodynamometer while the ophthalmic artery and its branches are observed through an ophthalmoscope. Pulsations of the arterioles appear when the diastolic pressure is reached and disappear once systolic pressure is

Table 3-2. Blood in the Cerebrospinal Fluid Arising from a Traumatic Tap Versus Subarachnoid Hemorrhage

Variable	Traumatic tap	Subarachnoid hemorrhage
Three-tube test	Progressive clearing or drop in hematocrit	No clearing
Appearance	Thready	Blood evenly mixed with CSF
Xanthochromia	Absent	Present, provided hemorrhage is at least 6–12 hours old
Red-cell ghosts	Absent	May be present
CSF pressure	Normal	Elevated with ruptured aneurysm
WBC count	Same proportion as blood (i.e., 1 WBC/700 RBC)	May be disproportionately high

WBC = white blood cell; RBC = red blood cell.

attained. Readings are compared to the brachial blood pressures on the same side and also to the reading on the opposite side. A difference of 10 percent between the two eyes suggests stenosis or occlusion of the ipsilateral internal carotid artery on the side with the lower reading. The technique is used much less frequently now because of the widespread availability of more accurate ultrasound techniques.

NEURORADIOLOGICAL AND RELATED PROCEDURES

Plain Skull X-ray Study

An inexpensive and simple test, plain skull x-ray studies remain a good way to evaluate the bones of the skull and sinuses. Routine views, preferably stereoscopic, are obtained in the lateral and anteroposterior projections, and special views such as Stenver's views are used for examining the internal auditory canals. A submental-vertex projection is used to visualize the foramina at the base of the skull. Tomograms of areas such as the pituitary fossa, internal auditory canals, and base of the skull allow more detailed assessment. Examples of findings revealed by a skull x-ray study are:

Suture diastasis and increased digital markings in children with raised intracranial pressure
Fusion of sutures in craniosynostosis
Discrete lesions of the bones of the calvarium produced by cysts, metastatic tumors, multiple myeloma, and so on
Skull fractures
Underdevelopment of the middle cranial fossa with temporal lobe atrophy due to early life damage
Enlarged sella with erosion of the floor in the presence of pituitary tumors or an empty sella
Shifted pineal gland with an intracranial mass lesion causing brain displacement
Intracranial calcifications from tumors (e.g., meningioma), arteriovenous malformations, aneurysms, or other lesions (e.g., granuloma)
Enlargement of various foramina with a neoplasm (e.g., acoustic neuroma or optic glioma)

Plain Spine (Vertebral Column) X-ray Studies

Plain x-ray films of the cervical (Fig. 3-2), lumbar, and, at times, thoracic (Fig. 3-3) vertebral column in the lateral and anteroposterior planes are indicated in the following situations:

1. Persistent neck or low back pain.
2. Significant trauma to the head or spine.
3. Possible metastatic disease to the spine (although radioisotope bone scanning is more sensitive).
4. Evidence of acute or chronic spinal cord compression.
5. Cervical or lumbosacral radicular pain or signs of root involvement. Oblique views are recommended for visualizing the foramina of nerve root exits. Findings include scoliosis, fractures, bony spurs impinging on root foramina, narrowing of the anteroposterior diameter of the cervical spinal canal caused by bony hypertrophy, narrowed intervertebral spaces due to disc degeneration, and involvement of vertebrae by metastatic tumors. Special views, at times in neck flexion and extension, are necessary for evaluating the cervicocranial junction and the odontoid process.

Cerebral and Arch Angiography

Cerebral and arch angiography can visualize the four major arteries supplying the brain, their points of origin, their intracranial and extracranial branches plus draining veins, and the sinuses.

To perform the procedure, a semirigid catheter is passed through a needle inserted into the femoral artery and guided up the aorta under fluoroscopic control. The catheter tip can be maneuvered selectively into the innominate, common carotid, or left subclavian arteries and then into the vertebral, internal, or external carotid arteries. An iodinated contrast agent is then injected under pressure through the properly positioned catheter. Direct punctures of the common carotid artery or retrograde injections into the brachial artery for imaging the vertebral arteries can be used in selected cases, rather than the femoral approach.

cranial circulation. A larger femoral catheter is used for evaluating the aortic arch and branching-off points of the major vessels. This can delineate many abnormalities, including: stenosis; occlusion or ulcerated atherosclerotic plaques at the origin of the major neck vessels; the diffuse vessel abnormalities common with atherosclerosis, arteritis, or spasm; occluded intracranial arterial branches or venous structures; aneurysms and arteriovenous malformations; midline shifts and displacement of vessels caused by mass lesions; and changes such as abnormal vasculature, early filling veins, stretching and displacement of vessels, and a capillary "blush" produced by brain tumors.

Subtraction techniques, in which background "noise" such as that created by bony structures is masked, and magnification are commonly used. However, angiography is associated with a complication rate of about 1 percent and its use in the elderly or patients with generalized atherosclerotic or significant cardiac disease should be carefully weighed. Possible sequelae consist of embolization precipitated by catheter manipulation that can lead to transient or permanent neurological deficits, occlusion of arteries at the puncture site as the result of hematoma formation or dissection, and transient neurological deficits (e.g., cortical blindness following vertebral artery injection) possibly related to the effect on the artery of injecting dye under high pressure.

Digital Subtraction Angiography

Digital subtraction angiography is a newer method of computerized vascular enhancement and can improve the contrast resolution offered by traditional arteriography. It has also made possible the intravenous injection of contrast agent for the evaluation of neck vessels, thereby lessening the invasiveness and risk of angiography. However, the spatial resolution of the technique is currently less than that achieved with conventional angiography and large quantities of dye are needed. It can be performed on an outpatient basis to evaluate extracranial occlusive disease. The patient must be able to cooperate so that swallowing artifacts can be

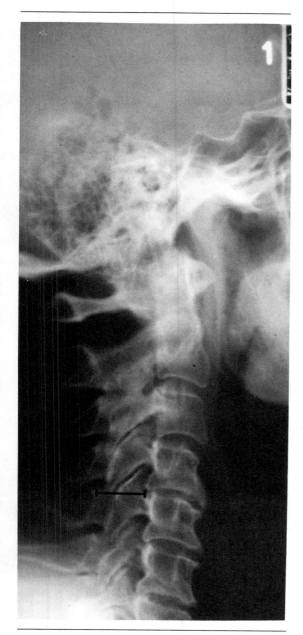

Fig. 3-2. *Lateral cervical spine x-ray study. The narrowest anteroposterior diameter of the spinal canal is meaured from the posterior part of the vertebral body (or protruding osteophytes) to the anterior part of the spinous process.*

Rapid serial x-ray images are recorded in the frontal and lateral projections over an 8- to 10-second interval to outline the arterial, capillary and venous phases of the extracranial and intra-

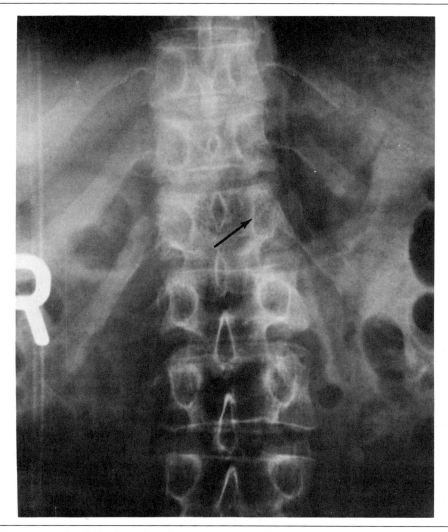

Fig. 3-3. *Plain x-ray study of the thoracic spine in a patient with subacute spinal cord compression and paraparesis. The flattening of the medial margin of the T12 pedicle* (arrow) *corresponded to the level of complete block shown by myelography. The patient underwent resection of a meningioma.*

avoided. The incidence of allergic reactions to the dye is greater than that with arteriography.

Myelography

To perform myelography, an iodinated contrast material (5 to 25 ml) is injected into the lumbar subarachnoid space under fluoroscopic control. The patient is tipped into the headdown position on a tilt table and the dye is run up to permit visualization of the spinal subarachnoid space and nerve root sleeves in the areas of interest. Posterior fossa cisternography may be performed if the dye is allowed to pass through the foramen magnum.

X-ray pictures are taken at appropriate levels. Oil must be removed through the needle at the end of the procedure, but, with the introduction of metrizamide, a water-soluble contrast agent, this is no longer necessary. Metrizamide yields the best results in the lumbar region, but relatively frequently complications such as seizures or an encephalopathy arise afterwards. The nonionic water-soluble contrast agent iopamidol is better tolerated than metrizamide.

Myelography is used to diagnose conditions that impinge on the spinal cord or roots, such as protruding or herniated discs, cervical spondylosis, lumbar stenosis, and epidural mass lesions, or lesions that produce spinal cord enlargement such as tumors and syringomyelia. The technique carries little risk to the patient other than that posed by LP. High-resolution spinal cord CT with or without contrast injection and MRI have now replaced myelography in the evaluation of many conditions.

Computed Tomography

In the short time since its introduction in 1973, CT has revolutionized neurological diagnosis. Its use has reduced the number of invasive neuroradiological procedures performed, eliminated the need for pneumoencephalography, greatly added to our understanding of a variety of neurological conditions, and contributed immeasurably to our ability to make precise clinical pathological correlations in vivo. As opposed to other techniques, CT allows direct visualization of intracranial soft tissues, in addition to bone, ventricles, cisterns and subarachnoid spaces, the orbits, sinuses, and even vessels (Fig. 3-4). With the newer high-resolution scanners, the spinal cord, brainstem, and sellar area can be well seen in several planes.

To perform CT, the patient lies supine and a thin x-ray beam is passed through the skull in a plane about 20 degrees above horizontal. Its absorption is then measured by a crystal detector. As the x-ray–detector assembly is rotated, absorption measurements are recorded with each degree of rotation and, using a computer, an **attenuation coefficient** is calculated for each small square (pixel) in the plane of interest. The attenuation coefficients are then used to construct a picture of the particular brain slice, with low-density structures such as the ventricles appearing black, high-density areas such as bone appearing white, and various shades of gray representing densities in between. Successive 10-mm-thick slices are taken

between the base of the skull and vertex to complete the axial series.

The intravenous injection of an iodinated contrast agent facilitates the detection of certain lesions either because of their vascularity or a breakdown in the blood-brain barrier. CT has been most valuable for the diagnosis of intracranial hemorrhage, cerebral infarcts, neoplasms, abscesses, traumatic brain lesions, edema, hydrocephalus, and atrophy.

Apart from occasional serious allergic reactions or renal impairment in diabetics related to the contrast agent, CT is safe and the radiation exposure to the patient is minimal. This makes it ideal for following the progression of a lesion.

Magnetic Resonance Imaging and Spectroscopy

MRI scanning has come into widespread clinical use over the past ten years and complements CT as a neuroimaging technique (Fig. 3-5 and Table 3-3). The complexity of the method, purchase and running costs of the equipment, the fact that about 5 percent of patients are too claustrophobic to undergo the procedure, and the difficulty of performing the test in uncooperative or seriously ill patients have limited its broader use. In addition, it cannot be used in patients with pacemakers or ferrous aneurysm clips. However, MRI scans provide exquisite anatomical detail and its sensitivity to certain early pathological changes far exceeds that of CT.

The patient is placed inside a magnetic field produced by a powerful (e.g., 1.5-tesla) superconducting magnet cooled with liquid helium. This causes freely moving hydrogen ions (protons) within water or fat to align themselves with the magnetic field. A specifically chosen short sequence of radiofrequency (RF) pulses is then administered through a coil placed around or over the surface of the body part of interest. The most popular pulse sequences have been termed the *spin-echo* and *inversion-recovery sequences*.

When exposed to the RF pulse, a certain number of protons align their magnetic fields against the prevailing magnetic field. When the RF signal is turned off, the protons return to a

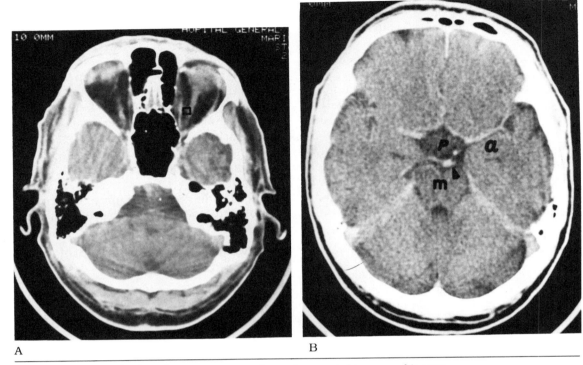

A   B

Fig. 3-4. *Four sample slices from a contrast-enhanced computed tomographic scan (axial view). (A)* Square = optic nerve. *(B)* p = *suprasellar cistern;* a = *temporal lobe (middle cerebral artery entering sylvian fissure is seen just above);* arrowhead = *basilar artery tip;* m = *midbrain.*

lower energy state while oscillating (precessing) about their axes. This emits a radio signal that is detected by a coil antenna. The intensity and time duration of this signal is determined by the number of mobile proteins and the characteristics of the surrounding molecules, and therefore can be used to extract anatomical information.

Gradient coils in the X, Y, and Z planes are used to superimpose another magnetic field on the main magnetic field in order to extract spatial information and calculate the signal intensity from each voxel (small cube) within the tissue slice being imaged. This requires special and complex calculations that are done by computer.

The rate of relaxation of the proteins is described by two time constants: the T_1 and T_2 relaxation times. T_1 (the spin-lattice relaxation constant) represents the time needed for the magnetic vector to return to 63 percent of its longitudinal length, and it generally varies between 0.5 and 3 seconds. T_2 (the spin-spin relaxation time) represents the time required for the protons to lose 63 percent of their transverse oscillatory movement and generally varies between 20 and 1,500 msec. The time to echo, which measures the delay before sampling the signal after the RF pulse is applied, and the repetition rate, which measures how rapidly the RF pulse is repeated, can be varied in such a way as to favor the T_1 or T_2 time constants in constructing an image. T_1-weighted images show excellent anatomical detail and CSF appears black. T_2-weighted images are fuzzier, show the CSF in white, and are more sensitive to pathological lesions that generally have an increased water content.

Besides providing images with a higher contrast resolution, MRI has several other advantages over CT. No adverse biological effects have been attributed to its use and patients are

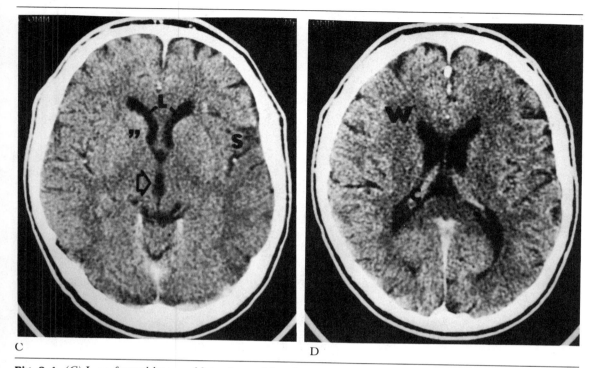

Fig. 3-4. *(C)* L = *frontal horns of lateral ventricles; "* = *internal capsule with caudate nucleus just above;* S = *sylvian fissure;* arrow = *third ventricle. (D)*W = *subcortical white matter appearing less dense than gray matter;* C = *choroid plexus.*

spared exposure to ionizing radiation. Images can be reconstructed easily from the data in any desired plane. Because it does not image cortical bone, this eliminates one of the main sources of artifact on CT—the base of the skull—thus allowing much clearer pictures of posterior fossa structures and the medial temporal areas. However, CT is superior to MRI for visualizing calcified intracranial lesions and abnormalities of the skull bones. MRI has proved particularly valuable for imaging the cervicomedullary junction and the spinal cord and roots, and may eventually replace myelography for this purpose.

Some of the main applications of MRI are for the early diagnosis of gliomas, determining the extent of tumor invasion, the early diagnosis of multiple sclerosis, the early diagnosis of cerebral infarction (particularly in the brainstem), the diagnosis of syringomyelia and syringobulbia, the detection of diffuse white matter changes in demented patients (Binswanger's disease), the early diagnosis of herpes simplex encephalitis, the delineation of lesions in head

trauma, and the preoperative localization of epileptic foci and lesions causing epilepsy.

Because the technique is so sensitive, unexpected areas of altered signal intensity whose clinical significance is unclear are frequently detected. Newer modifications in the MRI and CT technology have made it possible to obtain three-dimensional reconstructed images of the whole brain viewed in conjunction with the surrounding skull. This has proved invaluable to neurosurgeons in planning the optimal placement of a craniotomy to gain access to a lesion and has also permitted the diagnosis of subtle abnormalities in the surface anatomy of the brain (e.g., developmental gyral anomalies). More information from MRI can now be obtained with the use of paramagnetic intravenously administered contrast agents such as gadolinium diethylenetriaminepentaacetic acid, which is useful for differentiating tumor tissue from surrounding edema.

Magnetic resonance spectroscopy represents a sophisticated application of nuclear magnetic

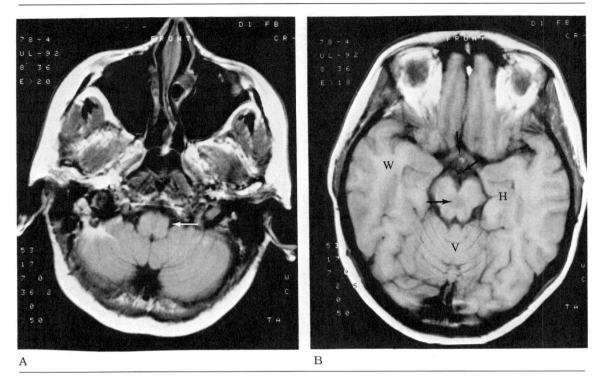

Fig. 3-5. T_1-weighted slices from normal MRI scan. (A) Horizontal arrow = medulla. (B) vertical arrow = optic chiasm; oblique arrow = flow void of basilar artery; W = white matter of temporal lobe; H = hippocampus and medial temporal structures; V = vermis of cerebellum.

resonance requiring high-field strengths that can determine the metabolism of brain or muscle in vivo. Phosphorus, sodium, and proton spectroscopy are possible. Various compounds and ions have been assessed experimentally, including magnesium, glucose, phospholipids, lactate, and neurotransmitters. The measurement of high-energy phosphorous compounds furnishes specific information on regional metabolic activity. The technique has been used mainly to investigate the potential mechanisms responsible for cell death during cerebral ischemia as well as to localize abnormalities in epileptic patients and to investigate brain tumors.

Magnetic resonance angiography is a noninvasive way of demonstrating intracranial arteries and veins. Rapidly flowing blood produces an absence of signal, or a "flow void." The technique is currently under development and cannot yet provide the resolution of conven-tional angiography. However, in certain patients who cannot undergo angiography because of difficulty or risk, it can serve as an alternative method for visualizing the intracranial vasculature.

Radionuclide Brain Scanning and Cisternography

A radioisotope (usually technetium 99m) injected intravenously can be picked up by scanning with special detectors over the scalp, and a picture generated based on the distribution of the agent within the vascular compartments. Lesions that cause a breakdown of the blood-brain barrier or that have a prominent vascular supply will appear as discrete "hot spots." The technique is useful for localizing tumors, infarcts, arteriovenous malformations, subdural hematomas, and brain abscesses. It poses no risk to the patient and the patient does not

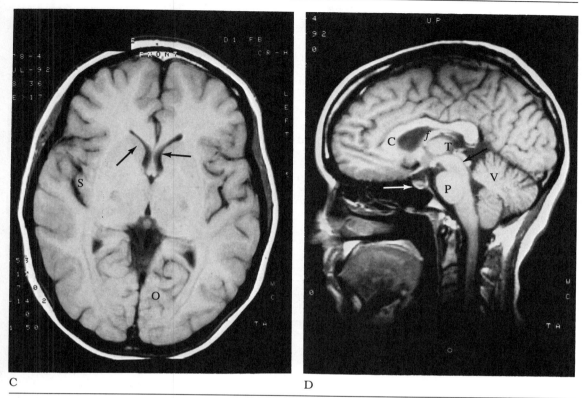

Fig. 3-5. *(C)* Horizontal arrow = *frontal horns, lateral ventricles;* oblique arrow = *caudate nucleus;* S = *sylvian fissure;* O = *occipital cortex. (D) Sagittal midline section. (C = corpus callosum;* f = *fornix;* T = *thalamus;* P = *basilar pons;* V = vermis of cerebellum;* horizontal arrow = *sella turcica;* oblique arrow = *sylvian aqueduct with tectum posterior.)*

have to remain perfectly motionless during the procedure. Dynamic scanning can be done to gain some idea of flow through the internal carotid arteries. However, these techniques have been largely supplanted by more modern neuroimaging procedures and single-photon emission CT (SPECT).

Radionuclide **cisternography,** employing radioiodinated serum albumin or labeled ytterbium injected into the lumbar subarachnoid space, is a method for examining CSF dynamics. By scanning over the head at various intervals following injection of the contrast agent, the path of the tracer can be followed through the basal cisterns and upward over the cerebral convexities (see Chapter 4). The technique is used most frequently for the diagnosis of normal-pressure hydrocephalus.

Ultrasonography

A variety of ultrasound techniques are now available that either produce an image of the vessels in the neck or measure flow within various extracranial vessels to show their patency. Doppler techniques make use of the Doppler principle, whereby ultrasound signals reflecting off moving objects (e.g., erythrocytes in flowing blood) show a shift in frequency that is proportional to the velocity of the moving object.

Continuous-wave or pulsed-wave Doppler probes are placed over arteries and both emit and record the ultrasound signal. Unlike angiography, these techniques cause no discomfort and pose no risk to the patient, making them useful for screening purposes (e.g., for asymptomatic neck bruits or before cardiac surgery).

Table 3-3. A Comparison of MRI and CT Scanning

	CT	MRI
Safety	X-ray exposure, needs special consideration in pregnancy	None, apparently safe in pregnancy
Cost of test	Moderately high	High
Artifacts	Beam-hardening artifacts near bone at base of skull	Not subject to artifacts near base of skull
Imaging of bone	+	Marrow only
Flexibility	Images in limited number of planes	Allows direct imaging in any plane
Spatial resolution	High	Very high
Ability to determine specific pathology	+	+ +
Usefulness in acutely ill patients	+	−
Usefulness in patients with cardiac pacemakers and metallic aneurysm clips	+	−
Functional information	Limited	MR angiography and spectroscopy capabilities

MRI = magnetic resonance imaging; CT = computed tomography; + = positive feature; + + = strongly positive feature; − = feature lacking.

They are also valuable for investigating patients with transient ischemic attacks, determining vessel patency after carotid endarterectomy, and observing the course of lesions. These techniques cannot distinguish total occlusion of an artery from a high-grade stenosis and have difficulty detecting ulcerated atherosclerotic plaques. Ideally, ultrasound techniques should be used in conjunction with other methods, such as ocular plethysmography and bruit analysis, for the acquisition of maximum information.

Of the various ultrasound techniques, the Doppler methods are the most widely used. Velocity of flow, turbulence, and direction of flow within the neck and periorbital vessels can be measured and the patency of a vessel inferred from this information. Reversal of flow within the ophthalmic artery is an important sign of severe stenosis or occlusion of the internal carotid artery. **B-mode ultrasound imaging** can render an actual picture of the extracranial vessels and may be done in conjunction with Doppler scanning.

Transcranial Doppler has been used increasingly to measure the velocity of intracranial vessels and has been promoted as a repeatable, safe, and inexpensive alternative to cerebral an-

giography under certain circumstances. In this method, a lower pulsed-wave ultrasound frequency is used, the probe is placed over the thinner temporal regions of the skull as well as the orbits and foramen magnum, and measurements are made at selected depths inside the skull. The examiner must have a certain amount of experience in order to successfully localize the arteries of interest and obtain maximal signals. In about 5 to 15 percent of patients, satisfactory recordings cannot be obtained from the "temporal windows." Anatomical variations may make it impossible to record signals from one anterior or posterior cerebral artery in certain individuals. Peak systolic, diastolic, and mean velocities are displayed and calculated, and three-dimensional color display of the major intracranial arteries is now possible with newer techniques. Pulsatility indexes can also be calculated. In general, narrowing of an artery due to stenosis or vasospasm produces increased flow velocity.

Transcranial Doppler has been used for identifying extracranial or intracranial stenosis of the internal carotid artery, detecting stenosis of the major intracranial branches of the internal carotid artery as well as the vertebral and basilar arteries, continuous intraoperative monitoring of the intracranial circulation, evaluating vaso-spasm following subarachnoid hemorrhage, screening for arteriovenous malformations, monitoring raised intracranial pressure, and aiding in the diagnosis of cerebral death.

Other Techniques

Positron Emission Tomography

Positron emission tomography (PET) is a sophisticated technique, used mainly for research purposes, that evaluates brain function by creating an image of the distribution of positron-emitting isotopes that are incorporated into various biologically active substrates such as drugs and ligands. Various neurotransmitter systems and pharmacological processes have been investigated using PET. Some of the most popular tracers have been [^{18}F]deoxyglucose for measuring glucose metabolism, ^{15}O-labeled oxygen for measuring oxygen metabolism, and ^{15}O-labeled water for determining regional cerebral blood flow. These and other positron-emitting isotopes have relatively short half-lives and an on-site minicyclotron is therefore required for their manufacture. In addition, the need for a team of experts in radiochemistry, and the like, make this a very expensive technique to perform.

PET scanning has been used to determine precisely which parts of the brain are activated in normal subjects during various motor, language, visual, and other sensory tasks. Cerebrovascular disease has been extensively studied by PET and it can detect early areas of ischemia before conventional neuroimaging techniques can reveal structural abnormalities. An increased oxygen extraction fraction is seen in areas of ischemia and PET can identify which areas are likely to show eventual infarction. The technique has been used in the preoperative evaluation of epileptic patients to help localize epileptic foci that show hypometabolism inter-ictally.

The specific diagnosis of degenerative diseases is an area where PET has been increasingly used. Presymptomatic patients with Huntington's disease exhibit reduced metabolism in the caudate nuclei before atrophy is seen on CT or MRI scans. In patients with early Alzheimer's disease, hypometabolism can be demonstrated in the superior parietal association areas. These changes gradually spread to involve the rest of the parietal and eventually the temporal lobes. A reduction in the 6-fluoro–L-DOPA uptake in the putamen can distinguish Parkinson's disease from other similar akinetic-rigid syndromes. Brain tumors have been explored in an attempt to identify metabolic or receptor peculiarities that could be exploited for therapy. PET can help distinguish more malignant grades of tumor and also radiotherapy-induced necrosis from that attributable to recurrent tumor.

This powerful technique has been used mainly as a research tool, but is also being used increasingly to provide complementary information to CT, MRI, magnetic resonance spectroscopy, and EEG in the clinical arena.

SPECT Scanning

SPECT utilizes principles similar to those of PET but is much less expensive to perform and more widely used clinically. The gamma rays emitted following the injection of specially developed radiotracers (e.g., [^{123}I]iofetamine and [^{99m}Te]hexamethylpropyleneamineoxime) are detected by specialized detectors placed around the scalp. The tracers cross the blood-brain barrier and are distributed proportionate to the cerebral blood flow. A cross-sectional image is then reconstructed. The technique is somewhat prone to technical artifacts and its resolution is lower than that of PET. Similar to PET, the technique has found clinical application in identifying the early or subtle areas of cerebral ischemia, localizing epileptic foci, and distinguishing multiinfarct dementia from Alzheimer's disease.

ELECTROPHYSIOLOGICAL TESTS

Electroencephalography

Electroencephalography (EEG) supplements the information provided by techniques such as CT and MRI because it provides data about brain function rather than structure (Table 3-

4). It is an innocuous and relatively inexpensive method that can be easily repeated as indicated. Advanced technology has allowed the extension of the EEG into areas such as computerized electrical brain mapping, combined EEG radiotelemetry–video monitoring, and EEG portable cassette monitoring.

A standard EEG makes use of 21 recording electrodes that are applied to the scalp and linked in various ways (montages). The EEG signal consists of minute (around 50 μV) brain potentials that represent fluctuating superficial dendritic potentials originating from cortical pyramidal cells, which are recorded, amplified, and traditionally inscribed on moving paper by a series of pens. Each pen is driven by a galvanometer that moves it up or down according to the potential difference on its two grids, each receiving input from one electrode. Newer computerized digital techniques allow raw EEG data to be recorded and stored in computer memory, then displayed on the computer monitor in any desired montage. "Paperless EEG" saves on cost and storage space and permits a much more flexible display of data. Each channel on the EEG record therefore represents a continuous record of the potential differences between two recording electrodes. A standard recording entails about 30 minutes, during which activation techniques such as hyperventilation and photic

Table 3-4. Advantages and Disadvantages of Electroencephalography

---

Advantages
  No patient risk, little discomfort
  Inexpensive
  Readily repeatable
  Widely available
  Can be done in acutely ill patients
  Gives information about brain function
Disadvantages
  Subject to physiological and electrical artifacts
  Few etiologically specific patterns
  Affected by physiological state (e.g., level of
    alertness, drugs, hypoglycemia)
  Limited spatial sampling (records only a portion
    of scalp activity and only from superficial
    cortical layers)
  Limited time sampling

---

stimulation with a stroboscopic light are used to elicit possible brain wave abnormalities.

In interpreting the EEG, the following are considered: the frequency of the predominant rhythms (background), amplitude, abnormal waves or wave groupings (e.g., bursts or paroxysms), right-left asymmetries, and abnormal responses to measures like eye closure, hyperventilation, and photic stimulation. The EEG potentials are classified according to frequency, as follows: 0.5 to 3 Hz (cycles per sec), delta; 4 to 7 Hz, theta; 8 to 13 Hz, alpha; and 18 to 35 Hz, beta. The normal resting adult rhythm, with the eyes closed in a relaxed state, is a sinusoidal-type alpha rhythm, which is synchronous and fairly symmetrical over both posterior head regions (Fig. 3-6). The following factors influence the EEG recording:

1. Level of consciousness—drowsiness, sleep (Fig. 3-7), coma, and anesthesia cause slowing.
2. Maturation—background rhythms are slower and less well organized in children.
3. Chemical environment—hypocapnia and hypoglycemia produce slowing.
4. Drugs—several tranquilizers and psychoactive drugs produce diffuse beta rhythms or slowing.
5. Pathological conditions:
   Focal slowing with destructive lesions
   Diffuse slowing occurs in the presence of metabolic disorders, raised intracranial pressure, and so on.
   Focal spikes or sharp waves are often associated with irritative lesions and scarring.
   Epileptiform (sharp and paroxysmal) activity or seizure patterns are seen in epilepsy. Although the EEG may help localize an intracranial lesion, its major application is in the diagnosis of epilepsy, metabolic encephalopathy, and certain conditions that manifest specific patterns.

Intensive EEG monitoring, with video recording, is used in patients with uncontrollable epileptic seizures, both to quantify and classify the seizures in patients with recurrent spells of uncertain origin and in the preoperative

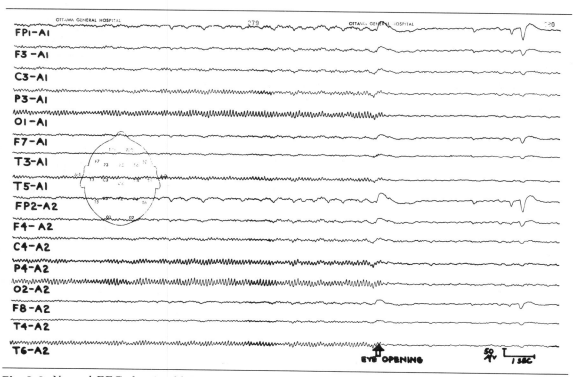

Fig. 3-6. *Normal EEG showing blocking of the sinusoidal background posterior alpha rhythm with eye opening.*

assessment of epileptic patients to determine where in the brain the seizures originate. For the latter purpose, patients are admitted to the hospital for continuous monitoring, often for several days. Outpatient intensive monitoring, which is done for 7 to 8 hours, is particularly useful for differentiating pseudoseizures and other nonepileptic spells from true epileptic attacks. For this approach to succeed, spells must be frequent (at least 1 to 2 per week) or reliably precipitated by specific stimuli or circumstances. Both cable telemetry and radiotelemetry techniques are in widespread use. In both methods, the EEG recording is displayed in a split-screen format along with a video picture of the patient, allowing precise EEG–behavioral correlations. Patients are comfortable during these prolonged recordings and are free to walk about from time to time, which does not interfere with the continuous nature of the recording. Both EEG and video signals are recorded on videocassettes for later playback and review.

Ambulatory EEG monitoring using small cassette devices is particularly useful in children who are having spells at school. Drawbacks to this method include: the number of recording channels is limited, there is no video signal, which can make interpretation of events difficult, and the signals are subject to artifact.

Brain electrical activity mapping makes use of digitally recorded EEG signals and computer technology to display the mean frequency spectra across the scalp utilizing a special color format. This technique can highlight certain trends, such as focal slowing or right-left differences in background frequency, which might not be readily evident on the standard EEG record.

Sensory Evoked Potentials

Very low-voltage potentials evoked by visual, auditory, or somatosensory stimuli (e.g., reversing checkerboard pattern, clicking noises,

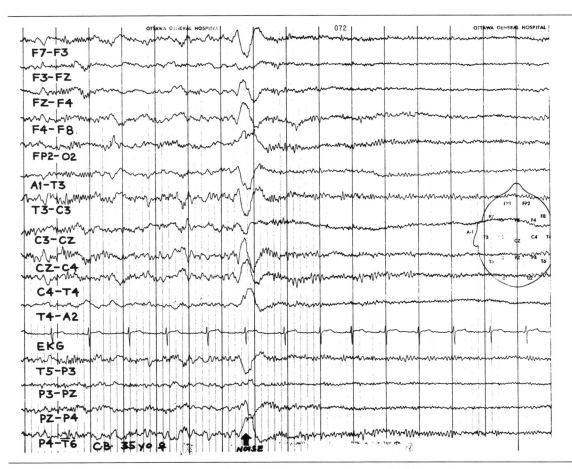

Fig. 3-7. *Normal EEG of stage II sleep showing a vertex transient provoked by noise, followed by an awake pattern.*

and electrical shocks delivered to the median or posterior tibial nerves, respectively) may be recorded from the scalp. Because of the tiny voltages involved, an averaging computer, which sums and enhances the potentials and is time-locked to a series of stimuli, is used to improve the signal-to-noise ratio. The latencies and amplitudes of the various evoked potential components are measured and compared between the two sides of the head and with normal values. Analysis of brainstem auditory evoked potentials recorded from the scalp allows specific conclusions to be drawn about the intactness of auditory pathways at various levels and can be used to assess hearing. Information can also be gained about overall brain functioning (e.g., in the diagnosis of cerebral death) and about lesions in specific sensory pathways which may not be apparent clinically, as in multiple sclerosis (see Chapter 25). The technique has also been used intraoperatively to monitor the integrity of neuronal pathways (e.g., eighth nerve function during the removal of acoustic neuromas).

Peripheral Nerve Conduction Velocities

Motor conduction velocities can be measured by stimulating a particular nerve at two points a measured distance apart and recording the latency of the responses over the corresponding muscle. The velocity of conduction over the nerve between the two points is then easily calculated (Fig. 3-8A). Terminal latencies can also be measured when the distal portion of a nerve (e.g., the median nerve at the carpal tunnel) is stimulated.

Sensory conduction is measured by applying special electrodes to a digit and recording proximally over the nerve (Fig. 3-8B). The values obtained are compared with standard normal velocities and between the right and left sides as well as with the values obtained from comparable nerves in the same patient. Nerve conduction velocity may be slowed or absent in patients with peripheral neuropathies (especially demyelinating) or with compressive or traumatic lesions. These techniques are most valuable for distinguishing neuropathies from myopathies, localizing a lesion to a par-

ticular nerve or part of a nerve, distinguishing demyelinating from axonal neuropathies, diagnosing subclinical neuropathic illness, and following the progress or response to therapy in patients with peripheral nerve lesions.

Electromyography

Concentric or monopolar needle electrodes can be inserted into various muscles to record information about the amplitude, duration, form, and abundance of spontaneous motor unit potentials and those occurring with various degrees of muscle contraction (Fig. 3-9), and this constitutes the technique of electromyography (EMG). Recent improvements in instrumentation allowing digital signal pro-

Fig. 3-8. *(A) The technique for measuring motor nerve conduction velocities in the median nerve of the forearm. The nerve is stimulated at two different sites and the latency to the onset of the compound muscle action potential is recorded each time. The distance between the two sites of stimulation is carefully measured.*

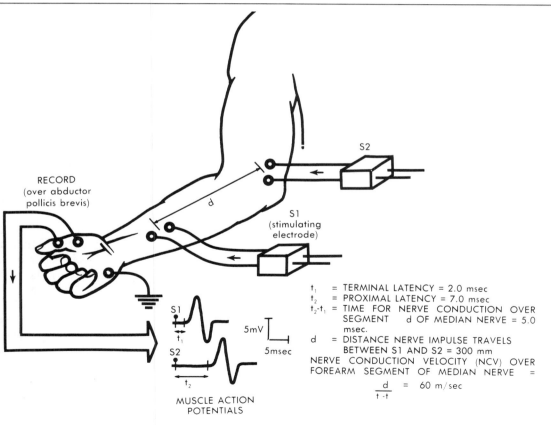

t_1 = TERMINAL LATENCY = 2.0 msec
t_2 = PROXIMAL LATENCY = 7.0 msec
t_2-t_1 = TIME FOR NERVE CONDUCTION OVER SEGMENT d OF MEDIAN NERVE = 5.0 msec.
d = DISTANCE NERVE IMPULSE TRAVELS BETWEEN S1 AND S2 = 300 mm
NERVE CONDUCTION VELOCITY (NCV) OVER FOREARM SEGMENT OF MEDIAN NERVE = $\frac{d}{t_2-t_1}$ = 60 m/sec

A

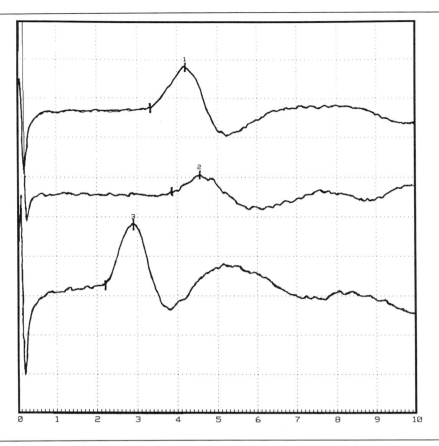

B

Fig. 3-8 *(Continued). (B) Sensory nerve conduction velocities measured across the wrist in the median nerve (top two tracings) and ulnar nerve (lower tracing). The median nerve responses were recorded over the first and lateral half of the fourth digits, and the ulnar nerve response, over the medial fourth digit. Stimulation was just above the wrist. The patient had a carpal tunnel syndrome, as shown by the increased latency and reduced voltage (second tracing) of median nerve responses. The calculated conduction velocity in the median nerve was 37.6 M/sec (normal, >50 M/sec). (Time scale is in milliseconds; amplitude = 10 μV/division.)*

cessing now permit data to be displayed in various ways and the easy calculation of a number of statistical measurements. EMG signals can also be listened to through a loudspeaker, and this information can supplement the visual interpretation of the recorded potentials. The amplitude, duration, and number of phases in the motor unit potentials are examined.

EMG is very useful for distinguishing neuropathies from myopathies, helping define the distribution of a denervating process (e.g., root versus nerve), aiding in the diagnosis of motor neuron disease, and identifying specific myopathic conditions such as myotonic dystrophy. The technique is used in conjunction with nerve stimulation to diagnose neuromuscular junction disorders such as myasthenia gravis. Single-fiber EMG using small recording electrodes and filtering techniques permits simultaneous recording from two or more nearby muscle fibers. *Jitter* is defined as a variability in the discharge time between two fibers and is increased in neuromuscular transmission disorders such as myasthenia gravis. Further discussion of nerve

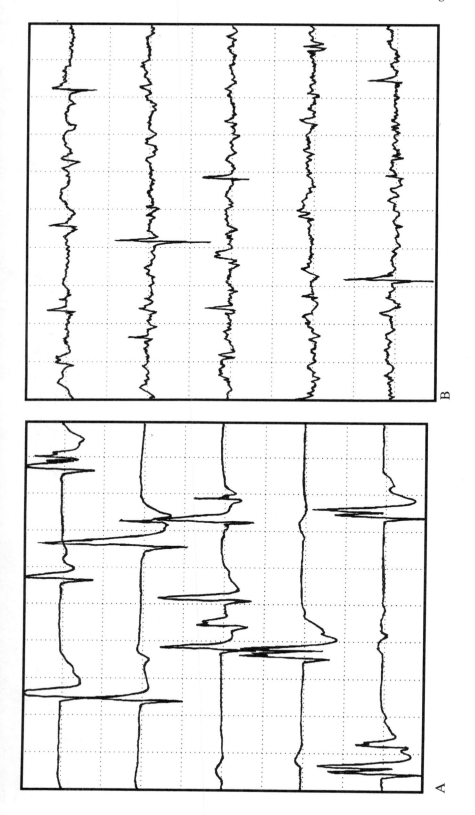

Fig. 3-9. *Electromyographic recordings. (A) Neurogenic (denervation) pattern showing high-voltage, long-duration polyphasic units and a reduced number of units with moderate effort. Recording was taken from the rectus femoris muscle in a patient with an L3–L4 disc herniation. (Sweep speed = 10 msec/division; gain = 2.0 mV/ division.) (B) Fibrillation potentials recorded from the orbicularis oculi muscle in a patient with Bell's palsy. This indicates axonal damage, denervation, and a likely prolonged recovery period. (Sweep speed = 10 msec/division; gain = 0.05 mV/ division.)*

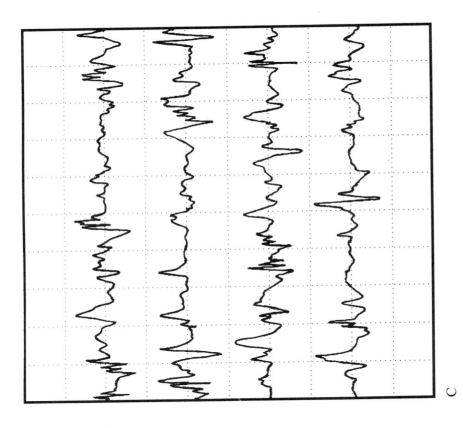

C

Fig. 3-9 *(Continued). (C) Myopathic pattern with low-amplitude, polyphasic, short-duration units and early recruitment of abundant units with minimal effort. (Sweep speed = 10 msec/division; gain = 0.5 mV/division.)*

conduction velocity studies and EMG is found in Chapters 15 and 16.

BIBLIOGRAPHY

Ackerman, R.H. Noninvasive diagnosis of carotid disease in the era of digital subtraction angiography. *Neurol. Clin.* 1:263–278, 1983.

Aminoff, M.J. (editor). Electrodiagnosis. *Neurol. Clin.* 3:471–697, 1985.

Aminoff, M.J. *Electrodiagnosis in Clinical Neurology*, 3rd ed. New York: Churchill Livingstone, 1992.

Aminoff, M.J. Evoked potential studies in neurological diagnosis and management. *Ann. Neurol.* 28:706–710, 1990.

Atlas, S.W. (editor). *Magnetic Resonance Imaging of the Brain and Spine*, New York: Raven, 1991.

Ball, J.B., Jr. et al. Complications of intravenous digital subtraction angiography. *Arch. Neurol.* 42:969–972, 1985.

Brody, A.S. New perspectives in CT and MRI imaging. *Neurol. Clin.* 9:273–286, 1991.

Buonanno, F.S. (editor). Neuroimaging. *Neurol. Clin.* 2:635–924, 1984.

Caplan, L.R., et al. Transcranial Doppler ultrasound: present status. *Neurology* 40:696–700, 1990.

Council on Scientific Affairs Report of the Panel on Magnetic Resonance Imaging. Magnetic resonance imaging of the central nervous system. *JAMA* 259:1211–1222, 1988.

Daly, D.D. and Pedley, T.A. *Current Practice of Clinical Electro-encephalography,* 2nd ed. New York: Raven, 1990.

Deyo R.A., Bigos, S.J. and Maravilla, K.R. Diagnostic imaging procedures for the lumbar spine. *Ann. Intern. Med.* 111:865–867, 1989.

Fishman, R.A. *Cerebrospinal Fluid in Diseases of the Nervous System,* 2nd ed, Philadelphia: Saunders, 1992.

Frackowiak, R.S.J. (editor). Positron emission tomography. *Semin. Neurol.* 9:275–402, 1989.

Gerard, G. and Rossi, D.R. (editors). Nuclear magnetic imaging of the nervous system. *Semin. Neurol.* 6:1–106, 1986.

Gilmore, R.L. (editor). Evoked potentials. *Neurol. Clin.* 6:649–951, 1988.

Gilmore, R.L. (editor). Neurophysiologic diagnostic studies. *Semin. Neurol.* 10:111–209, 1990.

Greenberg, J.O. Neuroimaging of the spinal cord. *Neurol. Clin.* 9:679–704, 1991.

Guberman, A. and Couture, M. *Atlas of Electroencephalography*. Boston: Little, Brown, 1989.

Gumnit, R.J. (editor). *Intensive Neurodiagnostic Monitoring* (Vol. 46, Advances in Neurology). New York: Raven, 1987.

Hankey, G.J., Warlow, C.P. and Sellar, R.J. Cerebral angiographic risk in mild cerebrovascular disease. *Stroke* 21:209–222, 1990.

Holman, B.L. and Tumeh, S.S. Single-photon emission computed tomography (SPECT): applications and potential. *JAMA* 263:561–564, 1990.

Kimura, J. Principles and pitfalls of nerve conduction studies. *Ann. Neurol.* 16:415–429, 1984.

Kimura, J. *Electrodiagnosis in Diseases of Nerve and Muscle: Principles and Practice.* Philadelphia: Davis, 1989.

Kinkel, W. Computerized tomography in clinical neurology. In R.J. Joynt (editor). *Clinical Neurology*. Philadelphia: Lippincott, 1991, Pp. 1–115.

Kinkel, W. Nuclear magnetic resonance imaging in clinical neurology. In R.J. Joynt (editor). *Clinical Neurology*. Philadelphia: Lippincott, 1991, Pp. 1–68.

Lee, S.H. and Rao, K.C. *Cranial Computed Tomography and MRI.* New York: McGraw-Hill, 1988.

Marton, K.I. and Gean, A.D. The spinal tap:

a new look at an old test. *Ann. Intern. Med.* 104:840–848, 1986.

Niedermeyer, E. and da Silva, L. *Electro-encephalography*, 2nd ed. Baltimore: Urban & Schwarzenberg, 1987.

Pearce, J.M.S. Hazards of lumbar puncture. *Br. Med. J.* 285:1521–1522, 1982.

Petito, F. and Plum, F. The lumbar puncture. *N. Engl. J. Med.* 290:225–226, 1974.

Petty, G.W., Wiebers, D.O., and Meissner, I. Transcranial Doppler ultrasonography: clinical applications in cerebrovascular disease. *Mayo Clin. Proc.* 65:1350–1364, 1990.

Shahani, B.T. and Young, R.R. Clinical electromyography. In R.J. Joynt (editor). *Clinical Neurology*. Philadelphia: Lippincott, 1991, Pp. 1–51.

Stevens, J.M., et al. Relative safety of intravenous digital subtraction angiography over the methods of carotid angiography and its impact on clinical management of cerebrovascular disease. *Br. J. Radiol.* 62:813–816, 1989.

Theodore, W.H. (editor). *Clinical Neuroimaging*. New York: Alan R. Liss, 1988.

Therapeutics and Technology Assessment Subcommittee of the American Academy of Neurology. Assessment: positron emission tomography. *Neurology* 41:163–167, 1991.

Tyner, F.S., Knott, J.R., and Mayer, W.B., Jr. *Fundamentals of EEG Technology. Clinical Correlations*, Vol. 2. New York: Raven, 1988.

Wagle, W.A. Neuroradiology. In R.J. Joynt (editor). *Clinical Neurology*. Philadelphia: Lippincott, 1991, Pp. 2–322.

4

Delirium and Dementia

DELIRIUM OR ACUTE CONFUSIONAL STATE

Delirium and *acute confusional state* are the neurologist's terms for what psychiatrists call an *acute organic brain syndrome*. Some distinguish delirium from acute confusional state by using the former to refer only to cases in which agitation is a feature. The syndrome is familiar to most physicians and one of the most common reasons for neurological consultation on hospital wards. These patients may initially be mistakenly admitted to psychiatric services with a diagnosis of acute psychotic reaction.

Definition and Pathogenesis

Strub defines the acute confusional state as: "a rapidly developing, yet fluctuating, behavior change that is characterized by altered arousal; inattention; incoherent speech, thought and action; global impairment of memory and intellectual processes; perceptual disturbances, in-cluding illusions and hallucinations; and marked emotional lability." Delirium may be thought of as the manifestation of relatively early and mild, acute or subacute brain failure. The causative agents are most commonly endogenous or exogenous toxins that produce a global metabolic impairment of brain function.

A deprivation of substrates for energy metabolism (oxygen and glucose), deficiency of vitamin cofactors, or direct interference with neurotransmitter action or neuronal membrane function may be responsible for its pathogenesis. If the underlying process is allowed to progress, stupor, coma, death, or irreversible brain damage frequently eventuates. Therefore, the early diagnosis and treatment of reversible disturbances is mandatory.

Clinical Picture

Although the syndrome can occur subacutely or acutely, it commonly appears when a minor metabolic upset, intercurrent infection, or change in environment precipitates decompensation in a patient already compromised by mild dementia or a previous brain insult. The elderly, mildly demented patient who becomes confused and paranoid and wanders at night in the hospital but was never a behavior problem at home is a familiar picture.

The symptomatology is fairly uniform regardless of the cause. Delirium tremens, hepatic encephalopathy, and hypoxic encephalopathy are typical examples. Early in the course, irritability, concentration difficulties, insomnia, and subtle intellectual and personality changes occur. With progression, attention deficits, frank disorientation, memory difficulties, global intellectual impairment, changes in the arousal level (withdrawal or agitation) which may fluctuate, perceptual derangements (hallucinations, usually visual and illusory—misinterpretations of actual sensory stimuli), and emotional disturbances (e.g., excessive lability and unprovoked panic) become apparent. There is frequently a paranoid flavor to the patient's thinking and hallucinations, although there may be a tendency to perceive the unfamiliar as familiar.

Commonly accompanying these mental deficits are speech disturbances, epileptic seizures, multifocal myoclonus, asterixis, autonomic disturbances (e.g., tachycardia, diaphoresis, and mydriasis), a gait disorder with a tendency to fall backward, hyperreflexia and other corticospinal tract signs, and respiratory alkalosis.

Etiology

The most common causes of delirium are listed in Table 4-1. In most instances, one or more factors are acting together. Although there is a wide variety of potential causes, toxic and metabolic disturbances are by far the most common.

Investigations

In view of the causes listed in Table 4-1, it is clear that laboratory investigations are often necessary to identify the underlying cause of delirium. However, in some situations, such as in postconcussion states, following a brief cardiac arrest that has produced hypoxic encepha-

lopathy, and in certain forms of intoxication, neither the neurological examination nor the laboratory evaluation will aid much in the diagnosis.

Initially serum electrolyte levels (including calcium and magnesium), the glucose concentration, blood urea nitrogen (BUN), liver function, and arterial blood gas levels should be assessed. An electrocardiogram and chest x-ray study should also be obtained early. If the diagnosis is still not clear after these investigations, a toxicological screen, urinalysis for the presence of porphyrins and porphobilinogen, and a computed tomographic (CT) scan followed by a lumbar puncture to rule out meningitis or subarachnoid hemorrhage should be obtained.

The electroencephalogram (EEG) will almost invariably show slowing of the background activity and possibly bifrontal bursts of rhythmic delta waves. In the event of psychoactive drug use, there is frequently excessive fast activity. Triphasic waves can be seen in the presence of hepatic, uremic, and at times other encephalopathies (Fig. 4-1). However, the chief uses of the EEG in this context are to distinguish an organic delirium from a psychiatric disorder, in which the EEG remains normal, and to follow the evolution of a metabolic encephalopathy.

Differential Diagnosis

An acute psychotic reaction or schizophrenic episode can resemble delirium but, in the former, orientation, calculation abilities, visuospatial functions, and the level of consciousness are usually well preserved. Hallucinations in this setting, when present, are more often auditory than visual and the signs of metabolic encephalopathy mentioned previously are lacking. A normal EEG is another important clue.

Occasionally a rapidly developing severe depression in an elderly person with pronounced psychomotor retardation and muteness may pose a diagnostic problem. In some cases, after laboratory results prove negative, one has to rely on the patient's response to antidepressant drugs or electroconvulsive therapy to make the diagnosis. An aphasia, particularly when speech is relatively fluent, may be mistaken for

Table 4-1. Causes of Delirium

Deprivation of oxygen, glucose, or cofactors
  Hypoxia
  Global ischemia (e.g., following cardiac arrest or
    severe hypotension)
  Severe anemia
  Hypoglycemia
  Cofactor (vitamin) deficiency (e.g., thiamine in
    Wernicke's encephalopathy)
Systemic organ failure
  Hepatic encephalopathy
  Uremic encephalopathy
  Pulmonary failure (CO_2 narcosis)
  Congestive heart failure
  Pancreatic encephalopathy (rare)
Endocrine and other metabolic disturbances
  Hypopituitarism
  Addison's, Cushing's disease
  Hypothyroidism, hyperthyroidism
  Porphyria
Electrolyte, acid-base, or osmolality disturbances
  Hyper- or hyponatremia
  Hyper- or hypocalcemia
  Hyper- or hypomagnesemia
  Acidosis or alkalosis
  Hyper- or hypoosmolality
Drugs and toxins
  Drugs
    Sedatives and hypnotics
    Tricyclic antidepressants, lithium
    Anticholinergics
    Antihistamines
    L-Dopa, bromocriptine, amantadine
    Anticonvulsant drugs
    Isoniazid, rifampin, penicillin, streptomycin,
      sulfonamides
    Digitalis, propanolol, antihypertensives

Oral hypoglycemics
Cimetidine
Various "street drugs"
Toxins: alcohol, methanol, ethylene glycol, glue-
  sniffing, solvents, insecticides
Drug withdrawal and alcohol withdrawal (delirium
  tremens)
Infections
  High fever (especially in children)
  Systemic infections such as pneumonia,
    septicemia, malaria
  Meningitis or encephalitis
  Acute HIV encephalopathy
Related to surgery and intensive care
  Following general surgery
  After cardiac bypass surgery
  ICU syndrome
Multifocal cerebral disease
  Multiple emboli (e.g., subacute bacterial
    endocarditis, fat embolism)
  Vasculitis (e.g., SLE)
  Acute hemorrhagic necrotizing leukoencephalitis
  Disseminated intravascular coagulation,
    thrombotic thrombocytopenic purpura
Other diffuse disturbances
  Post concussion
  Postictal (i.e., following epileptic seizures)
  Nonconvulsive status epilepticus
  Subarachnoid hemorrhage
  Encephalitis, meningitis
Focal cerebral disease (rarely)
  Right frontal or parietal infarct
  Limbic system infarct
Miscellaneous
  Heat stroke
  Remote effects of carcinoma

HIV = human immune deficiency virus; ICU = intensive care unit; SLE = systemic lupus erythematosus.

a confusional state. The characteristics of the patient's spoken and written language, especially if paraphasias or neologisms are present, are usually revealing.

Another rare condition that presents as an acute confusional state and may occasionally appear de novo in an elderly patient is nonconvulsive generalized status epilepticus ("petit mal status"). A slowing of mental processes and movements and an increased latency of response are characteristic of this condition. Diagnosis is based on the EEG demonstration of continuous or nearly continuous generalized spike waves or polyspike waves and the patient's prompt response to an intravenous injection of diazepam or lorazepam.

Management

One should attempt to make a specific diagnosis rapidly, especially considering the treatable or reversible conditions. Any correctable metabolic deficits should be reversed, but at times too-rapid treatment may provoke temporary worsening of the clinical state. Thiamine (50 mg intramuscularly [IM] and 50 mg intravenously [IV]) should be administered in suspected alcoholics. Specific treatments such as phy-

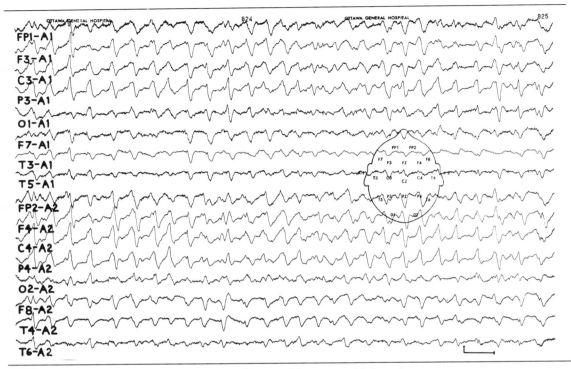

Fig. 4-1. *EEG showing triphasic waves in a 54-year-old woman with hepatic encephalopathy and chronic renal failure.*

sostigmine to counteract anticholinergic drug overdose, antibiotics for infection, and oxygenation and ventilation to reverse pulmonary failure should be undertaken. Close observation of vital and neurological signs is essential, at least until a specific diagnosis is determined.

In a case of severe agitated delirium, close attention must be paid to fluid and electrolyte imbalances, autonomic disturbances, and pulmonary function (e.g., avoidance of aspiration). Most such patients require the care of a constant attendant, especially at night when symptoms usually worsen. A family member, who can provide reassurance and a familiar presence, is often best for this purpose. The patient's room should be left partially illuminated at night. Physical restraints or sedation should only be used if necessary to protect the patient and prevent exhaustion. Haloperidol (5 or 10 mg IM) or a benzodiazepine in large doses (e.g., up to 1 gm of chlordiazepoxide per day in delirium tremens) can be given for sedation. Every attempt should be made to regulate

sleep, and a hypnotic such as chloral hydrate or oxazepam can be used for this purpose.

DEMENTIA

Dementia in the neurologist's vocabulary corresponds to the psychiatrist's *chronic organic brain syndrome*. It can be equated with chronic brain failure, leading in its most advanced stages to a comalike picture known as the persistent vegetative state, in which the patient has no meaningful contact with the environment. Dementia can be defined as a usually progressive, at times reversible, abnormal decline in cognitive functions that usually include a prominent memory deficit. It is differentiated from mental retardation by the fact that it entails a decline from a previously normal level. With an increasingly aged population, dementia has become more prevalent and is now believed to affect about 10 percent of the population over age 65, severely in about half of the cases. These figures are double for those over 80 years old. It has been estimated that Alzheimer's disease, the major cause of dementia, is the fourth leading cause of death. In only a small number of patients is dementia treatable or reversible, but, in view of the devastating nature of the illness and the high cost of long-term care, each patient deserves a full diagnostic evaluation that focuses on identifying possible treatable causes (Table 4-2 and Fig. 4-2).

Symptomatology: Cortical versus Subcortical Dementia

The onset of dementia is usually insidious, and, in its early phases, diagnosis depends on the patient's history, especially information provided by family members or associates. A dete-

riorating work performance; memory and word-finding difficulties; a tendency to get lost in formerly familiar surroundings; abandonment of previous interests; a tendency not to engage in conversation; and personality changes such as increased irritability, a loss of sense of humor, apathy, and depression can all be early indications of an advancing dementia. Inquiry should be made about the patient's ability to handle money, drive a car, and understand what he or she reads or sees on television.

There are two broad categories of dementia, cortical and subcortical (Table 4-3), although some patients do not clearly fit into either one of these categories. The clinical symptomatology depends on whether the pathological process affects mainly the cortical neurons or the basal ganglia as well as thalamic and upper

Table 4-2. Causes of Dementia in Adults

UNTREATABLE/IRREVERSIBLE

Primary degenerative
  Alzheimer's disease
  Pick's disease
  Huntington's disease
  Parkinson's disease
  Olivopontocerebellar degeneration
  Progressive supranuclear palsy
  Cortical-basal ganglionic degeneration
Infectious
  Creutzfeldt-Jakob disease
  Subacute sclerosing panencephalitis
  Progressive multifocal leukoencephalopathy
Metabolic
  Metachromatic leukodystrophy
  Kuf's disease
  Gangliosidoses

POTENTIALLY TREATABLE/REVERSIBLE

Infectious
  Chronic meningitis (cryptococcal)
  Syphilis (general paresis of the insane)
  HIV encephalopathy
Toxic
  Drugs (e.g., barbiturates, bromides, other sedative-hypnotics, anticholinergics, anticonvulsants, clonidine, methyldopa)
  Organic solvents
  Alcohol, methanol
  Heavy metals (lead, mercury, arsenic, thallium)
Vitamin deficiency
  Thiamine (Wernicke-Korsakoff syndrome)

  B_{12}
  Folate
  Niacin (pellagra)
Metabolic—endocrine
  Systemic organ failure (hepatic, renal, pulmonary)
  Dialysis dementia
  Hypocalcemia
  Hypercalcemia
  Other electrolyte imbalances
  Hypothyroidism
  Wilson's disease
Vascular
  Multiple infarcts (or lacunar state)
  Binswanger's disease
  Arteriovenous malformation with intracerebral steal phenomenon
  Severe stenosis of large neck vessels
  Vasculitis (e.g., collagen disease)
  Bilateral paramedian thalamic infarction
Space-occupying lesions
  Neoplasms (especially frontal or diencephalic)
  Subdural hematoma
  Cerebral abscess
Other
  Normal-pressure hydrocephalus
  Recurrent episodes of sleep apnea
  Other causes of recurrent hypoxia/ischemia or hypoglycemia
  Dementia pugilistica
  Uncontrolled epileptic seizures

HIV = human immune deficiency virus.

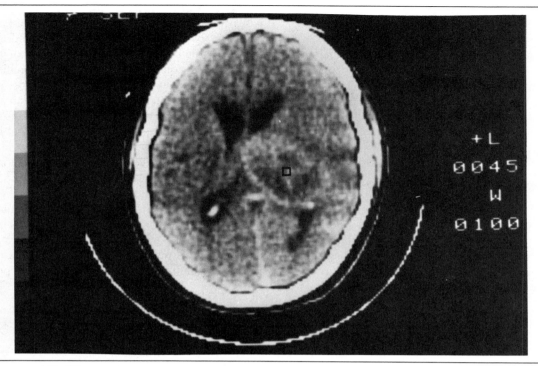

Fig. 4-2. *(A) CT scan.*

brainstem structures. Cortical dementias, such as Alzheimer's and Pick's disease, present with early memory deficits, and commonly patients show visuospatial deficits, aphasia, apraxia, and agnosia. Subcortical dementias, such as occur with progressive supranuclear palsy and Parkinson's disease, are characterized by a slowness of mentation, some memory disturbance, affective changes, and "dilapidation" of cognition as well as prominent extrapyramidal signs.

Specific Etiologies

Alzheimer's Disease

Alzheimer's disease was formerly classified as a presenile dementia with onset occurring before age 65. It is now recognized that senile dementia starting after age 65 is really the same disease pathologically and clinically and this form is now designated *senile dementia of the Alzheimer type.*

Pathophysiology and Etiology. The main pathological features of Alzheimer's disease consist of brain atrophy with neuronal loss, senile (neuritic) plaques located throughout the cortex, silver-staining neurofibrillary tangles found mainly within hippocampal neurons, and amyloid angiopathy affecting the capillaries and arterioles in the neocortex and meninges. Simplification of cortical neuronal dendritic branching, granulovacuolar degeneration in hippocampal neurons, and increased amounts of lipofuscin (aging pigment) are also seen. The degree of dementia has been correlated with the degree of synaptic loss, although some studies have shown a relationship to the density of "mature" neuritic plaques. An unanswered question is whether these changes, not different from those seen in the brains of nondemented older individuals, merely represent an acceleration of the aging process. More recently, a profound loss of cholinergic neurons from the nucleus basalis of Meynert has been shown.

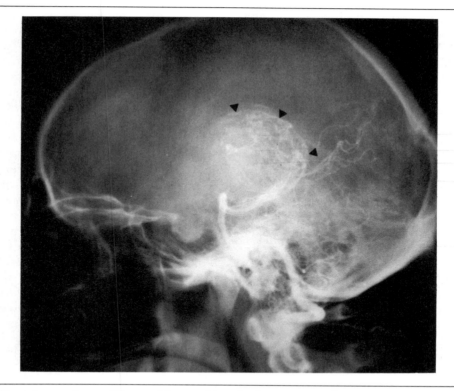

Fig. 4-2. *(B) angiogram from a 58-year-old man with a slowly progressive dementia due to a thalamic glioma. The tumor shows neovascularization* (arrowheads).

Table 4-3. Cortical Versus Subcortical Dementias

Characteristics	Cortical dementia	Subcortical dementia
Appearance	Alert, healthy	Abnormal (e.g., infirm)
Activity	Normal	Slow
Stance	Erect	Stooped, dystonic
Gait	Normal	Ataxic, festinating, dancing
Movements	Normal	Tremor, chorea, dyskinesia
Verbal output	Normal	Dysarthric, hypophonic, mute
Language	Abnormal (anomia, paraphasias)	Normal
Cognition	Abnormal (unable to manipulate knowledge)	Dilapidated
Memory	Abnormal (learning disorder)	Forgetful (retrieval disorder)
Visuospatial ability	Abnormal (construction disturbance)	Sloppy (due to movement disorder)
Emotional state	Abnormal (unaware, unconcerned)	Abnormal (apathetic, lacking drive)
Examples	Alzheimer's, Pick's disease	Progressive supranuclear palsy; Parkinson's, Wilson's, and Huntington's diseases

Adapted from J.L. Cummings and D.F. Benson, Subcortical dementia. Review of an emerging concept. *Arch. Neurol.* 41: 874–879, 1984.

Various other neurotransmitter systems and neuropeptides also show depletions. Although the changes in the brains of patients with Alzheimer's disease are widespread, their consistent focus in the enterorhinal cortex and perforant pathways to the hippocampus have suggested that the development of a functional disconnection between the hippocampus and neocortical as well as other subcortical areas may be the prime source of the memory deficit seen in Alzheimer's disease. Neurofibrillary tangles (Fig. 4-3), with electronmicroscopy features consisting of paired helical neurofilaments exhibiting a unique periodicity, are also seen in the amyotrophic lateral sclerosis–Parkinson's dementia complex that affects the Chomorro natives of Guam, as well as in patients with postencephalitic parkinsonism, dementia pugilistica (of boxers), and Down's syndrome (most of whom develop Alzheimer

changes after the age of 30). The neuritic plaques, which are extracellular, are composed of an amyloid core surrounded by degenerating neuronal cell processes or neurites with the same paired helical neurofilaments found in neurofibrillary tangles. Plaques may lie near microvessels surrounded by amyloid, although this is an inconsistent finding. The neurofibrillary tangles are intracellular structures but remain as a marker once the neuron has died. Each neurofilament has a diameter of about 10 nm and the half-periodicity of the helix is about 80 nm. Tau proteins, normally associated with microtubules, have also been identified in the outer portion of neurofibrillary tangles, and amyloid too is found in conjunction with these structures. Because identical sorts of tangles are encountered in a variety of disorders, they are considered to represent a relatively nonspecific reaction to a number

Fig. 4-3. *Microscopic view (original magnification, × 40) of silver-staining, flame-shaped neurofibrillary tangles* (oblique arrows) *surrounding a mature neuritic plaque* (P) *in the hippocampus of a patient with Alzheimer's disease. Vertical arrow indicates a neuron undergoing granulovacuolar degeneration.*

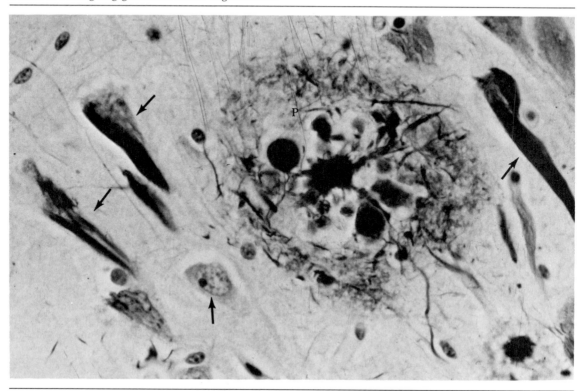

of pathogenetic factors leading to cytoskeletal injury and eventually neuronal death.

Currently, attempts to unravel the pathogenesis of the brain changes seen in Alzheimer's disease have focused on amyloid. Deposition of these abnormal peptide complexes occurs in various tissues in a number of disorders. The beta-amyloid found in plaques is identical to that found in microvessels in Alzheimer's disease and represents a 28–43–amino acid fragment of a larger protein, the beta-amyloid precursor protein, which is a transmembrane glycoprotein. Several lines of evidence now suggest that the deposition of abnormal quantities of beta-amyloid stemming from defective processing of the precursor protein lies at the heart of the pathogenesis of Alzheimer's disease. Whether it is derived from the blood and its accumulation represents an abnormal transport into the brain or whether it is produced in the brain itself is still unresolved.

Using modern molecular biological techniques, the gene for the beta-amyloid precursor protein has been localized to chromosome 21. This finding fits with the fact that trisomy 21 is found in patients with Down's syndrome, all of whom show Alzheimer changes in the brain by middle age. It is currently postulated that a mutation in the beta-amyloid precursor protein gene on chromosome 21 evokes abnormal metabolism of amyloid, which is then deposited in neurons and around vessels. The abnormal phosphorylation of tau proteins by amyloid then leads to tangle formation and neuronal death. A mutation in the amyloid precursor protein gene on chromosome 21 has been found in some patients with familial Alzheimer's disease. The role of genetic factors, potential environmental toxins such as aluminum, or perhaps even a virus or subviral particle in accelerating or precipitating this complex sequence of events is unknown. The realization that a central accumulation of amyloid may be the primary event in the degenerative changes responsible for Alzheimer's disease has spawned several therapeutic proposals.

Clinical Picture and Diagnosis. The onset of Alzheimer's disease may occur as early as age 40, but most cases arise in the elderly.

Alzheimer's disease accounts for up to 60 percent of the cases of dementia in patients over 65. Rare familial cases with dominant inheritance and early onset have been reported. The disease shows a female preponderance. Onset is insidious and progression is gradual. Memory impairment is usually the first symptom and patients may be aware of their deficits in the early stages, which may lead to a superimposed depression. With progression, the previously discussed signs of a cortical dementia appear and aphasic symptoms sometimes predominate. Language deficits may consist of impaired naming and comprehension, verbal paraphasias, empty speech, perseveration, and logorrhea (increased speech).

Primitive reflexes, extrapyramidal signs (rigidity, expressionless facies, and bradykinesia), and sphincter incontinence are later manifestations. Seizures or myoclonus may also occur in a minority of cases. Within an average of 8 years from onset, the patient becomes totally disabled and, in the terminal phases, is bedridden with quadriplegia in flexion, incontinence, muteness, and no meaningful contact with the environment. This end-stage picture is common to most dementing illnesses. The average survival from the time of onset is 8 to 10 years.

The diagnosis of Alzheimer's disease was formerly based on the exclusion of other identifiable causes of dementia. As the clinical picture has become better defined and neuroimaging and other special tests have become more widely used, however, the specificity of diagnosis has increased (Table 4-4). The EEG is often normal in the early phases of the disease but invariably shows slowing of the background rhythms as the condition progresses. Studies of regional cerebral blood flow and metabolism using positron emission tomography or single-photon emission computed tomography have revealed the existence of symmetrical deficits in the temporoparietal regions with relative sparing of other brain areas. Computed tomography (CT) and magnetic resonance imaging (MRI) show generalized atrophy as the disease advances, particularly affecting the medial temporal regions (Fig. 4-4).

The conditions most commonly mistaken for Alzheimer's disease are multiinfarct dementia,

Table 4-4. Clinical Diagnosis of Alzheimer's Disease

Main criteria
1. Dementia established by the clinical findings and confirmed by standardized neuropsychological testing
2. Deficits in two or more areas of cognition (e.g., memory, language function, praxis, visuomotor)
3. Progressive worsening of memory and other cognitive functions
4. Preservation of normal consciousness
5. Onset between ages 40 and 90 (usually after age 65)
6. Absence of systemic disorders or other brain diseases that could account for the progressive memory and cognitive changes

Supportive criteria
1. Progressive aphasia, apraxia, or agnosia
2. Impaired activities of daily living and altered patterns of behavior
3. Positive family history
4. Normal CSF, normal or minimally abnormal EEG, atrophy on CT or MRI scans with enlargement of the temporal horns of the lateral ventricles

CSF = cerebrospinal fluid; EEG = electroencephalogram; CT = computed tomographic; MRI = magnetic resonance imaging. Adapted from G. McKhann, et al., Clinical diagnosis of Alzheimer's disease: report of the NINCDS-ADRDA Work Group under the auspices of Department of Health and Human Services Task Force on Alzheimer's Disease. *Neurology* 34:939–944, 1984.

normal senescent forgetfulness, depressive pseudodementia, excessive sedative or hypnotic drug use in the elderly, and rarely primary progressive aphasia, subdural hematoma, or localized left temporoparietal lesions such as meningiomas. The prognosis and management of these conditions, many of which are reversible, differ considerably from those that pertain to Alzheimer's disease. Cortical-basal ganglionic degeneration, a rare degenerative disease (see Chapter 12), may occasionally be mistaken for Alzheimer's disease, but, in this disorder, asymmetrical limb involvement with dystonia, tremor, and myoclonus occur early along with generalized rigidity and bradykinesia, while apraxia and less commonly aphasia and dementia are late symptoms.

Management. Specific drug therapy of Alzheimer's disease has focused on increasing the brain acetylcholine level with a view toward reversing the memory loss likely due, at least in part, to a cholinergic deficit. Limited success has been achieved with the currently available agents.

Pick's Disease

Pick's disease is a rare condition that has also been classified as a presenile dementia. In it there is a strong tendency for atrophy to be concentrated in the frontal and temporal regions (lobar atrophy). Silver-staining Pick bodies in the neurons and ballooned neurons constitute the distinct histopathologic features. Familial cases are more common than they are in Alzheimer's disease and some patients have a concomitant motor neuron disease. Although the condition cannot be definitely distinguished from Alzheimer's disease on the basis of symptomatology, the early appearance of personality changes and deterioration of social behavior, early occurrence of the Klüver-Bucy syndrome (see Chapter 6), and the relative preservation of memory and visuospatial functions until late in the course are all more indicative of Pick's disease. Death typically occurs 2 to 15 years after onset.

Cerebrovascular Disease and Dementia

Cerebrovascular disease accounts for about 10 to 20 percent of the cases of dementia. The underlying abnormality in these cases is variable and, in fact, several pathogenetic mechanisms may be interacting in a complex manner. Multiple small lacunar infarcts throughout the basal ganglia and subcortical white matter (état lacunaire), subcortical and periventricular white matter degeneration likely due to small vessel disease, or multiple larger cortical infarcts, which may be embolic, can all produce dementia.

Hachinski has attempted to define the clinical features that would allow differentiation of multiinfarct dementia from Alzheimer's disease. The most salient of these are stepwise deterioration, residual neurological focal signs suggesting previous infarction, and known vascular disease such as severe hypertension or a cardiac source of embolization. When infarcts are seen on a CT scan in a demented patient,

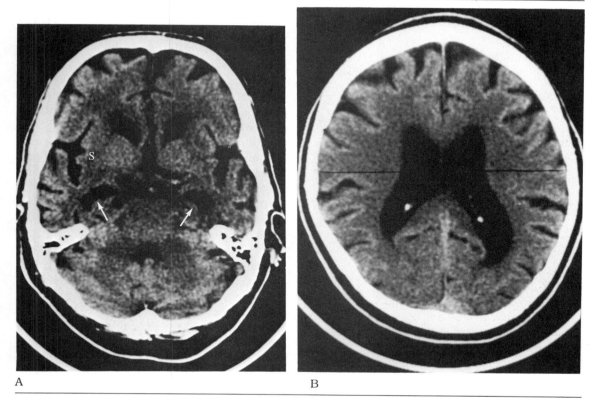

Fig. 4-4. *(A and B) CT scans showing cortical and especially temporal atrophy in a patient with advanced Alzheimer's disease. Arrows show enlarged temporal horns. (S = enlarged sylvian fissure.)*

this implies multiinfarct dementia. Hypertension is commonly the predisposing factor in these cases and its proper treatment may forestall further deterioration.

Recurrent bouts of hypotension, particularly in elderly or hypertensive patients who have a reduced capacity for antoregulation, may lead to ischemic white matter changes. Amyloid (congophilic) angiopathy can also produce white matter changes responsible for dementia and commonly occurs in patients with Alzheimer's disease. Rarely, severe stenoses or multiple occlusions of extracranial arteries may cause dementia resulting from global cerebral ischemia. Also rarely, discrete infarction in both paramedian thalamic areas can produce dementia along with a Korsakoff amnestic syndrome.

Binswanger's disease represents a form of subcortical sclerosis thought to have an ischemic etiology. It is now known that it is not a distinct pathological entity and has an unclear relationship to the white matter changes termed *leukoaraiosis* on neuroimaging studies. The MRI scan is even more sensitive for detecting small infarcts and is much more so for diffuse white matter changes (leukoaraiosis) (Fig. 4-5). However, these white matter changes bear an inconstant relationship to dementia.

Congophilic Angiopathy
Congophilic angiopathy is a rare entity that overlaps with Alzheimer's disease in both pathological and clinical terms. However, there is a striking amyloid deposition (which stains with Congo red) within the arterioles and capillaries of the neocortex and meninges as well as senile plaques. Patients may suffer massive intracerebral hemorrhage stemming from the weakening of vessel walls, and this can recur. When a subcortical frontal or occipital hemor-

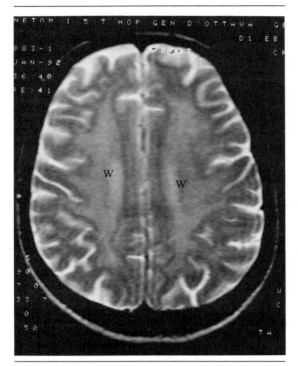

Fig. 4-5. *T_2-weighted MRI scan showing diffuse white matter changes* (W) *in a 76-year-old man with dementia presumably related to small-vessel disease.*

rhage occurs in a nonhypertensive older person with a preceding history of dementia, this diagnosis must be entertained. A familial form has been reported in Iceland and the Netherlands, which may present with intracerebral hemorrhage as early as the third or fourth decade. A genetic defect on chromosome 21 has been identified in some of these families.

Creutzfeldt-Jakob Disease

Formerly classified as a degenerative condition, Creutzfeldt-Jakob disease is a rare entity (incidence, approximately 1 case per million) that has now been proved to have an infectious origin and been successfully transmitted to monkeys and other species by the inoculation of tissue from affected patients. It has also been inadvertently transmitted in humans through corneal transplantation, the therapeutic use of contaminated human derived growth hormone, or the application of contaminated implanted depth electrodes during neurosurgical procedures.

The disorder is classified with kuru (an encephalopathy of New Guinea Fore natives) and scrapie (a disease of sheep) as a spongiform encephalopathy caused by widespread vacuolization that is seen microscopically in the cortex and basal ganglia as well as cerebellar gray matter. The vacuolization in neurons is accompanied by gliosis and neuronal loss without inflammatory changes. These conditions are considered unconventional slow-virus diseases because of their prolonged incubation period (up to 30 years) and the lack of classic pathological and cerebrospinal fluid (CSF) features typical of viral encephalitis.

Onset of the disease usually occurs during the fifth to seventh decades, but can begin earlier. Familial cases, some with accompanying motor neuron disease, have been reported. Interestingly, these familial cases, in which genetic alterations of prion protein handling have been implicated, are also transmissible to laboratory animals through the inoculation of affected brain tissue. Progression is usually rapid and patients exhibit dementia, extrapyramidal and pyramidal signs, cerebellar deficits, cortical blindness, a prominent startle response, and frequently myoclonus. Patients usually survive less than 1 year after the onset. CSF and CT findings are usually normal. In the middle stages of the illness, the EEG often shows periodic generalized sharp- and slow-wave complexes occurring approximately every second, with progressive disruption and slowing of the background rhythms (Fig. 4-6).

The **transmissible spongiform encephalopathies**, including Creutzfeldt-Jakob disease, have been extensively studied to characterize the nature of the infectious agent. Prusiner's group has named the agent a *prion* (proteinaceous infectious particle) and shown that it is not inactivated by conventional methods used to inactivate viruses. It does not appear to contain nucleic acid even though it multiplies in vivo.

The amyloid plaques found in the brains of patients with Creutzfeldt-Jakob disease and especially kuru appear to be composed of paracrystalline arrays of prion proteins. Prion protein is actually a normal cellular constituent that somehow undergoes posttranslational modification and polymerization into insoluble

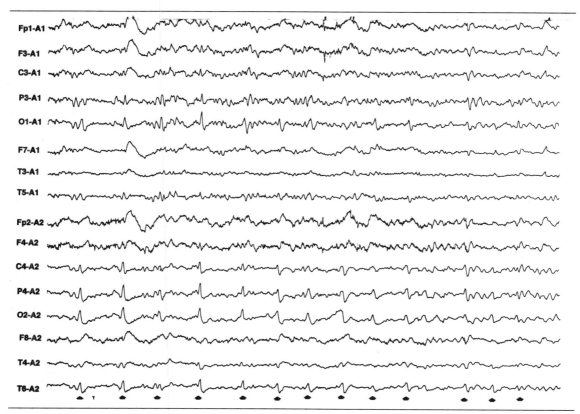

Fig. 4-6. *EEG showing simplification and slowing of the background rhythms as well as periodic complexes predominating in the right temporal area in a 64-year-old woman with autopsy-proved Creutzfeldt-Jacob disease.*

filaments that disrupt neuronal functioning. The mechanism underlying prion multiplication and cell-to-cell transmission is unknown. These novel infectious particles are found in two other animal diseases besides scrapie in sheep and goats: transmissible mink encephalopathy and chronic wasting disease of mule deer and elk.

Gerstmann-Sträussler-Scheinker syndrome (GSS) is another rare transmissible, usually familial, disorder thought to be caused by prions. It usually begins around the fourth to fifth decade, is more slowly progressive than Creutzfeldt-Jakob disease, and causes death within 1 to 11 years of onset. Cerebellar features or dementia may predominate but pyramidal signs, dysarthria, and gaze abnormalities are also found. Multicentric prion protein plaques are found in the cerebral and cerebellar hemispheres. There are overlaps between GSS and

familial Alzheimer's disease. A recently described condition, termed *fatal familial insomnia*, is also considered to stem from infection with prions. This disease is characterized by progressive insomnia, autonomic dysfunction, cerebellar signs, myoclonus, mild dementia, and selective atrophy of the anterior ventral and mediodorsal thalamic nuclei.

AIDS Dementia

Human immune deficiency virus (HIV) encephalopathy is a common cause of dementia in the 20- to 60-year-old age group. This diagnosis should be considered in patients in this age group who have been exposed to risk factors for AIDS. Dementia is the initial presenting feature in approximately 2 percent of adult patients with AIDS and in an even higher number of pediatric patients. Up to two thirds of the patients with AIDS exhibit a progressive cognitive decline. The syndrome has been termed the *AIDS dementia complex* because it is frequently accompanied by behavioral changes (apathy, withdrawal, or less commonly agitation) and motor symptoms (limb weakness and ataxia, writing and gait difficulties). In its early stages, concentration and memory deficits are seen along with slowed mentation. As the condition gradually progresses, more severe cognitive and memory impairment arises. Neuroimaging studies reveal diffuse brain atrophy and some patchy white matter degeneration. Direct invasion of the brain macrophages and neurons by HIV is responsible for this increasingly prevalent form of dementia.

Normal-Pressure Hydrocephalus

In 1965, Adams and colleagues drew attention to a dementia syndrome that was linked to an occult communicating hydrocephalus with normal lumbar CSF pressure. Some patients with this normal-pressure hydrocephalus (NPH) fully recovered following neurosurgical placement of a CSF shunt from the lateral ventricles to the peritoneal cavity that allowed the ventricles to shrink. The pathogenesis of the syndrome is unclear, but it can arise following subarachnoid hemorrhage, meningitis, or head trauma—all of which may produce scarring and impaired CSF flow through the subarachnoid spaces. Despite normal CSF baseline pressures, transient elevations of CSF pressure have been measured during rapid-eye-movement sleep in such patients.

A great deal of interest was generated by the report of this potentially treatable form of dementia, but initial enthusiasm for shunting waned when it was discovered that some seemingly typical patients showed little response to the procedure and that complications such as subdural hematoma, central nervous system (CNS) infection, seizures, and even death occurred in about one third of the patients who had shunts installed. More recent efforts have focused on devising criteria to identify those patients with NPH most likely to respond to shunting.

The classic clinical triad, not specific for NPH, consists of:

1. Mental change: usually a typical subcortical dementia, often the initial symptom, developing over weeks or months and at times fluctuating from day to day
2. Gait disturbance: an apraxic, wide-based, slow, unsteady gait ("as if stuck to the floor"), at times exhibiting spastic features
3. Urinary incontinence: tends to appear late

On examination, the patients frequently show parkinsonian features, primitive reflexes, leg spasticity, and hyperreflexia.

CT or MRI are now the best screening methods for detecting NPH. These scans show markedly dilated ventricles (including the third, fourth, and temporal horns) with little evidence of cortical atrophy (Fig. 4-7). Periventricular edema may also be seen. Dynamic CT scanning may be done to follow the route of metrizamide, which is injected into the lumbar space and then normally travels through the basal cisterns and over the convexity; this is impaired in NPH. Radionuclide cisternography is currently the best method for investigating CSF dynamics (Fig. 4-8). Classic findings in NPH are: (1) early ventricular filling (at 2 hours); (2) persistence of ventricular activity for 24 hours or more; and (3) no flow of radioisotope above the tentorium. Intermediate patterns of slow flow are also seen but are less specific for NPH.

The CSF infusion test involves infusing saline at twice the rate of CSF production while measuring the CSF pressure every 5 minutes for 60 minutes, or until the pressure reaches 500 mm H_2O. The plateau pressure and rate of rise of pressure are abnormally high in NPH. Artifacts, especially caused by faulty needle placement, must be avoided.

The EEG frequently shows slowing with high-amplitude bursts of delta activity. A lumbar puncture with drainage of CSF may produce a transient improvement in the clinical picture. Patients who show the classic clinical triad, and have a known cause for the NPH, symptoms of relatively short duration, without CT or MRI evidence of cortical atrophy, and classic findings on radionuclide cisternography, are the best candidates for a shunting procedure. Patient selection for shunting must be based on a combination of clinical and laboratory criteria. Rarely patients with an advanced dementia and disability will experience restoration of normal or near-normal functioning following a shunt procedure.

Depressive Pseudodementia

Pseudodementia, which is fully reversible, accounted for about 10 percent of the cases of dementia in a large series of patients. Many of the cognitive and affective symptoms of dementia and depression overlap, and certainly a concurrent depression frequently occurs in the early phases of dementia. Clues to the presence of a pseudodementia include a past history of psychiatric (depressive) illness, a relatively sudden onset, marked psychomotor retardation, absence of neurological signs (such as primitive reflexes), and specific deficits of higher cortical function such as aphasia and a tendency toward "near miss" answers or the reply "I don't know" on psychological testing. A successful trial treatment of antidepressant medication is often the best way to identify this disorder.

Investigations

Attention should be focused on possible treatable causes of the dementia (see Table 4-2).

A CT scan with contrast enhancement should be done early. Cortical atrophy will usually be well visualized on the CT scan, but there is a great deal of overlap between the appearance of sulci and ventricular size in elderly normals and in patients with atrophy

Fig. 4-7. *CT scans in a 48-year-old woman with normal-pressure hydrocephalus. (A) Preshunt scans showing enlarged ventricles without atrophy.*

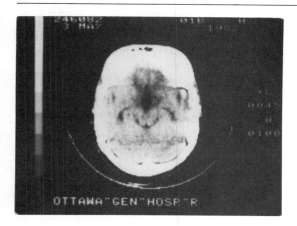
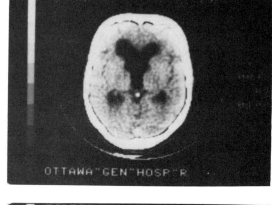
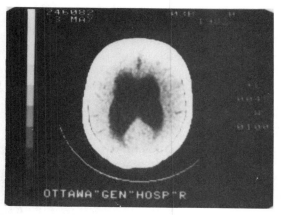
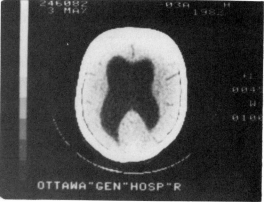

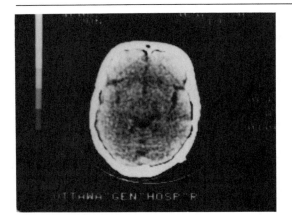
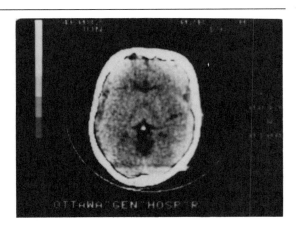
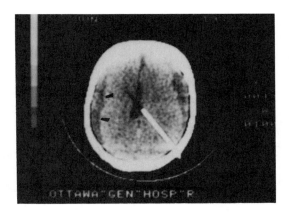
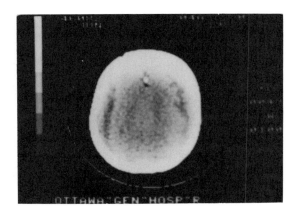

Fig. 4-7 *(Continued). (B) After a ventriculoperitoneal shunt was installed, there was a reduction in ventricular size but also a subdural hematoma* (arrows).

due to conditions like Alzheimer's disease. Nevertheless, severe cortical atrophy or very large ventricles, such as appear in NPH, can be helpful findings. Focal space-occupying lesions, multiple infarcts, the basal ganglia softenings seen in Wilson's disease, or the calcifications typical of parathyroid disorders may all be encountered. An MRI scan is even more sensitive for detecting these changes, particularly for small, deep lesions, as well as for medial temporal atrophy and diffuse changes in the white matter.

Serum B_{12} and folate levels, electrolyte concentrations (including calcium), CBC, liver profile, BUN, VDRL, HIV testing, and T_4 levels are ordered for screening purposes. In special circumstances, heavy metal levels,

serum ceruloplasmin and copper concentrations, a drug screen, and special tests for sphingolipidoses are indicated.

An EEG can provide valuable information because it usually shows abnormal slowing in patients with metabolic or toxic disorders, a space-occupying lesion, or NPH, but will often be normal in the early phases of Alzheimer's disease and other cortical dementias. The periodic complexes seen in Cruetzfeldt-Jakob disease may help confirm that diagnosis.

A Doppler examination can be used to effectively screen for any serious extracranial occlusive vascular disease. A routine lumbar puncture is indicated only when neurosyphilis or chronic meningitis are strong possibilities.

Formal neuropsychological testing can help

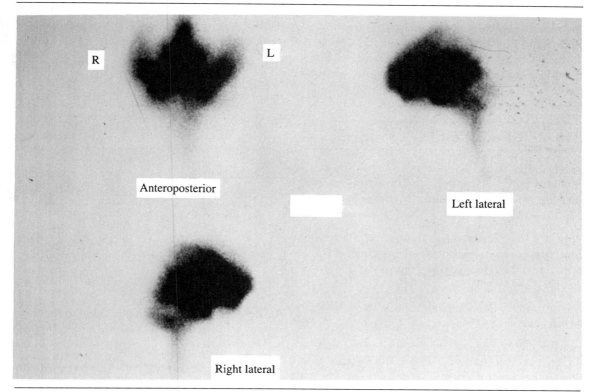

R   L

Anteroposterior

Left lateral

Right lateral

Fig. 4-8. *Radionuclide cisternography (radioactive iodinated serum albumin scan) in a patient with normal-pressure hydrocephalus showing activity remaining within the ventricular system after 24 hours. (R = right; L = left.)*

distinguish between an organic dementia and a depressive pseudomentia. In the former, there is usually a disparity between the performance and verbal scores on the Wechsler Adult Intelligence Scale, and there is evidence for specific higher function deficits (e.g., aphasia) in the cortical dementias. This testing is especially important in the diagnosis of early dementia in intellectually bright patients, in providing a baseline for the assessment of disease progression, and in making decisions such as whether patients can perform their work, look after their affairs, and live independently. Brain biopsy may be the only way of arriving at a diagnosis in certain cases and may be justified to allow the formulation of a more definite prognosis or for research purposes, but almost never uncovers an unexpected treatable condition.

Management of Irreversible Dementia

Awareness of the substantial psychological and economic burden that dementia can place on the family is essential. Counseling family members to be sure that the patient's affairs are managed by someone else and tactfully suggesting when it is time for the patient to be placed in a chronic care facility are important measures. The symptomatic management of agitation or sleeplessness can be achieved with drugs such as thioridazine, haloperidol, or chloral hydrate, but other stronger sedatives and minor tranquilizers should be avoided. Seizures must be treated appropriately and anticonvulsant medication levels monitored. The patient must be kept in as good a state of general health as possible through adequate nutrition and exercise. Day-care facilities that provide activities and respite care can be very helpful to the family and can also offer some pleasure to the patient. The patient's environment and routine should be kept as uniform and familiar as possible.

BIBLIOGRAPHY

Adams, R., et al. Symptomatic occult hydrocephalus with normal cerebrospinal fluid pressures, a treatable syndrome. *N. Engl. J. Med.* 273:117–126, 1965.

Albert, M.L., Feldman, R.G., and Willis, A.L. The "subcortical dementia" of progressive supranuclear palsy. *J. Neurol. Neurosurg. Psychiatry* 37:121–130, 1974.

Barrett, R.E. Dementia in adults. *Med. Clin. North Am.* 56:1405–1418, 1972.

Benson, D.F. Clinical aspects of dementia. In J.C. Beck (moderator). Dementia in the elderly: the silent epidemic. *Ann. Intern. Med.* 97:231–241, 1982.

Black, P. McL. Idiopathic normal-pressure hydrocephalus. *J. Neurosurg.* 52:371–377, 1980.

Brown, P. et al. Creutzfeldt-Jakob disease in France. II. Clinical characteristics of 124 consecutive verified cases during the decade 1968–1977. *Ann. Neurol.* 6:430–437, 1979.

Brown, P. Central nervous system amyloidoses: a comparison of Alzheimer's disease and Creutzfeldt-Jakob disease. *Neurology* 39:1103–1105, 1989.

Chui, H.C. Dementia. A review emphasizing clinicopathologic correlation and brain-behavior relationships. *Arch. Neurol.* 46:806–814, 1989.

Cummings, J.L. Cortical Dementias. In D.F. Benson and D. Blumer (editors). *Psychiatric Aspects of Neurologic Disease*, Vol. II. New York: Grune & Stratton, 1982, Pp. 93–120.

Cummings, J.L., and Benson, D.F. Subcortical dementia. Review of an emerging concept. *Arch. Neurol.* 41:874–879, 1984.

Cummings, J.L., and Benson, D.F. *Dementia: A Clinical Approach*, 2nd ed. Boston: Butterworth-Heinemann, 1992.

Guberman, A. and Stuss, D. The syndrome of bilateral paramedian thalamic infarction. *Neurology* 33:540–546, 1983.

Hachinski, V.C., Lassen, N.A., and Marshall, J. Multi-infarct dementia: a cause of mental deterioration in the elderly. *Lancet* 3:207–210, 1974.

Hachinski, V.C. The decline and resurgence of vascular dementia. *Can. Med. Assoc. J.* 142:107–111, 1990.

Hardy, J., and Allsop, D. Amyloid deposition as the central event in the etiology of Alzheimer's disease. *Trends Pharmacol. Sci.* 12:383–388, 1991.

Henderson, V.W., and Finch, C.E. The neurobiology of Alzheimer's disease. *J. Neurosurg.* 70:335–353, 1989.

Hsiao, K., and Prusiner, S.B. Inherited human prion disease. *Neurology* 40:1820–1827, 1990.

Hughes, C.P. Communicating Hydrocephalus in the Adult. In K. Nandy (editor). *Senile Dementia: A Biomedical Approach*. Amsterdam: Elsevier North-Holland, 1978, Pp. 209–222.

Johnson, R.T. Prion disease. *N. Engl. J. Med.* 326:486–487, 1992.

Katzman, R. The prevalence and malignancy of Alzheimer's disease. *Arch. Neurol.* 33:217–218, 1976.

Kokmen, E. Dementia—Alzheimer type. *Mayo Clin. Proc.* 59:35–42, 1984.

Mandybur, T.I., and Bates, S.R.D. Fatal massive intracerebral hemorrhage complicating cerebral amyloid angiopathy. *Arch. Neurol.* 35:246–248, 1978.

May, W.M. Creutzfeldt-Jakob disease. I. Survey of the literature and clinical diagnosis. *Acta Neurol. Scand.* 44:1–32, 1968.

McKhann, G., et al. Clinical diagnosis of Alzheimer's disease: report of the NINCDS-ADRDA Work Group under the auspices of

Department of Health and Human Services Task Force on Alzheimer's Disease. *Neurology* 34:939–944, 1984.

Medori, R., et al. Fatal familial insomnia, a prion disease with a mutation at codon 178 of the prion protein gene. *N. Engl. J. Med.* 326:444–449, 1992.

Nalbantglu, J. β-Amyloid protein in Alzheimer's disease. *Can. J. Neurol. Sci.* 18:424–427, 1991.

Okazaki, H., Reagan, T.J., and Campbell, R.J. Clinicopathologic studies of primary cerebral amyloid angiopathy. *Mayo Clin. Proc.* 54:22–31, 1979.

Palmert, M.R., et al. Soluble derivatives of the β-amyloid protein precursor in cerebrospinal fluid: alternatives in normal aging and in Alzheimer's disease. *Neurology* 40:1028–1034, 1990.

Price, R.W., Sidtis, J., and Rosenblum, M. The AIDS dementia complex: some current questions. *Ann. Neurol.* 23(suppl.):S27–S33, 1988.

Prusiner, S.B. Prions and neurodegenerative disease. *N. Engl. J. Med.* 317:1571–1581, 1987.

Robertson, K.R., and Hall, C.D. Human immunodeficiency virus–related cognitive impairment and the acquired immunodeficiency syndrome dementia complex. *Semin. Neurol.* 12:18–27, 1992.

Roos, R., Gajdusek, D.C., and Gibbs, C.J., Jr. The clinical characteristics of transmissible Creutzfeldt-Jakob disease. *Brain* 96:1–20, 1973.

Rumble, B., et al. Amyloid A4 protein and its precursor in Down's syndrome and Alzheimer's disease. *N. Engl. J. Med.* 320:1446–1452, 1989.

Siedler, H., and Malamud, N. Creutzfeldt-Jakob's disease. Clinicopathologic report of 15 cases and review of the literature (with special reference to a related disorder designated as subacute spongiform encephalopathy). *J. Neuropathol. Exp. Neurol.* 22:381–402, 1963.

Siu, A.L. Screening for dementia and investigating its cause. *Ann. Intern. Med.* 115:122–132, 1991.

Strub, R.L. Acute Confusional State, In D.F. Benson and D. Blumer (editors). *Psychiatric Aspects of Neurologic Disease*, Vol. II. New York: Grune & Stratton, 1982, Pp. 1–21.

Tanzi, R.E., St. George-Hyslop, P.H., Gusella J.F. Molecular genetic approaches to Alzheimer's disease. *Trends Neurosci.* 12:152–158, 1989.

Terry, R.D., and Katzman, R. Senile dementia of the Alzheimer type. *Ann. Neurol.* 14:497–506, 1983.

Terry, R.D., et al. Physical basis of cognitive alterations in Alzheimer's disease: synapse loss is the major correlate of cognitive impairment. *Ann. Neurol.* 30:572–580, 1991.

Van Hoesen, G.W., and Hyman, B.T. Hippocampal Formation: Anatomy and the Patterns of Pathology in Alzheimer's Disease. In J. Storm-Mathisen, J. Zimmer, and O.P. Ottersen (editors). *Progress in Brain Research*, Vol. 83. New York: Elsevier, 1990, Pp. 445–457.

Vinters, H.V., Miller, B.L. and Pardridge, W.M. Brain amyloid and Alzheimer's disease. *Ann. Intern. Med.* 109:41–54, 1988.

Yanker, B.A. and Mesulam, M.M. β-Amyloid and the pathogenesis of Alzheimer's disease. *N. Engl. J. Med.* 325:1849–1857, 1991.

Stupor and Coma

PATHOPHYSIOLOGY OF REDUCED LEVEL OF CONSCIOUSNESS

The two essential elements of consciousness are arousal and awareness. A normal level of alertness, awareness of the environment, and physiological variations of arousal (e.g., sleep) depend on the intact functioning of the **ascending reticular activating system** (ARAS) as well as the cerebral cortex. The ARAS is composed of cell bodies in the central reticular core of the upper brainstem (mainly midbrain) and their projections to widespread areas of the cerebral cortex via both thalamic and extrathalamic pathways. Acetylcholine and norepinephrine act as neurotransmitters or neuromodulators within this system.

Any lesion that interrupts the metabolic or structural integrity of the ARAS or enough of the cortical neurons receiving ARAS projections can cause coma. The ARAS is relatively susceptible to systemic metabolic imbalances and drugs and can also be disrupted by discrete lesions of the upper brainstem. Supratentorial expanding lesions that herniate through the tentorial notch, which is at the level of the midbrain, may also damage the ARAS. Metabolic or diffuse processes can also produce coma by causing widespread impairment of cerebral cortical neurons upon which the ARAS projects.

A corollary of these observations is that uncomplicated unilateral hemispheric lesions do not cause stupor or coma. Coma can be envisioned as the near final result of total brain failure and is frequently preceded by delirium or an acute confusional state (Chapter 4). In coma, cerebral blood flow and energy metabolism are markedly reduced.

DEFINITION OF COMA AND RELATED STATES

Coma can be defined as a state, usually with an acute or subacute onset and of relatively long duration, in which the patients show no meaningful response to environmental stimuli and from which (unlike sleep) they cannot be aroused. In a patient with stupor, there is a reduced level of alertness but the patient can be aroused to the point of showing some meaningful responses, such as fending off or moaning in response to painful stimuli.

Akinetic mutism ("coma vigil") is a form of coma in which the patient may lie with the eyes open and appear to look around but remain mute and immobile without any meaningful contact with the environment. In this setting, the lesion is either located around the third ventricle and involves the thalamus and hypothalamus, or it is in the cingulate gyrus and interrupts frontolimbic connections (e.g., spasm following a ruptured anterior communicating artery aneurysm).

The **persistent vegetative state** usually evolves from a coma due to a severe head injury or diffuse cerebral hypoxia following cardiac arrest that causes widespread cerebral cortical damage. Such patients have preserved brainstem reflexes, rudimentary movements, and, with stimulation, the eyes may open, indicating arousal, but higher-level cerebral responses or awareness are absent. The electroencephalographic (EEG) recording may be flat, or nearly so.

In the **locked-in syndrome**, which can be confused with coma, the patient is alert but mute and quadriplegic. The only movements are usually blinking and vertical eye movements. Ocular bobbing, or a quick downward and slow upward intermittent conjugate movement of the eyes, is frequently seen. The lesion in this disorder is in the ventral part of the pons (basis pontis), sparing the ARAS, and is commonly a hemorrhage or infarct (Fig. 5-1). Communication can often be established with the patient using an eye-blink code. It is important to distinguish it from coma because the patient is aware of what is said at the bedside. In a small proportion of cases, the syndrome is reversible.

Psychogenic unresponsiveness can be distinguished from coma by demonstrating voluntary avoidance responses (e.g., arm elevated above the head always falling away from the face), the preservation of nystagmus when oculovestibular responses are elicited by injecting ice

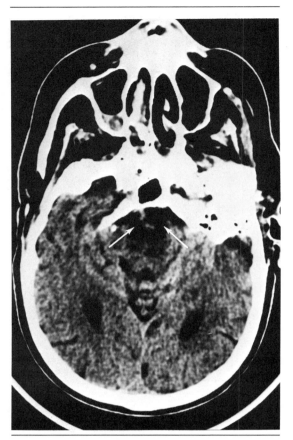

Fig. 5-1. *Unenhanced CT scan showing bilateral ventral pontine infarction* (arrows) *in a 60-year-old man with the locked-in syndrome.*

water into the external ear, or by a normal awake EEG. **Nonconvulsive generalized status epilepticus** (petit mal status) may occasionally present as a stuporous state and is confirmed by EEG.

ETIOLOGY OF COMA

The various causes of coma are outlined in Table 5-1. Drug intoxication and systemic metabolic disorders account for over half the cases encountered in hospitals. Head trauma, diffuse cerebral hypoxia and ischemia following cardiac arrest, and cerebrovascular disease (infarcts and hemorrhages) account for the majority of the remaining cases.

Table 5-1. Causes of Coma

FOCAL INTRACRANIAL STRUCTURAL LESIONS
Supratentorial
  Mass lesion with herniation
    Hemorrhage (intracerebral, subdural, epidural)
    Infarct
    Tumor
    Abscess
  Bilateral paramedian thalamic infarction
Infratentorial
  Brainstem
    Infarct
    Hemorrhage
    Tumor
    Abscess
    Central pontine myelinolysis
    Brainstem encephalitis
  Cerebellum
    Hemorrhage
    Infarct
    Tumor
    Abscess
  Extraaxial: posterior fossa subdural hematoma

DIFFUSE INTRACRANIAL LESIONS
Intraparenchymal
  Head trauma
  Encephalitis
  Multiple emboli
  Hypoxic-ischemic encephalopathy
  Vasculitis
  Hypertensive encephalopathy
  Disseminated intravascular coagulation
  Thrombotic thrombocytopenic purpura
  Acute disseminated encephalomyelopathy
  Acute hemorrhagic necrotizing
    leukoencephalopathy
  Heat stroke

Primarily extraparenchymal
  Meningitis
  Subarachnoid hemorrhage

METABOLIC DISORDERS
Systemic metabolic disorders
  Hepatic encephalopathy
  Reye's syndrome
  Uremia
  Dialysis dysequilibrium syndrome
  Pancreatic encephalopathy
  CO_2 narcosis due to pulmonary failure
  Metabolic acidosis
  Hyponatremia
  Hypercalcemia
  Hypocalcemia
  Hypomagnesemia
  Porphyria
Substrate or vitamin deficiency
  Hypoxia
  Hypoglycemia
  Wernicke-Korsakoff syndrome
  Vitamin B_{12} deficiency
Endocrine
  Diabetic ketoacidosis
  Nonketotic hyperosmolar hyperglycemic coma
  Myxedema coma
  Hyperthyroidism
  Addison's disease
  Hypopituitarism
Intoxication
  Drugs (e.g., depressants, salicylates, alcohol)
  Heavy metals
  Solvents (e.g., methanol, ethylene glycol)
Miscellaneous
  Postictal state
  Concussion

APPROACH TO DIAGNOSIS

General Approach

Rapid diagnosis is essential so that any specific conditions can be managed which, if left untreated, could lead to permanent brain damage. Initially, a rapid history and physical examination is performed, but attention is also paid to ensuring a patent airway, adequate oxygenation and a supply of glucose, and stabilization of blood pressure and cardiac rhythm. Clues should be sought that could distinguish metabolic disease (frequently reversible) from an intracranial structural abnormality, either supratentorial with rostral-caudal deterioration (often requiring neurosurgical intervention) or infratentorial (rarely requiring surgery or specific treatment measures unless there are cerebellar lesions such as hemorrhages).

Examination

In most patients, the diagnosis will be apparent from the history and examination findings alone. Serial observations are often essential to establish a diagnosis. A surprisingly complete neurological examination can be performed in the comatose patient, aside from language, strength, and most sensory testing. During the general examination, specific attention should be paid to neck suppleness, signs of head trauma (including Battle's sign, which consists of ecchymoses over the mastoid area with a basal skull fracture, as well as otorrhea and rhinorrhea), bite marks on the tongue suggesting a previous seizure, the stigmata of alcoholism or liver failure, needle marks suggesting drug abuse, and bullatous skin lesions that may occur with barbiturate and other drug overdoses.

The **respiratory pattern** is an important indicator of the level of central nervous system (CNS) dysfunction. Respiratory alkalosis with tachypnea accompanies many metabolic encephalopathies. Cheyne-Stokes respiration, with a crescendo-decrescendo pattern stretching over several seconds and periods of apnea between each cycle, indicates early bilateral hemispheric or diencephalic compromise. It is a frequent finding in metabolic encephalopathies but may also be seen in congestive heart failure and normal sleep. As the level of impairment descends, the breathing pattern may change from central neurogenic hyperventilation (very rapid breathing despite a normal partial pressure of oxygen), to apneustic breathing (sighing and long inspiratory pauses), to irregular ataxic breathing, and finally to apnea when the medullary respiratory centers are severely compromised.

The **level of alertness** is assessed by observing the patient's verbalization, blinking, and movements. Response to verbal stimuli and voluntary withdrawal or protective movements in response to noxious stimuli indicate stupor rather than coma. A useful noxious stimulus is a light tickle of the hairs in the nostrils, which may produce grimacing and head turning as well as fending-off arm movements when coma is light and motor responses are intact. Blinking in response to a hand clap is also good evidence for a relatively intact brainstem.

The cranial nerves are carefully assessed to discern the state of the brainstem structures, many of which lie near the ARAS. Funduscopy may reveal findings such as papilledema, retinal subhyaloid hemorrhages (in the presence of subarachnoid hemorrhage), or a congested appearance of the optic disc in the event of methanol poisoning. Special attention is given to the **pupillary responses** and **eye movements**, both dependent on midbrain and upper pontine structures. A unilateral dilated pupil is often indicative of uncal (mesial temporal) herniation caused by a supratentorial mass lesion. Small reactive pupils are characteristic of metabolic or pontine lesions. Midposition pupils that are unreactive to light usually indicate severe midbrain damage. Certain drugs such as glutethimide and atropinic agents, can cause coma with fixed dilated pupils.

Spontaneous gaze is examined. Roving, full conjugate eye movements usually indicate a metabolic encephalopathy. When spontaneous eye movements are absent, the oculocephalic (Doll's eye) reflexes are tested. In a stuporous or comatose patient with intact brainstem gaze centers, medial longitudinal fasciculus, and cranial nerves subserving extraocular movements, the eyes will move fully and conjugately in the opposite direction when the head is passively turned in a horizontal or vertical direction. Absence of this response indicates severe dysfunction at the pontine level. With more complete brainstem involvement, oculovestibular responses (deviation of the eyes toward the side of ice water irrigation of the external ear canal) are lost. Any blockage in the ear canal should be removed and up to 200 ml of ice water should be used in performing this test.

The corneal, nose tickle, and pinprick reflexes over the face are used to assess the fifth nerve. A corneomandibular reflex (see Chapter 2) elicited by a brisk stimulus to the center of the cornea indicates compromise of the upper brainstem and is frequently seen in patients with transtentorial herniation. Applying pressure over the styloid processes or a light nasal tickle may produce a grimace, thus allowing assessment of facial symmetry. If the patient puffs out one cheek during expiration, this can indicate unilateral facial weakness. The gag reflex (taking care not to produce vomiting) or response to suctioning can be used to test cranial nerves IX and X.

The rest of the neurological examination consists mainly of observing spontaneous movements and assessing muscle tone, reflexes, and motor responses to noxious stimuli. Particularly important are lateralizing signs (e.g., a unilateral Babinski response, unilateral flaccidity, and asymmetrical withdrawal to pain), bilateral corticospinal tract signs, and decorticate (arms flexed, legs extended) or decerebrate (arms extended and hyperpronated, legs extended) posturing. Decorticate posturing indicates corticospinal tract impairment at the diencephalic level, and decerebrate posturing points to impairment at the brainstem level. A lower extremity withdrawal response to painful stimulation of the feet may represent a spinal reflex and can occur even in the presence of brain death.

Rostral-Caudal Deterioration

Plum and Posner coined the term rostral-caudal deterioration to describe the progressive deterioration in cerebral and brainstem function that occurs with expanding supratentorial lesions producing downward herniation of either the mesial temporal lobe (uncus) or of the whole brainstem through the tentorial notch (central herniation). This condition presents a distinctive clinical picture: level of consciousness, respirations, pupillary responses, extraocular movements, and motor responses tend to be impaired in a fixed sequence, moving in phase as successively lower levels of the neuraxis become compromised (Table 5-2). Early recognition and reversal of the process are essential if permanent severe brainstem damage or death is to be prevented.

Clues to Metabolic Coma

The following clinical features indicate coma likely stemming from a metabolic cause:

1. Absence of focal or lateralizing neurological signs; however, their presence does not rule out metabolic coma and they are particularly common with hypoglycemia, hyperosmolar nonketotic states, and hepatic encephalopathy.
2. Signs of neurological dysfunction occurring simultaneously at different levels (e.g., very light coma with absent oculocephalic and oculovestibular reflexes).
3. Acute confusional state with hallucinations and seizures progressing to coma.
4. Multifocal myoclonus.
5. Hyperventilation with respiratory alkalosis.

Special Tests

Diagnostic studies in all patients with coma of unknown cause should include CBC; determination of serum glucose, electrolyte (including calcium and magnesium), BUN, amylase, arterial blood gas, serum B_{12}, T_4, and cortisol levels; liver function tests (including serum ammonia); and a drug screen. Urine should be tested for the presence of glucose, ketone bodies, and porphobilinogen.

An unenhanced computed tomographic (CT) scan should be done early to help identify supratentorial expanding lesions producing brain shifts and rostral-caudal deterioration. A normal CT scan precludes this possibility. Movement artifacts should be eliminated by sedating the patient if necessary. Intracerebral or subdural hemorrhages, abscesses, and tumors are usually obvious, but infarcts in the first 12 to 24 hours are often not visible on CT. The CT appearance of subarachnoid hemorrhage usually consists of blood outlining the brainstem and filling both the sylvian fissures and the cortical sulci (see Chapter 23). In meningitis, the subarachnoid spaces and basal cisterns may be enhanced by contrast material. Brainstem and cerebellar hemorrhages, or cerebellar infarcts, or central pontine myelinolysis may be visualized in the posterior fossa. Resolution is not usually sufficient to demonstrate brainstem infarcts unless they are large. A magnetic resonance imaging (MRI) scan may provide additional important information and is particularly useful for identifying herpes simplex encephalitis and brainstem pathology.

A lumbar puncture should be done once brain shifts or marked hydrocephalus have been ruled out by a CT scan. Meningitis, encephalitis, and subarachnoid hemorrhage are the main conditions for which a lumbar puncture can be a diagnostic aid.

The EEG is often extremely helpful diagnos-

Table 5-2. Neurological Changes in Rostral-Caudal Deterioration

	Cerebral or diencephalic	Upper brainstem	Lower brainstem
Level of consciousness	Stupor	Coma	Deep coma
Respiration	Cheyne-Stokes	Central neurogenic hyperventilation → apneustic breathing → ataxic breathing	Apnea
Pupils	Reactive or unilateral dilatation (uncal herniation)	Midposition and fixed or small (pontine)	—
Extraocular movements	Spontaneous roving eye movements or full oculocephalic responses	Absent oculocephalic responses	Absent oculovestibular responses
Motor responses	Decorticate	Decerebrate	Flaccid quadriplegia or slight lower extremity flexion to pain

tically, and relatively specific changes are seen in some metabolic disorders (e.g., triphasic waves with hepatic or uremic encephalopathy, and mixed fast and slow activity with sedative overdose), anoxic encephalopathy (e.g., burst suppression [Fig. 5-2]), herpes simplex encephalitis (periodic sharp and slow discharges), nonconvulsive generalized status epilepticus (generalized 2- to 4-Hz polyspike wave), subdural hematoma (focal voltage suppression and generalized slowing), brain abscess (focal high-voltage very slow waves), raised intracranial pressure (projected slow-wave bursts), and pseudocoma (normal awake EEG). A relatively normal EEG may be obtained in rare cases of true coma due to ventral pontine lesions or unresponsiveness due to basilar migraine. Brainstem auditory evoked potentials can be used to help distinguish intrinsic brainstem lesions from metabolic processes.

MANAGEMENT

Once vital functions are stabilized, attention should turn to obtaining a rapid specific diagnosis that will guide the planning of further treatment (Table 5-3). An intravenous (IV) glucose drip should be started and a bolus of 50 ml of 50% glucose should be given (if hyperosmolar hyperglycemic states have been ruled out) along

Table 5-3. Management of Acute Coma

1. Stabilize airway, blood pressure, and cardiac rhythm
2. Treat any severe injury
3. Determine whether coma is due to metabolic process (e.g., drug overdose or hypoglycemia) or to structural intracranial lesion on the basis of history, examination, and laboratory findings (e.g., standard blood tests and urine drug screen); administer 50 ml of 50% glucose and thiamine IV
4. Determine whether rostral-caudal deterioration with raised intracranial pressure is present; if so, treat immediately (see Chapter 20)
5. Perform CT (or MRI) scanning of head early
6. If diagnosis is still uncertain, do lumbar puncture followed by EEG
7. Treat any underlying causes as much as possible
8. If coma is persistent, pay meticulous attention to skin care, respiratory care, hydration and nutrition, deep vein thrombosis prophylaxis, bladder care, and so on

with thiamine (50 mg intramuscularly and 100 mg IV). Naloxone (0.4 to 1.2 mg IV) should be given if narcotic drug overdosage is a possibility. Physostigmine (2 to 4 mg IV) can be administered in cases of anticholinergic drug overdose. The management of drug overdose also consists of early gastric lavage and activated charcoal instillation and, in severe cases,

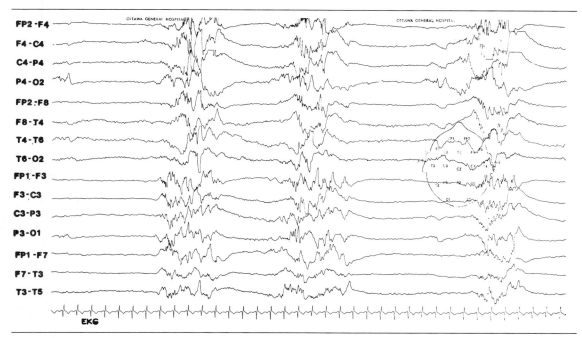

Fig. 5-2. *EEG showing suppression-burst pattern in a deeply comatose patient following severe head trauma. Note the periods of generalized background flattening lasting several seconds.*

hemodialysis. Other specific measures include reversing elevated intracranial pressure with mannitol and dexamethasone, controlling seizures with intravenous diazepam and phenytoin, correcting specific metabolic imbalances, treating hypoxia and ventilatory failure, and administering antibiotics for infection.

The institution of appropriate general supportive and nursing measures is essential in the comatose patient if complications such as aspiration, atelectasis, bedsores, muscle contractures, and pulmonary embolus are to be prevented. These measures include:

1. Keeping the patient in a semiprone position
2. Urinary catheterization
3. Nasogastric intubation with tube feedings as indicated in cases of prolonged coma
4. Oral airway, endotracheal intubation, or tracheostomy with frequent suctioning and airway care, as indicated
5. Frequent turning of the patient plus passive limb movements, chest physiotherapy, and skin care

6. Correction of extreme hyperthermia or hypothermia
7. Monitoring of vital functions
8. Antiembolic stockings and perhaps the administration of low-dose subcutaneous heparin

The Glasgow coma scale is useful for monitoring the neurological status of the patient (Table 5-4). The specific management of acute conditions associated with coma, such as meningitis, subarachnoid hemorrhage, and head injury, is discussed in later chapters.

PROGNOSIS

In a prospective, cooperative study of 500 patients who were in a coma for more than 6 hours arising from various causes (excluding trauma and drug intoxication), only 15 percent made a good initial recovery and there was a 76 percent mortality within the first month. A poor outcome is more likely when coma lasts longer

Table 5-4. Glasgow Coma Scale

Response	Scale
Eye opening	
Spontaneous	4
To sound	3
To pain	2
Never	1
Best verbal response	
Oriented	5
Confused	4
Inappropriate	3
Incomprehensible	2
None	1
Best motor response	
Obeys commands	6
Localizes	5
Flexion: normal	4
Flexion: abnormal	3
Extension	2
Nil	1

than 24 hours; there is a destructive brain lesion such as a hemorrhage, infarct, or contusion; or there are signs of severe brainstem impairment such as dilated and fixed pupils, absent reflex eye movements, absent corneal reflexes, or apnea. In the individual patient, prognosis must be formulated on the basis of a specific diagnosis and serial observations of neurological signs manifested over the first few days.

Brain Death

In recent years, much attention has been focused on the diagnostic criteria for determining brain death. Once brain death is established, the patient is considered medically and legally dead and this justifies the removal of life support systems from such patients, some of whom are potential organ donors. The criteria for brain death are:

1. Cessation of cerebral function as evidenced by deep coma as well as cerebral unreceptivity and unresponsivity. EEG or other laboratory confirmation may be used.
2. Absent brainstem function. This includes absent light, corneal, oculocephalic, oculovesticular, oculopharyngeal, and respiratory (apnea) reflexes.

3. Irreversibility. This implies that the cause of coma is known and reversible conditions such as drug overdose and hypothermia have been excluded. The patient must be observed for an appropriate period, usually 24 hours, to confirm that the cessation of all brain functions persists. An EEG, although helpful for establishing the diagnosis, is not essential. Other tests, such as radionuclide scans, magnetic resonance spectroscopy, cerebral angiography, and transcranial Doppler ultrasound studies, may at times be helpful in confirming brain death by showing absent cerebral blood flow and metabolism.

BIBLIOGRAPHY

Bertini, G., et al. Prognostic significance of early clinical manifestations in postanoxic coma: a retrospective study of 58 patients resuscitated after prehospital cardiac arrest. *Crit. Care Med.* 17:627–633, 1989.

Black, P. McL. Brain death. *N. Engl. J. Med.* 299:338–344; 393–401, 1978.

Guberman, A. Coma as a Neurological Emergency. In L.P. Ivan and D.A. Bruce (editors): *Coma, Physiopathology, Diagnosis and Management.* Springfield, IL: Thomas, 1982, Pp. 283–317.

Guidelines for the diagnosis of brain death. *Can. J. Neurol. Sci.* 13:355–358, 1987.

Levy, D.E., et al. Prognosis in nontraumatic coma. *Ann. Intern. Med.* 94:293–301, 1981.

Lewis, S.L. and Topel, J.L. Coma. In W.J. Weiner (editor). *Emergent and Urgent Neurology.* Philadelphia: Lippincott, 1992, Pp. 1–25.

Picton, T., et al. The Neurophysiological Investigation of Stuporous and Comatose Patients. In L.P. Ivan and D.A. Bruce (editors). *Coma, Physiopathology, Diagnosis and Management.* Springfield: Thomas, 1982, Pp. 31–70.

Plum, F. Organic Disturbances of Consciousness. In M. Critchley, J.L. O'Leary, and B. Jennett (editors): *Scientific Foundations of Neurology.* Philadelphia: Davis, 1972, Pp. 193–201.

Plum, F., and Posner, J.B. *The Diagnosis of Stupor and Coma*, 3rd ed. Philadelphia: Davis, 1980.

President's Commission for the Study of Ethical Problems in Medicine and Biomedical and Behavioral Research. *Guidelines for the Determination of Brain Death*. Washington, DC: 1981, Pp. 1–9.

Ropper, A.H. Lateral displacement of the brain and level of consciousness in patients with an acute hemispheral mass. *N. Engl. J. Med.* 314:953–958, 1986.

Ropper, A.H. (editor). Critical care. *Semin. Neurol.* 4:397–498, 1984.

Walker, A.E. An appraisal of the criteria of cerebral death: a summary statement: a collaborative study. *JAMA* 237:982–986, 1977.

Young, B., Blume, W., and Lynch, A. Brain death and the persistent vegetative state: similarities and contrasts. *Can. J. Neurol. Sci.* 16:388–393, 1989.

6

Aphasia and Other Localizing Disorders of Higher Brain Function

HEMISPHERIC DOMINANCE AND LATERALIZATION OF FUNCTION

Language function is localized in the dominant hemisphere, which is frequently correlated with handedness. In virtually all right-handers and about 60% of left-handers, the left hemisphere is dominant. Right hemisphere or bilateral dominance occurs in the remainder of left-handers. Evidence for the lateralization of language function has been gathered from many sources: studies that examined the effects of lateralized lesions or hemispherectomy on language, dichotic listening experiments (in which different stimuli are presented to each ear), observations of the effects of intracarotid amobarbital (Amytal) injection on speech (Wada test), evoked potential studies, anatomical interhemispheric differences, and investigations in patients who have undergone section of the corpus callosum and other interhemispheric commissures ("split-brain"). These last studies have shown that, even in left-brain–dominant individuals, the right hemisphere does have some rudimentary reading and reception capacities.

Hemispheric dominance in a given patient is inferred from his or her handedness (including foot and eye preference) and can be confirmed prior to neurosurgical procedures by the administration of intracarotid Brevital (an ultra-short-acting barbiturate) or Amytal, which produces transient contralateral hemiparesis and global aphasia when injected into the dominant hemisphere. Evidence of a substantial early life injury in one hemisphere may also suggest that the opposite hemisphere is dominant.

The nondominant (usually right) hemisphere is more specialized than the dominant hemisphere for control of visuospatial functions. The ability to read maps, perform maze-learning tasks, draw, and appreciate pattern or form (as with music) resides mainly in the right hemisphere, although lateralization is not usually as complete in these instances as it is for language functions. Recent evidence suggests that the right hemisphere may also play a major role in governing attention mechanisms and regulating emotional responses.

APHASIA AND ALEXIA

Aphasia is defined as a language disorder stemming from a cerebral lesion. Although prosody (speed, rhythm, inflection, and stress) or volume is frequently affected in aphasic speech, aphasia can be distinguished from other speech disorders, such as **dysarthria** (an articulation defect) or **dysphonia** (a voice defect), by the presence of an accompanying writing and reading disorder. Morphemes are the smallest meaningful units of words and comprise individual speech sounds known as phonemes. Aphasia may affect various aspects of language use: syntax (the grammatical structure of sentences), the lexicon (the collection of words), and the morphology of words. Words serving a purely grammatical function, such as *but* or *therein,* are more vulnerable to misuse than substantives in most types of aphasia. Deliberate or propositional speech, meant to communicate ideas, may be affected in some aphasias (e.g., global), whereas nondeliberate or automatic speech (e.g., expletives or counting) may be preserved. Other symbolic functions such as the use of sign language and numbers are also impaired in an aphasic patient.

When reading is affected (with or without aphasia), the term *alexia* (or dyslexia) is applied. If a lesion in the cortical language areas produces a markedly deficient oral language output (at times muteness) but comprehension and writing are preserved and there is no aphasic symptomatology, this is referred to as *aphemia.* This disorder is usually accompanied by a severe oral-buccal-lingual-facial apraxia and is due to a small lesion in Broca's area.

Pure word deafness is an inability to comprehend spoken language, but with intact reading, comprehension, and hearing abilities, and results from a lesion in the cortical auditory association pathways. Although an aphasic patient may be mute initially (especially if afflicted with global aphasia), there are other causes of muteness, such as refusal to speak, lesions of the cingulate gyrus or supplementary motor area,

and severe articulatory dysfunction resulting from brainstem lesions.

To diagnose aphasia, it is therefore necessary to test spoken or written language output or comprehension. It is also important to distinguish between confused or psychotic patients, whose use of language may be bizarre or inappropriate but without the paraphasic or grammatical errors seen in aphasia, and those with true aphasia who are often wrongly thought to be confused.

Paraphasias, or incorrect substitutions of words or parts of words, are particularly characteristic of aphasia, especially with lesions posterior to the rolandic fissure. There are two types: literal, or phonemic, paraphasias, which involve substitutions of sounds that may create words resembling the intended word (e.g., "umbroller" for "umbrella"), and verbal paraphasias in which an actual word is substituted that may be somewhat related in meaning to the original word (e.g., "foot" for "sock").

The language areas are anatomically clustered around the sylvian fissure of the dominant (usually left) hemisphere (Fig. 6-1). **Broca's area,** which is involved in programming speech output, lies in the frontal operculum in the posteroinferior frontal lobe anterior to the motor cortex areas that supply the tongue, lips, and larynx. **Wernicke's area,** which is related to speech reception and decoding, lies in the posterosuperior temporal gyrus near the primary auditory receiving area. A band of white matter, the **arcuate fasciculus,** running deep to the supramarginal gyrus and insula, joins these two areas. The supplementary motor area, the head of the caudate nucleus, and thalamus also play a role in language function, and some aphasias have been observed in patients with dominant lesions of these structures. Aphasic deficits have been specifically correlated with certain lesions in the subcortical white matter of the dominant hemisphere. Testing for aphasia in the spheres of fluency, comprehension, naming, repetition, writing, and reading has been covered in Chapter 2. Formal, standardized, comprehensive tests for assessing the nature of an aphasia, such as the Boston Diagnostic Aphasia Examination or the Western Aphasia Battery, are useful for both following the prog-

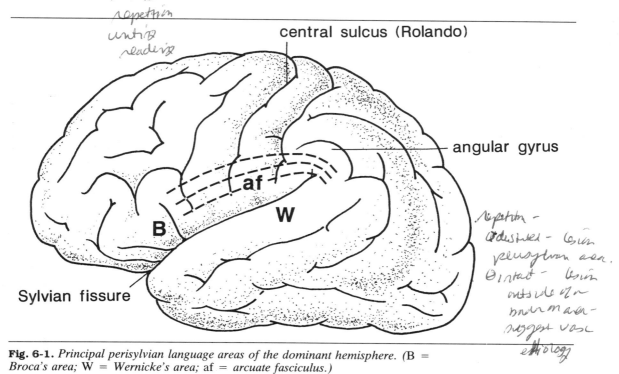

Fig. 6-1. *Principal perisylvian language areas of the dominant hemisphere. (B = Broca's area; W = Wernicke's area; af = arcuate fasciculus.)*

ress of aphasic patients and for planning appropriate therapy.

Although aphasic deficits, especially naming and word-generation problems, occur in widespread frontal and diffuse brain lesions and are often accompanied by dementia, there are specific aphasic syndromes that have a localizing value (Table 6-1). Studies correlating specific aphasic deficits with lesions, which have been localized fairly precisely by modern neuroimaging techniques, have largely confirmed the localizing significance of the classic aphasic syndromes. However, numerous interconnected brain areas likely govern each of the complex components of normal language function, and thus evidence from lesion studies must not be interpreted to imply that the destroyed area is the center responsible for a particular linguistic function. **Fluency,** or the ability to produce sentences of three to four words or more in a nonhesitant fashion and to speak at a rate of about sixty words per minute, is a primary consideration in classifying aphasia. In general, nonfluent aphasias indicate the existence of lesions anterior to the central fissure (prerolandic),

whereas fluent aphasias point to a postrolandic location. If a repetition disturbance occurs with aphasia, this implies that the lesion lies within the perisylvian area. Intact repetition is associated with lesions outside of or bordering on this area (transcortical aphasias), and suggests a vascular etiology. An example of the speech of a patient (Fig. 6-2) with a lesion near Wernicke's area follows:

Interviewer: "Is your name Mrs. Smith?"
Patient: "With who you."
Interviewer: "How are you feeling now?"
Patient: "Yes, I feel a lot better. The boys are coming to see me all the time."
Interviewer: "What's this [tie]?"
Patient: "It's a taff."
Interviewer: "This [watch]?"
Patient: "It's a tee. It comes every week once in a while like this one."
Interviewer: "Why did you come here?"
Patient: "I out with my son. Three of them

Table 6-1. Aphasic Syndromes

Type of aphasia	Spontaneous speech	Par-aphasias	Compre-hension	Repetition	Reading	Writing	Naming	Accompany-ing deficits	Pathology and cause
Broca's	NF (tele-graphic)	Minimal	N	↓	↓	↓	↓ (prompting helps)	Right hemiparesis, left apraxia	Broca's and surrounding area
Wernicke's	F	+ (mainly verbal)	↓	↓	↓	↓	↓	Usually none; may have field defect	Postero-superior left temporal gyrus, often embolic
Conduction	F	+ (mainly phone-mic)	N	↓	↓	Mildly ↓	↓	Often none; may have cortical sensory loss or mild right arm/face weakness	Arcuate fasciculus, left supra-marginal gyrus or left auditory cortex and insula
Global	NF (scant)	—	↓	↓	↓	↓	↓	Usually right hemiplegia	Large perisylvian or frontal and temporo-parietal combined

Transcortical mixed (isolation of speech area)	NF	Possibly	↓	Preserved, echolalia	↓	—	Watershed infarcts sparing perisylvian areas
Transcortical motor	NF (explosive)	Possibly	Good comprehension	Preserved	↓	Transient paresis	Superior or anterior to Broca's area
Transcortical sensory	F (scant)	+	↓	Preserved	↓	Transient paresis	Parieto-temporal junction surrounding Wernicke's area
Anomic	F	—	N	N	↓	—	Angular gyrus, diffuse; other diverse lesions (e.g., anterior temporal)

NF = nonfluent; F = fluent; N = normal; ↓ = reduced; + = present.
Adapted from D.F. Benson and N. Geschwind, The Aphasias and Related Disturbances. In A.B. Baker and L. H. Baker (editors). *Clinical Neurology*, Vol. 1. Philadelphia: Harper & Row, 1983, Pp. 1–18; and A.R. Damasio. Aphasia. *N. Engl. J. Med.* 326:531–539, 1992.

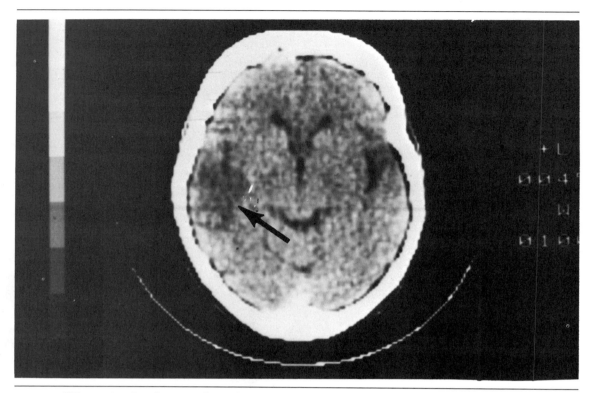

Fig. 6-2. *CT scan showing discrete infarct involving the posterior left temporoparietal area in a 64-year-old woman with a Wernicke-like aphasia.*

came here but I can't say what name they are. I know them."

Interviewer: "Touch your nose."

Patient: "Sure I have a nose here." (Patient touches it.)

Interviewer: "What are you doing in the hospital?"

Patient: "I go and see my sister and I go to see the boys. I don't know what else you're doing. You get a drink once in awhile."

The prognosis of aphasia is best in younger patients and left-handers with bihemispheric language function. The nature of the underlying disorder (e.g., vascular, neoplastic, or traumatic) also has a bearing on the prognosis (Fig. 6-3). In general, Broca's and conduction aphasias carry a better prognosis than Wernicke's aphasia. An intermittent type of treatable aphasia is that due to focal seizures involving the speech

areas. Aphasia may be the only manifestation in focal status epilepticus in the left temporoparietal area, and an electroencephalogram is required for diagnosis.

Primary progressive aphasia refers to an aphasic syndrome, presumably degenerative, that arises in the presenium and progresses over 5 to 10 years. This condition, which has an uncertain pathology, may be mistaken for Alzheimer's disease. Some patients, however, do show the pathologic characteristics of Alzheimer's disease. Degeneration is confined to the left perisylvian region and patients exhibit a nonfluent aphasia with phonemic paraphasic errors in the context of well-preserved memory as well as visuospatial and reasoning skills.

Speech therapy is of some value in aphasic patients, especially when comprehension is preserved, and at the very least helps the patient deal with the frequent prominent emotional difficulties involved.

Alexia is an inability to comprehend written

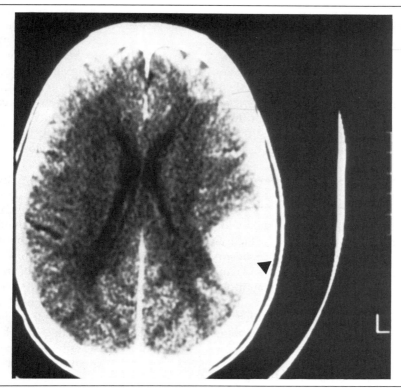

Fig. 6-3. *Contrast-enhanced CT scan showing left posterior temporal meningioma (arrowhead) in a 78-year-old woman presenting with aphasic transient ischemic attack–like episodes. EEG done during an episode showed no epileptic activity. The patient originally had word-finding difficulties and was thought to have early Alzheimer's disease.*

material as a result of brain damage. Reading difficulties may occur with various types of aphasias as well as with visual neglect, eye movement disorders, and visual agnosia. When alexia occurs without agraphia, writing is relatively well preserved and there is often a right homonymous hemianopia. The lesion responsible is usually an infarct that involves the dominant occipital lobe and posterior corpus callosum and is the result of a left posterior cerebral artery occlusion. Visual impulses from the intact right occipital cortex are thus disconnected from the left angular gyrus area. A lesion of the dominant angular gyrus is found in the context of alexia with agraphia.

APRAXIA

Apraxia (most commonly the ideomotor form) is an inability to perform learned skilled move-

ments but without a comprehension, attention, motor, or sensory deficit, or uncooperation (see Chapter 2). The apractic patient usually does not complain of specific problems, but, when sought, apraxia is quite commonly found in neurological patients. Several varieties have been distinguished, affecting either both hands (a lesion in the dominant posterior parietal area) or the left hand alone. In the latter case, the lesion responsible is frequently an infarct in the territory of the left middle cerebral artery, producing a right hemiparesis and extending into the anterior corpus callosum (territory of the anterior cerebral artery). This causes the right hemisphere premotor area to be disconnected from the left hemisphere areas where the command to move the arm was initially received, interpreted, and transmitted across the corpus callosum. Apraxia of the left hand may also arise with lesions of the right premotor area (limb-kinetic apraxia) or with pure corpus callosum lesions (callosal apraxia).

Dressing apraxia refers to a dressing difficulty that is not due to obvious motor or sensory deficits. Usually a nondominant parietal lesion is the source of the problem. **Constructional apraxia** is better termed *constructional difficulty* and may be seen in patients with either dominant or nondominant parietal lesions, although it is more common in the latter (Fig. 6-4).

AGNOSIA

The agnosias represent disorders of higher cortical integrative sensory function in which an object cannot be recognized in one sensory sphere even though primary sensation and naming ability are intact. There are tactile, auditory, and visual types of agnosia. Disorders such as astereognosis and agraphesthesia, which are forms of tactile agnosia, have already been discussed (Chapter 2). Pure word deafness is one form of auditory agnosia.

There are various subgroups of visual agnosia stemming from lesions of the visual association cortex. **Simultanagnosia** is characterized by the inability to interpret visually the significance of a whole object or picture of various objects despite adequate identification of its various components. **Prosopagnosia** is an inability to identify familiar faces or other familiar objects within a class (e.g., one's own car in a parking lot). These patients usually have bilateral parietotemporooccipital lesions.

A patient with **anosognosia** is unaware of a neurological deficit such as hemiplegia. Hemispatial neglect or hemiinattention to sensory stimuli frequently accompanies this disorder (Fig. 6-5). The denial or unawareness of visual loss that occurs in cortical blindness (Anton's syndrome) is an example of this disorder. These symptoms are most common with lesions of either inferior parietal lobe, but are more common and severe with right-sided (nondominant) lesions. Anosognosia is a frank denial of the deficit. This denial can range from an inappropriate unconcern regarding the hemiplegia, a frank denial of the deficit, failure to recognize a limb as the patient's own, or, in the extreme, an impression that the paralyzed side is someone else. Neglect may evoke a pseudoparesis in which the

Fig. 6-4. *Writing and drawing samples from a 79-year-old woman with severe alexia, agraphia, and constructional deficit with bilateral posterior temporoparietal infarcts. (A) Attempt to write "the dog" and (B) to copy a diamond.*

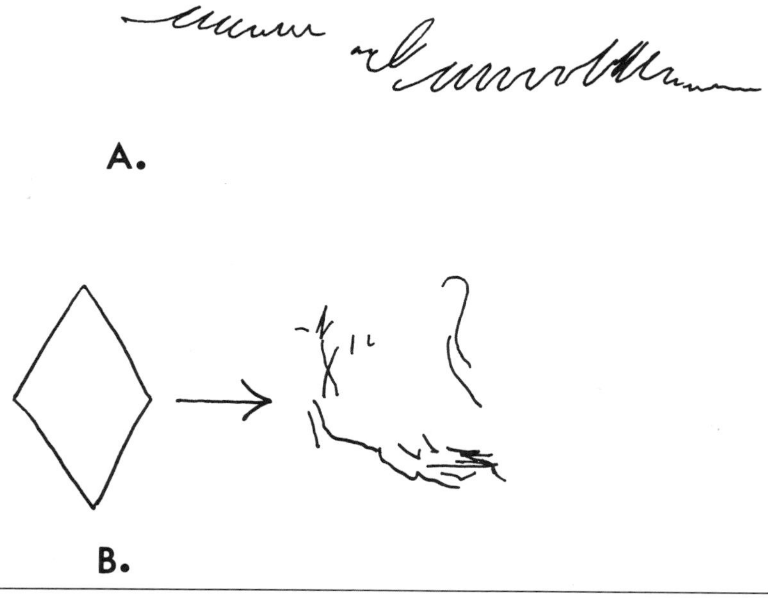

A.

B.

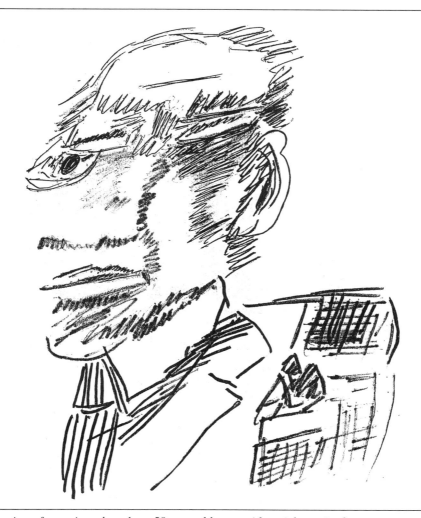

Fig. 6-5. *Drawing of examiner done by a 58-year-old man with a right parietal infarct. Note the neglect of the left hemispace indicated by much less detail on the left side of the drawing. The patient did not have a hemianopia.*

patient holds the limb immobile unless specifically urged to move it or both limbs simultaneously. When persistent in the stroke patient, neglect is a barrier to successful rehabilitation.

The possible signs manifested by a nondominant (right) parietal lesion may be summarized as follows (note that not all of the signs are specific to the nondominant hemisphere):

1. Left astereognosis and agraphesthesia, lack of two-point discrimination, and loss of other cortical sensory modalities

2. Left lower homonymous quadrantanopia (i.e., a visual field defect)

3. Reduced optokinetic nystagmus with tape moving to the right

4. Pseudoathetosis of the left arm observed either when testing for drift or when leaving the arm undisturbed

5. Cogan's sign, or spasticity of conjugate gaze (i.e., when closed eyes are forcibly opened, they deviate conjugately upward toward the side of the lesion)

6. Anosognosia, left hemispatial inattention,

and sensory extinction on double simultaneous stimulation

7. Impaired visuospatial abilities, including copying, construction, map-reading, drawing, and maze performance
8. Dressing difficulties
9. Motor impersistence (inability to sustain an action, such as keeping the arms elevated or the eyes closed, for any length of time)
10. Disturbance in the "pragmatics" of speech (e.g., inability to distinguish between variations in intonation or the emotional coloring of a sentence)

FRONTAL LOBE SYNDROME

The nature of frontal lobe symptomatology depends on whether the lesion involves the dominant hemisphere, in which case language disturbances are frequent, and whether it is confined to premotor association areas or extends far enough backward to involve the prerolandic motor cortex and produce hemiplegia. An acute lesion of the frontal gaze centers brings about a conjugate deviation of the eyes toward the side of the lesion, which is usually transient. The higher-function disturbances, best seen in the setting of the bifrontal involvement produced by surgical frontal leukotomy, large tumors, trauma, or degenerative dementing illnesses, can be summarized as follows:

1. Slowness of cognition and action
2. Apathy and loss of initiative and spontaneity
3. Loss of social concern and tact
4. Emotional lability and inappropriate jocularity
5. Inability to carry out planned activities and adapt strategies of action to changing circumstances (perseveration)
6. Gait disorder and incontinence

CALLOSAL SYNDROME

When surgical sectioning of the corpus callosum and interhemispheric commissures is performed for the control of epilepsy or the management of other callosal lesions such as tumors, abscesses, and Marchiafava-Bignami disease (a rare degenerative condition seen in alcoholics), subtle signs of hemispheric disconnection appear. Special testing can often reveal the following in right-handers:

1. Inability to report visual stimuli presented to the left visual field or auditory stimuli presented to the right ear
2. Inability to name points touched on the left side of the body or objects handled in the left hand
3. Left upper-extremity apraxia
4. Each hand operating at cross purposes with the other ("intermanual conflict"), also seen with some frontal lesions
5. Constructional difficulties with the right hand

These deficits are less prominent in the presence of a congenital **agenesis of the corpus callosum,** which may be accompanied by other developmental defects, mental retardation, and seizures.

GERSTMANN'S SYNDROME

The syndrome described by Gerstmann, and stemming from a lesion of the dominant posterior parietal area, is rarely seen either in its complete form or in isolation from other defects such as aphasia. The classic components of the syndrome are: agraphia, acalculia, right-left disorientation, and inability to identify fingers correctly (i.e., finger "agnosia").

AMNESIA

Memory is a complex function that is traditionally broken down into the following components: registration (depending on attention and perception mechanisms), retention (storage), and retrieval (recall). It is subserved by anatomical systems closely related to the limbic system, which plays an important role in mediating emotional and adaptive responses. The hippocampi and surrounding structures project through the fornices to the mamillary bodies, then to the mesial thalami via the mamillothalamic tracts. This circuit is vital to the process of learning. Two parallel systems, one involving the amygdala and the dorsal median nucleus of the thalamus and a second involving the hippocampus and anterior nucleus of the thalamus, may operate in normal memory function. The entorhinal cortex (parahippocampal gyrus) sends an important efferent projection, known as the *perforant pathway,* to specific areas of the hippocampus. This cortical area serves as a way-station that links areas of the cortex, with specific sensory and multimodality association functions, to the hippocampus. The perforant pathway also likely plays a vital role in memory.

A patient with amnesia has an impaired ability to learn or memorize and also to recall previously learned information. These are commonly called *short-term* and *long-term memory loss,* respectively, and frequently appear together, although their contribution may be disproportionate. In patients with pure amnesia, it is usually possible to localize a lesion to the bilateral hippocampal areas (Fig. 6-6), mamil-

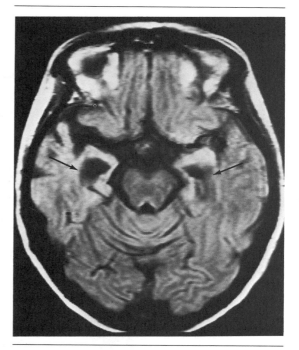

Fig. 6-6. T_1*-weighted MRI image from a 41-year-old woman with a marked amnestic defect appearing 17 years earlier following a difficult childbirth that required general anesthesia. The scan shows bilateral hippocampal ischemic lesions* (arrows) *and temporal lobe atrophy.*

Table 6-2. Amnesic Syndromes

Sudden onset—usually gradual but incomplete
    recovery
    Bilateral hippocampal infarction
    Bilateral paramedian thalamic infarction
    Trauma to diencephalon or mesial temporal
      regions
    Subarachnoid hemorrhage due to ruptured
      aneurysm
    Carbon monoxide poisoning and other hypoxic
      states
Sudden onset—transitory
    Temporal lobe seizures
    Post concussion
    Transient global amnesia
Subacute onset—usually incomplete recovery
    Wernicke-Korsakoff syndrome due to thiamine
      deficiency
    Herpes simplex encephalitis
    Tuberculous and perhaps other forms of
      granulomatous meningitis
Slowly progressive
    Diencephalic tumors
    Alzheimer's disease

Modified from M. Victor, The amnesic syndrome and its anatomical basis. *Can. Med. Assoc. J.* 100:1115–1125, 1969.

lary bodies, or the paramedian thalamic areas (dorsal median nucleus) or their interconnections (Fig. 6-7), but a memory deficit frequently constitutes a major part of the more global cognitive impairment seen in dementia. Patients with a primary complaint of memory difficulties commonly have other deficits, such as reduced concentration (often psychogenic) or word-finding (e.g., normal senescent forgetfulness) abilities, and therefore formal neuropsychological testing is recommended in most instances to help pinpoint the diagnosis and quantify the amnesia. Verbal memory is the skill usually tested, but auditory, visual, and somatosensory memory can also be tested and occasionally may be affected in isolation. There is a subtle relationship between agnosia and memory loss in these sensory spheres. Table 6-2 outlines the causes of amnesia.

The **Wernicke-Korsakoff syndrome** (see Chapter 29), found in chronic undernourished

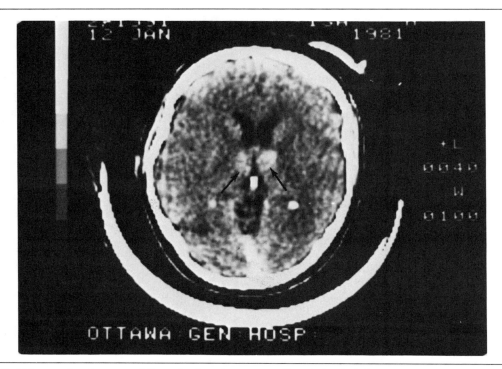

Fig. 6-7. *CT scan showing acute bilateral enhancing paramedian thalamic infarcts (arrows) in a 52-year-old man presenting in a transient coma with vertical gaze abnormalities. He was left with a permanent Korsakoff's amnestic syndrome. Ischemia in the territory of the bilateral subthalamothalamic perforating branches due to occlusion of a common stem arising from the posterior cerebral artery accounts for this syndrome.*

alcoholics and victims of other thiamine-deficiency states (e.g., prisoners of war, gastric carcinoma, or the severe persistent vomiting of pregnancy), has served as a model for the amnesic syndrome. Following recovery from their acute global confusional state, these patients exhibit a severely deficient learning ability, to the extent that they may not remember what they were shown or told seconds earlier. The memory deficit is more pronounced for verbal than nonverbal (e.g., maze-learning) material and, at times through prompting, it can be shown that there is some retention. There is also a patchy retrograde amnesia, with an inability to order events in time. This often gives rise to **confabulation,** or the tendency to fabricate responses (at times fantastic). The patients are frequently also apathetic and lacking in initiative. The essential lesion has been assigned to the dorsal medial nucleus of the thalamus.

Bilateral paramedian thalamic infarction also gives rise to a very similar amnestic syndrome.

Transient global amnesia is a not uncommon condition affecting middle-aged or elderly patients. It involves the sudden onset of a confusional state in a previously healthy person, with the patient commonly repeating questions such as "where am I?" and "what's happening?" When tested, the patient shows no ability to retain information and a marked retrograde amnesia, even though there are no other neurological signs. The state almost always resolves completely within several hours, leaving a permanent gap in the patient's memory for the period involved. The pathogenesis in most cases is thought to be vascular in nature, representing a transient ischemic attack of both hippocampal areas. It has been seen in patients with migraine, subdural hematomas, and craniopharyngioma, and also in patients at the time of cardiac catheterization, likely related to embolization when the catheter was flushed. Recurrences are rare, but a few cases of patients who eventually suffered a permanent memory deficit have been reported. In certain cases, an epileptic rather than vascular mechanism has been suggested.

KLÜVER-BUCY SYNDROME

Animals with bilateral ablations of the mesioanterior temporal areas, including the amygdala, exhibit a constellation of behavioral symptoms, including placidity and absence of anger or fear responses, hypersexuality, hyperbulimia (indiscriminate overeating), increased oral exploratory tendencies, a form of visual agnosia, and a tendency to react to visual stimuli with a stereotyped pattern of motor responses. Only rarely has the full syndrome been documented in human subjects, but fragments of it have been seen in patients after bilateral temporal lobectomy or herpes simplex encephalitis, or with Pick's or Alzheimer's disease.

BIBLIOGRAPHY

Albert, M. L., and Helm-Estabrooks, N. Diagnosis and treatment of aphasia. Part II. *J.A.M.A.* 259:1205–1210, 1988.

Albert, M. L., and Helm-Estabrooks, N. Diagnosis and treatment of aphasia. Part I. *J.A.M.A.* 259:1043–1047, 1988.

Alexander, M. P., Naeser, M. A., and Palumbo, C. L. Correlations of subcortical CT lesion sites and aphasia profiles. *Brain* 110:961–991, 1987.

Benson, D. F., and Geschwind, N. The Aphasias and Related Disturbances. In A. B. Baker and L. H. Baker (editors). *Clinical Neurology,* Vol. 1. Philadelphia: Harper & Row, 1983, Pp. 1–18.

Benson, D. F., and Stuss, D. *The Frontal Lobes.* New York: Raven, 1986.

Critchley, M. *The Parietal Lobes.* New York: Hafnar, 1966.

Damasio, A. (editor). Behavioral neurology. *Semin. Neurol.* 4:117–259, 1984.

Damasio, A. R. Aphasia. *N. Engl. J. Med.* 326:531–539, 1992.

Fisher, C. M., and Adams, R. D. Transient global amnesia syndrome. *Acta Neurol. Scand.* 40 (suppl. 9):7–82, 1964.

Geschwind, N. Disconnexion syndromes in animals and man. *Brain* 88:237–294; 585–644, 1965.

Guberman, A., and Stuss, D. The syndrome of bilateral paramedian thalamic infarction. *Neurology* 33:540–546, 1983.

Heilman, K. M., and Van Den Abell, T. Right hemisphere dominance for attention: the mechanisms underlying hemispheric asymmetries of inattention (neglect). *Neurology* 30:327–330, 1980.

Lhermitte, F. Human autonomy and the frontal lobes. Part II: Patient behavior in complex and social situations; the "environmental dependency syndrome." *Ann. Neurol.* 19:335–343, 1986.

Lhermitte, F., Pillon, B., and Serdaru, M. Human autonomy and the frontal lobes. Part I: Imitation and utilization behavior; a neuropsychological study of 75 patients. *Ann. Neurol.* 19:326–334, 1986.

Mesulam, M. M. (editor): *Principles of Behavioral Neurology.* Philadelphia: Davis, 1985.

Shuping, J. R., Rollinson, R. D., and Toole, J. F. Transient global amnesia. *Ann. Neurol.* 7:281–285, 1980.

Victor, M. The amnesic syndrome and its anatomical basis. *Can. Med. Assoc. J.* 100:1115–1125, 1969.

Weintraub, S., Rubin, N. P., and Mesulam, M. M. Primary progressive aphasia. Longitudinal course, neuropsychological profile and language features. *Arch. Neurol.* 47:1329–1335, 1990.

Epilepsy and Syncope

EPILEPSY

Pathophysiology

An **epileptic seizure** is an excessive and abnormal electrical discharge of brain neurons that is manifested by behavioral or electroencephalographic (EEG) changes, or both. **Epilepsy** is a brain disorder arising from many causes that leads to recurrent, usually spontaneous, epileptic seizures. Everyone is capable of having an epileptic seizure under the right circumstances (e.g., electroconvulsive therapy or strychnine intoxication), although individual seizure thresholds vary and are probably largely genetically determined. Most seizures arise from a focal area of brain damage, aberrant development, or metabolic impairment and these are termed *partial*. Other seizures appear to involve the whole brain at once and are termed *primary generalized*.

The physiological mechanisms underlying focal epileptogenesis are relatively well understood and seem to be basically similar independent of the focal process responsible (Table 7-1). At the cellular level, neuronal membranes in an epileptic focus undergo periodic spontaneous slow depolarizations with superimposed high-frequency bursts of action potentials known as *paroxysmal depolarizing shifts*. The synchronous activation of large numbers of neurons within an epileptic focus gives rise to the epileptic interictal spike recorded from the surface EEG. For these potentials to develop within the cerebral cortex, there must be a subpopulation of neurons possessing the intrinsic ability to support high-frequency firing (burst discharges), a loss of postsynaptic inhibitory control mechanisms, and a tendency for neurons to fire in synchrony resulting from increased excitatory coupling. These processes in turn depend on changes in the balance between the inward (Na^+ and Ca^{2+}) and outward (K^+) ionic currents that govern neuronal excitability. In recent years, alterations in the concentrations of the inhibitory neurotransmitter gamma-aminobutyric acid (GABA) or excitatory neurotransmitters such as glutamate and aspar-

Table 7-1. Possible Mechanisms in Epileptic
Seizures

1. Defect in the neuronal membrane, either in the
   transport of ions or in the properties of ion
   channels
2. Defect in the inhibitory mechanisms (failure of
   GABA-mediated recurrent inhibition)
3. Defect in the excitatory, glutamate-related
   systems
4. Defect in the modulatory systems governing
   excitatory and inhibitory function

GABA = gamma-aminobutyric acid.

tate have been implicated as major factors in
epileptogenesis. GABA serves as a transmitter
for inhibitory stellate interneurons in the cortex
and hippocampus. These interneurons limit the
ability of depolarizations to produce burst discharges and also the ability of pacemaker cells
to recruit adjacent cells into epileptic firing patterns. Convulsant agents such as penicillin
block GABA-mediated inhibitory postsynaptic
potentials. GABA agonists (e.g., muscimol),
GABA pro-drugs (e.g., progabide), GABA
transaminase inhibitors (e.g., gamma-vinyl
GABA), and benzodiazepines acting on specific receptors related to the GABA receptor
complex are all anticonvulsants that are effective in both animals and humans.

Recently, specific receptors that are linked
to the generation of excitatory postsynaptic potentials by glutamate and aspartate (the main
cortical excitatory neurotransmitters) have
been characterized, cloned, and sequenced.
Three types of receptors have been defined according to their selective excitation by either
N-methyl-D-aspartate (NMDA), kainate (a glutamate analogue), or alpha-amino-3-hydroxy-
5-methyl-4-isoxazolepropionic acid (AMPA).
A fourth receptor type is termed metabotropic
since it is not associated directly with ion channels and since excitation leads to the activation
of second messengers such as phospholipase C
within the cell. The receptor responding to
NMDA mediates slower, longer-lasting responses and the receptor-activated membrane
channels are calcium permeable. There is normally a voltage-dependent Mg^{2+} blockade of
NMDA receptor–associated channels. Because

of these properties, it is likely that activation
of these receptors underlies the development
of paroxysmal depolarizing shifts and burst generation. Excessive excitation of NMDA receptors may also cause "excitotoxic" neuronal
damage, which may result from epileptic seizures.

Other factors that seem to operate in the
genesis of epileptic foci in humans are the
formation of gliotic scars and partial deafferentation of neurons in the focus. The former may
lead to distortions of neuronal architecture,
alterations in the extracellular environment,
or possibly alterations in the way neurotransmitters are handled. Partial deafferentation of
the neurons may lead to neuronal hyperexcitability.

The concept of **kindling** has been studied extensively in experimental settings and may have
implications for human forms of epilepsy and
their treatment. In various animal models and
at various brain sites, especially limbic structures, when a subthreshold electric shock is applied repeatedly at regular intervals, this leads
to increasingly greater afterdischarges, both in
terms of duration and spread, and eventually
spontaneous seizures may occur. The substantia
nigra may also play a specific role in the kindling
process. These findings imply that even subclinical epileptic discharges in humans may produce
alterations that eventually lower the seizure
threshold. Some investigators have used these
observations to explain why epilepsy may
worsen over time in a particular patient, and
this has given rise to the concept that "seizures
breed seizures." Kindling has also been used to
explain the "mirror focus" that may eventually
form in the hemisphere opposite a unilateral
epileptic focus.

For a seizure to become apparent clinically,
the discharging neurons must recruit surrounding neurons into abnormal firing patterns.
Eventually the whole brain can become involved (secondary generalization) through
propagation via nonspecific thalamocortical
and interhemispheric pathways. Because abnormal neuronal firing underlies epileptic seizures, they are characteristically seen in the
context of lesions or conditions involving the
gray matter of the brain: the cortex, hippocam-

pus, basal ganglia and thalamus, amygdala, and possibly the reticular core of the brainstem.

The **aura,** which can precede a generalized seizure, is the clinical manifestation of an epileptic discharge within the focus and therefore is of value for determining where in the brain a seizure begins. The particular features of a focal (partial) seizure or of the aura (also a partial seizure) preceding a generalized seizure depend on the function of that part of the brain being irritated, or more rarely inhibited, by the epileptic discharge. For example, a focal epileptic discharge beginning in the area of the motor cortex controlling thumb movements will give rise to twitching of the thumb. As the discharge propagates along the motor strip and adjacent areas become involved, the twitching ascends sequentially to involve the whole hand, forearm, arm, shoulder, and face (jacksonian "march" or seizure).

Instead of beginning focally, an epileptic seizure may be generalized from the onset and seemingly involve all areas of the brain virtually simultaneously. The **corticoreticular theory** of generalized epilepsy is based on the concept that there is a complex interplay between cortical neurons and thalamic reticular pathways in both human generalized seizures and animal models of generalized seizures. When primary generalized seizures are caused by structural brain disease, the underlying disorder is frequently found to affect both cortical and subcortical areas, suggesting an alteration in the corticoreticular circuits. When a corticoreticular discharge is primarily inhibitory, a clinical absence seizure is the result; when excitatory, a generalized tonic-clonic (GTC) seizure occurs. The corticoreticular theory also explains the facilitatory effect of sleep and the inhibitory effect of sensory arousal as well as the effects of certain drugs on epileptic seizures.

One of the most important unanswered questions in the study of epilepsy is: given that the epileptic focus or tendency is a chronic abnormality, what immediate factors determine when a seizure occurs? Only in a small minority of cases can specific (e.g., sensory stimuli in the reflex epilepsies) or nonspecific (e.g., alcohol, sleep deprivation, and emotional upset) triggering mechanisms be identified.

Epidemiology and Etiology

Epilepsy affects between 1 and 2 percent of the population. This is probably an underestimate because some cases go undiagnosed and others are so benign that medical care is never sought. This incidence of seizures is greatest in the neonatal period. There are also peaks in the first and seventh decades. Approximately 60 percent of cases begin in childhood or adolescence and only 2 to 3 percent of the patients have onset after age 50. GTC, complex, and simple partial seizures are the most common types.

The etiology of epilepsy includes most brain disorders, but almost half of the cases are idiopathic (Table 7-2). The likelihood of a particular etiology depends on the age of onset and the seizure type. A specific detectable cause is much more likely in patients with partial seizures than in those with generalized seizures. Seizures in neonates are usually due to conditions such as birth hypoxia, trauma, intraventricular hemorrhage, meningitis, developmental central nervous system (CNS) anomalies, hypocalcemia, hypoglycemia, and pyridoxine deficiency. In adults, head trauma, brain tumors, metabolic abnormalities, drug and alcohol withdrawal, and arteriovenous malformations are prominent causes. In the elderly, cerebrovascular disease, tumors, and Alzheimer's disease are the most likely causes.

For unknown reasons, seizures due to cerebral damage incurred at birth may not begin until early adulthood. Additional epileptogenic factors such as hormonal facilitation may be required before a brain lesion can generate a seizure. Knowledge concerning the etiology of partial seizures has been gained from the pathological examination of material resected at the time of temporal lobectomy. In these cases, mesial temporal sclerosis (scarring presumably due to birth hypoxia or ischemia or to previous febrile seizures), hamartomatous lesions, cortical dysplasias, small tumors, and arteriovenous malformations account for the majority of identifiable lesions.

In general, epilepsy is inherited in 5 to 10 percent of the cases. The chance of epilepsy in the offspring of an epileptic mother is approxi-

Table 7-2. Etiology of Epilepsy

Infants and children	Adults
Idiopathic	Idiopathic
Birth and neonatal	Stroke
Vascular insults and anomalies	Head trauma
Congenital developmental brain anomalies and syndromes	Drug or alcohol abuse
	Brain tumors and vascular malformations
Inherited metabolic disorders	Infections
Head injuries	Congenital developmental brain anomalies
Infections	Inherited metabolic disorders
Tumors	Multiple sclerosis
Genetic	Alzheimer's disease

mately 3 percent and of an epileptic father, 1.7 percent. When one parent and one child have epilepsy, the risk for the next offspring rises to approximately 10 percent. Genetic factors have primarily been implicated in generalized corticoreticular epilepsy (especially childhood-onset absence attacks with a 3-Hz spike-wave in the EEG), which is thought to be inherited in a multifactorial manner. The EEG spike-wave trait is inherited in an autosomal dominant fashion and shows an age-dependent expressivity; it is most commonly seen in children between the ages of 5 to 15. Juvenile myoclonic epilepsy is another genetically based syndrome, which is most likely inherited in an irregular autosomal dominant fashion. Genetic influences are also thought to play some role in febrile seizures and possibly a minor role in posttraumatic seizures and complex partial seizures. Epilepsy is a major feature of several genetically determined autosomal recessive diseases, such as phenylketonuria and Tay-Sachs disease, as well as dominantly inherited disorders, such as tuberous sclerosis.

Classification of Seizures and Syndromes

The International Classification of Seizures (Table 7-3) has been formulated from the clinical features of the seizure (which are not always available) and the EEG features. Usually only interictal (between-seizure) EEG data are available, although at times actual seizures are recorded. The classification divides seizures

Table 7-3. International Classification of Seizures (modified)

Partial (focal) seizures (with or without secondary generalization)
  Simple
    Motor
    Sensory
    Autonomic
    Psychic
  Complex (with or without automatisms)
    Simple partial onset followed by impairment of consciousness
    Impairment of consciousness at onset
Generalized seizures
  Tonic-clonic
  Absence (typical or atypical)
  Myoclonic
  Clonic
  Atonic
  Tonic

into the two major categories: generalized and partial, thereby implying that the latter are almost always due to an underlying focal brain lesion. However, certain metabolic disorders such as hypoglycemia, hyperglycemic hyperosmolar nonketotic states, and hepatic encephalopathy can produce focal seizures in the absence of a detectable focal brain disorder. Generalized seizures may also be due to a focal brain lesion that precipitates such rapid generalization of the discharge that no aura occurs. When the clinical manifestation of a seizure is generalized but the EEG shows a focal epileptiform abnormality, it is classified as partial with secondary generalization. Many times several seizure types occur in the same patient.

There is no universally accepted classification of the epilepsies, but several syndromes (some of which are discussed later in this chapter) are well recognized. An epileptic syndrome is defined on the basis of the seizure types involved, age of onset, etiology, natural history, and prognosis (Table 7-4). A specific seizure type may be seen in several syndromes. For example, absence seizures can occur in Lennox-Gastaut syndrome, childhood absence epilepsy, epilepsy with myoclonic absences, juvenile absence epilepsy, and juvenile myoclonic epilepsy. The so-called **benign focal epilepsies of childhood** usually disappear by late childhood or adolescence, respond well to medication, and, despite focal EEG abnormalities, are not caused by structural brain lesions. Rolandic seizures with centrotemporal (sylvian) spikes and benign occipital epilepsy are included in this category. The latter syndrome has a poorly understood interrelationship with migraine. Besides facilitating the diagnosis of epilepsy, accurate classification allows the appropriate choice of initial antiepileptic drug treatment. For the most part, surgical therapy is reserved for patients with partial seizures.

Generalized Tonic-Clonic Seizure

A GTC seizure represents the common grand mal convulsion. An ictus begins with tonic contraction of the muscles, first in brief flexion and then in extension. The eyes roll back, the teeth are clenched (which may cause tongue biting), and the patient may utter a cry due to forced expiration. The patient loses consciousness from the onset and falls. There is then a brief vibratory phase consisting of a fine muscular tremor. During the clonic phase that follows, muscle contraction is interrupted by periodic relaxation, giving rise to jerking movements that are spaced farther and farther apart. Hypertension, apnea (often with cyanosis), tachycardia, mydriasis, increased sphincter and bladder tone, and increased salivation and bronchial secretions are some of the autonomic phenomena that appear during the tonic phase. In the postictal period, there is a brief tonic muscle contraction before complete flaccidity and relaxation supervene, and this lasts for several minutes. During this phase, the urinary sphincter relaxes and urinary incontinence occurs. Respirations become regular, although increased secretions and flaccidity of tongue and pharyngeal muscles may cause a partial obstruction. Babinski's signs are frequently present. The patient gradually recovers consciousness following a phase of confusion and may either be combative (especially if overrestrained) or pass into a prolonged sleep. Postictal headache is common. The active motor components of the seizure last about 60 to 90 seconds.

During a seizure, the patient should be protected against head injury, and, in the postictal phases, moved into a semiprone position, dentures removed, and any excess secretions or vomitus cleared from the oral cavity to prevent aspiration. It is not anatomically possible to swallow the tongue. Objects should not be forced into the mouth to prevent tongue biting once a seizure has begun.

The EEG may show a brief low-voltage fast discharge (desynchronization) at the onset of the seizure, which is followed by a buildup of rhythmic 10-Hz generalized sharp activity. However, these changes are frequently obscured by muscle artifact. As the clonic phase supervenes, the fast activity is increasingly punctuated by high-voltage slow waves. In the postictal phase, the EEG is flat briefly and shows delta activity, which may persist for hours. Interictally patients may show paroxysms of generalized 3-Hz spike waves.

Table 7-4. Epileptic Syndromes and Prognosis for Seizure Control

Good prognosis
  Benign focal epilepsies of childhood
    Benign partial epilepsy with rolandic
      (centrotemporal spikes) and sylvian seizures
    Benign occipital epilepsy
  Childhood absence seizures
  Juvenile myoclonic epilepsy (on valproic acid)
Poor prognosis
  West's syndrome (infantile spasms)
  Lennox-Gastaut syndrome
  Temporolimbic epilepsy
  Progressive myoclonus epilepsies
  Nonconvulsive generalized status epilepticus

Absence

The absence seizure (formerly called *petit mal*) represents an inhibition of cortical activity that causes a sudden suspension of movement and speech, blank stare, and unresponsiveness to stimuli. They are most common in the pediatric population and tend to disappear, along with the 3-Hz spike-wave EEG trait (Fig. 7-1), by age 20. Most absence attacks last for 5 to 10 seconds, but they may persist for 30 seconds or longer. The patient does not usually lose muscle tone or fall during an attack but may display rhythmic blinking or subtle clonic movements and at times minor tonic or atonic components (e.g., head drooping).

Automatisms, which are semipurposeful, often repetitive movements or vocalizations that the patient has no memory of later, are common if the attack lasts more than 15 seconds. Typical examples are lip smacking, repetitive swallowing or chewing, fumbling or picking movements, rubbing or patting, and opening and closing drawers or doors. One of the most characteristic features of absence seizures is their abrupt onset and cessation with no postictal confusion. Patients may be aware of a gap in their activity or that they have "missed something" but immediately resume whatever they were doing. The EEG tracing during a typical absence attack shows a rhythmic, approximately 3-Hz spike-wave burst with a generalized distribution, rapid onset, and offset. Atypical absence seizures are characterized by a more gradual onset or recovery, more pronounced motor features such as loss of postural tone, and a slower spike-wave discharge of approximately 2 Hz.

Other Generalized Seizures

Pure clonic, tonic, myoclonic, and atonic seizures are less common types of epilepsy. They are frequently seen, often in combination, in

Fig. 7-1. *EEG showing interictal 3-Hz, generalized spike-wave bursts in a 35-year-old woman with absence attacks.*

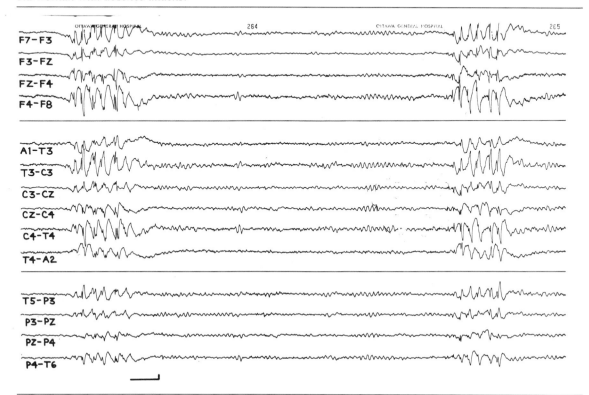

patients with the **Lennox-Gastaut syndrome.** This is a common epileptic syndrome of childhood that is often associated with mental retardation and atypical absence seizures, atonic seizures (causing sudden head drooping or falls), secondarily generalized tonic-clonic seizures, myoclonic seizures, and tonic seizures during sleep. Injuries due to falls are a frequent consequence of atonic or myoclonic seizures.

The EEG pattern consists of very frequent interictal bursts of generalized slow (approximately 2-Hz) spike waves (Fig. 7-2). The etiology also includes birth anoxia, tuberous sclerosis, congenital infections, phenylketonuria, and cerebral malformations.

West's syndrome is an infantile encephalopathy with onset usually around the age of 6 months. It is also due to various causes and consists of frequent myoclonic seizures (infantile spasms), developmental delay or regression, and a disorganized EEG pattern called *hypsarrhythmia*. The infantile spasms occur in clusters many times a day and often involve sudden flexion of the trunk and legs and extension of the arms in front of the body. This disorder carries an ominous prognosis because many of the children ultimately become mentally retarded or manifest the Lennox-Gastaut syndrome. Prolonged intravenous adrenocorticotropic hormone (ACTH) treatment, begun as soon as the diagnosis is established, has proved beneficial in some cases for seizure control, normalization of the EEG brain-wave activity, and improving the mental state, but side effects are common. In one major controlled study, patients on nitrazepam did just as well as those on ACTH.

Juvenile myoclonic epilepsy is a relatively common form of epilepsy that usually begins around puberty and probably has a genetic basis. In 17 to 49 percent of the cases, patients have close or distant relatives with epilepsy.

Fig. 7-2. *EEG showing interictal generalized, atypical spike-wave bursts (2–2.5 Hz) in an 18-year-old mentally retarded boy with Lennox-Gastaut syndrome.*

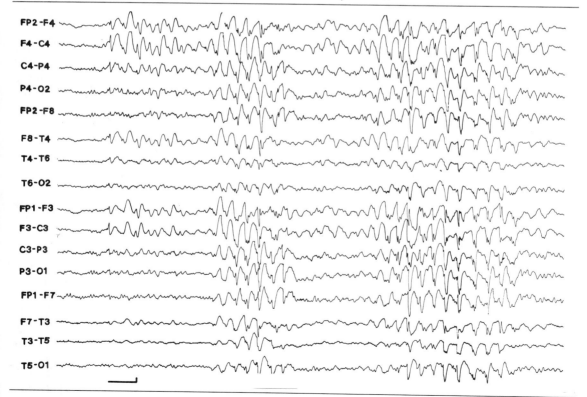

These patients experience myoclonus (usually of the upper extremities) for a period after awakening in the morning. The myoclonus may actually cause objects to fly out of their hands. They also experience GTC seizures and less frequently absence attacks upon awakening or shortly afterward. Nocturnal seizures also occur, and seizures are often provoked by sleep deprivation. The interictal EEG may reveal bursts of 4 to 6 Hz or generalized spike-wave activity as well as photosensitivity. The seizures and myoclonus usually respond well to valproate therapy, which often has to be continued indefinitely because the seizures do not remit.

Partial Seizures

Impairment of consciousness (defined as either a diminished responsiveness to stimuli or amnesia for the attack) distinguishes complex from simple partial seizures. **Simple partial seizures** may occur in any sensory modality, involve autonomic features, or consist of psychic phenomena such as déjà vu (feeling that an unfamiliar situation is familiar) or jamais vu (failure to recognize a familiar situation or environment). The ictal EEG is normal in most of these patients.

Complex partial seizures (formerly known as psychomotor seizures) frequently produce a dreamlike state rather than a complete loss of consciousness and rarely mimic a syncopal attack. An attack may be preceded by an aura (a simple partial seizure) and can consist of a rising epigastric sensation, nonspecific vague unusual feelings, perceptual distortions (e.g., macropsia or micropsia), an unpleasant odor, psychic phenomena such as déjà vu or jamais vu, or fear. Automatisms, which may be simple (discussed earlier) or consist of complex activities such as driving a car or cooking a meal "automatically," are frequent during the period of impaired consciousness, and rarely may last hours, leading to an epileptic fugue state which the patient cannot remember. It is important to distinguish these seizures from absence seizures (Table 7-5) because different drugs are indicated for their control. Complex partial seizures also carry a worse prognosis, and surgical therapy may be used in intractable cases.

Secondarily generalized tonic-clonic seizures often occur with complex partial seizures. The epileptogenic lesion commonly involves the mesial temporal structures (hippocampus and amygdala) and less often the mesial frontal, orbitofrontal, or occipital areas. The ictal symptoms stem from epileptic discharges within the limbic system and its projections, and only rarely can they provide lateralizing clues to the epileptic focus (e.g., aphasic symptoms in a left-sided focus with seizures spreading to the temporal neocortex).

Frontal lobe complex partial seizures, versus those originating from the temporal lobe, do not usually begin with a fixed stare and arrest of activity. Instead, patients manifest bizarre bimanual and bipedal activity and vocalizations, and the seizures occur more frequently at night. The ictal EEG pattern is quite variable. It may show fast activity, rhythmic slowing, or spike-wave activity over one temporal area or with a more generalized distribution. The interictal EEG is positive in up to 90 percent of the patients, provided activation techniques such as sleep deprivation are used and recording is done with nasopharyngeal or sphenoidal electrodes. Spike or sharp waves are seen over the anterior and mesial temporal areas, but may be recorded from lateral, midtemporal, or orbito-frontal areas in some patients (Fig. 7-3). Bilateral independent or synchronous discharges are frequent, but in most cases the focus in one temporal lobe is dominant.

Diagnosis

Seizure History and Neurological Examination

A detailed description of the first attack as well as typical subsequent attacks and any variations should be obtained. Data must be solicited from anyone who has observed the spells. Particular attention should be paid to precipitating factors (e.g., flashing lights, alcohol, emotional upset, and sleep deprivation), the presence of an aura, the patient's responsiveness during an attack, motor phenomena, automatisms, tongue biting, urinary incontinence, and behavior during the postictal period. The temporal profile of the attacks and any relationship to the time of day, meals, or menstrual periods should be

Table 7-5. Complex Partial versus Absence Seizures

Characteristics	Complex partial	Absence
Age incidence	Children or adult	Usually 5–20 yr
Onset	May have aura or simple partial onset	Abrupt
Duration	Minutes	5–30 sec
Automatisms	Frequent and often complex, often involve lower extremities or trunk	Frequent when seizure lasts more than 7 sec, rarely involve lower extremities or trunk
Postictal	Gradually subsiding confusion	None
Ictal EEG	Variable temporal generalized fast, slow or sharp waves	Generalized 2–4 Hz spike waves
Interictal EEG	Temporal spike or sharp waves	Generalized spike wave elicited by hyperventilation
CT scan	May show temporal lobe lesion or atrophy	Normal

Fig. 7-3. *EEG showing right and left independently occurring mesial temporal lobe interictal spikes (dots) in a 50-year-old man with complex partial seizures. Note that spikes are well recorded by nasopharyngeal electrodes* (PG1 *and* PG2), *but not over the surface of the scalp.*

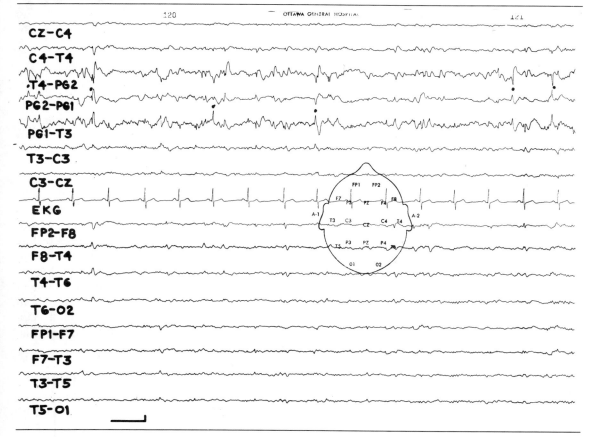

recorded. Specific questions should be asked about any tendency to daydream excessively or miss parts of conversations, olfactory hallucinations, and déjà vu or jamais vu phenomena. The birth and gestational history, a history of head trauma, reactions to immunizations, past meningitis or encephalitis, febrile convulsions in childhood, drug, alcohol, or volatile substance abuse, and a family history of epilepsy may suggest an etiology for the seizures. The recreational use of various drugs, including amphetamines, phencyclidine, and especially cocaine, has been associated with GTC seizures. Intravenous drug use and homosexual contacts raise the possibility of AIDS and its various cerebral complications as an explanation for the seizures. In one study of 100 patients with AIDS and seizures, 18 percent had a seizure or seizures as the first sign of CNS involvement by the HIV virus or various infectious or neoplastic processes. A full neurological functional inquiry and examination should be performed. During examination it is important to listen for intracranial bruits, inspect the skin for the areas of ashleaf depigmentation and adenoma sebaceum (Fig. 7-4) found in tuberous sclerosis as well as café-au-lait spots and cutaneous angiomata, and compare the two sides of the body (e.g., thumbnail size) for developmental asymmetries that might suggest a congenital brain lesion. If the patient reports that a particular maneuver such as hyperventilation can precipitate the attacks, this should be performed, preferably during EEG recording.

Electroencephalography

The EEG frequently furnishes strong evidence for the diagnosis of epilepsy by showing specific epileptiform patterns. Recording should always include the use of special activation procedures (e.g., sleep deprivation) and methods (e.g., nasopharyngeal electrodes) if the tracing is normal under standard conditions. Specific interictal patterns have already been discussed. Occasionally a seizure will be recorded by chance during EEG recording (Fig. 7-5). However, epilepsy represents a clinical diagnosis that can be rendered despite a negative EEG if there is a reliable description of the patient's spells. Furthermore, a patient can show a clearly epi-

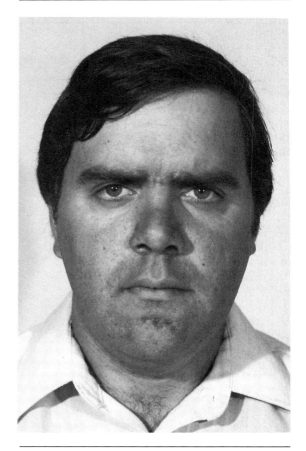

Fig. 7-4. *The only clinical clue to the cause of epilepsy in this 30-year-old university student was a small patch of adenoma sebaceum over the skin. The diagnosis in this patient was tuberous sclerosis.*

leptiform EEG but have no history of spells, and this finding, by itself, does not justify a diagnosis of epilepsy. The more EEGs obtained, the greater the likelihood of recording an intermittent interictal abnormality. Intensive EEG and video monitoring over prolonged periods is done in special centers to document the patient's spells when there is doubt about the diagnosis of epilepsy, the spells are intractable, or surgical therapy is being considered (Fig. 7-6).

Computed Tomography and Magnetic Resonance Imaging

Computed tomographic (CT) scans have shown unexpected abnormalities such as low-grade tu-

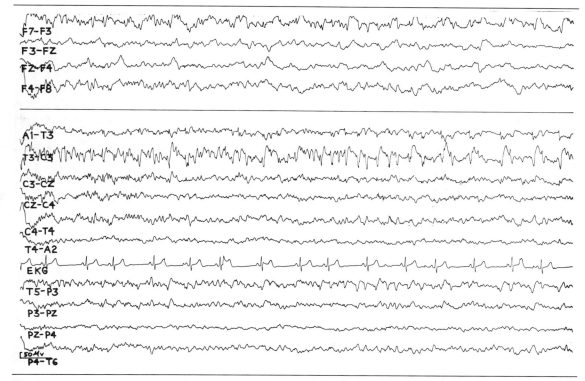

Fig. 7-5. *EEG showing the termination of an electrical seizure in the left temporal area (T3–C3) in a 30-year-old woman with a left temporal cavernous hemangioma.*

mors, cysts, arteriovenous malformations, infarcts, calcifications, and generalized or focal atrophy in 25 percent of epileptic patients who have no history of brain damage or neurological findings (Figs. 7-7 to 7-10). A CT scan should be obtained in all cases of epilepsy with an uncertain etiology, except in those patients with absence attacks who show 3-Hz spike waves on the EEG. Special planes of section have been used to better visualize mesial temporal structures.

Magnetic resonance imaging (MRI) is even more sensitive than CT for detecting small brain lesions responsible for epilepsy. Cortical dysplasias, cryptogenic vascular malformations, and small tumors in the temporal areas are much better visualized by MRI because the bones of the middle fossa are eliminated and various planes of section can be used. MRI reveals a significant lesion in approximately 20 percent of patients with complex partial seizures and a normal CT scan.

Other Studies

Single-photon emission computed tomographic scans are often a sensitive way of detecting epileptic foci, which show altered regional metabolism and blood flow. A 2-hour postprandial glucose and serum calcium determination is indicated in most cases. Antinuclear antibody levels should be measured in cases without an obvious cause, as seizures may be the initial manifestation in cerebral lupus. In children, certain studies for detecting metabolic disorders such as the aminoacidurias and lipidoses are frequently obtained. In cases of childhood epilepsy with myoclonus, skin and liver biopsy is done to facilitate the diagnosis of Lafora's body disease and other identifiable, usually hereditary, metabolic disorders.

Differential Diagnosis

Conditions that can cause or mimic transient recurrent impaired consciousness with or with-

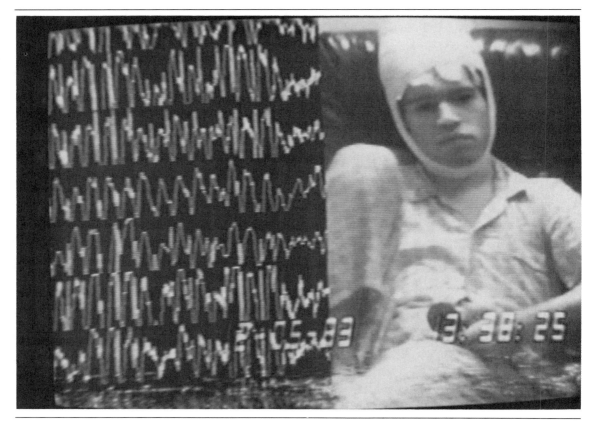

Fig. 7-6. *EEG telemetry combined with video intensive monitoring in an epileptic patient. Eight channels of the EEG are shown on one half of the screen and the video recording of the patient on the other half. Eight or more hours of recording are saved on videocassettes. This technique allows precise correlations to be made between the EEG and behavioral events.*

out abnormal motor and behavioral components include epilepsy, syncope, narcolepsy, transient ischemic attacks, hysterical pseudoseizures, dissociation-anxiety attacks, basilar migraines, and hypoglycemic attacks (Table 7-6). Differentiating true epilepsy from psychogenic pseudoseizures (Table 7-7) is particularly difficult, especially since both may occur in the same patient. Up to 15 percent of patients with intractable "epilepsy" are found to have psychogenic pseudoseizures. Actual observation or videotaping of the attack with simultaneous EEG recording can establish the diagnosis. This can best be accomplished in an EEG/video intensive monitoring laboratory. In many cases, pseudoseizures can be precipitated for recording purposes by placing a vibrating tuning fork on the patient's forehead and suggesting to the patient that this will provoke a spell.

A syncopal attack can be followed by an anoxic epileptic seizure, and such an event can be confused with epilepsy. However, the seizure is rarely of the full-blown tonic-clonic variety, is preceded by presyncopal sensations of lightheadedness and pallor, and usually has a short postictal phase (Table 7-8).

Management

Role of the Specialist
The initial evaluation of all cases and followup of complicated or uncontrolled cases should be undertaken by a neurologist, preferably one specializing in epilepsy.

Diagnosis and Classification

The diagnosis of epilepsy should be established and, if possible, the patient's seizures and epileptic syndrome classified. The cause of the epilepsy should also be sought.

Treatment Objectives and Patient Compliance

It must be borne in mind, and explained to the patient, that the ultimate goal of treatment is to eliminate seizures with minimal side effects. Uncontrolled seizures can cause brain damage, further lower seizure threshold, often be detrimental in social and vocational terms, and may expose the patient to injury or even death. Compliance with treatment must be frequently stressed to the patient.

Precipitating Factors

Any specific precipitating factors, such as sleep deprivation, alcohol, or excessive stress, should be identified and eliminated.

Initial Drug Selection: Monotherapy

Therapy is initiated using the least toxic drug effective for the specific seizure type (Table 7-9) and in the lowest possible doses. This therapeutic dose is attained gradually when carbamazepine, primidone, valproic acid, or clonazepam is used. Adequate time must elapse so that the drug's efficacy in reducing seizures can be assessed. Monotherapy is better for this purpose than the use of several anticonvulsants because additive toxicity, drug interactions, and undue cost are avoided and compliance and quality of life are maximized. Complete seizure control is achieved in up to 50 percent of patients on a single drug and about 70 to 80 percent of patients can be satisfactorily controlled.

Individualization of Therapy

Therapy must be individualized. For example, the greater expense of drugs like carbamazepine and valproic acid and the cognitive impairment or sedation caused by some can be

Fig. 7-7. *(A) Enhanced CT scan showing a right frontal arteriovenous malformation (arrow). The patient was a 42-year-old woman with a 25-year history of simple partial seizures involving left facial twitching.*

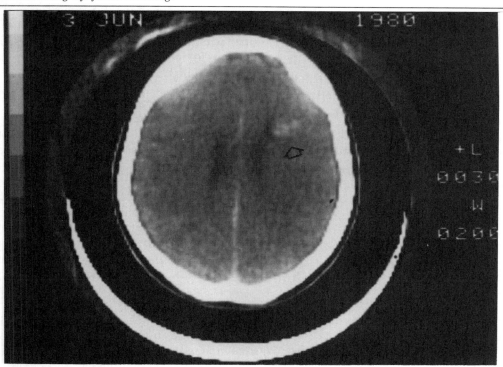

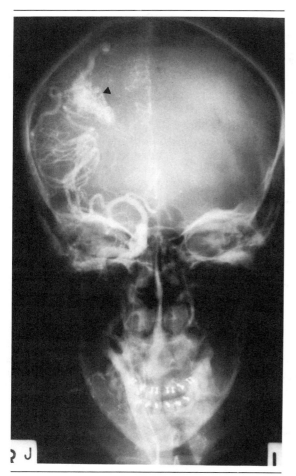

Fig. 7-7 *(Continued). (B) Cerebral angiogram from the same patient, showing the arteriovenous malformation* (arrowhead).

deciding factors in the detection of drugs. The acne, gum hyperplasia, and hirsutism sometimes produced by phenytoin make it an unwise first choice in adolescent girls. When long-term use over many years is anticipated in patients who are mentally active, carbamazepine or valproic acid may be preferable to phenytoin because their subtle effects on cognitive function appear to be less.

Additional Drugs

A second drug is substituted when an initial drug proves ineffective. However, polytherapy provides additional seizure control in only 10 to 20 percent of patients who do not respond to a single agent.

Use of Serum Levels

Only after appropriate serum levels are achieved and compliance confirmed should a drug be deemed ineffective in patients whose seizures remain uncontrolled. The therapeutic range is only a rough guide to dosage; seizures in many patients are controlled with subtherapeutic serum levels and others require and tolerate levels above the therapeutic range. When a patient's drug levels are subtherapeutic, a further dosage increase is likely to yield additional therapeutic benefit without undue toxicity. When the levels are at or above the upper limit of the therapeutic range, the opposite is concluded. It must be remembered that serum levels represent the total drug concentration, bound and free. Under certain circumstances, such as hypoalbuminemia, uremia, and drug interactions, the free drug level may be increased, leading to toxicity, despite overall levels that are regarded as therapeutic. In these circumstances, it may be useful to measure the free levels of those drugs possessing a relatively high protein-binding capacity. In addition, the metabolite levels of the parent drug, such as the 10,11-epoxide of carbamazepine or the phenylethylmalonamide metabolite of primidone, may correlate better with toxic or even therapeutic effects than the parent drug levels. Indications for measuring antiepileptic serum levels are listed in Table 7-10.

Drug Pharmacology and Pharmacokinetics

The practitioner must be familiar with the pharmacological and pharmacokinetic properties of the anticonvulsants prescribed (Table 7-11). Most of the drugs are rapidly and well absorbed. Antacids or nasogastric tube feedings may interfere with phenytoin absorption and gastrointestinal diseases may also affect absorption. Generally, the interval of drug administration is half the half-life, but doses may be given more frequently to prevent fluctuations in plasma levels, as the half-life of the drug in a given patient is usually known only within a broad range. A steady-state is reached within five half-lives following the initiation of a drug at its daily maintenance dose. At this point, the amount of drug eliminated during each dosing interval

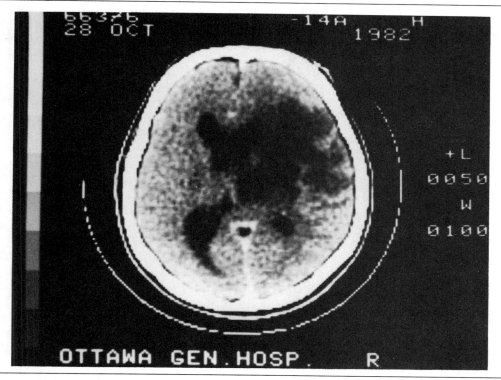

Fig. 7-8. *Enhanced CT scan showing a right frontal grade III astrocytoma with marked edema and shift of the ventricles to the left. The patient was a 29-year-old man with a 12-year history of seizures consisting of a focal twitching of the left side of the body and preceded by a hissing sound in the right ear. Neurological examination revealed no papilledema; the patient was fully alert. There was mild left lower facial weakness, a left upper extremity drift, and mild left-sided spasticity.*

is replaced by the next dose. Similarly, it takes approximately five half-lives for a drug to be completely eliminated from the body when it is discontinued or for a new steady-state to be reached with a change of dosage. A controlled-release form of carbamazepine (Tegretol-CR) is now available that produces less fluctuation in the serum levels during a 24-hour period and may reduce the intensity of transient toxic side effects.

Almost all of the antiepileptic drugs are metabolized by the hepatic microsomal mixed-oxidase enzyme system. A significant proportion of phenobarbital is excreted unchanged by the kidneys. Phenytoin has the peculiarity of shifting its pharmacokinetics from first-order (a linear dose–plasma level relationship) to zero-order kinetics at higher dose levels as hepatic enzyme systems become saturated. When zero-order kinetics are in force, very small increments in dose result in relatively large changes in the plasma level. As a result, when a patient is receiving, for example, 350 to 450 mg of phenytoin per day, an additional 25 mg per day may precipitate toxic blood levels. Carbamazepine tends to induce its own metabolism, such that the blood level usually declines after 2 to 5 weeks of therapy. Clonazepam and other benzodiazepines tend to lose their efficacy after a while in approximately one third of the patients because tolerance develops.

Stopping Drugs

When discontinuing a drug which a patient has been taking for a long time, it should be tapered over several months because otherwise seizures may rebound. This is particularly true for the barbiturates and benzodiazepines.

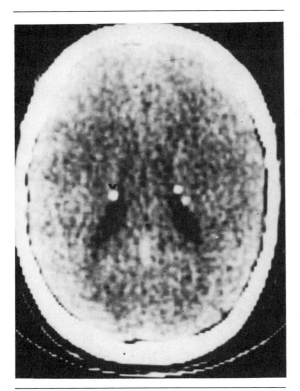

Fig. 7-9. *Unenhanced CT scan showing typical subependymal calcified glial nodules* (v) *in a patient with tuberous sclerosis and epilepsy.*

Drug Interactions

When two or more antiepileptic drugs are necessary, the drug interactions of the agents should be considered. Clinically important interactions include the inhibition of barbiturate metabolism by valproate or carbamazepine and the displacement of protein-bound phenytoin by valproate, thereby increasing the amount of free phenytoin. This may lead to transient phenytoin toxicity, but, because the rate of phenytoin metabolism is increased, the total phenytoin levels become reduced and the free phenytoin levels may not differ from the original levels. Carbamazepine is a potent inducer of the hepatic microsomal enzyme system, and for this reason, when combined with valproic acid, it may be difficult to achieve adequate serum levels of the latter. Combined valproic acid and carbamazepine treatment tends to lead to higher levels of 10,11-expoxide, the carbamazepine metabolite, and this constitutes a po-

tentially beneficial therapeutic effect. Other drugs, such as dicumarol, isoniazid, chloramphenicol, disulfiram, and aspirin, may cause an increase in the serum free or total phenytoin levels through displacement from protein binding or inhibition of metabolism. Cimetidine can inhibit the metabolism of phenytoin. Both erythromycin and verapamil can cause carbamazepine toxicity.

New or Soon-to-Be-Released Drugs

Clobazam, a 1,5-benzodiazepine with less sedating and stronger antiepileptic properties than conventional benzodiazepines, has been released for clinical use in Canada and Europe. It is well tolerated, free of serious side effects, and has a broad spectrum of action (especially in partial seizures with secondary generalization). Tolerance develops in about 10 to 20 percent of the patients and its efficacy has been unproved in monotherapy. Vigabatrin is a "suicidal" GABA-transaminase inhibitor that is available in Europe and reduces partial and secondary generalized seizures by 50 percent in approximately 50 percent of patients when used as an add-on agent. Lamotrigine is also available in Europe and is useful as an add-on agent for a variety of seizure types. Other drugs currently being developed for clinical use include gabapentin, stiripentol, felbamate, topiramate, and zonisamide.

Monitoring for Drug Toxicity

Periodic blood and liver function tests should be carried out to monitor the effects of most of the anticonvulsants on these systems. Hepatic and pancreatic function should be carefully watched during valproate therapy because cases of fatal liver toxicity or pancreatitis have arisen. However, liver abnormalities are not usually apparent prior to the sudden onset of massive liver damage and minor liver enzyme elevations of no clinical consequence are not infrequent. Recent findings indicate that severe hepatotoxicity does not occur in patients over 10 years old taking only valproic acid. Children under 2 years old on polytherapy are at greatest risk (approximately 1 per 1,000). Serum calcium and folate levels should be measured periodically in patients on phenytoin because osteoma-

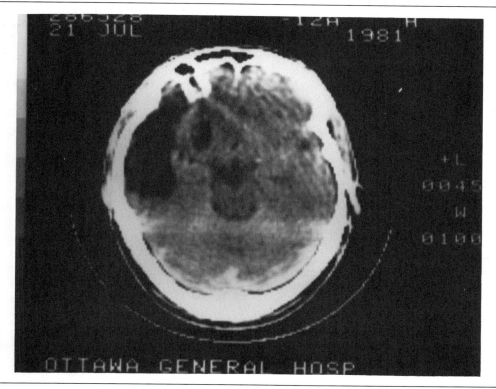

Fig. 7-10. *Enhanced CT scan in a 39-year-old, right-handed man who had had seizures since early childhood. The seizures are simple partial, occur once a month, and consist of a cold, shivering sensation that moves through his body, followed by brief generalized trembling without loss of consciousness. A left temporal arachnoid cyst is seen. Neurological findings and language function were normal.*

Table 7-6. Differential Diagnosis of Epilepsy

1. Syncope
2. Hysterical pseudoseizures
3. Anxiety–hyperventilation/panic attacks
4. Transient ischemic attacks
5. Migraine (especially vertebrobasilar or occipital)
6. Pheochromocytoma
7. Narcolepsy, sleep paralysis
8. Hypoglycemia
9. Paroxysmal dystonic or choreoathetotic disorders
10. Painful tonic spasms of multiple sclerosis

lacia and impaired folic acid absorption may occur. Carbamazepine may occasionally produce inappropriate antidiuretic hormone secretion with hyponatremia, but this is rarely clinically significant. At the initiation of therapy, idiosyncratic reactions may appear, such as skin rash (in 5 to 10 percent of patients). Some patients on long-term valproic acid therapy notice postural tremor of the hands and experience a substantial weight gain because it stimulates the appetite.

Difficult-to-Treat Seizures
Good seizure control is often difficult to achieve in patients with complex partial seizures and mixed myoclonic and atonic seizures of childhood (Lennox-Gastaut syndrome).

Use of Electroencephalography
The EEG should generally not be used to monitor the effectiveness of therapy, except in patients with absence seizures whose spike-wave

Table 7-7. Features Distinguishing Pseudoseizures from Generalized Convulsive Seizures

Features	Pseudoseizures	Epilepsy
PATIENT PROFILE		
Usual age of onset	Teens, young adult	Childhood, teens, young adult
Sex	F >> M	F = M
Intelligence	Often low	Variable
Psychiatric illness	Commonly extensive with history of personality disorder, suicide attempts	Common, especially with complex partial seizures
Emotionally traumatic event preceding onset of seizure disorder	Common	Uncommon
Past conversion reactions	Common	Uncommon
Family history of epilepsy	Uncommon	Relatively common
Antecedent etiological factor (e.g., birth trauma, head injury, febrile convulsions)	Uncommon	Relatively common
Response to anticonvulsants	None or worsening	Usually good
FEATURES OF ATTACK		
Precipitating factor	Emotional upset	Nonspecific (e.g., fatigue, alcohol)
Presence of others	Almost always	Alone at times
Suggestibility	Common	Absent

Table 7-8. Seizure versus Syncope

Features	Generalized tonic-clonic seizure	Syncope
Onset	Abrupt or a few seconds of aura, movements begin with loss of consciousness	Aura of pallor, nausea, sweating, lightheadedness, blurred vision, movements may occur 15–20 sec following loss of consciousness
Position	Any	Usually upright
Precipitating factors	Usually nonspecific	Emotional upset, pain, conditions provoking vasodilation
Motor phenomena	Tonic-clonic, intense	Tonic or myoclonic, brief
Duration	2–3 min	Less
Incontinence and tongue-biting	Common	Uncommon
Injury	Common	Rare
Pulse	Tachycardia	Bradycardia or arrest
Blood pressure	Hypertension	Hypotension
History of cardiac disease	None	Common
Interictal EEG	Usually abnormal	Normal

Table 7-9. Drugs of Choice for the Control of Various Types of Seizures

Seizure type	Drug		
	Primary	Secondary	Tertiary
Generalized tonic-clonic	Phenytoin Carbamazepine Valproic acid	Clobazam[a] Phenobarbital Primidone Vigabatrin[a] Lamotrigine[a]	Mephenytoin
Simple or complex partial	Carbamazepine Phenytoin	Valproic acid Clobazam[a] Vigabatrin[a]	Phenobarbital Primidone
Absence	Ethosuximide Valproic acid	Phenobarbital Clobazam[a]	Clonazepam
Myoclonic, atonic	Valproic acid Phenytoin	Clobazam[a] Ethosuximide Vigabatrin[a] Lamotrigine[a]	Clonazepam Nitrazepam
Photosensitive	Valproic acid		

[a]Not available in the United States.

Table 7-10. Indications for Determining Antiepileptic Serum Levels

1. Uncontrolled seizures—to allow dosage adjustments
2. Well-controlled seizures—to determine baseline therapeutic levels for future reference
3. To determine compliance
4. To identify the antiepileptic drug responsible for dose-related toxicity in a patient on several drugs
5. To gauge drug interactions
6. To carry out pharmacokinetic studies in special situations such as fast metabolizers, uremia, or pregnancy
7. To determine toxicity in infants or severely retarded patients who may not show or report the usual toxic symptoms
5. Poor absorption or rapid metabolism
6. Pseudoseizures in addition to real seizures
7. Antiepileptic drug toxicity (especially phenytoin and carbamazepine) which may rarely increase seizure frequency
8. An underlying metabolic, neoplastic, or degenerative brain disease

activity correlates somewhat with the clinical response.

Uncontrolled Seizures

When seizures are uncontrolled, the following possibilities must be considered.

1. Underdosage
2. Noncompliance
3. Wrong drug choice
4. Wrong diagnosis

Other Therapies

Alternative drugs, such as methsuximide, nitrazepam, and mephenytoin, can be considered in difficult cases. When medical therapy fails due to resistant seizures or intolerable toxicity, neurosurgical therapy can be considered.

Surgical Therapy

When optimal anticonvulsant therapy fails to control seizures, which are socially disabling, surgical therapy should be considered. For patients to be eligible for surgical intervention, the epileptic disorder should have persisted for at least 2 years, they should be capable of cooperating for the extensive preoperative evaluation and the operation itself, and in general there should be evidence that the seizures are arising from a potentially resectable focus. Recently partial or total section of the corpus callosum has been found to benefit some patients with intractable generalized seizures.

Table 7-11. Pharmacological Data on Principal Antiepileptic Drugs

Drug	Average adult dose and schedule	Therapeutic serum levels in mcg/ml and (μmol/L)	Half-life (hr)	Protein binding (%)	Principal side effects
Phenytoin (Dilantin)	150 mg qam 200 mg qhs	10–20 (40–80)	24 ± 12	90	Ataxia, blurred vision, sedation, gingival hyperplasia, hirsutism, folate deficiency, osteomalacia, rash, cognitive impairment
Carbamazepine (Tegretol, Tegretol CR)	300 mg qam 300 mg qpm 400 mg qhs	4–12 (20–50)	12 ± 3	70	Ataxia, diplopia, "drugged" feeling, rash, hepatic toxicity, blood dyscrasia, gastrointestinal upset, hyponatremia, headache, tremor
Valproic acid (Depakene, Depakote, Epival)	500 mg b.i.d. 500 mg qhs	50–100 (350–700)	12 ± 6	90	Gastrointestinal upset, tremor, sedation, behavioral disturbances, thrombocytopenia, alopecia, weight gain, rarely severe hepatic toxicity
Phenobarbital	120 mg qhs	20–40 (80–200)	96 ± 12	40–50	Sedation, hyperactivity in children, cognitive impairment
Primidone (Mysoline)	250 mg b.i.d. 250 mg qhs	3–8 (15–40 and 20–40 as phenobarbital)	12 ± 6	0–50	Sedation, cognitive impairment
Ethosuximide (Zarontin)	500 mg qam 500 mg qhs	40–100 (300–800)	30 ± 6	0	Sedation, blood dyscrasia, gastrointestinal upset
Clonazepam (Klonopin, Rivotril)	2 mg b.i.d. 2 mg qhs	0.005–0.07	20 ± 40	47	Sedation, behavioral abnormalities
Clobazam (Frisium)[a]	10 mg qam 20 mg qhs	Not defined	18 (clobazam), 42 (N-desmethyl-clobazam)	85	Sedation, ataxia, behavioral abnormalities, increased seizures
Vigabatrin (Sabril)[a]	1.5 gm b.i.d.	Not defined	5–7	0	Sedation, appetite change, nausea, depression, psychosis

[a]Not available in the United States.
qam = every morning; qhs = every night; qpm = every afternoon; b.i.d. = twice daily.

Such surgery is done at specialized centers that are equipped to carry out the extensive preoperative and intraoperative testing necessary to help localize the epileptic focus. At times it is necessary to record several spontaneous seizures from subdural electrode arrays or depth electrodes that are implanted for a prolonged period of time in hippocampal, amygdaloid, and other areas so that the epileptic focus giving rise to seizures can be identified. Other evidence, such as handedness, lateralized abnormalities revealed by neuropsychological testing, and foci of brain damage shown by CT, MRI, or positron emission tomographic scanning can point to an epileptic focus.

Speech lateralization must be determined preoperatively, usually through use of intracarotid amobarbital or methohexital injection, before a temporal brain resection can be safely undertaken. Anterior temporal lobectomy is the most commonly employed procedure, but recently selective amygdalohippocampectomy has also been advocated. In expert hands, the morbidity from the procedure is extremely low, the side effects are insignificant, and an excellent outcome with complete or nearly complete elimination of seizures, often off medication, is obtained in two thirds of the cases. Corpus callosotomy is being done increasingly for the management of secondarily generalized seizures and is especially effective in reducing drop attacks. It is estimated that surgical therapy for the control of epilepsy is greatly underutilized, but neurologists are recommending it increasingly early in intractable cases, before the often irreversible devastating psychosocial consequences develop.

Psychosocial Management

The social and psychological aspects of patient management should not be neglected. Reduction of stress may contribute significantly to seizure control in certain patients. The epileptic patient frequently carries a significant psychosocial burden because of the social stigma associated with epilepsy; the inconvenience, expense, and side effects of long-term medication; the inability to drive a car if seizures are uncontrolled; and the direct and indirect adverse effects of the seizures themselves. Adolescents frequently find their epilepsy poses a significant barrier to the achievement of independence. Specific personality traits, such as aggressiveness, hyperreligiosity, depression, a sober, humorless affect, and rarely a schizophreniform psychotic disorder, have also been noted in epileptics, particularly those with complex partial seizures (Table 7-12). The prognosis for ultimately leading a relatively normal adult life and for future vocational success mainly depends on the adequacy of seizure control, and may be significantly influenced by careful attention to patient education and the management of psychosocial factors by a trained health-care team. Some practical advice for the epileptic patient is listed in Table 7-13.

Prognosis

When judging the prognosis of epilepsy, one can consider the likelihood of remission off medication, the probability of complete or nearly complete seizure control with drugs, and the ultimate psychosocial adjustment of the patient. Some epileptic syndromes, such as childhood absence attacks or rolandic seizures with centrotemporal spikes, have a high probability of spontaneously remitting by late adolescence. Spontaneous remission in other syndromes,

Table 7-12. Behavioral and Psychiatric Changes in Epilepsy

Ictal
    Experiential phenomena during temporal lobe seizures
    Complex partial seizures simulating acute psychosis
    Ictal rage and aggression (extremely rare)
    Nonconvulsive generalized status or complex partial status epilepticus mimicking psychiatric syndromes
Postictal delirium
Interictal
    Personality traits possibly correlated with epilepsy (e.g., hyposexuality, viscosity, hypergraphia, excessive philosophical concern)
    Depression (periictal as well)
    Schizophreniform psychosis
    Social effects
    Medication effects

Table 7-13. Practical Advice for the Epileptic Patient

1. Avoid sleep deprivation and excessive alcohol use.
2. Avoid jobs that entail working at heights or near heavy machinery, flames, burners, or molten material. Certain careers such as fire fighter, airline pilot, bus driver, and truck driver are not recommended.
3. Never swim alone. Take showers sitting on a low stool rather than baths. Microwave cooking is preferable.
4. Most sports are permitted but those in which a sudden loss of consciousness would be dangerous, such as sky-diving, hang-gliding, rapid downhill skiing, mountain climbing, and scuba diving, are best avoided.
5. When a dose of medication is missed, it should be added to the next dose.
6. With phenytoin treatment, meticulous dental and gum care, as recommended by a dental hygienist or dentist, is necessary to prevent excessive tooth decay and gum problems.
7. Laws concerning driving vary, but generally do not allow driving a motor vehicle for 1 to 2 years after the last seizure. There may be exceptions for seizures that are strictly nocturnal, strictly simple partial, or related to discontinuation of anticonvulsant medication on a physician's advice.
8. First aid for a seizure consists of:
   a. Protecting the patient's head and body from injury
   b. Removing dentures, excessive secretions, and other foreign material from the mouth after the tonic and clonic phases
   c. Turning the patient into the semiprone position in the postictal period to prevent aspiration and blockage of the nasopharynx.

It is unnecessary to take the patient to the hospital after one or two uncomplicated seizures. However, if three or more seizures occur in brief a time or the patient does not regain full consciousness within a few hours, then he or she should be seen by a physician.

---

such as temporolimbic epilepsy or juvenile myoclonic epilepsy, is much less likely and many patients will require life-long medications. A newly diagnosed adolescent or adult patient with epilepsy on monotherapy has about a 75 percent chance of a 2-year remission within 8 years of the start of treatment. About 50 percent of all patients can eventually go without medication with prolonged remission.

During the first decade following diagnosis, epileptic patients exhibit a twofold increased mortality rate compared to the population as a whole. Some of the factors responsible are sudden death during a seizure, drowning, and suicide.

The psychosocial prognosis depends on such factors as the seizure type and frequency and the existence of neurological and intellectual deficits other than epilepsy. Interictal psychopathological conditions, including depression, personality disturbances, and rarely a schizophreniform psychosis, may develop in patients with long-standing epilepsy, especially of the temporolimbic type (see Table 7-12). The causes of these psychiatric disorders are multifactorial and include disrupted limbic system functioning due to seizures and subclinical epi-

leptic discharges, disturbed interpersonal relationships, the effects of underlying disorders on limbic structures, and, in some patients, the effect of antiepileptic drugs. In one study of complex partial seizures beginning in childhood, 50 percent of the patients were found to have school difficulties and subsequently behavioral or employment problems when surveyed after 5 years. The unfavorable prognosis in childhood temporolimbic epilepsy has prompted attempts to control seizures through the institution of early aggressive medical therapy, with surgery considered an option at an early stage in drug-resistant patients.

Special Situations

Febrile Seizures

Seizures occurring in the context of a specific or nonspecific febrile illness in infants or young children without evidence of an acute CNS problem such as meningitis, encephalitis, severe dehydration, Reye's syndrome, or lead encephalopathy are termed *febrile seizures*. They occur in approximately 4 percent of all children, usually between the ages of 6 months and 5 years. A third of the patients have one or more recurrences, usually within a year of the initial attack.

In patients with so-called simple febrile seizures, the subsequent occurrence of epilepsy is slightly higher than that in the population without febrile seizures. However, the risk for developing epilepsy increases if one or more of the following factors exist: (1) preceding neurological abnormalities in the child; (2) prolonged seizures (exceeding 15 minutes); (3) focal aspects to the seizure or postictal Todd's paralysis; (4) recurrent seizures within the ensuing 24 hours; or (5) a family history of afebrile seizures.

Because there is some evidence that prolonged febrile seizures or febrile status epilepticus may lead to brain damage and the later development of epilepsy, some have recommended the institution of prophylactic anticonvulsant therapy following an initial febrile convulsion, especially when the child is less than a year old, since the risk of recurrence is highest in this group. Both phenobarbital and sodium valproate are effective for this purpose, provided therapeutic blood levels are maintained. However, the frequent behavioral disorders seen in patients taking phenobarbital and the possibility of severe liver toxicity with the use of sodium valproate, plus a lack of evidence confirming that this therapy reduces the long-term risk of developing epilepsy, have generated controversy concerning this treatment philosophy. In addition, significant cognitive impairment has recently been documented in children receiving phenobarbital therapy for the prophylaxis of febrile convulsions.

If antiepileptic therapy is deemed advisable, perhaps because of an initial complicated febrile convulsion at an early age, then only continuous therapy with serum level monitoring can protect against recurrences, but the drug of choice is still not established. Another approach has been the intermittent rectal administration of diazepam or lorazepam at the time fever is noticed. As part of the initial evaluation of a child with a febrile convulsion, the cause of the fever must be sought and any preexisting or acute intracranial or systemic abnormality ruled out. Cerebrospinal fluid (CSF) should be examined in any child under 2 years old or when there are signs of meningeal irritation; an EEG and a CT scan should be obtained if there is any suspicion of an intracranial abnormality.

Epilepsy and Pregnancy

Epileptic seizures appearing for the first time in pregnancy may be due to the onset of a true epileptic disorder, intracranial hemorrhage, a brain tumor or vascular malformation becoming symptomatic, cortical venous thrombosis, or hyponatremia secondary to oxytocin intoxication. True gestational epilepsy, in which seizures occur only during pregnancies, is rare.

When a woman with epilepsy becomes pregnant, several considerations come into play. In general, pregnancy does not adversely affect seizure control, but seizures may increase in a small proportion of patients. GTC seizures and, in particular, status epilepticus can precipitate miscarriages. In many cases, the seizure increase stems from a decrease in the antiepileptic drug levels, which is most marked toward the end of pregnancy. Accelerated metabolism, reduced compliance, and diminished absorption probably all contribute toward lowering serum drug levels. For this reason, serum levels should be monitored monthly in the later stages of pregnancy and doses increased to maintain therapeutic blood levels. Ideally, free drug levels should be followed.

The possible teratogenicity of anticonvulsant drugs has received a great deal of attention recently. It is likely that phenytoin or barbiturate use during the first trimester of pregnancy is associated with a 5 to 10 percent (two- to three-fold increase) risk of malformation in the fetus, including cardiac anomalies, cleft lip and palate, and digital dysplasia. Carbamazepine was considered a relatively safe anticonvulsant and was often substituted for phenytoin or barbiturates prior to conception or early in the first trimester. However, the findings from recent studies have suggested that carbamazepine may be associated with an increased incidence of craniofacial defects, fingernail hypoplasia, and developmental delay. Spina bifida has been reported in about 0.5 percent of exposed fetuses. Valproic acid is associated with a 1 to 2 percent risk of spinal fusion abnormalities in the fetus, which can be detected by ultrasound and serum

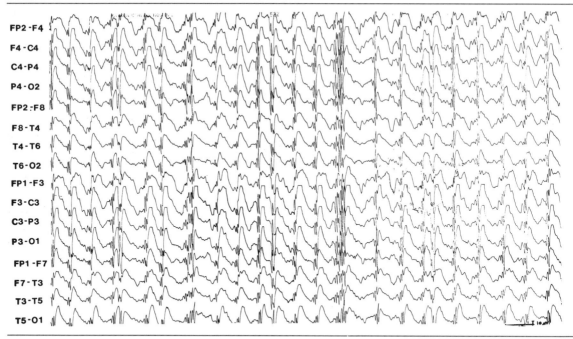

Fig. 7-11. *(A) EEG showing continuous generalized poly-spike-wave discharges during a prolonged bout (several hours) of nonconvulsive generalized status epilepticus. The patient was a 19-year-old man who had had several similar bouts of status epilepticus of unknown etiology over a 7-year period. During this episode, the patient appeared to be slowed down and mildly confused, but was able to walk around, answer questions, and carry out simple commands.*

alpha-fetoprotein measurements around 19 weeks of gestation. A relationship between antiepileptic teratogenicity and folate deficiency has been suggested.

Polytherapy, perhaps through the induction of specifically teratogenic metabolites, appears to be associated with a higher incidence of teratogenicity. Once the first trimester has elapsed, there is little rationale for changing drugs. Minimum effective doses of drugs should be used during pregnancy and unnecessary drugs eliminated. Phenytoin and phenobarbital produce a hemorrhagic tendency in the newborn, and therefore prophylactic vitamin K should be administered to babies born to mothers on these drugs and to mothers for 2 to 3 weeks preterm. Most of the anticonvulsants enter breast milk to a greater or lesser extent; however, the effects on the fetus are insignificant, aside from some sedation when barbiturates are involved.

Status Epilepticus

Status epilepticus is a prolonged epileptic state consisting of either a continuous seizure or series of seizures (without interictal recovery of consciousness) that lasts for more than 30 to 60 minutes. The minimum duration of continuous seizure activity qualifying as status epilepticus is somewhat arbitrary. Commonly, status epilepticus refers to a series of GTC seizures that can represent a life-threatening emergency. However, virtually any type of seizure may develop into status epilepticus. Simple partial motor seizures may occur for days or weeks in an uninterrupted fashion in an otherwise perfectly alert patient in the condition known as **epilepsy partialis continua. Complex partial status epilepticus** is extremely rare and may present as a series of complex partial seizures or as a fixed state of behavioral alteration resembling a confusional or psychotic state. An EEG showing a continu-

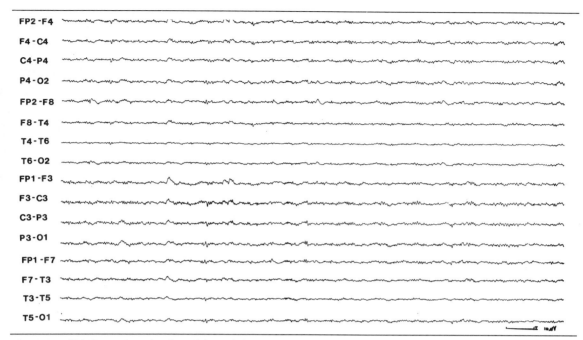

Fig. 7-11. *(B) Sixty seconds after 10 mg of diazepam was given intravenously. The status attack has been terminated, the patient is fully alert, and no further epileptic activity appears in the EEG.*

ous lateralized frontal or temporal epileptiform or slow pattern (which may not be seen with surface electrodes) confirms the diagnosis.

Nonconvulsive generalized status epilepticus and its subvariant **absence status epilepticus** present as a prolonged confusional state with slowness of responses lasting hours to days and a continuous generalized 2- to 4-Hz generalized spike-wave or poly-spike-wave pattern in the EEG recording (Fig. 7-11). Because this condition may appear de novo in nonepileptic elderly patients, it is frequently mistaken for a psychiatric disorder. It responds rapidly to intravenously administered diazepam.

Status epilepticus usually appears in the context of a previously known epileptic disorder, but may also be the first manifestation of epilepsy, particularly when an underlying structural brain lesion is responsible. GTC status epilepticus is more commonly seen in patients with brain tumors, CNS infections, metabolic abnormalities, and other identifiable causes for

their seizures than in patients with idiopathic epilepsy. In a known epileptic, the sudden withdrawal of antiepileptic medication, alcohol consumption or withdrawal, head injury, and neurosurgical procedures are some of the possible precipitating causes.

Alcohol withdrawal rarely produces status epilepticus unless there is a concurrent complicating factor such as head injury, hypoglycemia, electrolyte imbalance, or meningitis. Withdrawal seizures usually present as two or three GTC seizures taking place within a brief time, with onset about 18 to 24 hours after drinking is stopped. If status develops, it should be treated as outlined in Table 7-14.

GTC status is a medical emergency that requires intensive treatment and termination within 1 to 2 hours of onset to prevent cerebral damage and possible death consequent to the severe cerebral and systemic metabolic effects involved. Table 7-14 contains a suggested protocol for the management of GTC status.

Table 7-14. Protocol for Management of Generalized Tonic-Clonic Status Epilepticus

1. Secure an airway, remove dentures, and support respiration if necessary.
2. Treat hypotension and cardiac arrhythmias if present.
3. Start an intravenous (IV) with normal saline, obtain blood for the determination of electrolyte, glucose, BUN, calcium, and anticonvulsant levels, and inject 50 ml of 50% glucose. Draw arterial blood gases and start oxygen.
4. Monitor the electrocardiogram and vital signs frequently.
5. Intubate early rather than late to gain control of the airway (e.g., suctioning), prevent aspiration, and prepare for ventilatory support in the event of respiratory depression.
6. Rapidly obtain the patient's history and perform a physical examination, looking for:
   Signs of head injury
   Signs of raised intracranial pressure (papilledema)
   Signs of CNS infection (nuchal rigidity, fever)
   Lateralizing or focal neurological signs
   Signs of uremia, hepatic failure, alcoholism, drug abuse
7. Observe the features of seizures and conditions resembling status epilepticus:
   Decerebrate spasms
   Tetanic spasms (tetanus, strychnine)
   Hysterical pseudoseizures
   Choreoathetosis and dystonic reactions to drugs
8. Drug treatment. All drugs should be given intravenously, except valproate which may be given rectally. Paraldehyde may also be administered rectally, although the IV route is preferred. Drugs must be given in adequate recommended doses even if the patient is on antiepileptic medication.
   a. Initially **diazepam,** 2–5 mg/min IV to a total of 20 mg or until seizures stop. Monitor respirations and blood pressure. May repeat × 1 in 20 minutes PRN. **Lorazepam** (0.05 mg/kg) may be substituted and has a longer duration of action.
   b. Also initially (in the opposite arm) **phenytoin,** 20 mg/kg IV but not faster than 50 mg/min. This may be placed in Soluset with 100 ml N saline or administered with an infusion pump. Monitor blood pressure and electrocardiogram.
   c. If seizures persist, administer **phenobarbital** (5 mg/kg at 100 mg/min). Repeat × 2 PRN 20 minutes apart. The patient should be intubated by this time and may require ventilatory support.
   d. If seizures persist, start a **diazepam** drip (100 mg in 500 ml of 5% dextrose in water at 40 ml/hr) administered in a glass bottle or in a regular infusion set changed every 2 hours.
   e. If seizures persist for more than 60 to 90 minutes, initiate general anesthesia with **thiopental,** consisting of an initial bolus of 1.5 to 3 mg/kg followed by continuous infusion at 50 to 150 mg/hr. A second bolus may be necessary in the initial phases. EEG should be monitored frequently. Infusion may be stopped a few hours after seizures are controlled.
9. Treat hyperthermia with alcohol sponges and cooling blanket.
10. Obtain frequent blood gas measurements in prolonged status and treat acidosis with bicarbonate.
11. A search for the underlying causes of the status episode should be made as early as feasible, utilizing appropriate tests such as CT, MRI, lumbar puncture, and angiography.
12. In a prolonged intractable case, mannitol (20% solution IV, 250 ml initially) can be tried as well as dexamethasone (10 mg IV initially, followed by 4 mg q6h) to control possible raised intracranial pressure due to anoxia, increased cerebral blood flow, or underlying pathological processes.
13. Try not to overstimulate the patient with suctioning, injections, examination, and so on (except for what is essential) as this may trigger seizures.
14. Do not overtreat partial motor status epilepticus (epilepsy partialis continua) because it usually does not compromise vital functions, is rarely life threatening, and will usually resolve within several days. It is advisable to avoid the complications of drug-induced coma and respiratory depression in these cases unless vital functions are being compromised.

SPECIAL SITUATIONS
1. In the patient undergoing **alcohol withdrawal,** thiamine (50 mg IM and 50 mg IV) should be given.
2. In the **pediatric patient,** the doses are adjusted, as follows: phenytoin (20 mg/kg IV); phenobarbital (10 mg/kg IV, repeat in 10 minutes PRN); diazepam (0.3 mg/kg IV, repeat in 15 minutes PRN).

Table 7-14. (Continued)

3. In the event of **isoniazid intoxication,** the regimen should include large doses of pyridoxine IV.
4. In **porphyria,** along with the general treatment of high carbohydrate intake and hematin infusion, status epilepticus can be relatively safely managed with diazepam, paraldehyde, or bromides.
5. In patients also suffering from **eclampsia,** the regimen should include magnesium sulfate but drugs that would depress fetal functioning should be avoided.

SYNCOPE

Syncope, or fainting, is the sudden transient loss of consciousness with inability to maintain postural tone due to a reduction in cerebral perfusion or the oxygen supply. The common form of syncope, the vasodepressor or vasovagal attack, stems from a reflex bradycardia and loss of vascular tone producing a sudden drop in blood pressure. It usually occurs following a noxious stimulus such as venipuncture. With careful evaluation, including history and physical examination; measurement of blood pressure supine and erect; electrocardiography; 24-hour cardiac monitoring; special electrophysiological cardiac testing and cardiac catheterization when indicated; and EEG, CT, and cerebral angiography when indicated, a specific diagnosis can be reached in about half of such patients. When obtaining the history, attention should be focused on whether the episodes occur in the recumbent or upright position, or both, and any relationship to exercise, eating, coughing, micturition, emotional upset, and preceding palpitations. In about half of the patients who receive a specific diagnosis, a cardiac cause is implicated, including various arrhythmias, aortic stenosis, or pulmonary hypertension. According to one study, about 14 percent of all patients with syncope die within 12 months of presentation and the mortality is double that in those with an identifiable cardiac cause.

The various causes of syncope are listed in Table 7-15. Only a very small number of patients have a primary neurological or cerebrovascular cause for their syncope, such as vertebrobasilar ischemia, subclavian steal, intermittent obstructive hydrocephalus, and, very

Table 7-15. Etiology of Syncope

Vasodepressor syncope (common faint)
Cardiogenic
  Arrhythmias (various)
  Obstructive
    Aortic stenosis
    Dissecting aortic aneurysm
  Pulmonary hypertension and pulmonary embolus
Situational
  Cough syncope
  Micturition syncope
  Defecation syncope
  Swallow syncope
Carotid sinus hypersensitivity
Orthostatic hypotension
  Hypovolemia
  Drug-induced
  Idiopathic in adolescents (often athletic males)
  Autonomic neuropathies (e.g., diabetes)
  Other (e.g., Shy-Drager syndrome)
Sudden hypoxia due to various causes
Transient brainstem ischemia
  Vertebrobasilar migraine
  Subclavian steal
  Takayasu's (pulseless) disease
  Vertebrobasilar ischemia due to other mechanisms
Reflex with glossopharyngeal or trigeminal neuralgia
Obstructive hydrocephalus

rarely, a hypothalamic tumor. Cough syncope in some patients is due to a partial herniation of the cerebellar tonsils through the foramen magnum, as occurs with an Arnold-Chiari malformation, which causes compression of the lower brainstem and then fainting when intrathoracic and intracranial pressure is increased by coughing.

Patients with vertebrobasilar migraine may be subject to syncopal attacks at the time of their headaches or independently. An epileptic seizure may rarely mimic a syncopal attack (e.g., atonic or certain complex partial seizures), but a brief anoxic seizure that occurs secondary to a syncopal attack is more commonly misdiagnosed as epilepsy. The differential diagnosis has been dealt with earlier in this chapter (see Table 7-8).

Both trigeminal and glossopharyngeal neuralgia can give rise to sudden fainting spells. Although a patient with syncope is often referred to a neurologist for evaluation, in most cases the neurologist's role is confined to taking an adequate history, performing a neurological examination, ordering an EEG if there is any question of a seizure, and then referring the patient for cardiology assessment. Sometimes having a family member observe the patient for pallor, hyperventilation, or clonic movements and monitor the pulse for any irregularities of rate or rhythm will yield information that clarifies the nature and cause of obscure attacks of transient loss of consciousness.

The *breathholding spells* seen in infants and young children are nonepileptic syncopal phenomena. Such children begin with crying, usually after a spanking or fall, and the spells are accompanied by apnea, cyanosis or pallor, bradycardia or asystole, and at times opisthotonos and a few clonic movements. The spells first start to occur around 1 year of age and cease before age 6. They probably stem from familial hyperactive vagal reflexes and may also accompany migraine attacks in childhood.

BIBLIOGRAPHY

Epilepsy

Aicardi, J. The problem of the Lennox syndrome. *Dev. Med. Child. Neurol.* 15:77–81, 1973.

Ajmone-Marsan, C. Clinical Electrographic Correlations of Partial Seizures. In J. Wada (editor). *Modern Perspectives in Epilepsy,* Montreal: Eden Press, 1978, Pp. 76–98.

Alldredge, B. K., Lowenstein, D. H., and Simon, R. P. Seizures associated with recreational drug abuse. *Neurology* 39:1037–1039, 1989.

Aminoff, M. J., and Simon, R. P. Status epilepticus. Causes, clinical features and consequences in 98 patients. *Am. J. Med.* 69:657–666, 980.

Anderson, V. E., et al. (editors). *Genetic Basis of the Epilepsies.* New York: Raven, 1982.

Annegers, J. F., et al. Factors prognostic of unprovoked seizures after febrile convulsions. *N. Engl. J. Med.* 316:493–498, 1987.

Berkovic, S. F., et al. Progressive myoclonus epilepsies: specific causes and diagnosis. *N. Engl. J. Med.* 315:296–305, 1986.

Berkovic, S. F., et al. Concepts of absence epilepsies: discrete syndromes or biological continuum? *Neurology* 37:993–1000, 1987.

Browne, T. R., and Feldman, R. G. *Epilepsy. Diagnosis and Management,* Boston: Little, Brown, 1983.

Caveness, W. F., et al. The nature of posttraumatic epilepsy. *J. Neurosurg.* 50:545–553, 1979.

Currie, S., et al. Clinical course and prognosis of temporal lobe epilepsy. A survey of 666 patients. *Brain* 94:173–190, 1971.

Dam, M., and Gram, L. (editors). *Comprehensive Epileptology,* New York: Raven, 1991.

Delgado-Escueta, A. V., et al. Management of status epilepticus. *N. Engl. J. Med.* 306: 1337–1340, 1982.

Delgado-Escueta, A. V., et al. (editors). Status Epilepticus. Mechanisms of Brain Damage and Treatment. *Adv. Neurol.* Vol. 34, 1983.

Delgado-Escueta, A. V., Janz, D., and Beck-Mannagetta, G. (editors). Pregnancy and teratogenesis in epilepsy. *Neurology* 42(suppl. 5), 1992.

Delorenzo, R. J., and Towne, A. R. Epilepsy. *Curr. Neurol.* 9:27–76, 1989.

Dodrill, C. B., et al. Psychosocial problems among adults with epilepsy. *Epilepsia* 25:168–175, 1984.

Dreifuss, F. E. The differential diagnosis of

partial seizures with complex symptomatology. *Adv. Neurol.* 11:187–197, 1975.

Dreifuss, F. E., et al. Infantile spasms: comparative trial of nitrazepam and corticotrophin. *Arch. Neurol.* 43:1107–1110, 1986.

Engel, J. E., Jr. (editor). *Surgical Treatment of the Epilepsies.* New York: Raven, 1987.

Engel, J. E., Jr. *Seizures and Epilepsy.* Philadelphia: Davis, 1989.

Farwell, J. R., et al. Phenobarbital for febrile seizures. Effects on intelligence and on seizure recurrence. *N. Engl. J. Med.* 322:364–369, 1990.

Gastaut, H., et al. Childhood epileptic encephalopathy with diffuse slow spike-waves (otherwise known as "petit mal variant") or Lennox syndrome. *Epilepsia* 7:139–179, 1966.

Giordani, B., et al. Improvement in neuropsychological performance in patients with refractory seizures after intensive diagnostic and therapeutic intervention. *Neurology* 33:489–493, 1983.

Gloor, P. Generalized epilepsy with spike-and-wave discharge: a reinterpretation of its electrographic and clinical manifestations. *Epilepsia* 20:571–586, 1979.

Gomez, M. R., and Klass, D. W. Epilepsies of infancy and childhood. *Ann. Neurol.* 13:113–124, 1983.

Guberman, A. Psychogenic pseudoseizures in non-epileptic patients. *Can. J. Psychiatry* 27:401–404, 1982.

Guberman, A. The role of computed cranial tomography (CT) in epilepsy. *Can. J. Neurol. Sci.* 10:16–21, 1983.

Guberman, A., et al. Nonconvulsive generalized status epilepticus: clinical features, neuropsychological testing and long-term follow-up. *Neurology* 36:1284–1291, 1986.

Hauser, W. A., Ng, S. K. C., Brust, J. C. M. Alcohol, seizures and epilepsy. *Epilepsia* 29(suppl. 2): 566–578, 1988.

Hauser, W. A. (editor). *Current Trends in Epilepsy: A Self-Study Course for Physicians.* Bethesda: National Institutes of Health, 1988.

Holtzman, D. M., Kaku, D. A., and So, Y. T. New-onset seizures associated with human immunodeficiency virus infection: causation and clinical features in 100 cases. *Am. J. Med.* 87:173–177, 1989.

Janz, D., et al. (editors). *Epilepsy, Pregnancy, and the Child.* New York: Raven, 1982.

Jeavons, P. M., Bower, B. D., and Dimitrakoudi, M. Long-term prognosis of 150 cases of "West syndrome." *Epilepsia* 14:153–164, 1973.

Jennett, B. Post-traumatic epilepsy. *Adv. Neurol.* 22:137–147, 1979.

Jones, K. L., et al. Pattern of malformations in the children of women treated with carbamazepine during pregnancy. *N. Engl. J. Med.* 320:1661–1666, 1989.

Kotagal, P., et al. Complex partial seizures of childhood onset—a five-year follow-up study. *Arch. Neurol.* 44:1177–1180, 1987.

Kutt, H. Interactions between anticonvulsants and other commonly prescribed drugs. *Epilepsia* 25(suppl. 2):S118–S131, 1984.

Levy, R. H., et al. *Antiepileptic Drugs,* 3rd ed. New York: Raven, 1989.

Lombroso, C. T. Sylvian seizures and mid-temporal spike foci in children. *Arch. Neurol.* 17:52–59, 1967.

Lüders, H., and Lesser, R. P. (editors). *Epilepsy—Electroclinical Syndromes.* London: Springer-Verlag, 1987.

Mathieson, G. Pathologic aspects of epilepsy with special reference to the surgical pathology of focal cerebral seizures. *Adv. Neurol.* 8:107–138, 1975.

Mattson, R. H., et al. Comparison of carbamazepine, phenobarbital, phenytoin, and primidone in partial and secondarily generalized tonic-clonic seizures. *N. Engl. J. Med.* 313:145–151, 1985.

McIntyre, H. B. *The Primary Care of Seizure Disorders: A Practical Guide to the Evaluation and Comprehensive Management of Seizure Disorders*. Boston: Butterworths, 1982.

Nelson, K. B., and Ellenberg, J. H. Prognosis in children with febrile seizures. *Pediatrics* 61:720–727, 1978.

O'Donohoe, N. V. *Epilepsies of Childhood*. London: Butterworths, 1979.

Penry, J. K. (editor). Valproate monotherapy in the treatment of epilepsy. *Am. J. Med.* 84(suppl. IA):1–41, 1988.

Penry, J. K., and Newmark, M. E. The use of antiepileptic drugs. *Ann. Intern. Med.* 90:207–218, 1979.

Penry, J. K., Porter, R. J., and Dreifuss, F. E. Simultaneous recording of absence seizures with video tape and electroencephalography. A study of 374 seizures in 48 patients. *Brain* 98:427–440, 1975.

Porter, R. J., Penry, J. K., and Lacy, J. R. Diagnostic and therapeutic re-evaluation of patients with intractable epilepsy. *Neurology* 27:1006–1011, 1977.

Porter, R. J., and Theodore, W. H. (editors). Epilepsy. *Neurol. Clin.* 4:495–700, 1986.

Rasmussen, T. Surgical treatment of complex partial seizures: results, lessons, and problems. *Epilepsia* 24(suppl. 1):565–576, 1983.

Reynolds, E. H., and Trimble, M. R. *Epilepsy and Psychiatry*. Edinburgh: Churchill Livingstone, 1981.

So, E. L., and Penry, J. K. Epilepsy in adults. *Ann. Neurol.* 9:3–16, 1981.

Stevens, J. R. Psychiatric aspects of epilepsy. *J. Clin. Psychiatry* 49(suppl. 4):49–57, 1988.

Theodore, W. H., Porter, R. J., and Penry, J. K. Complex partial seizures: clinical characteristics and differential diagnosis. *Neurology* 33:1115–1121, 1983.

Thomas, J. E., Reagan, T. J., and Klass, D. W. Epilepsia partialis continua. *Arch. Neurol.* 34:266–275, 1977.

Trimble, M. R. The interictal psychoses of epilepsy. In D. F. Benson, D. Blumer (editors). *Psychiatric Aspects of Neurologic Disease*. Vol. 2. New York: Grune & Stratton, 1982, Pp. 75–91.

Troupin, A. S. The measurement of anticonvulsant agent levels. *Ann. Intern. Med.* 100:854–858, 1984.

Van Buren, J. M., et al. Surgery of temporal lobe epilepsy. *Adv. Neurol.* 8:155–196, 1975.

Wilson, D. H., Reeves, A. G., and Gazzaniga, M. S. "Central" commissurotomy for intractable generalized epilepsy: series two. *Neurology* 32:687–697, 1982.

Yerby, M. S. Problems and management of the pregnant woman with epilepsy. *Epilepsia* 28(suppl. 3):529–536, 1987.

Syncope

Day, S. C., et al. Evaluation and outcome of emergency room patients with transient loss of consciousness. *Am. J. Med.* 73:15–23, 1982.

Kapoor, W. N., et al. A prospective evaluation and follow-up of patients with syncope. *N. Engl. J. Med.* 309:197–204, 1983.

Lombroso, C. T., and Lerman, P. Breath-holding spells (cyanotic and pallid infantile syncope). *Pediatrics* 39:563–580, 1967.

Noble, R. J. The patient with syncope. *JAMA* 237:1372–1376, 1977.

Ross, R. T. *Syncope*. Philadelphia: Saunders, 1989.

Sleep Disorders

PHYSIOLOGY

On the basis of the electroencephalogram (EEG) and other measures, sleep has been shown to consist of two distinct phases: **rapid-eye-movement** (REM) and **non-rapid-eye-movement** (NREM) sleep. NREM sleep is further divided into four successively deeper stages. In stage 1, the EEG shows low-amplitude, mixed-frequency activity and there are slow rolling eye movements. Sleep spindles with a frequency of 12 to 16 Hz (see Fig. 3-7) as well as high-voltage discharges called *K complexes* appear in the EEG during stage 2. High-voltage delta waves progressively dominate the EEG recording throughout stages 3 and 4, comprising slow-wave sleep.

During REM sleep, there is a low-voltage, mixed-frequency (desynchronized EEG) pattern that also contains triangular 3- to 5-Hz sawtooth waves. Hippocampal sinusoidal waves of 5 to 10 Hz are seen continuously during REM sleep. Phasic bursts of rapid conjugate eye movements occur in REM sleep and the electromyographically (EMG) recorded activity and the tone of most muscles are reduced or absent, reflecting inhibition from the brainstem centers. Subjects often show hyperventilation, tachycardia, and fluctuations in blood pressure. Dreaming is, for the most part, associated with REM sleep.

From the time of sleep onset, there is a progressive descent and reascent through stages 1 to 4 over a 70- to 100-minute period followed by a REM burst. This cycle repeats itself approximately every 90 minutes, with slow-wave sleep becoming less abundant and REM periods more prolonged as the night progresses (Fig. 8-1). REM periods average about 15 minutes and account for about 20 percent of the total sleep time. Infants and young children spend a disproportionate amount of time in stages 3 and 4 sleep and the elderly show relatively decreased amounts of slow-wave sleep, frequent awakenings, and less total sleep time.

This exquisitely balanced architecture of normal sleep is controlled by interconnected

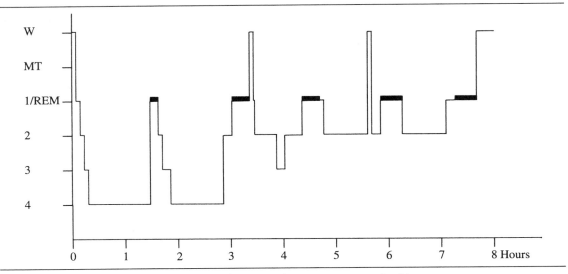

Fig. 8-1. *Computer-generated sleep-staging histogram in a young, normal subject. Note the decreased depth of sleep and lengthening REM periods as the night progresses. (W = awake; MT = movement time.)*

centers located in the upper brainstem, diencephalic regions, and the basal forebrain that are responsible for initiating and regulating sleep. The locus ceruleus and nuclei in the pontine tegmentum are involved in the production of REM sleep through the influence of a noradrenergic mechanism. Pontogeniculate-occipital waves are correlated with the eye movements and dream imagery that occur in REM sleep. The nuclei of the median raphe of the pons, operating through the influence of a serotonergic mechanism, are associated with slow-wave sleep. Hypothalamic and nonspecific thalamic areas also play a role in sleep regulation. Sleep spindles arise from oscillatory activity within the thalamus playing upon the cortex. Degenerative lesions of the thalamus may produce insomnia and a marked sleep disturbance. These two sleep systems have a close relationship to the ascending reticular activating system that governs wakefulness. Although sleep involves a reduction in the neuronal activity of the neuronal circuits promoting wakefulness, it is an active rather than a passive state, with heightened activity in certain brainstem and diencephalic areas.

Patients can be studied in sleep laboratories by means of polysomnography, which includes the simultaneous recording of the EEG, EMG (the mentalis muscle), eye movements (extraoculogram [EOG]), electrocardiogram (ECG), and respirations during sleep (Fig. 8-2). The findings yielded by such recordings in conjunction with clinical data have helped define the following major categories of sleep disorders: disorders of initiation or maintenance of sleep (insomnias), disorders of excessive daytime somnolence, disorders of the sleep-wake schedule, and dysfunctions associated with sleep, sleep stages, or partial arousals (parasomnias).

INSOMNIAS

Transient insomnia is common when an individual is experiencing emotional stress, pain, or changes in routine. When insomnia persists for weeks, an underlying cause should be sought. In certain cases, polysomnography shows that patients complaining of insomnia are actually sleeping normal amounts. However, insomnia is best defined according to the patient's perceived need for more nocturnal sleep in order to function optimally during the day, and not by the amount of sleep actually obtained. Conversely, there are habitual short sleepers who

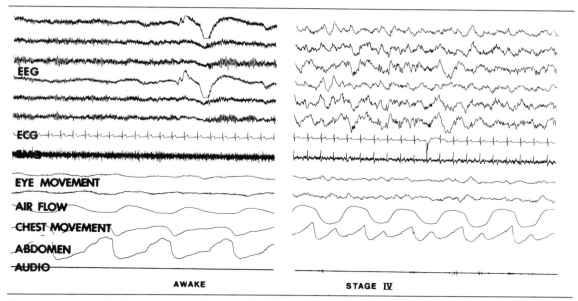

Fig. 8-2. *A normal polysomnogram showing the awake state and stage IV sleep. Note that the EEG tracing appears compressed because it is run at half-normal speed (15 mm/sec).*

sleep less than 4 hours a night and yet feel rested during the day.

Depression is often the source of early morning wakening. Alcohol, sedative, hypnotic, and stimulant drug abuse or withdrawal from these agents is a relatively common cause of insomnia. Most hypnotic agents generally lose their effectiveness after 1 month, cause a disorganization of the sleep architecture including a suppression of REM sleep, and can lead to sleep-disrupting withdrawal effects. Treating this ensuing insomnia with further hypnotic agents only compounds the problem. Sleep apnea is discussed later in this chapter.

Certain neurological conditions such as fatal familial insomnia (see Chapter 4) or Wernicke-Korsakoff syndrome can produce insomnia by destroying the thalamic nuclei responsible for promoting synchronized sleep. **Periodic limb movements during sleep** may occur in a wide variety of sleep disorders and can interfere with sleep. These movements, usually confined to the legs, are stereotyped and highly periodic, occurring approximately every 20 to 30 seconds and mostly found in NREM sleep. They are distinct from "sleep starts," a variety of nocturnal myoclonus often experienced by normal subjects when falling asleep and involving the trunk as well as the legs.

The **restless legs syndrome** may occur during the day but is often worse during or confined to the time in bed. These patients have an indescribable discomfort in their legs, creating an urge to move them or get up and walk. Some of these patients have an underlying peripheral neuropathy or their symptoms are related to the ingestion of drugs such as phenothiazines or L-dopa. The symptoms may interfere with falling asleep and may also recur throughout the night. There is also a high incidence of regular periodic movements during sleep in these patients. Treatment for this condition may be difficult, although occasionally benzodiazepines such as clonazepam in combination with tricyclic antidepressants are successful.

A spectrum of brief nocturnal spells with arousal from stage 3 or 4 sleep, bizarre dystonic limb movements, autonomic activation, and at times vocalizations have recently been described. These spells often occur several times a night. They have been termed *paroxysmal arousals, nocturnal paroxysmal dystonia,* or *episodic nocturnal wanderings,* depending on their length and complexity. Although the EEG pattern is normal during these spells in most patients, they are considered to represent epileptic seizures, likely arising from mesial frontal structures, and may respond to carbamazepine treatment. Occasional cases may represent an unusual movement disorder of basal ganglionic origin.

DISORDERS OF EXCESSIVE SOMNOLENCE

Sleep is considered excessive when it occurs at times during the day when the patient would rather be awake or inappropriately in circumstances requiring wakefulness. Excessive daytime sleepiness stemming from a transient disturbance of nighttime sleep is not considered pathological. The hypersomnolent patient feels tired throughout much of the day, may nap excessively, is often difficult to arouse in the morning, and has an overall increase in the sleep time during a 24-hour period.

The **Multiple Sleep Latency Test** quantitates how quickly a patient falls asleep under favorable circumstances and includes EEG monitoring during five daytime trials conducted in the sleep laboratory. Normal subjects have a mean sleep latency of 10 to 20 minutes. A mean latency of 5 to 10 minutes indicates mild to moderate hypersomnolence, and less than 5 minutes, severe hypersomnolence.

Hypersomnias can generally be categorized as narcolepsy, sleep apneas, idiopathic hypersomnia, or periodic hypersomnias, or due to the prolonged use of CNS depressant drugs or stimulants or to a variety of psychiatric, neurological, and medical conditions (Table 8-1). The previously mentioned conditions that cause chronic insomnia are also associated with excessive daytime sleepiness.

Narcolepsy

Narcolepsy is the prototype of a primary sleep disorder occurring in otherwise healthy persons. It is encountered in about 0.07 percent of the population. Many cases are undiagnosed, with the excessive sleepiness wrongly attributed to psychological factors. The hallmark of the

Table 8-1. Conditions Producing Excessive Daytime Sleepiness

Miscellaneous sleep disorders
  Narcolepsy
  Disturbed nocturnal sleep due to periodic limb movements or sleep apnea (may be secondary to medical or neurological disorders)
  Idiopathic hypersomnia
Neurological disorders
  Encephalitis (e.g., encephalitis lethargica, African trypanosomiasis, chronic mesodiencephalic encephalitis)
  Head injury
  Raised intracranial pressure
  Brain tumors affecting the mesodiencephalic junction area
  Bilateral paramedian thalamic infarction
  Kleine-Levin syndrome
  Parkinson's disease
  Multiple sclerosis
  Myotonic dystrophy
Psychiatric disorders
  Depression and depressive phase of manic-depressive illness
  Personality disorders
  Conversion hysteria
  Schizophrenia
Medical disorders
  Chronic pulmonary failure with hypercapnia
  Uremia
  Hepatic encephalopathy
  Hypothyroidism
  Overuse of sedative drugs or withdrawal from stimulants

condition is irresistible sleep attacks that frequently occur under inappropriate circumstances such as while driving, eating, and conversing. The attacks may occur abruptly, but they are preceded by extreme sleepiness in three quarters of the patients. Most commonly, there are several attacks per week and often several per day. The usual attack lasts about 1 to 10 minutes, after which the patient awakens feeling refreshed. There is usually a refractory period of one to several hours before the next attack. Many narcoleptics are drowsy between sleep attacks, and fragmented nighttime sleep is also common. In fact, narcoleptics may not spend more time sleeping than normal subjects in a 24-hour period.

Sleep attacks are but one of the symptoms comprising the so-called **narcoleptic tetrad,** which also includes cataplexy, sleep paralysis, and hypnagogic hallucinations. **Cataplexy** is a sudden generalized or partial loss of mainly axial muscle tone causing the patient to fall, knees to buckle, or head to droop, and lasts for seconds to several minutes. Laughter, surprise, or strong emotion characteristically can precipitate the episode. Cataplexy most often occurs at different times from the sleep attacks. It is found in about 90 percent of the cases of narcolepsy and usually begins to appear several years or even decades after the onset of sleep attacks. **Sleep paralysis** is a temporary inability to move, which the patient is aware of, appearing in the transitional state between sleep and wakefulness. It occurs most commonly when patients are falling asleep. **Hypnagogic hallucinations** are vivid, often terrifying, auditory or visual hallucinations that are usually experienced while falling asleep and often in conjunction with sleep paralysis. These last two symptoms are also seen in nonnarcoleptics, but in this instance more commonly upon awakening in the morning. The complete tetrad is found in only about 10 percent of narcoleptic patients. Although the pattern of sleep attacks remains constant throughout life, the other components of the tetrad may abate with age.

The pathogenesis of narcolepsy is related to an abnormal intrusion of REM sleep fragments into the waking state. The sleep attacks are actually REM episodes in most cases and in all cases that include cataplexy. The cataplexy and sleep paralysis stem from the muscle inhibition and the hypnagogic hallucinations from the dreaming that occur during normal REM sleep. Whether isolated brief NREM sleep attacks should be classified as narcolepsy or as a form of idiopathic hypersomnia is still unsettled. Studies have shown a strong familial component in narcolepsy, suggesting a multifactorial mode of inheritance. This has been supported by the virtual 100 percent association found between narcolepsy and the HLA-DR2 haplotype. A history of irregular sleep habits in many narcoleptics is also thought to have a possible bearing on the pathogenesis. Many cases seem to arise after a period of sleep deprivation or disruption in the habitual sleep patterns. Rare cases of narcolepsy secondary to CNS trauma, infection, or hypothalamic tumors have been reported. The diagnosis of narcolepsy is based on the history of irresistible brief sleep attacks, often with cataplexy occurring at separate times. Hypersomnolence can be confirmed by the Multiple Sleep Latency Test. A large percentage of narcoleptics exhibit a sleep-onset REM period at night or during daytime siesta EEG recordings. Two or more recordings may be necessary to demonstrate these features.

Narcolepsy is an extremely disabling disease, usually beginning in the second decade and persisting without remission for the lifetime of the patient. Automobile and household accidents, underachievement, and severe social restrictions are prevalent in affected patients.

CNS stimulants, of which methylphenidate (10–30 mg t.i.d. given in the morning, noon, and midafternoon on an empty stomach) is the current favorite, can lessen the number of sleep attacks and improve alertness. However, side effects of nervousness, appetite suppression, and addiction make this treatment less than ideal. Tricyclic antidepressants such as clomipramine or monoamine oxidase–inhibiting drugs such as phenelzine often lessen the episodes of cataplexy and the attendant symptoms.

Idiopathic Hypersomnia and the Kleine-Levin Syndrome

Idiopathic hypersomnia, either presenting as exaggerated daytime sleepiness alone or in combination with excessively sound nighttime sleep and "sleep drunkenness" following awakening in the morning, is often a familial condition. CNS stimulants may help these patients.

The Kleine-Levin syndrome is a rare periodic condition usually encountered in adolescent boys that is associated with excessive amounts of sleep lasting days or weeks, a voracious appetite, and abnormal sexual behavior. Some patients are mentally retarded and others harbor brain lesions around the hypothalamus. Most patients exhibit otherwise normal behavior and the attacks tend to disappear with time. The condition in most cases is considered an idiopathic hypothalamic-limbic system disturbance. Periodic hypersomnia may also rarely occur in females related to menstruation.

Sleep Apneas

The sleep apneas are a group of conditions that have recently sparked intense interest. In these disorders, breathing stops for over 10 seconds on average more than ten times per hour of nighttime sleep. By monitoring chest wall movements, nasal air flow, arterial blood gases, EKG, EEG, EMG, and EOG, three types of sleep apnea have been distinguished.

In **central apnea,** respiratory movements cease because of diaphragmatic arrest. In **obstructive apnea,** there is upper airway obstruction and the absence of nasal air flow is associated with increased respiratory effort. **Mixed apnea** is an obstructive apnea preceded by nonobstructive apnea. CNS lesions, such as infarcts affecting the respiratory centers in the medulla, or neuromuscular conditions, such as poliomyelitis or myotonic dystrophy, may give rise to central sleep apnea. However, obstruction of the upper airway tract arising from numerous conditions causing upper airway malformation or oropharyngeal muscle dysfunction (Table 8-2) is a much more common cause.

Physiological changes, such as muscle flaccidity, occurring in REM sleep in particular, tend to compound an already existing subobstructive state by allowing the tongue and jaw muscles to fall backwards and the pharyngeal walls to come into apposition.

Most patients with sleep apnea are male. The presenting complaint is usually daytime hypersomnolence consequent to the frequent nocturnal arousals caused by apneic episodes, of which the patient is usually unaware. Loud snoring, pauses in respiration, and excessive movements are often reported by the bed partners of these patients. However, in some cases, snoring is not a feature and the spectrum of the disorder has been extended to include patients with only mild increases in upper airway resistance who experience repeated nocturnal arousals. Headache upon awakening in the morning, personality changes, depression, intellectual deterioration, systemic and pulmonary hypertension, transient cardiac arrhythmias, and stroke are possible consequences of this syndrome.

During a prolonged apneic spell, severe oxygen desaturation is common, there is often a severe elevation of blood pressure, and cardiac arrhythmias including cardiac arrest may occur. Sudden death during sleep is a definite risk in the more severe cases. An audio recording of the patient's respirations during sleep at home may aid in the diagnosis, but, for the confirmation and determination of the type of sleep apnea, polysomnography (EEG, EMG, EKG, EOG, and respiratory and blood gas monitoring) should be done in a sleep laboratory.

Alcohol and bedtime hypnotics must be strictly avoided in these cases because they aggravate the apnea. Weight loss is mandatory. In the obstructive cases, permanent tracheostomy (which is opened only during sleep) has brought about immediate relief of symptoms. Drugs such as clomipramine and medroxyprogesterone acetate may be somewhat beneficial in mild cases. Further treatment may include such measures as maxillofacial surgery or uvulopalatopharyngoplasty, depending on the nature of the underlying problem. The administration of air through the nose under continuous positive pressure during sleep has been the most well tolerated and effective therapy. Diaphragmatic pacing has been tried in some cases of central sleep apnea.

Table 8-2. Conditions Associated with Obstructive Sleep Apnea

Obesity
Hypognathism
Tonsillar and adenoid hypertrophy
Large tongue
Maxillomandibular deformities
Congenital palatopharyngeal abnormalities
Chronic obstructive pulmonary disease
Hypothyroidism
Acromegaly

OTHER SLEEP-RELATED DISORDERS

Disorders of the sleep-wake schedule can arise in patients whose circadian rhythms are, for some reason, out of phase with the usual 24-hour sleep-wakefulness rhythms imposed by society. This occurs transiently in jet lag and in shift workers, but normally quickly resolves. However, some patients suffer a more chronic, unexplained aberrant synchronization of their internal rhythms with the usual 24-hour cycle and find themselves constantly alert and unable to fall asleep at the correct time in the evening and awaking with difficulty at the right time in the morning. These patients' habitual sleep and waking rhythms can be gradually readjusted to the clock when necessary.

The **parasomnias** include several disorders, such as somnambulism (sleep walking), night terrors (pavor nocturnus), and enuresis (bed wetting), that occur nocturnally but in the context of otherwise normal sleep. These disorders are more common in children, frequently disappear in adulthood, and are specifically related to stages 3 and 4 NREM sleep rather than to REM sleep. A partial arousal from deep sleep, of unknown cause, is thought to be responsible for the problem, although psychological mechanisms are implicated in some cases.

BIBLIOGRAPHY

Broughton, R. J. Narcolepsy. In M. J. Thorpy (editor). *Handbook of Sleep Disorders*. New York: Dekker, 1990, Pp. 197–216.

Broughton, R. Sleep disorders: disorders of arousal? *Science* 159:1070–1078, 1968.

Coleman, R. M., et al. Sleep-wake disorders based on a polysomnographic diagnosis. A national cooperative study. *JAMA* 247:997–1003, 1982.

Coleman, R. M., Pollack, C. P., and Weitzman, E. D. Periodic movements in sleep (nocturnal myoclonus): relation to sleep disorders. *Ann. Neurol.* 8:416–421, 1980.

Critchley, M. Periodic hypersomnia and megaphagia in adolescent males. *Brain* 85:627–656, 1962.

Culebras, A. (editor). The neurology of sleep. *Neurology* 42(suppl. 6):6–94, 1992.

Gillin, J. C., and Byerley, W. F. The diagnosis and management of insomnia. *N. Engl. J. Med.* 322:239–248, 1990.

Guilleminault, C., and Dement, W. (editors). *Sleep Apnea Syndromes*. New York: Liss, 1978.

Hauri, P. *The Sleep Disorders* (2nd ed.) (Scope monograph). Kalamazoo: Upjohn, 1977.

Kales, A., et al. Narcolepsy-cataplexy. I. Clinical and electrophysiologic characteristics. *Arch. Neurol.* 39:164–168, 1982.

Kales, A., and Kales, J. D. Sleep disorders. Recent findings in the diagnosis and treatment of disturbed sleep. *N. Engl. J. Med.* 290:487–499, 1974.

Kaplan, J., and Staats, B. A. Obstructive sleep apnea syndromes. *Mayo Clin. Proc.* 65:1087–1094, 1990.

Kessler, S., Guilleminault, C., and Dement, W. A family study of 50 REM narcoleptics. *Acta Neurol. Scand.* 50:503–512, 1974.

Kimoff, R. J., Cosio, M. G., and McGregor, M. Clinical features and treatment of obstructive sleep apnea. *Can. Med. Assoc. J.* 144:689–695, 1991.

Krueger, B. R. Restless legs syndrome and periodic movements of sleep. *Mayo Clin. Proc.* 65:999–1006, 1990.

Kryger, M., Roth, T., and Dement, W. *Principles and Practice of Sleep Medicine*. Philadelphia: Saunders, 1989.

Parkes, J. D. *Sleep and Its Disorders*. London: Saunders, 1985.

Richardson, J. W., Fredrickson, P. A., and Lin, S. C. Narcolepsy update. *Mayo Clin. Proc.* 65:991–998, 1990.

Roth, B. *Narcolepsy and Hypersomnia*. Basel: Karger, 1980.

Thorpy, M. J., and the Diagnostic Classification Steering Committee. *International Classi-fication of Sleep Disorders: Diagnostic and Coding Manual.* Rochester, MN: American Sleep Disorders Association, 1990.

Thorpy, M. J., and McGregor, P. A. The use of sleep studies in neurologic practice. *Semin. Neurol.* 10:111–122, 1990.

Zarcone, V. Narcolepsy. *N. Engl. J. Med.* 288:1156–1166, 1973.

Headache, Facial Pain, and Cranial Neuralgias

HEADACHE

Approximately 10 to 20 percent of the population experiences recurrent headaches, although in only a small proportion is the problem severe enough to require medical attention. Patients frequently regard headaches as an ominous sign, and therefore the physician's first task is to arrive at a definitive diagnosis, both to reassure the patient and also to identify those rare cases with a serious underlying disorder. An accurate detailed headache history, including any contributing psychological factors, and careful examination, plus the use of selected laboratory tests, frequently allows the headache to be classified into one of three broad categories: (1) vascular (usually migraine); (2) muscle contraction (tension); or (3) extracranial or intracranial, structural or inflammatory conditions. A fourth category, rarely seen, is psychogenic headache in which the pain is akin to a conversion symptom. Table 9-1 presents a more detailed classification of headaches.

Pathogenesis of Headache

The various pain-sensitive structures within the intracranial cavity consist of the dura mater (region of the middle meningeal artery, dural sinuses and entering veins, falx, and tentorium), the middle meningeal artery, the arteries at the base of the brain and their major branches, and branches of the sensory nerves. Brain tissue itself is insensitive to pain. The periosteum of the skull; skin, fascia, muscles, arteries, and nerves of the scalp; and mucosa of the sinuses are also pain sensitive.

The first division of the trigeminal nerve mediates pain sensitivity mainly over the anterior and middle cranial fossae. The ninth and tenth nerves as well as sensory branches from C2 and C3 supply much of the posterior cranial fossa. Consistent with this innervation, pain from supratentorial lesions tends to be referred to the anterior scalp and vertex, and that from infratentorial lesions is often felt in the occipital, mastoid, or nuchal areas.

Intracranial lesions may produce pain by ex-

Table 9-1. Classification of Headaches

Vascular
  Migraine
    Common (without aura)
    Classic (with aura)
    Hemiplegic
    Ophthalmoplegic
    Basilar
    Other with neurological symptoms (e.g.,
      ophthalmic)
  Cluster
  Acute, symptomatic (e.g., fever, carbon
    monoxide, hangover, vasodilator drugs)
  Hypertensive (including pheochromocytoma)
  With vascular occlusive disease
  Temporal arteritis
Muscle-contraction (tension)
Cranial structural or inflammatory disease
  Intracranial mass lesions with or without raised
    intracranial pressure
  Pseudotumor cerebri
  Meningeal irritation (e.g., meningitis,
    subarachnoid hemorrhage)
  Diseases of the eye, ear, nose, throat, teeth, or
    temporomandibular joints
  Destructive or inflammatory lesions of the skull
    or sinuses
Psychogenic headache
Low-pressure (e.g., post lumbar puncture) headache

erting traction on or displacing pain-sensitive structures such as the venous sinuses and dural septa. Direct pressure, destruction, or inflammation involving other pain-sensitive structures may also cause headache. These mechanisms can be responsible for tumor headaches or they can also arise through direct tumoral involvement of the sensory nerves, before an elevation of intracranial pressure.

"Low-pressure" headache, such as occurs following lumbar puncture and resulting from a downward shifting of the brain, is also due to a traction mechanism. Dilatation or inflammation of intracranial vessels may also provoke pain. Meningitis causes the direct inflammation of sensory nerve endings. Dilatation of extracranial and meningeal arteries may be responsible for the pain experienced in vascular headache, although in migraine there is a superimposed component of sterile inflammation surrounding the arteries, which is mediated by histamine and pain-producing vasoactive peptides.

Inflammation of extracranial arteries, as occurs in temporal arteritis, also brings about pain. The sustained contraction of muscles about the head and neck stemming from various causes stimulates nerve endings and constricts arterioles within the muscles, leading to ischemic pain.

Subtypes of Headache

Migraine

Pathophysiology and Etiology. The pathogenesis of migraine is not fully understood but is generally attributed to a defect, possibly inherited, in the neurovascular control mechanisms that causes an excessive reactivity of cranial arteries to various stimuli. During the aura phase of a classic or hemiplegic migraine attack, there is a general as well as focal reduction in the cerebral blood flow likely due to the vasoconstriction of brain arterioles mainly in areas corresponding to the particular neurological symptoms. There may also be a more widespread systemic vasoconstriction precipitating such symptoms as pallor. The ensuing headache is accompanied by an extracranial vasodilatation that can be seen, felt, and measured in the form of increased pulsations in the superficial temporal and other external carotid branches. These dilated arteries are frequently tender because of the effects of locally concentrated vasoactive pain-sensitizing substances such as histamine, bradykinin, substance P, and serotonin on the tissue.

What triggers the chain of events ultimately leading to a migraine headache is still unknown. An increase in platelet aggregability with a release of serotonin and decline in plasma levels has been documented during migraine attacks. This may lead to or derive from alterations in brainstem and hypothalamic serotonin levels that affect both central pain and autonomic control mechanisms. A dampened vasoconstrictive effect of serotonin peripherally could explain the extracranial vasodilatation that takes place during a migraine attack.

The importance of **serotonin** in the pathophysiology of migraine is also corroborated by the fact that the administration of drugs releasing serotonin can trigger migraine and many of the abortive or preventive drugs for migraine act on $5HT_1$ or $5HT_2$ receptors, both centrally and at the level of the nervous adventitial plexus surrounding meningeal and extracranial arteries.

Electrical stimulation of the periaqueductal gray region of the central brainstem has brought to light the possible importance of central brainstem structures in triggering the abnormal vascular response of migraine, in that some patients who underwent stimulation in this area developed typical migraine headaches for the first time. This region contains the dorsal raphe nucleus, which is rich in serotonin and important for the regulation and control of pain impulses entering the spinal cord and trigeminal pathways. Projections from the dorsal raphe of the midbrain to cerebral arteries as well as to visual centers of the brain could constitute the route that mediates the alterations in cerebral blood flow and visual phenomena of migraine.

The observation that stimulation of the trigeminal nuclei in the pons of experimental animals can elicit dilation of intracranial meningeal arteries over the surface of the brain with a perivascular extravasation of plasma proteins has given rise to the **trigeminovascular hypothesis.** The concentrations of vasoactive, pain-enhancing peptide substances such as substance P also increased around vessels. A vicious circle phenomenon may thus evolve, whereby the released nociceptive substances cause further excitation of trigeminal afferents leading from vessels. Vasodilatation would then be an epiphenomenon and not the cause of the headache per se. Serotonin agonists, such as sumatriptan, can block this process.

The pathophysiological mechanism that initiates the sequence of events leading to a clinical migraine is still unknown. Some experts have attributed migraine attacks to the "noise" within the brainstem neurovascular control circuit. The cortex has come under increased scrutiny as a possible initiator of the process. In the classic form of migraine, the anterior spread of oligemia at 2 to 3 mm per minute advancing from the occipital region resembles a phenome-

non, long-known in animals, termed the *spreading depression of Leao*. In this phenomenon, there is a spreading wave of reduced electrical activity in the exposed or damaged cortex of animals. Recent magnetic resonance spectroscopy studies performed in migraine patients have shown that their extracellular magnesium level is reduced, which may correlate with this phenomenon. However, the role of spreading depression remains uncertain.

Clinical Picture and Diagnosis. Migraine is by far the most common form of recurrent, severe headache prompting neurological consultation. Migraine is a syndrome that varies widely in its manifestations from patient to patient, and these often change in a given patient. The headache proper may be accompanied by many other symptoms, including drowsiness, mood changes, irritability, diuresis, as well as visual and focal neurological symptoms. Its most characteristic features are: (1) recurrent vascular-type headaches (i.e., throbbing; increased by stooping or straining; worsened by conditions causing vasodilatation such as exercise, alcohol, and fever; and lessened by circumstances prompting vasoconstriction such as ergot ingestion); (2) onset in early life, often in childhood; (3) usually a hemicranial distribution; (4) accompanying gastrointestinal upset; and (5) a family history in about 60 percent of the cases. Other common features are an aura or prodromal period that may consist of nothing more than irritability, fatigue, or trouble concentrating; a tendency to occur premenstrually; photophobia; aversion to loud noises and strong odors during the headache; and a history of unexplained cyclic vomiting or motion sickness in childhood (Table 9-2). Migraine frequently appears upon awakening in the morning and commonly lasts for several hours.

Migraine without aura, known as **common migraine,** exhibits no specific neurological symptoms before or during the headache. **Migraine with aura,** or **classic migraine,** consists of a gradually developing visual aura that precedes the headache and lasts for 15 to 30 minutes. Scintillating scotomata (described as flashing lights, stars, sparkles, flashbulbs popping, and the like), fortification spectra (zigzag lines), and

Table 9-2. Diagnostic Criteria for Migraine

Historical features
  Usual onset in childhood or adolescence
  Family history in two thirds of patients
  Exacerbations premenstrually or while on oral
    contraceptives
  History of motion sickness
Characteristics of attacks
  Provoked by circumstances promoting
    vasodilation (e.g., alcohol, exercise, fever,
    coitus, vasodilating drugs)
  Duration 4–72 hours (untreated)
  Headache typically unilateral, pulsating, and
    intense
  Usually accompanied by nausea with or without
    vomiting, photophobia, sonophobia, and
    irritability
  Visual or neurological aura in classic migraine
  Response to ergot preparations or sumatriptan

various other visual distortions and phenomena may occur in half of or throughout the visual fields. A full-blown hemianopia may develop. Other transient nonvisual symptoms such as hemiparesis or hemisensory loss may also precede the headache as an aura.

In **hemiplegic migraine,** which is either sporadic or inherited as an autosomal dominant trait, hemiplegia with or without other signs such as hemisensory loss, hemianopia, and aphasia appears as an aura but may persist during and even outlast the headache. If the diagnosis of migraine has been well established using the criteria cited earlier and the patient is young, investigations can be confined to an enhanced computer tomographic (CT) scan, which should reliably rule out the existence of an arteriovenous malformation (Fig. 9-1).

If transient ischemic attacks (TIAs) are a consideration in the differential diagnosis, either because of the patient's older age or the headache proper is an insignificant aspect of the patient's problem, a fuller vascular investigation is indicated. Even in younger patients with recent-onset attacks of headache accompanied by neurological signs, a CT, ultrasound examination of neck vessels, and careful cardiac evaluation is called for. One useful distinguishing feature of the neurological symptoms that appear during a migraine attack is that they tend

to progress from one body area to another over the course of several minutes, but this does not happen in TIAs.

A lesser intense focal neurological symptomatology may supervene on occasion in patients with common migraine. Several personal cases have been documented of young women with common migraine who, during the middle stages of pregnancy, for the first time experienced focal neurological symptoms with their migraine (classic migraine). This likely arises because of the changed hormonal environment involved.

Ophthalmoplegic migraine, which is rare, usually begins in childhood and typically consists of recurrent bouts of fairly complete third nerve paralysis ipsilateral to a hemicranial headache that precedes the ophthalmoplegia by several hours or days. These patients should generally undergo angiography to rule out a posterior communicating artery aneurysm, which can produce similar recurrent symptoms.

Basilar migraine (of Bickerstaff) is most common in children and adolescents, and, in it, the migraine attack is preceded or accompanied by prominent neurological symptoms such as vertigo, ataxia, dysarthria, facial paresthesias, stupor, and blurred or dimmed vision or even blindness. Recurrent confusional episodes in childhood, at times with little or no headache, may be due to basilar migraine. If loss of consciousness occurs, this may be confused with epilepsy. Some cases of transient global amnesia in adults have also been attributed to migraine.

A **complicated migraine** represents any variety of migraine in which an attack includes a prolonged neurological deficit (e.g., hemiplegic or ophthalmoplegic migraine) or a stroke ensues. A CT scan may demonstrate a small infarct, usually in the deeper areas of the brain, after a particularly severe migraine attack with a persistent focal neurologic abnormality. Prolonged deficits are relatively common in sufferers of ophthalmoplegic migraine, but rare in other types. When persistent hemiplegias or other fixed deficits arise in a patient with common, classic, or hemiplegic migraine, every attempt should be made to exclude other causes of stroke. A prolapsed mitral valve leaflet may give rise to emboli to the brain and its incidence has been reported to be increased in migraine sufferers.

Carotodynia is a recurrent pain and tenderness felt over the carotid artery, in the neck or in the face. It is usually observed in migraine sufferers and is noted at times separate from their headaches.

Management. Reassuring the patient that there is no brain tumor or other serious intracranial disorder causing the migraine attacks is often important at the outset. A skull x-ray study is also frequently a reassuring measure and may unexpectedly reveal the presence of calcified lesions, sinus infection, a shifted pineal gland, or other evidence of raised intracranial pressure which would account for the headaches. A CT scan should be done in intractable cases.

An electroencephalogram (EEG) frequently shows paroxysmal sharp and slow activity in the temporal and posterior head areas during a migraine attack. In so-called dysrhythmic migraine the EEG changes may be epileptiform. In patients with basilar migraine who present with syncope, such EEG changes may wrongly be interpreted to suggest epilepsy.

In all cases, trigger factors, which may vary from case to case (Table 9-3), should be identified and dealt with if possible. This may involve, for example, advising the use of another method of contraception besides birth control pills (which should be avoided in migraineurs), eliminating certain foods from the diet, the consumption of which the patient notices is consistently related to the onset of a migraine attack, or recommending the adoption of a less hectic life-style or less stressful job.

Acute attacks may often be aborted by mild analgesics such as aspirin or acetaminophen, often in combination with codeine, when taken early during the aura or prodromal phase. The nausea and vomiting is treated with oral metoclopramide (10 mg) or dimenhydrinate (50 mg), administered orally or by rectal suppository, with each dose of analgesic. Preparations containing ergotamine tartrate (1 or 2 mg), often in combination with caffeine, should be tried in patients whose migraine attacks do not

Fig. 9-1. *(A) Enhanced CT scan.*

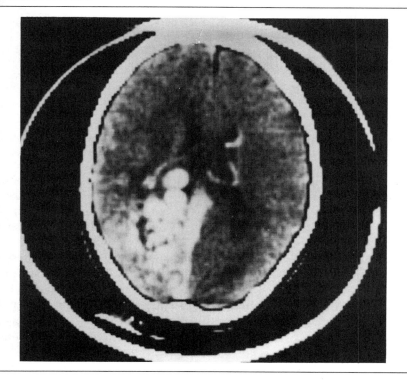

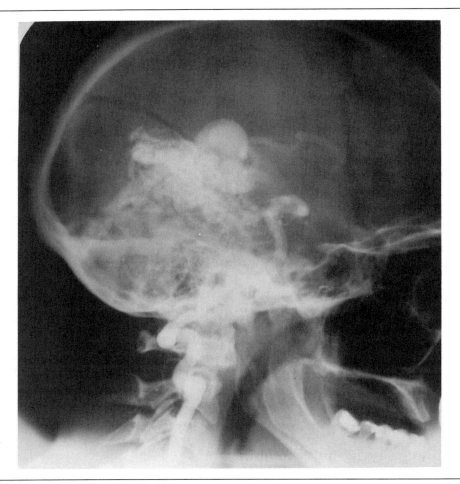

Fig. 9-1 *(Continued). (B) Angiogram showing left occipital arteriovenous malformation in a 22-year-old woman seen because of headaches that resembled classic migraine, with an aura of scintillating scotomata in the right visual field. Headaches were throbbing and responded to ergot but were always left sided. There was a loud bruit over the left mastoid and a right peripheral homonymous visual field deficit.*

respond to mild analgesics and if their headaches show some warning before they reach their full intensity. These preparations may not be tolerated when taken orally because of gastrointestinal upset, which they can aggravate, but can also be taken sublingually or by rectal suppository. Rectal absorption is often superior to that achieved by the oral route. Reduced gastrointestinal motility during a migraine attack may also interfere with the effectiveness of oral medication.

Ergot, which is a vasoconstrictor and may also act directly on the brain, must be taken at

the first sign of an impending attack, preferably during the aura phase. In classic, hemiplegic, or basilar migraine it is probably best not to use it during the focal aura, even though studies have shown that it does not reduce cerebral blood flow. An initial oral dose of 1 to 2 mg is taken and repeated every half hour to a maximum of 6 mg until the headache disappears. It is unusual for subsequent doses to be effective if the initial one or two tablets have not been so. The weekly dose of ergotamine should be limited to about 14 mg.

Ergot is contraindicated in the context of

Table 9-3. Trigger and Exacerbating Factors in Migraine

Stress or following stress

Sleep deprivation or excess

Exercise

Coitus

Hormonal
 Premenstrual
 Oral contraceptives
 Pregnancy

Fever

Head trauma

Vasodilator drugs (e.g., nitroglycerin)

Caffeine withdrawal

Alcohol

Foods containing tyramine (e.g., strong cheeses),
 phenylethylamine (e.g., chocolate), or nitrites
 (e.g., hot dogs)

---

pregnancy, severe hypertension, and coronary or peripheral arterial disease. Dependence may occur and prolonged overuse may lead to ergotism, with severe peripheral vasoconstriction causing distal paresthesias and ischemic ulcerations of the fingers and toes. These changes are usually reversible once the drug is stopped. Headache may also occur as a symptom of ergot withdrawal, leading to the vicious cycle of worsening headache and ergot overuse. Restricting the use of ergotamine to two or fewer days per week will lessen the likelihood of dependency.

Dihydroergotamine is a useful parenteral preparation that lacks the arterial vasoconstrictive properties of ergotamine and produces less nausea and physical dependence. The patient can inject it subcutaneously or intramuscularly in a dose of 0.25 to 0.5 mg. It can also be given intravenously and may abort the headache within minutes. The presence of nausea and vomiting may necessitate the simultaneous administration of metoclopramide or domperidone.

The recent release of the $5HT_{1D}$-receptor agonist sumatriptan (Imitrex) represents an important development in the treatment of severe acute attacks of migraine or cluster headache. Although it is a vasoconstrictor, its selective action on receptors that are largely confined to extracranial vessels means that it lacks some of the side effects seen with ergot substances. It can be given by subcutaneous self-injection or orally, has a rapid onset of action, and will abort the headache in up to 80 percent of patients even hours after onset. Side effects are minimal but the drug is expensive.

Intravenously administered chlorpromazine (12.5–25 mg) is frequently successful in aborting acute migraine attacks. The hypotensive side effect may be avoided by preloading with 500 ml of N saline. Nonsteroidal antiinflammatory drugs such as naproxen sodium (275 mg, one or two tablets at the onset of headache) or ibuprofen (400–800 mg at the onset of headache) are useful agents in certain patients who do not respond to regular analgesics. Prophylactic medication should be tried in patients with headaches that are frequent and severe enough to interfere with work, school, and other activities (Table 9-4). An arbitrary cutoff of more than four disabling headaches per month is often used as the criterion for deciding when to institute continuous medication.

Even when prophylactic medication is taken, patients may still require analgesics or ergotamine to abort any attacks that may yet occur. The patient must understand that prophylactic agents should be taken regularly, whether or not headaches occur, and that there may be a latency of several weeks before they begin to act. Amitriptyline, working up to a dose of 75 to 150 mg taken at bedtime, is the most effective prophylactic agent for both migraine and tension headaches. Its action is independent of its antidepressant effect. Frequently it can be discontinued after 3 to 6 months of treatment without disabling headaches returning for an extended period.

Should amitriptyline prove ineffective, other agents that can be tried include propranolol, flunarizine, verapamil, pizotyline (not currently available in the United States), methysergide, and monoamine oxidase inhibitors such as phenelzine (see Table 9-4). The dose of pizotyline and methysergide should be built up gradually to allow the patient to develop tolerance to its sedating effects. Amitriptyline, methysergide, and pizotyline appear to act mainly on $5HT_2$ receptors in the brain. The calcium channel blocker flunarizine may take 6 to 12 weeks

Table 9-4. Drugs for Prophylaxis of Migraine

Drug	Action	Trade name	Usual daily dose (mg)	Side effects
Amitriptyline[a]	Decreases presynaptic monoamine uptake centrally	Elavil	75	Sedation, dry mouth, weight gain, constipation
Propranolol[b]	Beta-blocker	Inderal, Inderal LA	80–320	Lethargy, insomnia, constipation, light-headedness, bradycardia, hypotension, worsening of asthma
Metoprolol, atenolol	Cardioselective (beta₁) beta-blockers	Lopressor, Tenormin		Like propranolol; may be used cautiously in asthmatics
Pizotyline[c]	Serotonin antagonist	Sandomigran	1.5–6	Leg pains, weight gain
Cyproheptadine	Serotonin antagonist, antihistamine	Periactin	12–24	Sedation, weight gain
Methysergide	$5HT_2$ antagonist, vasoconstrictor	Sansert	2–8	Nausea, muscle cramps, insomnia, weight gain, edema, peripheral (rarely retroperitoneal) pulmonary or cardiac fibrosis if used for more than 5–6 mo.
Flunarizine[c]	Centrally acting calcium-channel blocker	Sibelium	10	Depression, increased appetite, sedation, extrapyramidal symptoms
Verapamil	Calcium-channel blocker	Isoptin	240–480	Constipation
Belladona-ergot phenobarbital preparations	Vasoconstrictor, sedative	Bellergal spacetabs	1 tablet b.i.d.	Blurred vision, dry mouth, drowsiness
Phenelzine	MAO inhibitor	Nardil	45	Hypertensive crises, precipitated by strong cheeses, red wines, nuts, beans, chocolate, avocado, etc.
Naproxen sodium	Nonsteroidal antiinflammatory	Anaprox, Naprosyn	550 b.i.d.	Gastrointestinal bleeding or irritation

[a] Doxepin, desipramine, or nortriptyline may be substituted.
[b] Nadolol or timolol may be substituted.
[c] Not available in the United States.
MAO = monoamine oxidase.

to become fully effective. Its use is contraindicated in patients with a personal or family history of depression. Relaxation therapy, biofeedback, and various other measures to reduce stress should be employed when pharmacological treatment proves ineffective, or in conjunction with drug treatment in difficult cases. The supportive role of the physician and other health-care team members, including counselors, psychologists, and in some cases psychiatrists, should not be underestimated. In some intractable cases, a phase of continuous, disabling, resistant headache lasting for weeks may supervene. In many such patients with chronic daily headache, a gradual reduction of prolonged analgesic use combined with changes in life-style and counseling will foster significant improvement.

Status migrainosus poses a true challenge to the physician. Hospitalization for several days with the judicious use of analgesics, sedatives and prophylactic agents, and steroids, along with sympathetic handling of the patient's conflicts and sources of stress, is the best approach to management. A regimen of dihydroergotamine IV given every 8 hours for 48 hours has broken the cycle in some cases. Removing patients from their environment and providing adequate sleep for a few weeks is also often sufficient to break the vicious cycle of headaches.

Cluster Headache

Unlike migraine, cluster headache exhibits a relatively stereotyped picture (Table 9-5).

Table 9-5. Diagnosis of Cluster Headache

Male predominance
Onset in young adults
Clustering of attacks
Unilateral periorbital/temporal pain
Extremely intense, brief (<1 hr) headache
Rhinorrhea, tearing and congestion of the eye,
 oculosympathetic paralysis (ptosis, miosis)
Tendency for nocturnal occurrence, often around
 the same time
Provocation by alcohol consumption
Tendency to pace during the headache

There is a 5 to 1 male to female predominance and it tends to begin between the ages of 20 to 40. Its name derives from the fact that the headaches tend to occur in clusters or bouts lasting from one to several weeks with interspersed headache-free periods, often lasting several months. However, there may not be headache-free intervals in the chronic variety of cluster headache.

Typically, during a cluster period, the headache occurs once or twice per day and, peculiarly, often at the same hour, frequently awakening the patient from sleep with clocklike regularity. The pain is excruciating, with a boring or stabbing quality; it is also nonthrobbing and almost always located around or behind one eye. It may radiate to the forehead, temple, face, teeth, gums, or ear. During a given cluster attack, the pain is usually confined to one side but may later shift to the other side. The pain rapidly builds up and then abates, with each episode tending to last about one hour, making the use of ordinary analgesics of little value. Other symptoms include tearing and congestion of the eye, nasal stuffiness (rhinorrhea), flushing, photophobia of the involved eye, a partial Horner's syndrome (miosis or ptosis), and nausea in about 50 percent of the cases. Patients are typically restless during the attack, preferring to pace. One of the most characteristic features is the tendency for a headache to be precipitated by the consumption of even small amounts of alcohol during a cluster period.

Although the clinical picture is relatively stereotyped and straightforward, cluster headache is frequently misdiagnosed and many patients are initially seen by ear, nose, and throat specialists or by dentists. The symptoms of intermittent sinus obstruction may resemble cluster headache, although the pain is less severe and tends to respond to measures reducing sinus congestion.

The pathogenesis is unclear. Familial cases do occur but are uncommon. Management is difficult in certain cases but every effort should be made to provide relief from what some have described as "the worst pain that man can suffer." Ergotamine (1 or 2 mg), given sublingually or by another route at the onset of the attack, prophylactically 1 hour before the expected time of the attack, or regularly three times a day is often effective. Sumatriptan given subcutaneously, although an expensive agent, is one of the most effective medications for aborting acute attacks. The inhalation of 100% oxygen (5–8 L/min) by mask for 5 to 10 minutes is another useful measure for aborting attacks. Preventive treatment can also be tried using verapamil, pizotyline (2 mg t.i.d.), methysergide (2 mg t.i.d. or q.i.d.), prednisone (40 mg per day), or lithium carbonate (900 mg per day; blood levels, 0.3–1.2 mEq/L). Prednisone should be tapered over a 3-week period. Lithium has proved most effective in controlling the chronic, unremitting variety of cluster headache.

Chronic Paroxysmal Hemicrania

Chronic paroxysmal hemicrania (CPH) is a rare variety of vascular headache that was originally described by the Norwegian neurologist Ottar Sjaastad. The headache somewhat resembles cluster headache, but there is a marked female predominance, the attacks occur during the day as well as at night, and the pain is distributed over the whole hemicranium and face (maximal around the eye and temple) and almost always occurs on the same side. Multiple, brief (1–45 min), and extremely painful attacks occur each day. As in cluster headache, there may be ipsilateral rhinorrhea or nasal obstruction, tearing, and a mild Horner's syndrome. The patient may experience nausea and vomiting in the more severe attacks. One of the most striking features of this disorder is its rapid, complete, and relatively specific response to the antiinflammatory agent indomethacin.

Cerebrovascular Disease and Hypertension

Vascular headache, often with an acute onset appearing in an elderly patient, may occur in the presence of significant occlusive disease in the carotid or vertebrobasilar system (Fig. 9-2). The postulated mechanism responsible is dilatation of extracranial collateral vessels such as branches of the superficial temporal artery that supply the internal carotid by reverse flow through the ophthalmic artery. Impaired central autoregulation due to ischemia may be a causative factor. Headaches may occur during TIAs in up to 40 percent of the patients, at the onset of neurological deficit in an acute cerebral infarction, or without any neurological deficit in severe stenotic disease of arteries in the neck.

The headache usually has a throbbing quality and may be quite severe and persistent. It has been postulated that late-life migraine equivalents may account for some of the transient neurological or visual symptoms in older individuals, with or without accompanying headaches. These patients may have a past history of migraine, lack the usual concomitant vascular or cardiac factors predisposing to TIAs, and, as unlike TIAs, present with neurological deficits that spread to adjacent areas of the body over several minutes, as in hemiplegic migraine. Acute pain is also felt over the carotid or vertebral arteries in the neck along with dissections of those vessels.

As is well known, subarachnoid hemorrhage presents with a severe, explosive headache accompanied by nuchal rigidity, nausea, and vomiting. A "sentinel" headache, which has a similar behavior but is less severe and prolonged, may occur when there is leakage of blood prior to the full-scale rupture of an aneurysm.

A very similar explosive headache is also seen in migraine attacks and may include nuchal rigidity resulting from the secondary contraction of neck muscles.

When extensive, intracerebral hemorrhage precipitates a sudden severe headache, either stemming from leakage into the subarachnoid spaces and subsequent meningeal irritation or from raised intracranial pressure. Arteriovenous malformations commonly produce headaches that are usually consistently unilateral, but otherwise may display all of the characteristics of common or classic migraine. An intracranial bruit, asymmetry of body development, seizures, or a visual field defect may offer clues to their presence.

Uncomplicated hypertension does not usually cause headaches. However, headaches with a typical early morning onset may occur when blood pressure is very high. Uncontrolled hypertension may also aggravate a preexisting migraine problem.

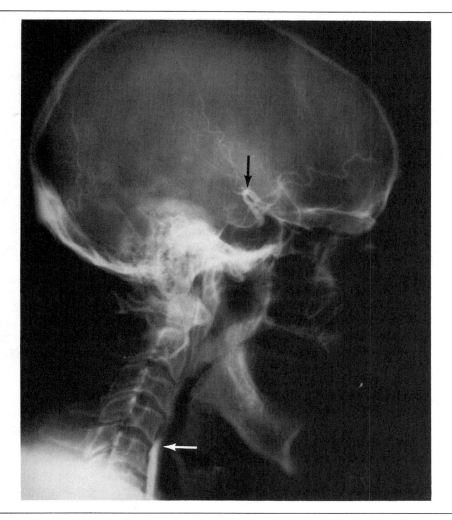

Fig. 9-2. *Angiogram in a 62-year-old man who was seen because of severe right temporal throbbing headaches but who had no neurological deficits. The horizontal arrow indicates the site of a complete internal carotid artery occlusion. The vertical arrow shows the carotid siphon filling retrograde from the ophthalmic artery.*

Pheochromocytoma is known to produce severe, sudden, and brief headaches accompanied by a sudden rise in blood pressure, pallor, sweating, tachycardia, and tremor.

Temporal Arteritis

Temporal arteritis, better termed *giant-cell arteritis,* affects females in three quarters of the cases and occurs in patients over 50, with the prevalence increasing in older age groups. Although uncommon, this disorder is important

because, if the diagnosis is missed and steroid therapy not instituted early, irreversible visual loss or other serious consequences may eventuate. The condition may stem from an autoimmune disturbance, and the characteristic pathological changes that affect the medium and large arteries consist of: (1) an inflammatory infiltrate of lymphocytes, plasma cells, macrophages, and the like, throughout the vessel wall; (2) disruption of the internal elastic lamina; (3) multinucleated giant cells concentrated in the region of the internal elastic lamina; and (4) intimal thickening due to fibroblast proliferation.

Headache is the major presenting symptom of temporal arteritis and consists of an intermittent, severe, boring, superficial pain felt mainly over one temporal region but at times on both sides. Tenderness over the area may interfere with sleeping or wearing a hat. Another symptom is jaw claudication that increases during chewing. Two thirds of the patients also have **polymyalgia rheumatica,** which consists of muscle pain and stiffness that particularly involve the shoulder girdle, neck, and hip girdle symmetrically. These patients are also systemically ill with malaise, weight loss, fever, night sweats, anorexia, and anemia.

Visual loss due to involvement of the posterior ciliary or rarely central retinal arterial branches of the ophthalmic artery is the most feared complication, occurring in over 50 percent of untreated cases. Rarely is visual loss the presenting symptom, but it may occur with dramatic suddenness at any time after headaches start to occur. Attacks of amaurosis fugax (transient monocular blindness) may foreshadow permanent visual loss.

Steroid treatment will usually prevent visual loss but will do little to reverse established blindness. The loss of vision becomes bilateral in a significant number of untreated cases. Other areas that may be involved by the disease process include the aorta, which may lead to dissection or rupture; cranial nerves III, IV, VI, or VIII, presumably due to vasa nervorum involvement; facial arteries, producing pain in the face; major cerebral arteries (especially the vertebral), leading to strokes or confusional states; and coronary arteries, causing myocardial infarction.

Palpation of the superficial temporal arteries in patients with temporal arteritis typically reveals a tender, pulseless, cordlike artery (Fig. 9-3). There may be redness, swelling, hair loss, and muscle atrophy over the inflamed area. The erythrocyte sedimentation rate (ESR) is usually markedly elevated, almost always within the range of 50 to 100 mm/hr. The diagnosis is confirmed by the findings from temporal artery biopsy. Because the pathological lesions may be

segmental, the biopsy specimen may be normal. For this reason, a relatively long segment of the artery should be sampled, with serial sections obtained and frozen sections done at the time of biopsy to allow immediate biopsy of the contralateral temporal artery if results are negative. Angiography, if performed, may show a beaded irregular appearance or missing branches in the distribution of the external carotid artery.

Treatment should be initiated with prednisone (80 mg per day in divided doses) as soon as the diagnosis is suspected and blood for ESR is drawn. Full-dose treatment should be maintained for about 4 weeks followed by gradual tapering to the lowest dose that will keep the patient symptom-free and the ESR less than 20 mm/hr. Treatment should be continued for a minimum of 6 months. Following the institution of steroids, headaches and systemic symptoms usually resolve rapidly and the ESR returns to normal limits within 3 to 6 weeks.

Muscle Contraction (Tension) Headache

Tension headache is a very common form of headache that possesses the following features that distinguish it from migraine and other vascular headaches. It is usually experienced as a nonthrobbing squeezing or weightlike sensation, is usually bioccipital, bifrontal, or bandlike in distribution, often continues for long periods, and lacks prominent gastrointestinal symptoms. The headache is often worse toward the end of the day. It occurs in circumstances that predispose to the chronic contraction of nuchal and scalp muscles, such as neck trauma (e.g., whiplash injury), cervical spondylosis or arthritis, the prolonged maintenance of fixed neck postures such as when working at a desk, and a tense, anxious personality. The neck, occipital, and shoulder muscles are often tender and patients commonly cannot relax various muscles on request. These headaches are best managed by conservative measures, including reassurance, use of non–narcotic-containing analgesics, hot or cold compresses and massage applied to nuchal muscles, relaxation techniques, and measures that help the patient manage stress and underlying conflicts. Psychiatric consultation and formal psycho-

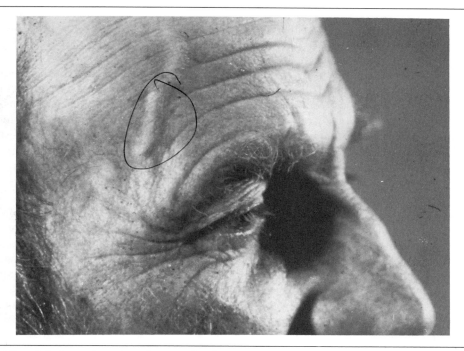

Fig. 9-3. *Dilated, indurated, and tender superficial temporal artery in a man with biopsy-proved temporal arteritis.*

therapy is indicated only when there is a significant psychopathologic component besides the headaches.

Brain Tumor Headache

Headache caused by traction or distortion of pain-sensitive structures appears relatively early in at least one third of patients with brain tumor. When lateralized, the side on which a headache occurs is usually the side affected by the tumor. Headache features that arouse suspicion of a brain tumor, but are by no means exclusive to a neoplastic process, include: an intermittent nonthrobbing headache that becomes more severe over the ensuing weeks and months, a tendency to occur nocturnally or upon awakening in the morning, and exacerbation when bending, straining, or coughing.

Headache precipitated exclusively by coughing suggests the existence of a posterior fossa mass. When intracranial pressure becomes elevated, the headache is often more continuous and is accompanied by severe vomiting and obtundation. A sudden, severe, brief headache often precipitated by a change in posture from lying to standing, or vice versa, and accompanied by severe vomiting, ataxia, and obtundation is seen in conjunction with tumors or cysts interfering with cerebrospinal fluid (CSF) pathways, such as colloid cysts of the third ventricle or midline cystic cerebellar tumors.

Investigation of the Headache Patient

Patients with uncomplicated headaches whose diagnosis is relatively certain and neurological findings are negative require no special tests. In migraine patients, an EEG may show paroxysmal sharp and slow waves, often in the temporal and posterior head regions, providing further confirmation of the diagnosis. Any patient with headache and accompanying focal neurological or visual symptoms or headache that does not respond to treatment should have an enhanced CT scan and a Doppler examination of the neck vessels to search for tumors, arteriovenous malformations, or extracranial arterial occlusive disease. Angiography is reserved for patients with ophthalmoplegic or hemiplegic symptoms or for late-onset intractable vascular headaches. A lumbar puncture (following CT scan) should also be done in most cases of intractable headaches when the diagnosis is unclear or when pseudotumor cerebri is suspected, although there have been rare instances when the CSF pressure has been normal in patients with pseudotumor cerebri. An ESR should be measured in all patients with onset of headaches after age 50. Hypothyroidism may also precipitate headaches and, for this reason, thyroid studies are worthwhile. An antinuclear antibody test should be done to screen for systemic lupus erythematosus in patients with unexplained headaches.

There are several circumstances that should alert the clinician to the possibility of an underlying serious cranial disorder (Table 9-6). However, a sudden explosive headache, which is a characteristic of intracranial hemorrhage, may also be seen in the context of migraine, viral meningitis, and a sudden increase in intracranial pressure, such as may occur with a colloid cyst of the third ventricle causing acute obstruction of CSF flow within the ventricles.

CRANIAL NEURALGIAS AND OTHER CAUSES OF FACIAL PAIN

Trigeminal Neuralgia

Trigeminal neuralgia (tic douloureux) is a sudden, brief, extremely severe, and lancinating pain that is experienced within the distribution of one or more branches of the fifth nerve on one side of the face. The second and third divisions of the trigeminal nerve are most commonly involved, and only rarely is the ophthalmic division involved alone. The condition becomes bilateral in about 2 to 3 percent of the cases. Characteristically the pain is elicited by merely touching or blowing on a trigger zone, often located somewhere around the nasolabial fold. The trigger zone may be remote from the actual area of the pain and, in rare

cases, has been located in a finger or toe. Eating, talking, swallowing, and yawning also frequently set off paroxysms of excruciating pain and, for this reason, the patient may be reluctant to eat, talk, or shave. The pain occurs in self-limited bouts lasting seconds or minutes, although there may be a continuous burning facial discomfort in the interim. After several days or weeks, the pain may remit spontaneously, only to recur at a later date and eventually become constant. The condition is mostly seen in older age groups, and female sufferers outnumber males by 3 to 2.

In the idiopathic form of trigeminal neuralgia, examination reveals no objective evidence of fifth nerve dysfunction. The pathogenesis of this condition is still not established, despite Janetta's recent evidence that vascular compression of the trigeminal root in the posterior fossa is seen at surgery in most patients. The offending vessel in this disorder, which is not usually abnormal on angiograms, may be the superior cerebellar artery, anterior inferior cerebellar artery, a tortuous basilar artery, or a pontine vein. Other theories attribute the disorder to the degeneration of fibers in the gasserian ganglion with advancing age that causes "short-circuiting" or "cross-talk," centrally impaired pain integration, the transmission of internal carotid artery pulsations to the ganglion (which is close anatomically), kinking and stretching of the nerve due to a worsening basilar impression

Table 9-6. Signs of a Potentially Serious Underlying Etiology for Headache

Sudden, explosive onset of severe headache
Newly appearing headache gradually worsening over weeks and months
Nocturnal headache awakening the patient from sleep
Late-onset headache (over age 50)
Headache that is always on the same side
Neurological or visual symptoms outlasting the headache
Loss of consciousness with a headache
Headache appearing or disappearing abruptly with changing posture from lying to standing, or vice versa
Cough or exertional headache

with increasing age, or persistent herpes virus within the ganglion.

Trigeminal neuralgia may occur secondary to various conditions, but, in these cases, a trigger zone is not usually found and a sensory deficit may be present. Aneurysms, tumors (e.g., cerebellopontine angle tumor or meningioma near the trigeminal ganglion), sphenoid sinusitis, and a preceding trigeminal sensory neuropathy are potential causes. Paget's disease with basilar impression has been known to produce tic in association with hemifacial spasm. Multiple sclerosis is found in about 4 percent of the cases of trigeminal neuralgia and a plaque at the root entry zone of the fifth nerve in the pons is the underlying lesion. These patients tend to have bilateral tic and the condition appears at a younger age than the idiopathic variety.

Most patients with trigeminal neuralgia whose history is typical and who have no neurological deficits need no further investigations beyond a skull x-ray study (including basal views) and a CT scan. Medical treatment is effective in over 80 percent of the cases, at least in the short term (Table 9-7). Carbamazepine, prescribed in the same doses as those used for epilepsy (600–1200 mg/day), is the drug of choice. The dosage must be built up slowly from an initial dose of 100 mg twice daily, because patients are prone to experience sedation and confusion when taking the drug, especially the

Table 9-7. Management of Trigeminal Neuralgia

Medical
  Carbamazepine (200–400 mg t.i.d.)
  Phenytoin (300 mg/day)
  Amitriptyline (75–125 mg/day)
  Baclofen (30–60 mg/day)
Surgical
  Extracranial
    Percutaneous radiofrequency coagulation of
      trigeminal ganglion
    Percutaneous glycerol injection into
      retrogasserian area
    Nerve branch avulsions or phenol injections
    Stereotaxic medullary trigeminal tractotomy
  Intracranial
    Microvascular trigeminal root decompression
    Posterior fossa selective retrogasserian
      rhizotomy

---

elderly. It is also important that the drug be taken after meals or food ingestion to prevent gastrointestinal irritation. Rarely, severe blood dyscrasias or hepatotoxicity arise. Less effective alternative agents are phenytoin, amitriptyline, mephenesin, or baclofen.

Many patients ultimately require a surgical procedure to achieve pain relief, and this should not be delayed when pain is uncontrolled because some patients have been driven to suicide by the excruciating nature of the disorder. Percutaneous radiofrequency coagulation of the ganglion using an approach through the foramen ovale has yielded good long-term results, allows some preservation of touch over the face, and avoids the need for a craniotomy. However, the procedure is painful and requires patient cooperation. The percutaneous injection of glycerol into the retrogasserian area is a recently introduced variation on this technique.

Microvascular decompression of the roots in the posterior fossa through the insertion of a sponge between the vessel and roots is a technique popularized by Janetta. Good long-term results are seen with this method and the destruction of intact sensory pathways is avoided. Some surgeons prefer to first try an initial avulsion or phenol injection of a peripheral branch of the fifth nerve when the pain is restricted to a discrete area. Other methods include a selective posterior fossa retrogasserian rhizotomy, a percutaneous stereotaxic medullary trigeminal tractotomy, and a neuroaugmentation procedure in which electrical stimulation is administered transcutaneously or through implanted electrodes within the gasserian ganglion or its central projections. Because some patients may be dissatisfied with the resultant facial numbness brought about by ablative procedures, some surgeons perform a temporary percutaneous alcohol block of the ganglion to test the patient's tolerance for the resultant effects.

Glossopharyngeal Neuralgia

Glossopharyngeal neuralgia is a rare disorder resembling trigeminal neuralgia in its intensity and the shocklike quality of the pain. The pain involves the throat and tonsillar area, and at times is felt deep within the ear. The trigger area, which may be activated by touch or swallowing, is usually around the tonsillar area. Symptomatic forms may be due to intracranial neuromas or meningiomas, carcinoma of the pharynx, arterial compression of the ninth nerve, or peritonsillar abscess. Some of the patients experience a reflex bradycardia or cardiac arrest due to pain-induced vagal stimulation, which may lead to syncope, anoxic seizures, and rarely sudden death.

Carbamazepine, or the other drugs mentioned for the treatment of trigeminal neuralgia, is frequently effective, but section of the ninth nerve intracranially may ultimately be required. Pacemakers can be implanted to prevent syncopal attacks.

Postherpetic Neuralgia

Following an acute vesicular herpetic infection that involves the face, most often in the V1 (ophthalmic) distribution and in elderly patients, a small percentage of patients are left with a severe, burning pain in the area, often triggered by contact with the skin. There is usually some sensory loss and scarring within the affected area. The pain can be very intractable, but may respond to carbamazepine, tricyclic antidepressants, or phenothiazines. Other treatments include the topical application of capsaicin cream, ethylchloride spray, or the use of either a hand vibrator or a transcutaneous nerve stimulation apparatus. Most cases remit spontaneously within several months. (See also Chapter 19.)

Occipital Neuralgia

Rarely the greater occipital nerve (C2) can be involved with a shocklike neuralgic pain that radiates up from the base of the neck unilaterally toward the vertex. Pressure over the nerve may trigger the pain. Neuralgia-like symptoms and paresthesias within the C2 distribution have been observed in adolescents and young adults with disorders of the upper cervical spine that often lead to excessive mobility of C1 on C2. These patients should therefore undergo thorough x-ray examination of their upper cervical spine, including open-mouth views of the odon-

toid and lateral views in flexion and extension. In the presence of occipital neuralgia, infiltrating the greater occipital nerve with local anesthetics may yield some relief, and in rare cases section of the nerve is effective. However, medical management with carbamazepine or amitriptyline should be tried first.

Raeder's Syndrome

A persistent severe headache in the supraorbital area combined with an oculosympathetic paralysis (ptosis and miosis) is called *Raeder's syndrome,* or paratrigeminal neuralgia. The disorder may be confused with cluster headache and in fact may be due to migraine. However, lesions such as meningiomas or aneurysms around the region of the carotid artery where it lies near the gasserian ganglion may give rise to this clinical picture. The oculosympathetic fibers follow the internal carotid artery intracranially. When a lesion is responsible for the syndrome, there is often sensory loss within the V1 distribution.

Temporomandibular Joint Syndrome

A host of symptoms ranging from typical vascular or muscle contraction headaches to neuralgic facial pains, ear pain, vertigo, and hearing loss have been attributed to a pathologic condition or dysfunction of the temporomandibular joints. The combination of pain in the ear or preauricular area, tenderness over the muscles around the joint, and limitation and clicking upon jaw opening suggest temporomandibular joint dysfunction. Dentists tend to overdiagnose this condition and recommend treatment for malocclusion in headache patients, usually to no avail.

Atypical Facial Pain

When pain about the face does not fit into any of the previously described categories and is not due to dental disease, sinusitis, tumors of the head and neck, or other structural lesions, it is termed *atypical facial pain.* Many of these patients will respond to amitriptyline, regardless of whether there is evidence for an underlying depression.

BIBLIOGRAPHY

Appenzeller, O. Temporal arteritis. *Postgrad. Med.* 56:133–140, 1974.

Appenzeller, O. Cerebrovascular aspects of headache. *Med. Clin. North Am.* 62:467–480, 1978.

Bickerstaff, E. R. Basilar artery migraine. *Lancet* 1:15–17, 1961.

Blau, J. N. (editor). *Migraine: Clinical and Research Aspects.* Baltimore: Johns Hopkins University Press, 1987.

Bradshaw, P., and Parsons, M. Hemiplegic migraine. A clinical study. *Q. J. Med.* 34:65–72, 1965.

Carter, J. E. Ophthalmic and neuro-ophthalmic aspects of headache and head pain. *Neurol. Clin.* 1:415–443, 1983.

Couch, J. R. (editor). Facial pain. *Semin. Neurol.* 8:255–338, 1988.

Couch, J. R., Ziegler, D. K., and Hassanein, R. Amitriptyline in migraine prophylaxis. *Arch. Neurol.* 36:695–699, 1979.

Diamond, S. (editor). Headache. *Med. Clin. North Am.* 75:521–797, 1991.

Dugan, M. C., Locke, S., and Gallagher, J. R. Occipital neuralgia in adolescents and young adults. *N. Engl. J. Med.* 267:1166–1177, 1962.

Edmeads, J. Complicated migraine and headache in cerebrovascular disease. *Neurol. Clin.* 1:385–397, 1983.

Edmeads, J. Cerebral blood flow in migraine. *Headache* 17:148–152, 1977.

Ekbom, K. A clinical comparison of cluster headache and migraine. *Acta Neurol. Scand.* [Suppl.] 41:1–48, 1970.

Fisher, C. M. Late-life migraine accompaniments as a cause of unexplained transient ischemic attacks. *Can. J. Neurol. Sci.* 7:9–17, 1980.

Friedman, A., Harter, D. H., and Merritt, H. H. Ophthalmoplegic migraine. *Arch. Neurol.* 7:320–327, 1962.

Graham, J. Methysergide for prevention of headache. Experience in five hundred patients over three years. *N. Engl. J. Med.* 270:67–72, 1964.

Janetta, P. Arterial compression of the trigeminal nerve at the pons in patients with trigeminal neuralgia. *J. Neurosurg.* 52:381–386, 1980.

Kudrow, L. Cluster headache: new concepts. *Neurol. Clin.* 1:369–383, 1983.

Lance, J. W. A concept of migraine and the search for the ideal headache drug. *Headache* 30(suppl.):17–28, 1990.

Lance, J. W., and Anthony, M. Some clinical aspects of migraine: a prospective survey of 500 patients. *Arch. Neurol.* 15:356–361, 1966.

Lance, J. W. *The Mechanism and Management of Headache,* 4th ed. Boston: Butterworths, 1983.

Marbach, J. J. Arthritis of the temporomandibular joints. *Am. Fam. Physician* 19:131–139, 1979.

Moskowitz, M. A. The visceral organ brain: implications for the pathophysiology of vascular head pain. *Neurology* 41:182–186, 1991.

Moskowitz, M. A., et al. Pain mechanisms underlying vascular headaches. *Rev. Neurol.* (Paris) 145:181–193, 1989.

Nelson, R. F. BC-105—a new prophylactic agent for migraine—four years' experience in seventy-five patients. *Headache* 13:96–103, 1973.

Olesen, J., et al. Timing and topography of cerebral blood flow, aura, and headache during migraine attacks. *Ann. Neurol.* 28:791–798, 1990.

Pearce, J. M. S. Migraine: a cerebral disorder. *Lancet* 2:86–89, 1984.

Peroutka, S. J. The pharmacology of current antimigraine drugs. *Headache* 25:5–11, 1990.

Peroutka, S. J. Migraine. In M. V. Johnston,

R. L. Macdonald, and A. B. Young (editors). *Principles of Drug Therapy in Neurology*. Philadelphia: Davis, 1992, Pp. 161–177.

Prensky, A. L. Migraine and migrainous variants in pediatric patients. *Ped. Clin. North Am.* 23:461–471, 1976.

Price, R., and Posner, J. Chronic paroxysmal hemicrania. A disabling headache responding to indomethacin. *Ann. Neurol.* 3:183–184, 1978.

Raskin, N. H. The pathogenesis of migraine. *Curr. Opin. Neurol. Neurosurg.* 2:209–211, 1989.

Raskin, N. H., and Appenzeller, O. *Headache* (Vol. 19, Major Problems in Internal Medicine). Philadelphia: Saunders, 1980.

Raskin, N. H. *Headache* (Vol. 10, Current Neurology). Chicago: Mosby–Year Book, 1990, Pp. 195–219.

Riley, T. L. Muscle-contraction headache. *Neurol. Clin.* 1:489–500, 1983.

Saper, J. R. Chronic headache syndromes. *Neurol. Clin.* 7:387–412, 1989.

Silberstein, S. D. (editor). Intractable headache: inpatient and outpatient treatment strategies. *Neurology* 42(suppl. 2):5–51, 1992.

St. John, J. N. Glossopharyngeal neuralgia associated with syncope and seizures. *Neurosurgery* 10:380–384, 1982.

The Subcutaneous Sumatriptan International Study Group. Treatment of migraine attacks with sumatriptan. *N. Engl. J. Med.* 325:316–321, 1991.

Weber, R. M., and Reinmuth, O. M. The treatment of migraine with propanolol. *Neurology* 22:366–369, 1972.

Welch, K. M. A. Migraine: a biobehavioral disorder. *Arch. Neurol.* 44:323–327, 1987.

Wolff, H. G., Goodell, H., and Hinkle, L. E., Jr. The pathophysiology of headache. *Int. J. Neurol.* 3:287–314, 1962.

10

Dizziness and Vertigo

The vestibular system provides information concerning: (1) the subjective awareness of angular and linear body motion and spatial orientation; (2) coordination of eye movements with head movements through the vestibuloocular reflex (VOR), which allows one, for example, to read a road sign while in motion; and (3) maintenance of posture through vestibulospinal reflexes. The maintenance of balance, posture, and coordination of movements depends on input to the central nervous system from three main sources: vision, proprioception (tendon and joint receptors), and vestibular sensation. An unaccustomed discrepancy in the afferent signals from these sources or more commonly a disparity in the vestibular input between sides may give rise to a subjective sensation of disorientation in space, or in more severe cases **vertigo,** which is a false illusion of movement of oneself or the environment.

Vertigo, with its accompanying autonomic symptoms, is a distressing condition that may lead to a state of panic and chronic phobic anxiety. Imbalance without vertigo may also result from a disturbance in the efferent systems involved with posture maintenance and movement. Structures that may be involved include the cerebellum, basal ganglia, corticospinal tracts, vestibulospinal tracts, and the neuromuscular apparatus. A disturbance in the VOR produces nystagmus, abnormal saccades, and oscillopsia (an illusion that stationary objects are moving back and forth or oscillating).

ANATOMY OF THE VESTIBULAR SYSTEM

The bony labyrinth is contained in the petrous portion of the temporal bone on each side. It is filled with perilymph, which has a relatively high sodium concentration and surrounds the membranous labyrinthine structures. These latter structures consist of the **vestibular apparatus** (three semicircular canals oriented in different planes and the otolith sacs—the utricle and saccule) and the **cochlea,** which is the primary organ of hearing and connects to the saccule.

These structures are filled with endolymph, which has a relatively high potassium concentration. At the point where each semicircular canal joins the utricle is a bulbous expansion (ampulla) that houses the cupula and cristae— sensory receptors which respond mainly to angular acceleration. The three **semicircular canals** are oriented so that the two horizontal (lateral) canals (lying in a plane 30 degrees above the horizontal when the head is in the primary position) and each superior and contralateral posterior pair act together.

In the normal state, when the resting input from one horizontal canal decreases due to movement, there is a corresponding increase in input from its opposite member. The otolith sacs contain maculae possessing sensory hair cells that are embedded in a gelatinous substance. These sacs relay information mainly concerning linear acceleration but also code information about the direction and amplitude of head translation as well as orientation to gravity.

The **vestibular division** of the eighth cranial nerve conveys impulses from the vestibular apparatus to the brainstem via a first-order neuron that synapses in Scarpa's ganglion within the internal auditory canal. The nerve crosses the cerebellopontine angle where it lies near the seventh nerve and enters the brainstem near the pontomedullary junction to synapse in the four vestibular nuclei lying in the floor of the fourth ventricle.

The superior and medial nuclei are involved in VORs via the medial longitudinal fasciculus that runs between the sixth and contralateral third nerve nuclei. These vestibular nuclei connect to the opposite pontine gaze center, which, when excited, causes ipsilateral conjugate eye deviation. The lateral (Deiter's) nucleus influences muscle tone and postural reflexes through vestibulospinal and reticulospinal pathways. The spinal (descending) nucleus projects mainly to the flocculonodular lobe and vermis of the cerebellum. The nuclei also have autonomic projections and connect rostrally through the thalamus to cortical centers in the temporal and adjacent parietal lobes. Blood supply to the peripheral vestibular system is furnished by the **internal auditory artery,** which is a branch of the anterior inferior cerebellar artery.

PATHOPHYSIOLOGY

Physiologically, firing patterns of the vestibular nerve or nuclei can be analyzed in terms of **tone** (the resting firing rate) and **gain** (the ratio of output to input when the head is moved). Either of these aspects may be affected when there are vestibular lesions, and the nature of the vestibular symptoms depends on which of the two functions is mainly disturbed. An imbalance in vestibular tone between sides results in vertigo, impulsion (a sensation of linear movement), or a sensation of tilt as well as nystagmus. Gain-related abnormalities lead to movement-induced vertigo. Central compensation is much more rapid in response to imbalances of tone than to disorders of gain. The latter relies on visual information and may take months or years to resolve, thus causing symptoms to persist during body or head movements or a change of position.

Disturbances in the VORs give rise to the most obvious objective sign of vestibular dysfunction—**nystagmus.** Nystagmus is defined as to-and-fro or torsional involuntary oscillations of the eyes. The most common form of vestibular nystagmus is jerk nystagmus, which has both fast and slow components. With body movement or rotation in one direction, there is normally a vestibular-mediated, slow "tonic" deviation of the eyes in the opposite direction, followed by a quick corrective component as the limits of gaze are reached. The fast component arises from contralateral frontal cortical gaze centers. A pathological imbalance in the vestibular input, perceived as body motion, similarly precipitates nystagmus.

The direction of the nystagmus is named according to the direction of the fast component. Most peripheral vestibular lesions are destructive and produce nystagmus *away* from the lesion, but, in certain instances, such as in inflammatory disorders or some stages of Meniere's disease, the affected side may be stimulated. Nystagmus toward the affected ear may also be seen in the recovery phases due to adaptation.

Other consequences of an acute destructive labyrinthine lesion are vertigo, usually with a rotatory component *away* from the side of the lesion; a tendency to fall toward the side of the lesion; gait ataxia; and secondary autonomic effects consisting of nausea, vomiting, pallor, sweating, and anxiety. Oscillopsia, which is a subjective visual sensation of to-and-fro movement in the environment, may accompany the nystagmus.

Because any head movement worsens the side-to-side discrepancy of vestibular input due to a gain imbalance when one labyrinth is totally or relatively inactive, movement usually exacerbates the vertigo and other symptoms. For this reason, affected patients prefer to keep their heads still. In the presence of bilateral vestibular destruction, there may be little vertigo but gait ataxia may be the major symptom, emerging particularly when visual cues are removed, such as when getting up in the middle of the night. The system possesses a very strong adaptive capacity and, in the presence of an acute peripheral lesion, symptoms normally markedly abate within several days. Because this habituation may depend on the existence of adequate cerebellar function, patients with concurrent cerebellar lesions may never be able to adapt. Elderly patients are also much slower to adapt to the effects of vestibular lesions. Certain types of physiological vertigo, such as motion sickness, height vertigo, and visual vertigo, are due to a mismatch between the visual or somatosensory and the vestibular information.

CLINICAL PICTURE AND DIAGNOSIS

Patients complaining of dizziness are extremely common in general neurological and otolaryngological practice. The term *dizziness* is nonspecific and may be used to refer to such widely disparate symptoms as unsteadiness of gait, blurred vision, mental confusion, presyncopal sensations, or true vertigo. In true vertigo, patients experience a definite hallucination of motion, either of themselves or their environment.

Although rotatory sensations are most common, stemming from lesions of the semicircular canals, drifting (with otolith lesions), rocking (like the motion of a ship), or vague feelings of unsteadiness may also result from vestibular disorders. Patients should be encouraged to describe their dizziness in definite terms, such as lightheadedness, faintness, a drunken feeling, fogginess of thinking, or loss of balance. It is often useful to ask patients to compare their symptoms to that experienced as a child when they would whirl around and then suddenly stop.

The precipitating factors often provide important clues to the nature of the symptom. Vertigo that is precipitated by head movement, rolling over in bed, or sudden changes of posture from lying to standing (or vice versa) arises from a vestibular origin. However, head turning or extension may also cause vertebral artery compression in an older person, which in turn may produce transient brainstem ischemia with vertigo, usually accompanied by other symptoms. Assuming the upright posture may also elicit a dizzy, faint feeling due to orthostatic hypotension. Loud noises can precipitate vertigo in patients with labyrinthine perilymph fistulas (disruption of the labyrinthine membrane usually at the oval or round windows) or Meniere's disease. Sudden increases in middle ear pressure, such as occur with sneezing or when doors are slammed, may also provoke vertigo in patients with a fistula. In anxious individuals who find themselves in stressful circumstances, hyperventilation can be a common cause of dizziness, and this can be diagnosed by having the patient hyperventilate for 3 minutes to determine whether this precipitates the symptoms.

Other important factors that may have a bearing on the etiology of vertigo are a history of head trauma; the existence of hypertension, cardiac disease, or generalized or cerebrovascular disease; a history of migraine; and the ingestion of ototoxic drugs.

Once the presence of true vertigo is established, it is then necessary to distinguish peripheral vertigo from central vertigo and to identify a specific cause (Table 10-1). Peripheral vestibular lesions that involve the vestibular end-organ or eighth nerve constitute the vast major-

Table 10-1. Causes of Pathologic Vertigo

VESTIBULAR

External and middle ear
  Impacted cerumen
  Eustachian tube dysfunction
  Otitis media
  Tumors (e.g., cholesteatoma, glomus tumors)
  Otosclerosis
Inner ear
  Benign positional paroxysmal vertigo
    (?cupulolithiasis)
  Meniere's disease
  Viral neural labyrinthitis
  Labyrinthitis (acute suppurative, syphilis, Lyme's
    disease)
  Toxic (e.g., quinine, streptomycin)
  Post trauma
  Occlusion of labyrinthine blood supply
  Labyrinthine fistula
  Cogan's syndrome
Eighth nerve
  Acoustic neuroma
  Other cerebellopontine angle tumors (e.g.,
    meningioma, metastatic)
  Viral neural labyrinthitis (vestibular neuronitis)
  Infectious, inflammatory (e.g., herpes zoster,
    syphilis)
  Ischemic neuritis (e.g., diabetic)
Central

Supratentorial
  Epilepsy (temporal lobe)
  Psychogenic (with or without hyperventilation)
Infratentorial
  Multiple sclerosis
  Vertebrobasilar insufficiency
  Medullary/cerebellar infarction (e.g., lateral
    medullary syndrome)
  Migraine
  Spinocerebellar degenerations
  Syringobulbia
  Basilar impression
  Arnold-Chiari malformation
Other
  Toxic (heavy metals, anticonvulsants, alcohol,
    sedatives)
  Infectious, parainfectious
  Benign paroxysmal vertigo of childhood
  Hypothyroidism

NONVESTIBULAR

Visual
  With diplopia
  Post cataract surgery
Somatosensory
  Peripheral neuropathy
  Deep cervical lesions

ity of cases. These disorders are usually benign and transient. Central lesions involve the brainstem, cerebellum, or rarely the temporal lobes and pose a much more serious problem. The distinction is made on the basis of several factors (Table 10-2), the most important of which are the quality of the vertigo and the nature of the accompanying symptoms.

Central vertigo is rarely of the rotatory variety and usually lacks the severity and prominent accompanying autonomic symptoms (e.g., nausea and vomiting) seen with peripheral vestibular lesions. Symptoms pointing to auditory or middle ear involvement, such as tinnitus, hearing loss, recurrent ear infections, or discharge, strongly suggest a peripheral cause. Vertigo is

Table 10-2. Features Distinguishing Central from Peripheral Vertigo

Signs and symptoms	Peripheral vertigo[a]	Central vertigo[b]
Severity of vertigo	Marked	Mild
Direction of nystagmus	Mainly unidirectional, fast-phase opposite lesion	Bi- or unidirectional
Vertical nystagmus	Never present	May be present
Tinnitus and/or deafness	Often present	Usually present
Signs of brainstem dysfunction	Absent	Often present

[a]Lesions involve the vestibular end-organ or eighth nerve.
[b]Lesions involve the brainstem, cerebellum, and rarely the temporal lobes.

rarely the only symptom manifested by central lesions; usually there are also brainstem or cerebellar symptoms such as diplopia, total loss of vision or gray-outs, facial numbness, dysarthria, dysphagia, weakness, ataxia, or loss of consciousness. However, patients with peripheral vertigo may also lose consciousness, arising because of a vasovagal syncopal attack secondary to the concomitant autonomic stimulation. Epileptic vertigo may also present with loss of consciousness following a vertiginous aura. The vertigo seen with central lesions tends to be persistent and continuous, whereas that seen with peripheral lesions is usually intermittent and recurrent and attacks may be as brief as a few seconds or minutes. The clinical picture presented by lesions of the labyrinth, vestibular nuclei, and vestibular cerebellum may be indistinguishable.

Positional and Positioning Vertigo

Positional vertigo, which occurs when the patient's head is in certain positions (e.g., supine with the head turned to one side or standing with the head extended), and positioning vertigo, which is precipitated by changes in body or head position, usually indicate labyrinthine dysfunction and are most commonly seen in the syndrome of benign positional paroxysmal vertigo (BPPV). This syndrome may occur as a sequel to head trauma or stem from the presence of loose degenerated otoconia from the utricular macula lying on the cupula of the posterior semicircular canal—cupulolithiasis. Although central lesions such as metastatic tumors of the cerebellum or developmental anomalies of the hindbrain (Fig. 10-1) may also produce positional vertigo, its characteristics in this context differ from those of the peripheral variety.

In patients with positional or positioning vertigo, the clinician tries to reproduce their symptoms, along with positional nystagmus, by first having them assume and maintain the supine, supine right lateral, supine left lateral, and supine with head hyperextended position for 30 seconds each. Then the examiner can use the Nylen (or Hallpike-Dix) maneuver, which consists of abruptly throwing the patient backward from a sitting position with the legs extended

to a supine position, with the head supported and turned to one side hanging over the edge of the table. Initially, the patient keeps the head and eyes to the right. The test is then repeated (following a 5-minute interval if the result is positive) with the patient's head and eyes kept to the left. In the presence of positional vertigo-nystagmus of the peripheral type, 3 to 30 seconds will elapse before vertigo and nystagmus arises. In addition, the vertigo is usually quite severe and distressing, it fatigues after about 30 seconds, and repetition of the test will reveal some habituation, with the symptoms becoming progressively less pronounced. Characteristically a burst of mixed upbeat-torsional nystagmus is observed. Abruptly sitting the patient up will often elicit vertigo and nystagmus in the opposite direction. Positional vertigo-nystagmus of the central type may appear immediately upon throwing the patient backward. It is also less severe, continues as long as the patient is held in the head-hanging position, and the response to repeated testing will be undiminished.

Other Relevant Clinical Findings

Several other aspects of the physical and neurological examination may also provide useful information about vestibular function. To search for **past-pointing,** patients extend their arms and place their fingertips opposite those of the examiner's. With the eyes closed, the arms are elevated above the head and then returned to the starting position. If there is a vestibular lesion, the patient's arms may deviate to the side of the lesion. To perform the **sharpened Romberg** test, the patient attempts to stand with one foot directly behind the other and the arms folded across the chest. Patients with vestibular lesions have difficulty keeping their balance in this position when the eyes are closed. Patients with cerebellar lesions have difficulty even with eyes open. The patient can be asked to walk slowly forward then backward in the heel-to-toe position (**tandem gait**). The patient's performance will be poor if their vertigo is due to cerebellar or vestibular lesions.

The **fistula test** is performed by compressing the air column in the external canal by pressing

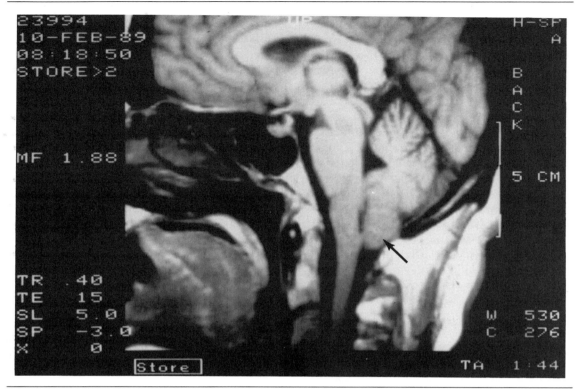

Fig. 10-1. *MRI scan from a 46-year-old woman with long-standing positional vertigo and normal neurological findings. This sagittal view shows the cerebellar tonsils lying below the foramen magnum, indicating an occult mild Arnold-Chiari malformation* (arrow).

on the tragus or by insufflating air through a specially equipped otoscope. A sudden experience of vertigo suggests a fistula located between the perilymph and middle ear spaces, which may be congenital or acquired as the result of head trauma, barotrauma, or infection.

VOR gain can be evaluated using the ophthalmoscope to determine whether the optic disc remains stable as the head is gently oscillated. Visual acuity is tested while the patient's head is moved gently back and forth, and should also not change, provided the VOR is intact. The head shaking test is done to look for nystagmus in patients who have compensated unilateral vestibular lesions and no spontaneous nystagmus. In this test, patients shake their heads as quickly as possible for about 20 cycles, and nystagmus is sought, with patients wearing Frenzl's glasses to facilitate detection.

Tests of Vestibular Function

Caloric Testing

Caloric testing is normally done in the laboratory in conjunction with electronystagmography (ENG), which furnishes a quantitative permanent record and also allows evaluation of oculomotor function. The test is done either with the patient supine and the head elevated 30 degrees or sitting with the head extended back 60 degrees, which brings the horizontal canal into a vertical position to promote the maximal effect of convection currents. The ear canal is checked to make sure there is free access to the eardrum and no perforation. Cold water (30°C) and warm water (44°C) are successively infused into each ear with 5 minutes elapsing between tests. Twenty milliliters is injected over 20 seconds and the duration of the nystagmus is recorded. In normal individuals, because the effect of the cold water mimics a destructive labyrinthine lesion, nystagmus occurs toward the opposite side and lasts for 80 to 120 seconds. Warm water elicits nystagmus in the opposite direction. Although the nystagmus may be easily observed, the patient wears Frenzl's glasses (20-diopter lenses mounted in goggles), which eliminate visual fixation and have an internal light source. This facilitates quantification of the nystagmus and the patient cannot then use visual fixation to reduce the nystagmus. If patients do not exhibit nystagmus with 20 ml of water, larger quantities of water or a few milliliters of ice water should be tried.

The duration of the nystagmus and amplitude are reflections of vestibular responsiveness. When nystagmus fails to develop or lasts at least 30 seconds less with both cold and hot water irrigation compared to the opposite ear, this is deemed **canal paresis.** An excitability difference of 25 percent or more indicates some disorder within the peripheral vestibular system. If there is a **directional preponderance,** this implies that the nystagmus tends to predominate toward the right or the left independently of the ear irrigated. The direction of the nystagmus is usually toward a central lesion and away from a peripheral vestibular lesion. Combinations of canal paresis and directional preponderance can occur.

Besides providing an objective test of vestibular function, caloric testing allows the patient to experience true vertigo, which may help clarify the nature of his or her own dizziness. A mini ice-water caloric test (using 0.5 ml) can be performed at the bedside (preferably with the patient wearing Frenzl's glasses) to detect a pronounced vestibular underresponsiveness. Conventional vestibular tests cannot detect lesions of the vertical semicircular canal or otolith organs, however, and therefore cannot be used to exclude a vestibular disorder.

Electronystagmography

Electrodes placed at the outer canthi of each eye and above and below one eye can record eye movement potentials arising from the positive charge carried by the cornea in relation to the retina. Spontaneous and evoked nystagmus

as well as pursuit and saccadic eye movements can be recorded in this fashion. The speed of the slow phase of the nystagmus can also be measured and the effects of removal of fixation by eye closure are easily determined. ENG cannot detect torsional nystagmus, which is commonly observed in patients with BPPV, and therefore negative findings cannot be considered to exclude a peripheral vestibular disorder.

Other Tests

Various **audiometric tests,** including pure-tone audiometry, stapedius reflex measurement, speech discrimination, and brainstem evoked response audiometry, can indicate whether a hearing deficit in a patient with vertigo is cochlear, retrocochlear, or central in origin.

Brainstem auditory evoked responses provide sensitive objective information about auditory pathways, which may be affected together with vestibular pathways.

Patients can be placed in specialized **rotating chairs** and their ENG responses recorded during different maneuvers. This can measure vestibular function objectively and evaluate the adaptive process following vestibular injury.

Some Specific Syndromes

Benign Positional Paroxysmal Vertigo

BPPV is one of the most common causes of intermittent vertigo. It may be caused by infection, head trauma, or cupulolithiasis. The latter condition refers to displacement of degenerated otoconia material from the utricular macula onto the cupola of the posterior semicircular canal. Symptoms characteristically occur when the patient changes body or head position, such as when rolling over in bed, bending over, and straightening up or extending the neck. The characteristic burst of brief upbeat-torsional nystagmus following the test for postural vertigo confirms diagnosis. A negative test result and a normal ENG, which does not record torsional nystagmus, do not rule out the disorder, however. Between attacks, many patients experience a vague sensation of dysequilibrium or unsteadiness. Vestibular exercises have been beneficial in a high percentage of patients by promoting gradual adaptation to the disorder.

(handwritten margin notes: ① 30–50 yo; ② hearing loss; ③ tinnitus; vertigo b/f by 6–12mo; sense pressure/fullness in ear)

Meniere's Disease

Meniere's disease usually appears between the ages of 30 and 50 years. In fully developed cases, besides attacks of vertigo, patients also suffer hearing loss (for low-pitched tones initially) and tinnitus, although vertigo may precede hearing problems by 6 to 12 months. Fifteen to twenty percent of the cases are bilateral. The attacks of vertigo, which normally last from 1 to 24 hours, are often preceded by a sensation of fullness in the involved ear. Nystagmus is usually toward the affected side (irritative) early in the attack but away from the involved ear (paralytic) later. The condition is also known as *endolymphatic hydrops* because it is caused by an overaccumulation of endolymph, which may lead to ruptures in the membranous labyrinthine structures.

(handwritten left margin: Mngt ① bed rest ② elim tobacco ③ sedation ④ antiemetics)

Management of the acute attack involves bed rest, elimination of tobacco use, sedation (e.g., diazepam, lorazepam, or promethazine), and the administration of antiemetics and anti–motion sickness drugs, delivered orally, parenterally by rectal suppository, or transdermally (e.g., dimenhydrinate, scopolamine, or droperidol). Diuretics, a low-salt diet, antihistamines, and vasodilators have also been recommended as part of treatment, and are perhaps of some long-term benefit in the prevention of attacks.

Various surgical interventions have been devised for the treatment of intractable incapacitating vertigo. A labyrinthectomy can be performed when the disease is unilateral, of more than 2 years' duration, and hearing is severely and irreversibly impaired (since it will be lost postoperatively). Other procedures include endolymphatic-subarachnoid shunts and section of the vestibular nerve.

Vestibular Neuronitis

(handwritten: ① follow viral infxn ② hearing preserved ③ tinnitus)

Vestibular neuronitis (viral neural labyrinthitis) refers to the condition of recurrent bouts of vertigo experienced following a viral (usually upper respiratory) infection. Such patients may also exhibit hearing problems or tinnitus. Many of these patients have no clear-cut antecedent history of viral illness and the cause is therefore presumptive. Recurrent bouts of vertigo, often precipitated by postural changes, may stretch over the course of several months. Long-term

(handwritten bottom: Mngt — ① meclizine + betahistine. scopolamine)

use of agents such as meclizine or betahistine may reduce the frequency and duration of attacks. Transdermal scopolamine may also be useful for treating acute attacks. However, these agents may interfere with the natural central adaptive process.

(handwritten: ① tinnitus + hearing impair precede vertigo)

Acoustic Neuroma

A slow-growing benign tumor, acoustic neuroma (schwannoma) usually forms on the vestibular division of the eighth nerve within the internal auditory canal. Tinnitus and hearing impairment (especially speech discrimination deficits that are manifested as difficulties understanding on the telephone) usually precede the vertigo. When it appears, the vertigo is usually mild and continuous, and the patient's gait is unsteady. The tumor tends to involve the seventh and then the fifth cranial nerves as it grows out of the canal into the cerebellopontine angle. Early reduction of the corneal reflex and sensation over a portion of the external ear canal may be detected.

As the tumor enlarges, there is lower cranial nerve involvement, brainstem compression, and raised intracranial pressure. The protein level in the cerebrospinal fluid may be substantially elevated in the presence of larger tumors. Bilateral acoustic neuromas are virtually confined to cases of neurofibromatosis.

Early diagnosis is essential if the tumor is to be removed via a retrolabyrinthine, rather than intracranial, approach; this offers the best possibility for the preservation of hearing and seventh nerve function. Audiometry usually demonstrates sensorineural hearing loss, with speech discrimination and tone decay most affected. There is no recruitment as there is in Meniere's disease, and Békésy audiometry most commonly shows a type IV pattern. Brainstem auditory evoked potentials also show fairly distinctive changes early in the course. Caloric testing reveals the existence of an underactive canal. Plain radiographs of the skull with Stenver's views often show widening, "trumpeting," and erosion of the medial aspect of the internal auditory canal. Tomograms are often necessary to demonstrate these changes. An enhanced computed tomographic (CT) scan readily detects all but very small tumors (Fig. 10-2). Use of air or metrizamide with the CT scan improves the rate of detection. However, the most sensitive test is a T_1-weighted gadolinium-enhanced magnetic resonance imaging scan with cuts through the cerebellopontine angle.

Cerebrovascular Disease

Transient ischemic attacks or infarcts within the vertebrobasilar system can produce vertigo, but almost always in combination with other brainstem or cerebellar signs. Vertigo is one of the components of the lateral medullary syndrome.

Postural vertigo may occur at the onset of a cerebellar infarction within the posterior inferior cerebellar artery territory. Signs of homolateral limb ataxia accompany the vertigo. Sudden onset of vertigo with or without deafness may rarely stem from occlusion of the internal auditory artery or its divisions, resulting from embolization, atherosclerotic disease in the basilar system, or vasculitis.

Multiple Sensory Deficits

Particularly in elderly and diabetic patients, a combination of visual, proprioceptive, and ves-

Fig. 10-2. *(A) CT scan showing a large enhancing right acoustic neuroma* (T) *in a 60-year-old woman with a 1- to 2-year history of progressive gait ataxia, brief spasms of the right face when she stood up, and recent-onset headache. She had gradually become deaf in that ear and experienced progressively worsening vertigo over the same period. She had been told she had Meniere's disease. Examination revealed deafness in the right ear, vertical and horizontal nystagmus worse on left gaze, a right fifth nerve sensory loss, and a tendency to fall to the right.*

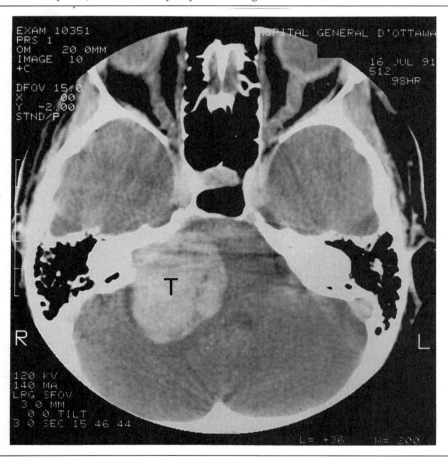

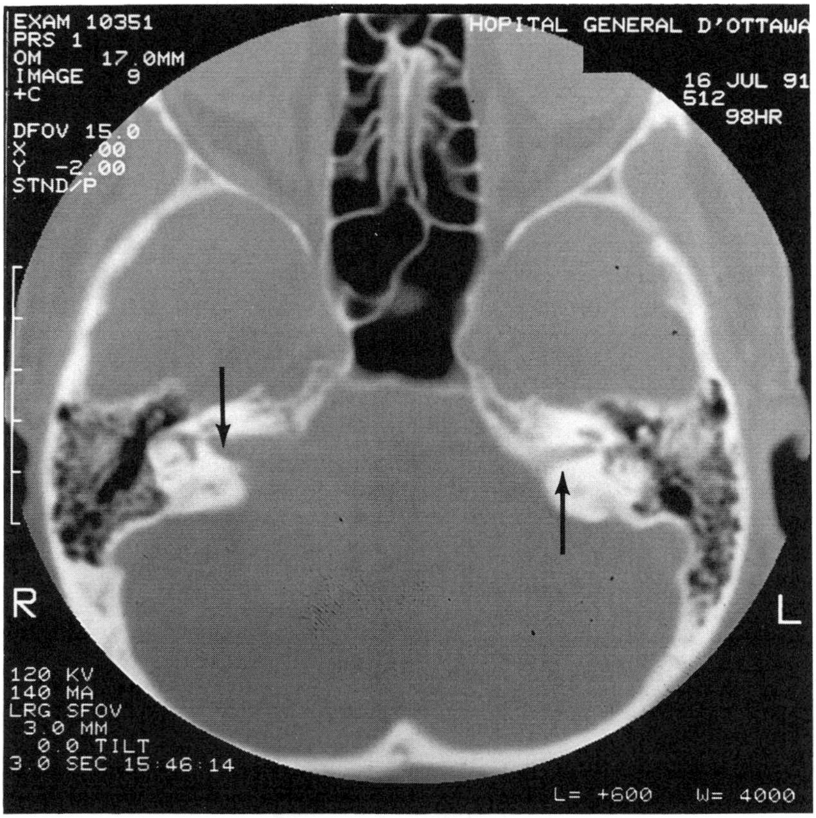

Fig. 10-2. *(B) CT scan with bone windows* (arrows) *revealing widening of the internal auditory canal on the side of the tumor, virtual proof of an acoustic neuroma.*

tibular dysfunction can lead to vertigo, gait instability, and possibly falls.

MANAGEMENT

Specific causes of vertigo, some of which have been dealt with, require appropriate medical or surgical treatment. Acute bouts of disabling vertigo are managed as described for Meniere's disease. However, it is important to avoid prescribing sedative and other medication, if possible, to allow patients to adapt to their symptoms.

Patients with persistent positional vertigo can learn to avoid the positions or movements that precipitate their attacks. Desensitization should be attempted by having patients do a series of graded vestibular exercises. These specific movements may actually displace the offending calcific material from the posterior semicircular canal. If a patient can fixate visually on an object during vertiginous attacks of peripheral origin, this may reduce the vertigo. Vestibular nerve sectioning may be used as a last resort in the treatment of intractable persistent cases of positional vertigo. Due to the extremely distressing nature of the symptom, some patients with severe vertigo live in dread of their next attack. Phobic anxiety may then develop, which itself requires specific psychological management.

BIBLIOGRAPHY

Arenberg, I. K., and Smith, D. B. (editors). Diagnostic neurology. *Neurol. Clin.* 8:199–481, 1990.

Baloh, R. W. The dizzy patient: treatment options. In V. Hachinski (editor). *Challenges in Neurology*. Philadelphia: Davis, 1992, Pp. 15–27.

Baloh, R. W., Honrubia, V., and Jacobson, K. Benign positional vertigo: clinical and oculographic features in 240 cases. *Neurology* 37:371–378, 1987.

Baloh, R. W., Jacobson, K., and Honrubia, V. Idiopathic bilateral vestibulopathy. *Neurology* 39:272–275, 1989.

Barber, H. O. Diagnostic techniques in vertigo. *J. Vertigo* 1:1–16, 1974.

Barber, H. O., and Sharpe, J. A. *Vestibular Disorders*. Chicago: Mosby–Year Book, 1988.

Brandt, T., and Daroff, R. B. The multisensory physiological and pathological vertigo syndromes. *Ann. Neurol.* 7:195–203, 1980.

Brandt, T. Man in motion: historical and clinical aspects of vestibular function. A Review. *Brain* 114:2154–2157, 1991.

Daroff, R. B. Vertigo. *Am. Fam. Phys.* 16:143–150, 1977.

Drachman, D. A., and Hart, C. W. An approach to the dizzy patient. *Neurology* 22:323–334, 1972.

Hain, T. C., and Zee, D. S. The dizzy patient: diagnostic approaches. In V. Hachinski (editor). *Challenges in Neurology*. Philadelphia: Davis, 1992, Pp. 3–14.

Henriksson, N. G., et al. A synopsis of the vestibular system. *Sandoz Monogr.* 1972, Pp. 1–65.

Troost, B. T., and Patton, J. M. Exercise therapy for positional vertigo. *Neurology* 42:1441–1444, 1992.

Wolfson, R. J., et al. Vertigo. *Ciba Found. Symp.* 34:2–32, 1982.

Neuroophthalmology

Neurological and muscular diseases frequently cause oculomotor, pupillary, or visual disturbances. These neuroophthalmological signs can often be used to aid in the precise localization of lesions. The ability to detect objective neuroophthalmological abnormalities allows precise documentation of the lesion progression. Tests now in widespread use include orbital computed tomographic (CT) scanning or magnetic resonance imaging, plotting of visual fields, electrooculography (or electronystagmography), electroretinography, retinal fluorescein angiography, and visual evoked potentials. The neuroophthalmological bedside examination is covered in Chapter 2. This chapter emphasizes the major neuroophthalmological symptoms and their diagnostic significance.

EYE MOVEMENTS AND THEIR DISORDERS

Normal Eye Movements

A complex and finely regulated nervous and muscular system is responsible for acquiring and maintaining a visual image on the macula of each retina during fixation, pursuit, and saccades. As one visually pursues a slowly moving object or quickly initiates saccades to shift fixation from one object to another, normally both eyes move smoothly and conjugately, such that the visual axes are aligned, and there are no readily apparent extraneous movements or oscillations. Saccades are initiated in part by the **frontal eye fields** located on each side anterior to the motor strip. Axons from these neurons descend in the internal capsule and cross in the oculomotor decussation of the midbrain to reach the contralateral pons, from where the final common pathway for pursuit and saccades originates.

The **superior colliculi** also play a role in saccadic gaze. Burst cells responsible for the generation of horizontal saccadic eye movements lie in the **parapontine reticular formation** (PPRF). These cells project to the abducens nucleus, which contains motor neurons that innervate the ipsilateral lateral rectus muscle and interneurons that decussate in the **medial longitudinal fasciculus,** and then ascend to innervate the contralateral medial rectus.

The brainstem centers for vertical gaze lie more rostrally and dorsally around the meso-diencephalic junction. The critical structure involved in vertical eye movements is the rostral interstitial nucleus of the medial longitudinal fasciculus. In a fashion analogous to the PPRF, burst cells responsible for generating vertical saccades are located in this nucleus.

Upgaze commands ascend to cross in the posterior commissure and pretectal area and downgaze commands pass directly downward to the third and fourth nerve nuclei. Pursuit commands descend from higher cortical centers to the ipsilateral pontine nuclei. The parietal lobes play an important role in governing smooth pursuit, as evidenced by the impairment of ipsilateral smooth pursuit seen in patients with parietal lobe lesions. Cells in the occipital striate cortex also influence pursuit gaze.

Because the anatomical systems involved with pursuit and saccadic gaze are partially separated, rarely either of these systems may be selectively impaired. A partially separate vergence system is responsible for the dysconjugate movements seen during normal convergence or divergence. Vestibular inputs also produce reflex eye movements to compensate for head or body movements (see Chapter 10). The actions of cranial nerves III, IV, and VI supplying the extraocular muscles are dealt with in Chapter 2.

Diplopia

Diplopia, or double vision, if real, is virtually always a sign of a defect either in the innervation of the extraocular muscles or in the muscles themselves. Although central diplopia has been described, it is extremely rare, and therefore diplopia generally signifies a lesion affecting the midbrain, pons, cranial nerves III, IV, and VI, or the extraocular muscles.

An **internuclear ophthalmoplegia** (INO) (see later discussion) may or may not give rise to diplopia. Monocular diplopia is either psychogenic in origin or arises because of abnormalities of the ocular media, especially the lens. Affected patients can usually describe whether the two images are separated in the horizontal or vertical planes, in which particular direction

of gaze the diplopia is maximal, and whether the diplopia is worse on near gaze (third or fourth nerve palsy) or distant gaze (sixth nerve palsy).

Misalignment of the visual axes may be readily apparent or so subtle that special techniques, such as a Maddox rod, are needed to detect it. The red glass test (see Chapter 2) is a helpful bedside technique for determining which particular nerve or muscle is involved. An intermittent diplopia (e.g., myasthenia gravis), the head tilt that occurs in the opposite direction to the side of a fourth nerve palsy, and ptosis or pupillary dilatation that may accompany a third nerve palsy are helpful clues to diagnosis. Patients with long-standing misalignment of the eyes due to strabismus do not complain of diplopia and usually exhibit full eye movements when each eye is tested individually.

Palsies of Cranial Nerves III, IV, or VI

Individual cranial nerves supplying the extraocular muscles may be compromised within the brainstem at the level of their nuclei or between the nucleus and point of emergence from the brainstem. They may also be affected within the posterior cranial fossa or at the level of the tentorium as they cross the subarachnoid space, within the cavernous sinus, as they pass through the superior orbital fissure, or within the orbit itself. Disease that affects the extraocular muscles, such as ocular myasthenia or dysthyroid ophthalmopathy or intraorbital disease, can cause eye movement abnormalities that at times mimic the ocular manifestations of individual nerve palsies.

Third Nerve
Lesions of the third nerve produce various combinations of ptosis, pupillary dilatation, and ophthalmoplegia with the eye in a down-and-out position. The two third nerve nuclei in the midbrain tegmentum consist of various subnuclei lying near the midline. These subnuclei provide ipsilateral innervation to their respective muscles, except for the superior rectus, which receives a contralateral supply. The

levator palpebri are supplied bilaterally by a midline subnucleus, and therefore a discrete midbrain lesion can cause bilateral ptosis, which rarely occurs in isolation. The Edinger-Westphal nucleus supplying the pupil is located anterosuperiorly.

A third nerve lesion at the nuclear level or involving its fibers as they course forward in the midbrain is usually due to a vascular lesion, although neoplasms and trauma are also considerations. Other accompanying neurological signs, such as a contralateral hemiplegia (Weber's syndrome) or contralateral ataxia and intention tremor (Benedikt's syndrome), point to the existence of an intrinsic midbrain lesion.

An expanding aneurysm at the junction of the posterior communicating and internal carotid arteries is a strong possibility in the context of any acutely or subacutely appearing painful third nerve palsy. Third nerve impairment may occur before actual rupture or leakage. Pupillary involvement is almost always seen when oculomotor paralysis is complete. Diabetic or hypertensive vascular disease may precipitate an infarct of the third nerve that tends to involve the central portion of the nerve and spare the more peripheral pupilloconstrictor fibers. Pain is a frequent but not invariable accompaniment of this disorder. Complete recovery within three months is the rule. Rarely pupillary sparing has been reported with infiltrative or lymphomatous lesions. When the pupil is intact in the presence of an otherwise complete acute or subacute third nerve palsy, patients can be spared the need of undergoing angiography, provided they recover within 3 months and there is evidence of diabetes or vascular disease as the source of the problem. The third nerve may also be affected by trauma, neoplasms, or inflammatory processes (e.g., syphilis or meningitis) at various points along its course. Cavernous sinus lesions such as tumors and aneurysms may lead to isolated third nerve involvement.

Ophthalmoplegic migraine begins in childhood and occurs in the context of a well-developed migraine syndrome, typically appearing when the headache has reached its zenith or is receding. Transtentorial herniation of the uncus of the temporal lobe due to an expanding supra-tentorial mass elicits the early appearance of third nerve palsy together with initial pupillary dilatation, which is explained by the fact that the third nerve courses along the edge of the tentorial notch. Within the anterior cavernous sinus or superior orbital fissure, the nerve divides into two branches. A lesion that involves the superior division produces superior rectus weakness and levator palsy (ptosis).

Fourth Nerve

The fourth nerve crosses in the dorsal midbrain and supplies the contralateral superior oblique muscle. The eye may be elevated at rest in the presence of a fourth nerve palsy. Diplopia is worsened either when the head is tilted toward the side of the palsy or by contralateral gaze. Characteristically the head is held tilted toward the side opposite the palsy with the faced turned toward the same side and the chin depressed. Head trauma, which can be relatively minor, is the most common cause of a unilateral or bilateral fourth nerve palsy. Diabetes, other vascular diseases, and neoplasms are additional causes.

Sixth Nerve

A lesion of the sixth nerve nucleus produces an ipsilateral gaze palsy plus a lateral rectus palsy (Fig. 11-1). Because the seventh nerve wraps around the sixth nerve nucleus within the pons, intrinsic pontine vascular lesions may affect these nerves together, at times in conjunction with a contralateral hemiplegia. The sixth nerve is commonly involved by a neoplastic process (e.g., nasopharyngeal, sinus, or metastatic carcinoma), especially at the base of the skull as it ascends along the clivus. Pontine gliomas or cerebellopontine angle tumors may also produce sixth nerve lesions.

An isolated sixth nerve palsy may occur in combination with elevated intracranial pressure (e.g., pseudotumor cerebri), but in this instance has no localizing value. Mastoiditis and otitis causing inflammation at the apex of the petrous bone and sixth nerve involvement in combination with hearing impairment comprises **Gradenigo's syndrome.** The sixth nerve may also be involved in patients suffering from dia-

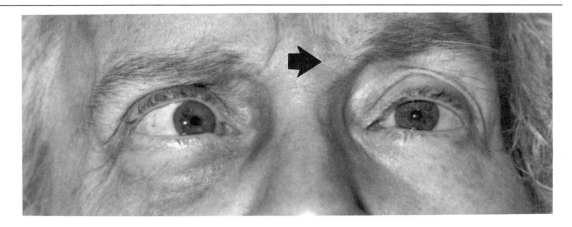

Fig. 11-1. *Left sixth nerve palsy and ptosis in a patient with a cordoma of the clivus invading the cavernous sinus. The patient is attempting to gaze to the left. Note the asymmetrical position of the light reflex with respect to the pupil.*

betes, aneurysms, head trauma, Wernicke's encephalopathy, or multiple sclerosis.

Basal skull films, CT or magnetic resonance imaging, a glucose tolerance test or 2-hour postprandial glucose test, VDRL, cerebrospinal fluid (CSF) analysis, and, in some cases, angiography are part of the investigation of an isolated sixth nerve palsy. Full investigation of an isolated painless sixth nerve palsy is not necessary in an elderly patient unless there is no resolution after 3 months.

Duane's syndrome is a congenital abnormality consisting of horizontal ocular movements that produce limited abduction, and may be confused with a sixth nerve palsy. The upper lid in such patients shows an apparent elevation with attempted abduction and apparent depression with adduction. Forced duction tests may reveal restricted abduction, but aberrant lateral rectus innervation is thought to be responsible in most cases.

Cavernous Sinus Syndromes

Structures traversing the cavernous sinus include the third, fourth, and sixth cranial nerves, the first two divisions of the fifth nerve, sympathetic fibers supplying the pupil, and the carotid artery. Various combinations of these structures may be impaired when there are le-

sions in this area. Parasellar tumors, carotid aneurysms, carotid-cavernous fistulas (spontaneous, posttraumatic, or secondary to ruptured aneurysms), metastatic and invasive tumors originating from the base of the skull (e.g., nasopharyngeal carcinoma), and thrombosis resulting from inflammatory lesions and hypercoagulable states may all be responsible. Besides the neurological signs, proptosis, orbital chemosis, and an orbital bruit (with carotid-cavernous fistulas) may be seen. Specialized CT and angiographic techniques are often necessary to visualize this region.

Tolosa-Hunt Syndrome

Idiopathic recurrent painful ophthalmoplegia due to a nonspecific granulomatous infiltration around the cavernous sinus or superior orbital fissure comprises the Tolosa-Hunt syndrome. The diagnosis is one of exclusion, because lymphomatous and leukemic infiltrations, infectious meningeal involvement, collagen disease, and aneurysms may manifest a similar clinical picture. It may be necessary to perform meningeal biopsy to help confirm the diagnosis. Angiography may reveal narrowing of the intracavernous portion of the carotid artery and there may be a mild CSF pleocytosis and protein elevation. Ipsilateral sellar erosion and concurrent seventh nerve involvement have been reported. Steroids, which are prescribed once specific causes have been excluded, typically bring about a good response.

Eye Movement Abnormalities with Intrinsic Pontine and Other Posterior Fossa Lesions

Pontine versus Frontal Gaze Palsy

Damage acutely incurred in the frontal gaze center causes the eyes to deviate toward the side of the lesion, away from an accompanying hemiplegia. The saccadic palsy encountered in these cases is usually temporary and tends to remit, with recovery of full consciousness. Pontine gaze palsies are often bilateral, asymmetrical, and rarely isolated. They cause eye deviation away from the side of the lesion and tend to last much longer than the frontal palsies. The various causes of pontine gaze palsies include pontine infarcts, hemorrhages, gliomas, abscesses, Wernicke's encephalopathy, and multiple sclerosis.

Internuclear Ophthalmoplegia

A lesion of the medial longitudinal fasciculus impairs adduction in the ipsilateral eye and causes nystagmus in the contralateral eye on gaze away from the side of involvement. It is called *internuclear* because the lesion lies between the sixth and opposite third nerve nuclei. Convergence is usually intact, thus ruling out a third nerve lesion as the source of the adduction deficit. At times this syndrome may be subtle but can be detected as an asymmetry seen during optokinetic nystagmus (OKN) with slowed adduction and decreased amplitude of the fast phase. Asymmetries of nystagmus observed during cold water caloric testing or by electrooculography may also reveal its existence. There is usually no diplopia. The most common cause in the elderly is brainstem infarction, but in younger patients the syndrome strongly suggests multiple sclerosis. Trauma and neoplasms are other causes. Although an INO is a strong indication of an intrinsic brainstem lesion, it can occasionally be associated with metabolic disorders such as hepatic encephalopathy and

can be mimicked closely in patients with myasthenia gravis.

Other Eye Movement Abnormalities

Wall-eyed bilateral INO is a bilateral exotropia (i.e., manifest outward eye deviation) that occurs in conjunction with a bilateral INO. Pontine infarction or demyelination are the usual causes.

"One and a half" syndrome is produced by a lesion involving the PPRF and ipsilateral medial longitudinal fasciculus that causes impairment of all horizontal conjugate eye movements, except for abduction of the contralateral eye.

Ocular bobbing consists of a conjugate involuntary recurrent downward movement of the eyes and is seen in patients with acute pontine lesions who are in a comatose or locked-in state. Horizontal eye movements are absent. In these patients there is usually a rapid downward movement with a slower return to the neutral position. Monocular bobbing and reverse (upward) bobbing may also be seen.

Skew deviation represents a misalignment of the eyes observed in the vertical plane that is not due to a lesion of the third or fourth cranial nerves. Vertical diplopia results. The lesion responsible is thought to be located in the pons, usually on the side of the higher eye, but may also be in the cerebellum.

The **sylvian aqueduct syndrome (Parinaud's syndrome)** includes a vertical gaze palsy, paresis of convergence, convergence-retraction nystagmus combined with pupillary hyporeactivity, and light-near dissociation. The lesion responsible, often a tumor such as a pinealoma, a vascular lesion, or hydrocephalus, is located at the midbrain tectum level.

Progressive Supranuclear Palsy

In supranuclear, as opposed to nuclear or infranuclear gaze palsies, voluntary and saccadic eye movements are affected, whereas various reflex eye movements such as the oculocephalic movements and Bell's phenomenon (i.e., upward eye deviation with forced eye closure) are relatively preserved. Progressive supranuclear palsy

(PSP) is an idiopathic syndrome with a prevalence of 1.4 per 100,000. It is also known as the Steele-Richardson-Olszewski syndrome. It should be considered in the differential diagnosis of patients with suspected Parkinson's disease and exhibits a fairly stereotyped clinical picture. Onset usually occurs in the sixth or seventh decade, and there is a 2 to 1 male-to-female predominance. Gait disturbance with falling is often the earliest symptom. Patients show a progressive paralysis of gaze mechanisms, beginning with early downgaze impairment and often leading to a total absence of voluntary gaze. Blepharospasm may occur as well.

Occasional patients do not exhibit apparent eye signs, or do so very late in the course. In addition, there is commonly an axial dystonia (with a tendency for the neck to be held hyperextended), pseudobulbar features with marked dysarthria, corticospinal tract involvement, mild parkinsonian symptoms, and a mild subcortical dementia.

CT and magnetic resonance imaging show marked atrophy of the midbrain tegmentum with relative sparing of the peduncles. Patients survive an average of 5 to 10 years. High doses of L-dopa may be somewhat beneficial, and patients have occasionally responded to dopamine agonists such as bromocriptine. Walking aids, speech therapy, diet modification, and botulinum toxin to treat the blepharospasm can all help improve the patient's quality of life.

The pathological features are characteristic; electron microscopy shows neurofibrillary degeneration, but straight filaments are seen instead of the twisted tubules seen in Alzheimer's disease. Many subcortical locations are involved, including the globus pallidus, subthalamic nuclei, red nucleus, substantia nigra, periaqueductal gray matter, midbrain tectum, reticular formation of the pons and midbrain, median raphe, locus ceruleus, vestibular nuclei, and dentate nuclei. Disorders that can cause progressive supranuclear impairment of gaze include progressive supranuclear palsy (Steele-Richardson-Olszewski), olivopontocerebellar degeneration, neoplasms of the mesodiencephalic junction, Huntington's chorea, Whipple's disease of the central nervous system, ataxia telangiectasia, Wilson's disease, and lipid storage diseases.

Progressive External Ophthalmoplegia

Progressive external ophthalmoplegia (PEO) is a clinical entity stemming from multiple causes that consists of the gradual symmetrical impairment of eye movements and ptosis without pupillary involvement. Some specific conditions producing this picture are: myasthenia gravis, thyroid ophthalmopathy, Refsum disease, Bassen-Kornzweig disease, myotonic and oculopharyngeal dystrophy, and the Miller-Fisher variant of the Guillain-Barré syndrome. PEO is a common feature of a heterogeneous group of both myopathic and neurogenic degenerative disorders. Many of these patients manifest other neuromuscular or systemic abnormalities (the ophthalmoplegia-plus syndrome).

One relatively well defined subgroup is the **Kearns-Sayre syndrome,** in which PEO begins before age 20 and is associated with atypical pigmentary retinal degeneration, heart block, elevated CSF protein levels, and frequently short stature and mental retardation. Ragged red fibers are seen on trichrome-stained muscle biopsy specimens and electron microscopy reveals mitochondrial abnormalities. This condition belongs to a group of genetic disorders known as the *mitochondrial encephalomyopathies,* and is characterized by deletions in the mitochondrial DNA. Maternal inheritance is a characteristic of these syndromes, which is in keeping with the fact that mitochondrial DNA is inherited through the mother. Ragged red fibers are a nonspecific finding and have also been seen in the context of other mitochondrial disorders as well as myopathies such as polymyositis. Prophylactic cardiac pacemakers should be implanted in these patients because of the risk of sudden fatal cardiac arrhythmias.

NYSTAGMUS AND RELATED EYE MOVEMENT DISORDERS

Nystagmus results from an abnormality in the slow phase of eye movements (see also Chapters 2 and 10). Therefore, the initial phase of nystagmus is a slow eye movement. The corrective phase may either be a slow eye movement (pendular nystagmus) or a fast eye movement (jerk nystagmus). Nystagmus may give rise to symptoms of blurred vision or oscillopsia, but most commonly goes unnoticed by the patient. Electrooculography has been used to analyze nystagmus and other involuntary eye oscillations and has revealed that this is an exceedingly complex subject. Only a few specific types are mentioned here and the following ones are special forms of nystagmus and extraneous ocular movements that possess some localizing significance.

The **gaze-paretic form of nystagmus** is fairly coarse and maximal when gazing in the direction of gaze weakness, with the fast component toward the side of gaze weakness. It arises from gaze paresis stemming from a cerebellar hemisphere lesion that possibly secondarily affects the gaze-holding network in the pons. **Vertical upbeat nystagmus** is seen in the presence of brainstem lesions, lesions of the anterior vermis of the cerebellum, and drug toxicity (e.g., phenytoin). **Convergence-retraction nystagmus** consists of a rhythmic retraction of the eyes into the orbit with convergence movements provoked by upward gaze (e.g., by looking at a downward moving OKN tape). It is not actually a true nystagmus. The lesion responsible is situated around the sylvian aqueduct and usually compresses the midbrain-pretectal region.

Downbeat nystagmus is often best seen when the patient's eyes are looking downward and laterally. The causative lesion is frequently located around the foramen magnum and affects the medulla or cerebellum. This form of nystagmus is most typically seen in the context of an Arnold-Chiari malformation, basilar impression, or cerebellar degenerations.

Rebound nystagmus is that elicited when a patient is gazing from the lateral position toward the midline. It occurs on re-fixation after a prolonged lateral gaze, and the fast phase is in the direction opposite the preceding lateral gaze. The lesion responsible is cerebellar.

In **periodic alternating nystagmus**, there is a regular cycling, first to one side for 1 to 2 minutes then, after a brief interval without nystagmus, jerking to the opposite side for 1 to 2 minutes. The lesion is in the brainstem or cerebellum.

Opsoclonus consists of chaotic involuntary conjugate multidirectional eye movements ("dancing eyes") that are seen most typically in association with ataxia and myoclonus in children with or without an underlying neuroblastoma. Brainstem-cerebellar encephalitis, underlying carcinoma and amitriptyline overdose, may also cause it. Opsoclonus, ocular dysmetria, and flutterlike oscillations are thought to reflect varying degrees of cerebellar abnormalities.

PTOSIS

Ptosis is an abnormal drooping of the eyelid, in which, according to the criteria of Caplan, the eyelid covers more than one third of the cornea, it measures more than 8 mm in vertical dimension, or the drooping is greater than that previously observed. A lesion anywhere along the third nerve tends to produce ptosis, which is bilateral in patients with nuclear lesions. Ptosis is also one of the signs of Horner's syndrome (see later discussion). Neuromuscular disorders, including myasthenia gravis, muscular dystrophies, and various myopathies, are also common causes of ptosis. Senile and traumatic changes in the supportive tissue of the eyelid may lead to ptosis. In addition, cerebral hemispheric lesions such as an infarct unusually precipitate bilateral, contralateral, or rarely ipsilateral ptosis.

PUPILLARY ABNORMALITIES

Control of Pupillary Function

Pupilloconstrictor fibers of the iris receive parasympathetic cholinergic innervation from the **Edinger-Westphal nucleus** by means of the third nerve. These fibers synapse in the ciliary ganglion lying at the apex of the orbit and reach the iris via the short ciliary nerves. Sympathetic noradrenergic innervation to the eye is responsible for active pupillary dilatation and widening of the palpebral fissure.

The **cephalic sympathetic supply,** including oculosympathetic innervation, consists of a three-neuron chain that begins in the posterior hypothalamus. The first neuron descends dorsolaterally in the brainstem and cervical spinal cord to synapse in the intermediolateral cell columns at the C7–T2 levels. The second neuron leaves the nervous system via ventral spinal roots and ascends in the sympathetic chain to synapse in the superior cervical ganglion, approximately at the level of the carotid bifurcation. The third neuron reaches the iris and Müller's muscle by ascending along the internal carotid artery, then traverses the cavernous sinus and the ciliary ganglion as the long ciliary nerves. Sympathetic fibers to the face that supply the sweat glands and arterioles travel with the external carotid artery.

Afferent Pupillary Defects

The pupil of a blind eye does not react to light directly but will show a consensual constriction response when light is shone in the opposite eye. This is known as an **amaurotic pupil.**

Lesions of the retina and the optic nerve can produce a difference in light input in the two eyes, known as a **Gunn pupil.** This can be detected by swinging a light from eye to eye. When present, there is bilateral pupillary dilatation or poor initial constriction rather than the expected brisk constriction when the light is swung onto the affected eye.

Normally the pupillary constriction responses to light and accommodation (focusing on a near object) are about equal. However, in the presence of lesions in the pretectal region of the midbrain, where impulses are received from the optic tract and relayed to the Edinger-Westphal nucleus, the light reflex may be totally or partially abolished even though the near reflex is preserved. This phenomenon, known as **light-near dissociation,** may appear in patients with diabetes mellitus, encephalitis, tumors and compressive lesions of the midbrain, multiple sclerosis, Wernicke's encephalopathy, bilateral retinal or optic nerve lesions, and classically in neurosyphilis as the **Argyll-Robertson pupil.** This pupil is typically small, irregular in outline, and often asymmetrical. It may appear early in neurosyphilis and is most closely associated with tabes dorsalis.

Efferent Pupillary Defects

Large Pupil

A large pupil may be seen in patients with a **third nerve lesion.** The causes are discussed earlier in this chapter. The pupillary dilatation tends to precede other signs of a third nerve lesion with transtentorial herniation, making it an important finding.

Certain **drugs,** such as LSD and other hallucinogens, antihistamines, glutethimide, anticholinergic agents, and dopamine, produce mydriasis when taken or administered in large doses. The deliberate or accidental topical ocular application of anticholinergic agents (especially among medical personnel) may cause unilateral mydriasis that lasts for several days. A transdermal scopolamine patch for the treatment of motion sickness applied to the mastoid region can also produce unilateral mydriasis. A 1% solution of pilocarpine applied to the eye will not constrict a mydriatic pupil caused by pharmacological blockade but will constrict large pupils resulting from other causes, except for direct trauma, which is usually obvious. Patients with botulism have bilaterally dilated fixed pupils.

Direct trauma to the eye can cause pupillary dilatation by damaging the nerve endings or iris sphincter muscle itself.

The **Adie's pupil** is typically large and responds to light poorly, and only after prolonged exposure. In the dark, some dilatation occurs after 30 to 60 minutes. However, there is usually complete, although slow, constriction on attempted accommodation. The presenting complaint may be anisocoria or blurred vision that is experienced when focusing on near objects, as there is frequently an accompanying accommodative defect. The opposite pupil often eventually becomes involved. About half the patients with a tonic pupil also have areflexia in the lower limbs—Adie's syndrome. The defect in these patients is at the level of the ciliary ganglion or short ciliary nerves and is usually idiopathic. A viral ciliary ganglionitis has been postulated as the cause in some cases.

Denervation hypersensitivity of the pupil can be shown by instilling 0.1% pilocarpine into the eye, which provokes marked constriction of an Adie's pupil but does not affect the normal pupil, nor usually a dilated pupil due to third nerve damage.

Small Pupil

Horner's syndrome in its complete form consists of miosis, ptosis of the upper eyelid, elevation of the lower lid ("upside-down" ptosis), and absence of sweating over the ipsilateral hemiface (Fig. 11-2). The anisocoria in Horner's syndrome is increased in dim light, unlike that of a parasympathetic (third nerve) lesion, which is worsened by bright light. Involvement anywhere along the sympathetic pathways from the hypothalamus to the long ciliary nerves (see earlier description) can theoretically produce a Horner's syndrome, and it represents an important localizing sign. With central involvement (e.g., lateral medullary infarction), neurological signs of brainstem involvement frequently appear. Postganglionic Horner's syndrome implies third-order neuron involvement (i.e., after the superior cervical ganglion) and patients have normal facial sweating. It is commonly seen in patients suffering from a cluster headache and also occurs in patients with Raeder's syndrome or lesions of the internal carotid artery, such as dissection. Trauma or infiltrative lesions of the lower brachial plexus affecting the C7–T2 roots can cause a preganglionic Horner's syndrome. Tumors of the apex of the lung can infiltrate the ascending sympathetic fibers and the sympathetic chain, also giving rise to a preganglionic Horner's syndrome. Various causes of Horner's syndrome are listed in Table 11-1.

The miosis and ptosis of Horner's syndrome may be subtle. However, the instillation of 10%

Table 11-1. Causes of Horner's Syndrome

Central (first-order neuron)
  Brainstem infarct (e.g., lateral medullary)
  Brainstem tumor
  Syringobulbia/syringomyelia
Peripheral
  Second-order neuron (preganglionic)
    Cervical rib
    Cervical trauma, infection, or neck tumor
    Brachial plexus trauma or neoplastic infiltration
    Carcinoma of the apex of the lung
    Internal jugular vein catheterization
    Improper placement of a chest tube
  Third-order neuron (postganglionic)
    Cluster headache
    Internal carotid aneurysm or dissection
    Tumor at the base of the skull
    Carotid inflammatory disease
    Basal skull fracture
    Raeder's syndrome
    Cavernous sinus thrombosis

Fig. 11-2. *A left Horner's syndrome in a 56-year-old man who had carcinoma of the gallbladder and invasion of the left brachial plexus. The patient also had intractable pain, sensory loss, and weakness in the left C7–T1 distribution.*

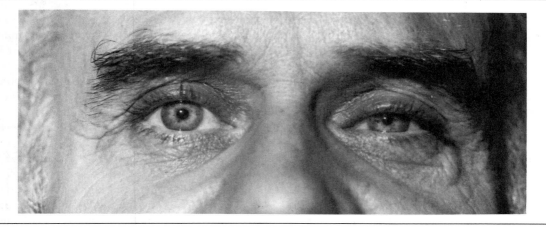

cocaine into both eyes will aggravate the anisocoria in Horner's syndrome because the involved eye cannot dilate significantly. One
percent hydroxyamphetamine (Paredrine) is
used to distinguish preganglionic and central
involvement, which are often due to a serious
disorder, from postganglionic involvement,
which is almost always due to relatively benign
lesions. Pupillary dilatation occurs only with
first- or second-order neuron involvement, because in third-order neuron involvement the
supply of norepinephrine is depleted. This
transmitter is necessary to the drug's action.

Other causes of bilaterally small pupils include miotic drops, narcotic medication, pontine hemorrhage or infarct, Argyll-Robertson
pupils, and, in later years, bilateral Adie's pupils.

DISORDERS OF THE OPTIC NERVE AND DISC

Papilledema and its distinction from papillitis
are discussed in Chapter 2. **Optic atrophy,**
which may affect only a portion of the disc, can
be seen with pregeniculate lesions and occurs
as a consequence of severe papilledema, optic
neuritis, ischemic optic neuropathy, optic nerve
trauma, optic nerve degenerative lesions, and
optic glioma.

Leber's hereditary optic atrophy is a maternally inherited form of gradual optic nerve degeneration that mainly affects males, with onset
usually between ages 18 and 25. It is due to a
defect in mitochondrial DNA. Visual loss can
occur subacutely, and, in most cases, the second
eye becomes involved within 12 months of the
first. Central vision may be lost in both eyes
simultaneously. Cardiac conduction abnormalities can occur in some pedigrees. Other forms
of hereditary optic atrophy, either exhibiting
dominant inheritance or associated with juvenile diabetes mellitus and deafness, have been
reported.

Optic neuritis is a condition consisting of inflammatory, toxic, infectious, or demyelinating
lesions of the optic nerve. Papillitis may also
occur and give rise to funduscopic findings of
disc congestion. The term *optic neuropathy* is

more general and used by some to refer to all
cases except those due to infectious or demyelinating causes. Retrobulbar neuritis is a form
of optic neuritis that affects the optic nerve far
enough posterior to the globe that the disc looks
normal on funduscopy. Central visual loss (central scotoma) and a subacute reduction in visual
acuity progressing over a few to several days is
the hallmark of optic neuritis. Poor color vision
and especially desaturation of red is a frequent
early symptom. In many cases, the disc appears
grossly normal in the acute stages but subtle
congestion may be apparent. Orbital CT scanning may show optic nerve swelling. After several weeks, there may be pallor of the whole
disk or its temporal portion where the papillomacular bundle enters. A painful globe (especially with eye movements), phosphenes (light
flashes) induced by rapid eye movements, and
headache are other possible symptoms. Visual
acuity returns to normal or near normal in the
vast majority of cases. A Marcus-Gunn pupil
or subtle defects in color vision, contrast sensitivity, visual fields, or visual evoked potential
abnormalities may be residual evidence of a
previous bout of optic neuritis. These abnormalities are particularly helpful in patients with
suspected multiple sclerosis when evidence for
disseminated white matter lesions is being
sought.

The causes of optic neuritis are listed in Table
11-2. Thirty to fifty percent of the cases without
an obvious cause exhibit other signs of multiple
sclerosis on follow-up, sometimes after an interval of many years. Whether these idiopathic
cases that do not develop other signs of white
matter involvement are in fact cases of monophasic multiple sclerosis remains an unanswered question, but the findings from
epidemiological studies have suggested that
these cases likely represent an entity distinct
from multiple sclerosis. In one study, 85 idiopathic cases were observed for a median of 12.9
years; 33 of the patients subsequently developed multiple sclerosis. Significant risk factors
were younger age, abnormal CSF findings at
the onset, and early recurrence of optic neuritis.

The treatment of optic neuritis is generally
unsatisfactory, although significant visual improvement occurs in most cases. A recent study

Table 11-2. Causes of Optic Neuritis and Optic Neuropathy

Demyelinating disease
  Multiple sclerosis
  Devic's variant of multiple sclerosis
  Postinfectious
Toxic
  Drugs
  Tobacco-alcohol amblyopia
  Heavy metals (lead, arsenic, antimony)
  Methanol
Nutritional
  B_{12} deficiency
Leber's hereditary optic atrophy and other
  hereditary optic atrophies (Behr's disease)
Infectious
  Tuberculosis
  Syphilis
  Cytomegalovirus in patients with retinitis (usually
    HIV infection)
  Toxoplasmosis
  Cryptococcosis
  Progressive multifocal leukoencephalopathy
Ischemic
  Vasculitis
  Systemic lupus erythematosus
  Temporal arteritis
  ?Polyarteritis nodosa
  Ischemic optic neuropathy (often associated with
    hypertension)
  Diabetes
Traumatic
Compressive or infiltrative
  Optic nerve meningioma
  Optic glioma
  Pituitary tumors
  Leukemia or lymphoma
  Eosinophilic granuloma
Miscellaneous
  Sarcoidosis

has shown that patients given a 3-day course of intravenous high-dose methylprednisolone followed by 11 days of oral prednisone recover slightly faster and have a better visual outcome after 6 months. In cases with a specific cause such as tuberculosis, treatment is directed at the underlying cause.

Ischemic optic neuropathy may be due to specific forms of vasculitis, such as systemic lupus erythematosus or temporal arteritis, but in the vast majority of cases is idiopathic. About half of the patients are hypertensive, and it has been suggested that the syndrome arises from a lacunar infarct of the anterior portion of the optic nerve, which is supplied by the posterior ciliary arteries. Patients are usually between 55 and 70 years of age. There are often no premonitory symptoms, and, unlike optic neuritis in multiple sclerosis, the visual loss is sudden. The visual loss progresses over days in a minority of cases, and the degree of loss is quite variable. Recovery is usually minimal. An ischemic papillopathy is readily appreciated on ophthalmoscopy, and is seen as disc swelling and pallor with surrounding flame-shaped hemorrhages. Field defects vary from altitudinal, quadratic, or arcuate defects to central scotomata. The opposite eye becomes involved in about 40 percent of the cases, often after an interval of years.

Central retinal artery occlusion occurs in the presence of various hypercoagulable states as well as atherosclerosis. Patients suffer profound and irreversible loss of vision and the retina becomes white and edematous because of infarction. The macula, by contrast, appears reddish because of the intact choroid circulation supplying the outermost retinal layers.

Compressive and infiltrative optic nerve lesions must always be ruled out initially in any case of a progressive or even subacute visual loss that does not resolve within 6 weeks. Optic nerve meningiomas, optic gliomas, and pituitary tumors are often easily detected by tomograms of the optic canals and appropriate CT scans. More diffuse infiltrative lesions such as lymphomas can exhibit optic nerve enlargement on CT scans, but exploration and biopsy may be required for definitive diagnosis. A trial of steroids will bring about improved vision as commonly or more commonly in patients with tumors affecting the optic nerve than it will in patients with optic neuritis stemming from various causes.

LESIONS OF AFFERENT VISUAL PATHWAYS; VISUAL FIELDS

The visual field of each eye can be accurately mapped by a technique known as *perimetry*. Normally the fields extend 100 degrees temporally, 60 degrees nasally, 60 degrees superiorly, and 70 degrees inferiorly. The physiological blind spot, corresponding to the retinal deficit produced by the optic nerve head, is about 15 degrees temporal to fixation. A tangent screen can be used to map the central 30 degrees of vision. Visual field deficits, especially scotomata (islands of relative or complete visual loss surrounded by areas of normal vision), have characteristic forms, depending on which part of the visual pathway is affected (Fig. 11-3).

Prechiasmatic Lesions

The optic nerve consists of axons of retinal ganglion cells that enter the optic disc as distinct nerve fiber bundles. From the temporal retina, each bundle arises from an arcuate retinal area. The papillomacular bundle carries impulses from the macula, where visual acuity is maximal, and enters the temporal portion of the optic nerve head. Lesions of the optic nerve anterior to the chiasm produce monocular visual field defects. These may consist of complete blindness in one eye, a central scotoma, altitudinal defects (characteristic of ischemic optic neuropathy or glaucoma), or arcuate scotomata, when individual nerve fiber bundles are involved. These defects generally respect the horizontal meridian. Bilateral symmetrical visual loss and centrocecal scotomas are seen with tobacco-alcohol amblyopia.

Chiasmatic Lesions

At the optic chiasm, which lies just above the sella turcica, the optic nerve fibers from the nasal retinae (i.e., temporal visual fields) cross over while the temporal retinal fibers remain ipsilateral. Fibers supplying the superior visual fields pass inferiorly through the chiasm, and therefore compressive lesions from below (e.g., pituitary adenoma) initially produce a bilateral superior temporal quadrantanopia before progressing to a full bitemporal hemianopia. Because the crossing nasal fibers swing slightly forward in the contralateral optic nerve before proceeding backward in the optic tract, a lesion of the posterior optic nerve near the chiasm (junctional defect) produces a central scotoma in the eye involved and a temporal field defect in the opposite eye.

Retrochiasmatic Lesions

The optic tracts run between the chiasm and the lateral geniculate nucleus of the thalamus where the visual fibers first synapse. The geniculocalcarine optic radiations first pass through the posterior portion of the internal capsule in close association with the motor and sensory fibers, and then traverse the parietal (inferior field fibers) and temporal (superior field fibers) lobes before reaching the primary occipital visual receiving area. The visual (striate) cortex occupies the upper and lower lips of the calcarine sulcus.

The retrochiasmatic pathway becomes progressively more topographically arranged as it proceeds posteriorly. Retrochiasmatic lesions produce homonymous hemianopia, in that they involve the same half-field in each eye and respect the vertical meridian. The term *hemianopia* implies that the whole half-field is involved, although the deficit may be denser superiorly or inferiorly. Altitudinal hemianopias, which are seen with retinal ischemia, involve the upper or lower half-field of one eye. The term *quadrantanopia* refers to the involvement of only one visual quadrant. Defects are said to be congruous when their size and shape in each eye is equivalent.

Lesions of the optic tract and lateral geniculate are rare in isolation and tend to produce incongruous homonymous hemianopic defects. Temporal lobe involvement, including the fibers that loop forward lateral to the temporal horn of the lateral ventricle (Meyer's loop), produces a superior quadrantanopia which is usually incongruous. Parietal lobe lesions lead to more congruous inferior quadrantanopias. Occipital lobe lesions manifest extremely congruous defects. Unusual and characteristic field defects can result from discrete occipital lesions because: (1) the peripheral fields are represented more anteriorly in the visual cortex and the central fields more posteriorly; (2) macular vision is probably represented bilaterally; and (3) the extreme temporal field of each eye is represented contralaterally without a corres-

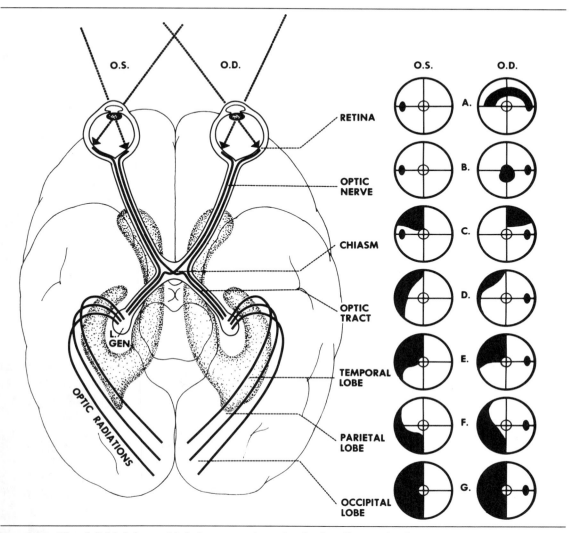

Fig. 11-3. *Visual field defects with lesions at various sites in the afferent visual pathways. A = arcuate scotoma respecting the horizontal meridian with a retinal lesion; B = central scotoma with optic nerve lesion; C = bitemporal upper quadrantanopia with chiasmatic lesion (e.g., pituitary adenoma); D = noncongruous homonymous defect with optic tract lesion; E = contralateral upper homonymous quadrantanopia with temporal lobe (Meyer's loop) lesion; F = contralateral inferior homonymous quadrantanopia with parietal lobe lesion; G = contralateral homonymous hemianopia with occipital lobe lesion, but with macular sparing and preservation of central vision. (O.S. = left eye; O.D. = right eye; L. gen. = lateral geniculate nucleus.)*

ponding nasal field segment coming from the opposite eye. Homonymous macular scotomata, homonymous hemianopias with macular sparing, and the exclusive involvement or sparing of the temporal crescent of the contralateral eye are some examples of these defects.

Cortical Blindness (Anton's Syndrome)

Total blindness with preserved pupillary light responses, unawareness or denial of blindness, tendency toward confabulation, and at times a

Korsakoff's amnesia and visual hallucinations are manifested by patients with bilateral occipital lesions involving the visual cortex accompanied by more diffuse cortical involvement. Vertebrobasilar ischemia, which can be a complication of vertebral angiography, and trauma are the most common causes.

EXOPHTHALMOS AND THYROID OPHTHALMOPATHY

Exophthalmos, or proptosis, is the abnormal protrusion of the globe, which may be unilateral or bilateral. The distance between the cornea of each eye and the lateral orbital rim can be measured by an exophthalmometer and in normal subjects ranges between 12 and 21 mm. A difference of 2 mm between eyes is considered abnormal.

The examiner can best see proptosis by standing behind the seated patient and looking down over the globes from above. The globe should be palpated and gentle retrodisplacement attempted. Conditions such as orbital pseudotumor, certain mass lesions of the orbit, and thyroid ophthalmopathy offer resistance with this maneuver, unlike soft tumors, such as hemangiomas or arteriovenous malformations of the orbit. An orbital bruit is observed in conjunction with arteriovenous malformations and carotid-cavernous fistulas. A pulsating exophthalmos may appear with carotid-cavernous fistulas or bony defects of the orbit secondary to trauma or neurofibromatosis. The proptosed eyeball may also be displaced upward, down-

Fig. 11-4. *Contrast-enhanced CT scan with orbital cuts in a 26-year-old man with Graves' disease. The patient had an elevated T4 level, right proptosis, and limited eye movements on the right. (A) Proptosis and thickening of the medial and lateral rectus muscles* (arrows) *compared to the opposite side.*

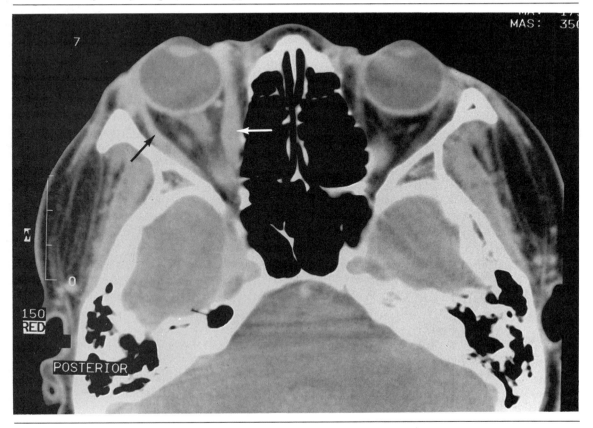

ward, or to one side, suggesting an orbital mass lesion in a particular quadrant and not thyroid ophthalmopathy, which produces a nondeviating exophthalmos. Pain commonly accompanies the exophthalmos in conditions such as orbital pseudotumor and orbital cellulitis. Vascular congestion and inflammation of the periorbital tissues (the "red orbit" syndrome) are seen in conjunction with conditions such as thyroid ophthalmopathy, orbital pseudotumor, orbital cellulitis, and carotid-cavernous fistula. Unilateral exophthalmos should always prompt a search for an orbital mass lesion, although thyroid ophthalmopathy is the most common cause of both unilateral and bilateral exophthalmos in adults.

Other conditions that are associated with bilateral exophthalmos are Wegener's granulomatosis, leukemia and metastatic neuro-blastoma in children, and carotid-cavernous fistulas. Loss of visual acuity prior to the development of exophthalmos is typical of tumors of the optic nerve, such as optic gliomas. The patient's age is particularly important when considering the cause of exophthalmos. Certain conditions such as thyroid ophthalmopathy, orbital pseudotumor, or carcinoma of the sinuses are found almost exclusively in adults, whereas others, such as metastatic neuroblastoma and orbital rhabdomyosarcoma, are encountered chiefly in the pediatric age group.

The evaluation of the patient with exophthalmos should include orbital CT scanning in the axial and coronal planes, which can provide details of bony structures, the globe, the optic nerves, and soft tissues, including vascular structures and the extraocular muscles (Fig. 11-4). The technique affords the objective verifica-

Fig. 11-4. *(B) Enlargement of the superior orbital vein* (arrow).

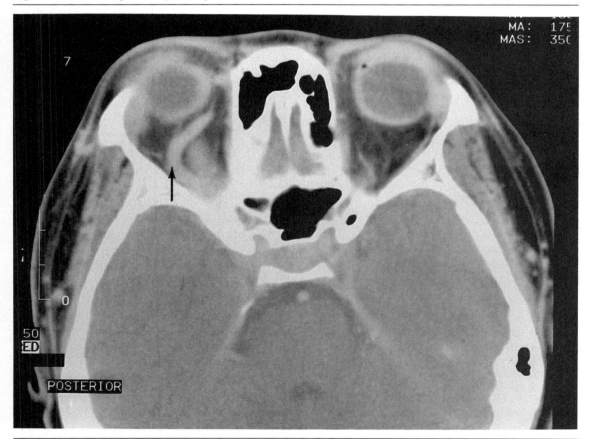

tion of both the presence and degree of proptosis and also yields valuable clues to etiology. Plain x-ray studies of the skull, orbital structures, and sinuses, as well as orbital ultrasound, angiographic, and venographic evaluation, also play a role in the assessment of selected cases of exophthalmos. The major causes of exophthalmos are listed in Table 11-3.

Exophthalmos appears at a relatively advanced stage in thyroid ophthalmopathy due to **Graves' disease.** A subtle stare due to lid retraction and lid lag can be elicited when the patient looks down slowly from an upward gaze, and these constitute earlier manifestations. As the condition progresses, ocular motility disorders due to extraocular muscle interstitial

Table 11-3. Etiology of Exophthalmos

Thyroid ophthalmopathy
Tumor
  Intraorbital
    Cavernous hemangioma or lymphangioma
    Meningioma
    Optic glioma (P)
    Lymphoma and leukemia
    Metastatic
    Orbital rhabdomyosarcoma (P)
    Neuroblastoma (P)
    Retinoblastoma
    Lacrimal gland tumor
    Neurofibroma
    Dermoid and epidermoid (P)
    Malignant melanoma
  Intracranial
    Meningioma
  Sinuses
    Carcinoma
    Mucocele
Inflammatory
  Orbital pseudotumor
  Orbital cellulitis (P)
  Wegener's granulomatosis
  Sarcoidosis
Vascular
  Carotid-cavernous fistula
  Orbital varix
Miscellaneous
  Trauma to orbital roof
  Retroorbital hematoma (posttraumatic)
  Neurofibromatosis with bony defects of orbit
  Encephalocele of orbit
  Fibrous dysplasia

(P) = mainly in pediatric age group.

edematous inflammatory infiltration (especially inferior and medial rectus) cause diplopia, and orbital edema and vascular congestion also appear. Compression of the optic nerve or exposure keratitis of the cornea may lead to visual loss.

It is well known that the course of the eye disease in thyroid ophthalmopathy is often independent of the status of the thyroid disease. Although most patients are hyperthyroid, a small fraction show normal thyroid function. Evaluation in these patients consists of a full battery of thyroid function tests, CT scanning, which can demonstrate enlargement of the extraocular muscles, and, in some cases, forced duction tests. This last test is done by grasping the anesthetized muscle with a special forceps and attempting to move the eyeball. If the eye cannot be displaced in this manner, then the limitation of eye movements is due to mechanical restriction and not paralytic muscle involvement. Restoring the patient to a euthyroid state may diminish the ophthalmopathy, but steroid treatment, radiotherapy, or surgical orbital decompression may be necessary to preserve vision or for cosmetic reasons. Some cases will regress spontaneously over 1 to 2 years.

BIBLIOGRAPHY

Ash, P. R., and Keltner, J. L. Neuro-ophthalmic signs in pontine lesions. *Medicine* 56:304–320, 1979.

Beck, R. W., et al. A randomized, controlled trial of corticosteroids in the treatment of acute optic neuritis. *N. Engl. J. Med.* 326:581–588, 1992.

Beck, R. W., and Smith, C. H. The neuro-ophthalmic examination. *Neurol. Clin.* 1:807–830, 1983.

Berenberg, R. A., et al. Lumping or splitting? "Ophthalmoplegia plus" or Kearns-Sayre syndrome? *Ann. Neurol.* 1:37–54, 1977.

Boghen, D. R., and Glaser, J. S. Ischaemic optic neuropathy: the clinical profile and natural history. *Brain* 98:689–708, 1975.

Bosley, T. M., and Schatz, N. Clinical diagnosis of cavernous sinus syndromes. *Neurol. Clin.* 1:929–953, 1983.

Caplan, L. R. Ptosis. *J. Neurol. Neurosurg. Psychiatry* 37:1–7, 1974.

Carroll, W. M., and Mastaglia, F. L. Leber's optic neuropathy: a clinical and visual evoked potential study of affected and asymptomatic members of a six generation family. *Brain* 102:559–580, 1979.

Cohen, M., and Lessell, S. A prospective study of the risk of developing multiple sclerosis in uncomplicated optic neuritis. *Neurology* 29:208–213, 1979.

Drachman, D. A. Ophthalmoplegia plus: the neurodegenerative disorder associated with progressive external ophthalmoplegia. *Arch. Neurol.* 18:654–674, 1968.

Ellenberger, C., Keltner, J. L., and Stroud, M. H. Ocular dyskinesia in cerebellar disease: evidence for the similarity of opsoclonus, ocular dysmetria and flutter-like oscillations. *Brain* 95:685–692, 1972.

Glaeser, J. S. (editor). *Neuro-ophthalmology,* 2nd ed. Philadelphia: Lippincott, 1990.

Grossman, R. I., and Lynch, R. M. Neuroimaging in neuro-ophthalmology. *Neurol. Clin.* 1:831–857, 1983.

Grove, A. S. Jr. Evaluation of exophthalmos. *N. Engl. J. Med.* 292:1005–1013, 1975.

Hamburger, J. I., and Sugar, H. S. What the internist should know about the ophthalmopathy of Graves' disease. *Arch. Intern. Med.* 129:131–139, 1972.

Jackson, J. A., Jankovic, J., and Ford, J. Progressive supranuclear palsy: clinical features and response to treatment in 16 patients. *Ann. Neurol.* 13:273–278, 1983.

Jacobs, L., Munschauer, F. E., and Kaba, S. E. Clinical and magnetic resonance imaging in optic neuritis. *Neurology* 41:15–19, 1991.

Keane, J. R. Oculosympathetic paresis: analysis of 100 hospitalized patients. *Arch. Neurol.* 36:13–15, 1979.

Kline, L. B. The Tolosa-Hunt syndrome. *Surv. Ophthalmol.* 27:79–95, 1982.

Lessell, S. Optic neuropathies. *N. Engl. J. Med.* 299:533–536, 1978.

McCrary, J. A., and Smith, J. L. Neuro-ophthalmological evaluation of the neurosurgical patient. In J. R. Youmans (editor). *Neurological Surgery.* Philadelphia: Saunders, 1973, Vol. 1, Pp. 371–408.

Moraes, C. T., et al. Mitochondrial DNA deletions in progressive external ophthalmoplegia and Kearns-Sayre syndrome. *N. Engl. J. Med.* 320:1293–1335, 1989.

Nadeau, S. E., and Trobe, J. D. Pupillary sparing in oculomotor palsy: a brief review. *Ann. Neurol.* 13:143–148, 1983.

Newman, N. J. Leber's hereditary optic neuropathy. *Ophthalmol. Clin. North Am.* 4:431–448, 1991.

Rucker, C. W. The causes of paralysis of the third, fourth, and sixth cranial nerves. *Am. J. Ophthalmol.* 61:1293–1298, 1966.

Rush, J. A., and Younge, B. R. Paralysis of cranial nerves III, IV and VI. *Arch. Ophthalmol.* 99:76–79, 1981.

Sandberg-Wollheim, M., et al. A long-term prospective study of optic neuritis: evaluation of risk factors. *Ann. Neurol.* 27:386–393, 1990.

Selhorst, J. B. The pupil and its disorders. *Neurol. Clin.* 1:859–881, 1983.

Sergott, R. C. Neuro-ophthalmic evaluation of the red orbit syndrome. *Neurol. Clin.* 1:897–908, 1983.

Shults WT (editor). Neuro-ophthalmology. *Ophthalmol. Clin. North Am.* 4:431–648, 1991.

Smigiel, M. R., Jr. Exophthalmos: the more commonly encountered neurosurgical lesions. *Mayo Clin. Proc.* 50:345–355, 1975.

Thompson, H. S. Adie's syndrome: some new observations. *Trans. Am. Ophthalmol. Soc.* 75:587–626, 1977.

Thompson, H. S. Diagnosing Horner's syndrome. *Ophthalmol. Trans.* 83:840–842, 1977.

Troost, B. T. Neuro-ophthalmology. In S. H. Appel (editor). *Current Neurology*. New York: Wiley, 1981, Vol. 3, Pp. 454-502.

Younge, B. R., and Sutula, F. Analysis of trochlear nerve palsies: diagnosis, etiology, and treatment. *Mayo Clin. Proc.* 52:11–18, 1977.

Zackon, D. H. Neuro-ophthalmology. *Prim. Care* 9:679–696, 1979.

12

Parkinson's Disease and Parkinsonism

BASAL GANGLIA PHYSIOLOGY AND PHARMACOLOGY

The basal ganglia are subcortical paired gray matter nuclei that include the caudate and putamen (which make up the striatum), globus pallidus, subthalamic nucleus, certain thalamic nuclei, and the substantia nigra (lying in the midbrain) that function in concert to aid in the control and coordination of cortical motor output. The basal ganglia interconnections are shown in simplified form in Figure 12-1.

The striatum receives widespread cortical inputs and sends information back to the cortex via the internal segment of the globus pallidus through the ventral anterior and ventral lateral nuclei of the thalamus. Other neurons within these same thalamic nuclei serve as a major relay between cerebellar deep nuclei and the cerebral cortex. The influence of the basal ganglia on spinal motor activities is thought to result entirely from inputs to the cerebral cortical neurons giving rise to the corticospinal tract.

Another major circuit consists of the **nigrostriatal pathway**, which arises in the pars compacta of the substantia nigra, and the **striatonigral pathway**, which enters the pars reticularis of the substantia nigra. The nigrostriatal pathway uses dopamine as a neurotransmitter and exerts an inhibitory influence on striatal function. It is the cells in the pars compacta of the substantia nigra giving rise to this pathway that are affected in the idiopathic or postencephalitic form of parkinsonism; this causes a dopamine deficiency state at the striatal level. It is estimated that Parkinson's disease becomes evident once about 80 percent of the cells within the substantia nigra are lost. The mesolimbic forebrain bundle and the tuberoinfundibular system also use dopamine as a neurotransmitter.

Several types of **dopamine receptors** have been identified. The D_1 receptor subtype is limited to the stimulation of the enzyme adenylate cyclase as a second messenger. Stimulation of the D_2 receptors does not alter or lower cyclic adenosine monophosphate (AMP) levels and

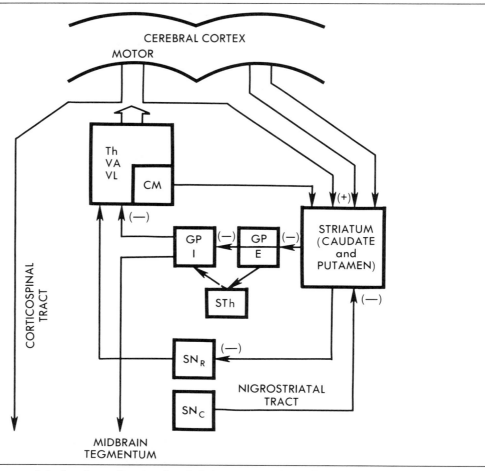

Fig. 12-1. *Diagram of the basal ganglia, showing their interconnections, afferents, and efferents. (GPE = globus pallidus, external segment; GPI = globus pallidus, internal segment; SN_C = substantia nigra, pars compacta; SN_R = substantia nigra, pars reticularis; STh = subthalamic nucleus; Th = thalamus; VA = ventral anterior nucleus; VL = ventral lateral nucleus; DM = centromedian nucleus.)*

they are more closely linked with the occurrence of Parkinson's disease. Symptoms of parkinsonism also result when striatal dopamine receptors are blocked pharmacologically (e.g., by phenothiazines).

In addition, there are other transmitters or neuromodulator substances that normally operate in the basal ganglia. **Glutamate** is thought to be the excitatory neurotransmitter of the corticostriatal tract. **Gamma-aminobutyric acid** is an inhibitory transmitter used by neurons within the striatum as well as the striatonigral pathway. Some of these same neurons also utilize enkephalin and other peptides as neuro-

modulators or neurotransmitters. Other interneurons within the striatum make use of acetylcholine as a neurotransmitter. An alteration in the striatal dopaminergic–cholinergic balance is considered an important event in the genesis of parkinsonian symptoms.

PARKINSON'S DISEASE

James Parkinson accurately described the features of "the shaking palsy" in 1817. Parkinson's disease is an idiopathic degenerative condition that possesses many of the same clinical features seen in secondary forms of parkinsonism (Table 12-1).

Pathology and Pathophysiology

Degeneration of the pigmented neuromelanin-containing neurons of the pars compacta of the substantia nigra, locus ceruleus, and dorsal motor nucleus of the vagus is the pathological hallmark of Parkinson's disease (Fig. 12-2). Lewy bodies are found within the neurons of these areas and consist of eosinophilic round inclusions. There is also nerve cell loss in the

Table 12-1. Causes of Parkinsonism

Idiopathic Parkinson's disease
Drugs
  Phenothiazines
  Butyrophenones
  Metoclopramide
  Reserpine
  Flunarizine
  Alpha-methyldopa
  Lithium
  Amiodarone
Toxins
  Manganese
  MPTP
  Carbon monoxide
  Carbon disulfide
  Amyotrophic lateral sclerosis–parkinsonism-
    dementia of Guam (cycad)
Brain Tumors
Trauma (dementia pugilistica)
Encephalitis
  Von Economo's encephalitis
  Venezuelan
  Japanese B
  Western equine
Cerebrovascular disease: lacunar state
Akinetic/rigid syndromes with parkinsonian features
    (Parkinson's plus)
  Progressive supranuclear palsy
  Huntington's disease
  Striatonigral degeneration
  Corticobasal ganglionic degeneration
  Olivopontocerebellar degeneration
  Normal-pressure hydrocephalus
  Alzheimer's disease
  Wilson's disease
  Hallervorden-Spatz disease
  Shy-Drager syndrome
  Familial calcification of the basal ganglia (Fahr's
    disease)

globus pallidus and mild diffuse cortical atrophy.

One of the early clues to the biochemical defect that occurs in Parkinson's disease was the demonstration of reduced levels of dopamine in the striatum of affected patients, compared to controls, and in the contralateral striatum of patients with hemiparkinsonism, compared to the opposite side (Fig. 12-3). The norepinephrine and serotonin concentrations are also reduced in the basal ganglia of patients with Parkinson's disease.

Animal models of involuntary movement disorders were developed by administering either dopamine-depleting drugs such as reserpine or other drugs that interfere with dopamine synthesis. Reserpine-induced bradykinesia could be reversed in mice by giving D,L 3,4-dopa. It was also widely recognized that central dopamine receptor–blocking drugs such as phenothiazines or butyrophenones commonly evoke parkinsonism as a side effect.

A clue to the possible pathogenesis of the nigral cell death in Parkinson's disease was provided by the discovery of the toxin MPTP (1-methyl-4-phenyl-1,2,3,6-tetrahydropyridine). This substance, which produces severe parkinsonism in patients who use it as "synthetic heroin," selectively destroys nigrostriatal dopaminergic neurons in humans, nonhuman primates, and rodents.

Epidemiology

About 1 percent of the population over 50 years of age is affected by Parkinson's disease. Although juvenile forms rarely occur, the usual age of onset is after 50, with the prevalence climbing steadily for older age groups. Familial aggregates are occasionally encountered, but the inheritance patterns and incidences in these cases are still unknown. Concordance studies conducted among twins have suggested that genetic factors are of little importance.

Clinical Picture

The clinical features of Parkinson's disease are summarized in Table 12-2. The first symptom

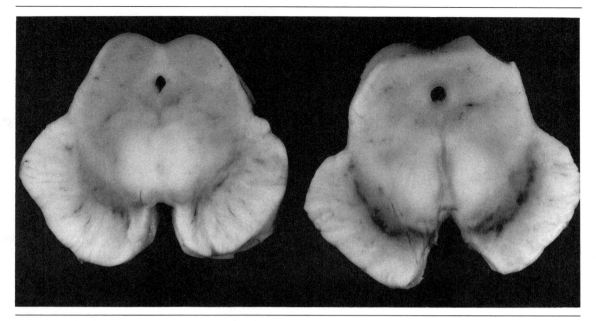

Fig. 12-2. *Depigmentation and atrophy of the substantia nigra in the midbrain of a patient with Parkinson's disease (left), as compared to a normal control (right).*

is usually **tremor**, which initially is often unilateral in one hand (Fig. 12-4) and then spreads to the opposite upper extremity, lower extremities, and the neck. The classic tremor consists of a "pill-rolling" motion of the hand, which is more pronounced at rest and exhibits a frequency of three to five cycles per second. In some patients, the tremor is exacerbated at the beginning or end of a movement or when the limbs are sustained in a particular posture (e.g., arms held outstretched), termed *postural tremor*. The tremor worsens under conditions of emotional stress or fatigue but completely disappears during sleep, as do virtually all involuntary movements, except for palatal myoclonus, some tics, and epileptic activity.

Bradykinesia, or slowness in initiating and carrying out movements, is the most disabling symptom of parkinsonism and its severity is the best predictor of the patient's degree of response to L-dopa. Axial movements such as turning over in bed are particularly difficult in advanced cases. **Rigidity** of either a cogwheel or lead-pipe variety worsens as the disease progresses and patients may assume fixed dystonic postures such as extreme truncal flexion. **Loss of postural reflexes**, including normal righting reflexes, may explain the tendency for patients to fall, seen early in the disease. The **gait disorder** in parkinsonism, when fully developed, includes a flexed posture (Fig. 12-5) with reduced or absent arm-swing (loss of associated reflexes), small steps (marche à petits pas), shuffling, and festination (an acceleration as if the person is trying to catch up to the center of gravity), and turning en bloc (i.e., body and head together).

The immobile and expressionless facies of parkinsonism (Fig. 12-6) with reduced blinking and seborrhea over the brow and at times drooling (sialorrhea), the monotonous quiet voice, the paucity of spontaneous movements, and general immobility complete the characteristic clinical picture.

Despite the relatively stereotyped appearance in fully developed cases, the diagnosis may not be readily apparent at initial presentation. A tendency to fall, generalized weakness, deterioration of handwriting with small letters (micrographia), depression, generalized aches, stiffness, and loss of olfactory sensation may all be early symptoms.

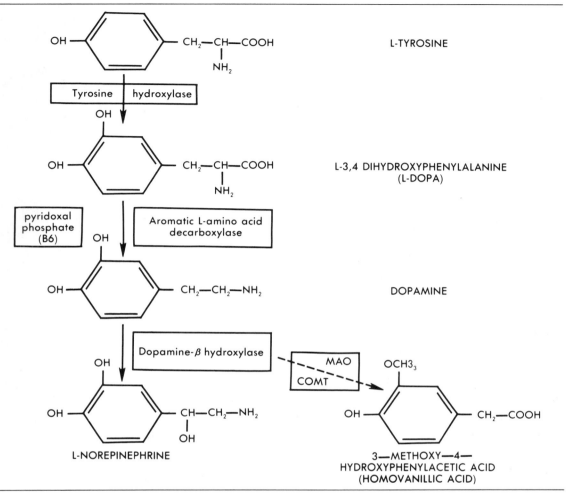

Fig. 12-3. *Pathway for dopamine synthesis and catabolism in the brain. (MAO = monoamine oxidase; COMT = catechol-o-methyl transferase.)*

A subtle decrease in arm-swing with walking, reduced facial expression, intermittent tremor in one hand, or cogwheel rigidity on moving the wrist passively in a circular manner, revealed by having the patient form a fist using the opposite hand, may be some of the early physical findings. In more advanced cases, the diagnosis is usually obvious at a glance. The glabellar tap sign (Myerson's sign) is elicited by tapping the glabellar region repetitively. Patient's with Parkinson's disease cannot suppress a blink each time the region is tapped. Fine rapid alternating limb movements are typically slow and very difficult to perform. Up-gaze is often limited and saccadic eye movements may have a jerky

quality. Rarely, Babinski's signs may be present but deep tendon jerks are not usually altered.

Autonomic features such as orthostatic hypotension, constipation, urinary hesitancy, and increased sweating are frequent problems. Depression is also prevalent and may partially stem from the underlying central disturbance in neurotransmitter function. The dementia, which is now considered to be relatively common as the disease advances, is a subcortical dementia (see Chapter 4), but the cause is uncertain. Some patients have concurrent Alzheimer's disease. As in Alzheimer's disease, the brains of patients with Parkinson's disease show degeneration of the cholinergic neurons that

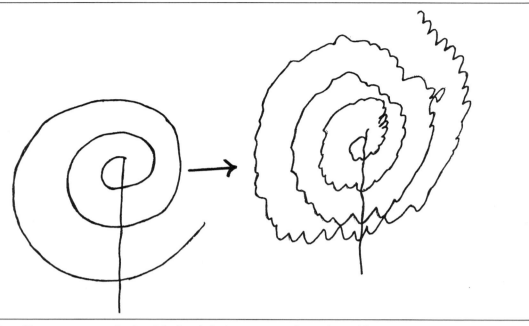

Fig. 12-4. *Tremor apparent in the right hand during attempt of a patient with Parkinson's disease to copy a spiral.*

project from the nucleus basalis of Meynert to the cerebral cortex. Although atrophy is a relatively common finding on the computed tomographic (CT) scans of patients with Parkinson's

Table 12-2. Diagnostic Features of Parkinson's Disease

Cardinal features
    Rigidity
    Resting tremor
    Bradykinesia
    Loss of postural reflexes (gait instability)
Other features
    Micrographia
    Reduced synkinesis (e.g., reduced arm-swing
        when walking)
    Gait disorder (flexed posture, short shuffling
        steps, festination, turning en bloc)
    Hypomimia (masked facies)
    Reduced blinking
    Reduced voice volume
    Glabellar tap sign
    Seborrheic dermatitis
Usually normal laboratory tests and neuroimaging
        procedures
    CT or MRI scan (may show atrophy)
    Serum ceruloplasmin

disease, its presence does not correlate well with the existence or degree of dementia.

Management and Prognosis

The various approaches to the treatment of Parkinson's disease are outlined in Table 12-3.

L-*Dopa*

The natural course of Parkinson's disease is one of relentless progression, and severe disability or death occurs within 14 years of onset in three quarters of the patients. Modern treatment has significantly improved this outlook, however.

Because Parkinson's disease presents a striatal dopamine deficiency state, this prompted efforts to replenish the striatal dopamine supply. Dopamine could not be used because it cannot cross the blood-brain barrier. Attempts to administer the precursor of dopamine, dopa, initially in a mixture of L and R racemic forms, failed because it caused severe nausea and vomiting. Finally, Cotzias and colleagues achieved a dramatic breakthrough in patients with advanced idiopathic Parkinson's disease by administering L-dopa in gradually increasing

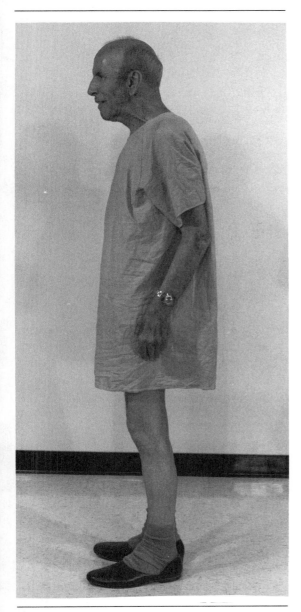

Fig. 12-5. *Flexed posture in a patient with moderately severe Parkinson's disease.*

doses up to several grams per day. The drug was also found to be effective in the treatment of postencephalitic parkinsonism. This event marked the beginning of a new era in clinical neuropharmacology and stimulated the search for correctable neurotransmitter disturbances in other neurological conditions. L-dopa is now the mainstay of therapy in most cases of Parkin-

son's disease. Rather than prescribing it in mildly affected patients, however, many neurologists advocate reserving L-dopa for later use because patients may experience a standard interval of about 3 to 5 years during which the L-dopa is maximally effective before the appearance of disabling side effects (see later discussion). Whether the use of L-dopa actually predisposes to the earlier development of dyskinesias and motor fluctuations is still debated.

Anticholinergic agents such as trihexyphenidyl (Artane), benztropine (Cogentin), procyclidine (Kemadrin), ethopropazine (Parsidol), or antihistamines such as diphenhydramine (Benadryl) were for many years the mainstay of therapy in Parkinson's disease. These agents are only mildly effective and are now used mainly to ameliorate the tremor or rigidity in mild cases. The anticholinergics produce side effects such as dry mouth, constipation, urinary retention, exacerbation of glaucoma, and hyperthermia in a hot environment, and may cause memory impairment and a confusional state. Amantadine hydrochloride (Symmetrel), an antiviral agent, in doses of 100 mg b.i.d. is more effective. It acts to increase striatal dopamine release from presynaptic sites and probably has some anticholinergic effect as well. Nightmares, psychosis, and livedo reticularis of the lower extremities are potential side effects of its use. The decision to treat at all or which agent to employ depends on the degree of disability, the patient's job or physical requirements, potential side effects, and the cost of the medication.

L-dopa is generally combined with a peripheral dopa-decarboxylase inhibitor (carbidopa in Sinemet in a proportion of 250/25, 100/25, or 100/10 and benserazide in Madopar), which prevents the conversion of L-dopa to dopamine outside the central nervous system. About 100 mg of carbidopa per day is needed to saturate the peripheral dopa-decarboxylase enzyme system. This makes more L-dopa available for central use and thus permits the use of lower average daily doses of 1 gm or less. With this strategy, certain side effects of L-dopa such as orthostatic hypotension can be avoided, and the severity of the nausea and vomiting (due mainly to the dopamine effect on the medullary chemoreceptor trigger zone that lies outside the blood-

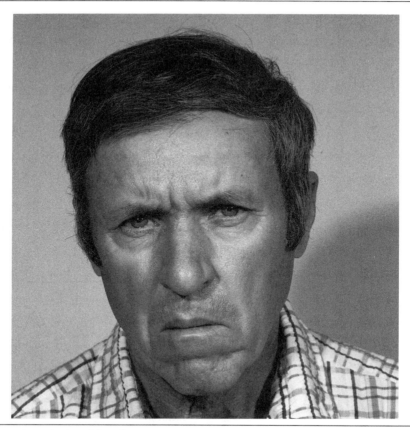

Fig. 12-6. *Hypomimia (reduced facial expression) in a man with early Parkinson's disease.*

brain barrier) seen with L-dopa administration alone is reduced. Pure carbidopa can be added to the regimen in patients suffering from persistent nausea. However, the dopa-decarboxylase inhibitor does not prevent or reduce the major side effects of psychosis (seen especially in demented patients) and disabling dyskinesias (various involuntary movements—choreiform, akathisia, and respiratory grunts). Other side effects from its use include insomnia, nightmares, drowsiness, and hypertension. The drug is contraindicated in patients with severe cardiovascular disease or malignant melanoma.

The normal starting dose of Sinemet is usually 100/25 mg b.i.d., with a gradual increase to 250/25 mg q.i.d. Higher doses are unlikely to be more beneficial. The patient should be maintained on the lowest possible dose compatible with a reasonable degree of functioning.

Because L-dopa has a half-life of 0.75 to 1.5 hours and a variable absorption, there may be marked fluctuations in performance during the day due to variations in plasma level. The response can be "smoothed out" by having patients take the drug every 2 hours. At times it is necessary for patients to take a dose immediately upon awakening to ensure optimal functioning in the morning. A controlled-release form of Sinemet is now available and provides more constant postsynaptic dopaminergic stimulation, thereby lessening the fluctuations in motor performance and dyskinesias.

After several years on L-dopa, as the disease progresses, most patients reach a stage of diminishing efficacy; large swings in performance, which may be sudden (the on-off phenomenon), start to occur, along with severe dyskinesias that patients must learn to tolerate

Table 12-3. Treatment of Parkinson's Disease

L-Dopa preparations
    L-Dopa + carbidopa
    L-Dopa + benserazide
    Controlled release preparation
    Continuous administration by IV infusion
      (investigational)
Direct-acting dopaminergic agents
    Bromocriptine
    Pergolide
Monoamine oxidase inhibitor
    Selegiline (deprenyl)
Amantadine hydrochloride
Anticholinergic agents
    Trihexyphenidyl
    Benztropine
    Procyclidine
Adjuvant agents
    Tricyclic antidepressants
    Domperidone
Physiotherapy

if they are to enjoy some mobility. Some of these sudden fluctuations in performance probably relate to the erratic absorption of L-dopa due to its interaction with amino acids from ingested proteins or to competition for blood-brain barrier transport sites from other amino acids, leading to poor penetration into the brain. These problems are reduced when controlled-release Sinemet is used. Studies are now under way to examine new ways to administer L-dopa (e.g., by continuous intravenous infusion) that might avert these problems. There is currently no ready solution to this difficult situation. A brief "drug holiday," while the patient is hospitalized, may temporarily restore responsiveness to the drug. A modified weekend drug holiday has also shown some success in outpatients. Recently the direct-acting ergot alkaloid dopaminergic agents bromocriptine and pergolide have been introduced into the treatment strategy for Parkinson's disease. Gradually adding one of them to the regimen, at the same time reducing the dose of L-dopa (about 50 percent), often diminishes the end-of-dose "wearing-off" reactions and dyskinesias.

Other Agents
Bromocriptine has a longer half-life than L-dopa and can be taken four times per day. It acts primarily on D_2 receptors. However, it is expensive and frequently causes side effects consisting of mental changes, psychosis, hypotension, gastrointestinal upset, and edema. Dyskinesias are also seen, particularly in patients who have previously received L-dopa. When combined with L-dopa, it is generally effective in doses of 25 to 80 mg per day, which have to be achieved gradually.

Pergolide acts on both D_1 and D_2 receptors and there is some evidence suggesting that, besides providing symptomatic therapy, it may retard progression of the disease. The usual doses are 1 mg t.i.d. and its side effects are similar to bromocriptine's. Some patients who do not respond to a particular dopamine agonist do respond to another.

The nausea, vomiting, or cardiac effects seen with these agents may be less with **domperidone**, a peripherally acting dopamine receptor blocker. **Deprenyl** (Selegiline), a monoamine oxidase-B inhibitor, may be of use when added to L-dopa for patients suffering from end-of-dose wearing-off phenomena with prominent akinesia. There is also some evidence that it may, in fact, slow the rate of deterioration in patients with Parkinson's disease ("neuroprotective effect") and should therefore be of use early in the disease. Free-radical scavengers such as **tocopherol** may also have a neuroprotective effect. None of these drugs has yet replaced L-dopa as the initial choice of therapy for moderately severe Parkinson's disease. Studies are in progress to evaluate the long-term effects of low doses of L-dopa combined with either a dopamine antagonist or Selegiline starting in the early phases of the disease.

Nonpharmacological Measures
Physical therapy, which provides both psychological and physical benefits, should not be neglected as an important mode of treatment in Parkinson's disease. One of the important features in the management of these patients is a careful assessment of the degree of disability at each visit, which should be performed consistently at the same time in relation to the previous drug dose. Simple maneuvers such as having the patient turn over in a lying position, walk a fixed distance while being timed, write

a few sentences, or complete a drawing are useful for documenting the patient's progress. Various disability rating skills have also been devised.

Patients must also be taught to keep careful daily records of the times they are mobile or experience side effects in relation to medication intake. Depression, which is common, may be managed with a tricyclic antidepressant. Other problems such as constipation and sialorrhea may require symptomatic treatment.

Stereotaxic surgery is still used occasionally for the treatment of Parkinson's disease in patients with unilateral involvement who respond poorly to medication. A lesion made in the ventrolateral nucleus of one thalamus may control severe contralateral tremor and to a lesser degree rigidity, but has no effect on the bradykinesia. Bilateral surgery is contraindicated because it frequently produces severe dysarthria. More recently, the transplantation of human adrenal medulla cells or fetal dopaminergic cells into the striatum has shown promising results in some patients.

OTHER TYPES OF PARKINSONISM

Postencephalitic

During 1916 to 1926, a worldwide pandemic of encephalitis lethargica (von Economo's) arose that was due to an unidentified virus. About one half of the survivors exhibited progressive parkinsonian signs, often after a latency period of several years following recovery from the encephalitis. Some cases were presumed to have resulted from a subclinical attack of encephalitis. These cases, which are extremely rare today, often exhibited features atypical of idiopathic Parkinson's disease. Onset frequently occurred in the third or fourth decade, as opposed to the sixth or seventh decade typical of Parkinson's disease. These patients often had cranial nerve palsies and marked dystonic features, and some had oculogyric crises. These crises consist of the involuntary upward deviation of the eyes with lid retraction lasting from seconds to hours and causing a great deal of

discomfort. Blepharospasm, sialorrhea, and seborrhea were prominent symptoms.

Pathological examination of the neural tissue in these cases revealed that there were no Lewy bodies but there were neurofibrillary tangles, similar to those seen in patients with Alzheimer's disease, in the substantia nigra and in other areas of cell degeneration. The substantia nigra in these cases shows a more uniform cell loss than that seen in Parkinson's disease. These patients may benefit from L-dopa therapy and usually respond to small amounts of the drug. Rarely a similar parkinsonian picture, often characterized by extreme rigidity, can arise following a bout of encephalitis caused by specific viruses such as Japanese B, western equine, or Venezuelan.

Drug-Induced

Dopamine-depleting drugs such as reserpine and dopamine postsynaptic receptor–blocking agents such as the phenothiazines, butyrophenones, and metoclopramide (Maxeran) can cause parkinsonism as a side effect. Aliphatic phenothiazines, with a high antipsychotic potency, and haloperidol are the most likely agents to give rise to this problem. Other drugs, such as alpha-methyldopa, lithium, and amiodarone, have also been rarely implicated. In fact, drug-induced parkinsonism is the most common form of parkinsonism seen today and is an extremely prevalent condition on psychiatric wards. Tremor is usually not a major feature in these patients, but akathisia, which is a restless sensation in the legs and an inability to sit still, is often prominent. Withdrawal of the drug, although not always possible with antipsychotic agents, may not produce remission of these symptoms for several months in some cases. Treatment with anticholinergic drugs such as benztropine or trihexyphenidyl is often effective and, in intractable cases, L-dopa has been used. However, an exacerbation of the preexisting psychosis is likely.

Toxin-Induced

Parkinsonism may develop in manganese miners following prolonged exposure to and inhalation of manganese dust. Akinesia and gait imbalance dominate the clinical picture. Intoxication with substances such as carbon monoxide, carbon disulfide, and cyanide may also cause fairly selective basal ganglia destruction and parkinsonism. Recently, MPTP has been shown to produce a severe parkinsonian syndrome with many of the clinical and pathological features of Parkinson's disease. This illness, like true Parkinson's disease, responds to treatment with L-dopa.

Amyotrophic Lateral Sclerosis—Parkinsonism-Dementia of Guam

A relatively high incidence of a unique form of parkinsonism in which patients also suffer from dementia and, in the terminal stages, from amyotrophic lateral sclerosis has been noted among the Chamorro natives of the Mariana Islands of the South Pacific. This disease has been termed the *ALS-PD complex of Guam*. Although it is often familial in origin, no clear-cut inheritance pattern has been determined. The pathological findings of widespread neurofibrillary tangles affecting various subcortical structures, hippocampal areas, and anterior horn cells has prompted a great deal of study of this entity. Evidence has been uncovered that neurotoxicity resulting from ingestion of the cycad plant, a traditional native food, may be responsible for the ALS-PD complex. The incidence of the disorder has been steadily declining since consumption of the cycad plant has decreased. Other geographic isolates have manifested a similar syndrome, and there is a rare North American form of familial or sporadic ALS-PD complex that lacks the extensive neurofibrillary degeneration found in the Guamanian variety.

Calcification of the Basal Ganglia

Familial calcification of the basal ganglia (Fahr's disease) is an autosomally dominant inherited disorder without any derangement of the serum calcium level. These patients may exhibit signs of typical parkinsonism as well as psychiatric and other neurological disturbances. Patients with hypocalcemia due to hypoparathyroidism or pseudohypoparathyroidism frequently show basal ganglia calcifications and rarely may manifest parkinsonian features.

Vascular Disease

The existence of "atherosclerotic parkinsonism" has long been debated. Patients, usually hypertensive, with multiple lacunar infarcts affecting the basal ganglia (as well as other areas) may show marked rigidity and bradykinesia, gait difficulty, and expressionless facies. In addition, corticobulbar and corticospinal tract signs are prominent. L-dopa is ineffective in these patients.

Brain Tumors

Although tumors of the basal ganglia may rarely give rise to signs of parkinsonism, the intracranial tumors seen in parkinsonian patients are located elsewhere, such as in the cerebellum. It is generally not necessary to search for an intracranial neoplasm in a patient who exhibits a typical picture of Parkinson's disease.

Specific Degenerative Conditions with Parkinsonian Features (Parkinson's Plus)

A number of pathologically and clinically distinct conditions with extrapyramidal features may be mistaken for Parkinson's disease, even though other "atypical" features, such as corticospinal tract signs, cerebellar ataxia, profound early dementia, marked eye movement impairment, pronounced automatic features, or family history, point to another diagnosis. The list of such disorders includes olivopontocerebellar degeneration, progressive supranuclear palsy, the rigid form of Huntington's disease, Wilson's disease, Alzheimer's disease, Hallervorden-Spatz disease, Creutzfeldt-Jakob disease, the Shy-Drager syndrome, and striatonigral degeneration.

Striatonigral degeneration may resemble Parkinson's disease quite closely, but tremor is uncommon. In this disorder, the putamen shows prominent cell loss and atrophy but the substantia nigra is only mildly affected.

Patients with **severe depression** may also superficially appear as though they have Parkinson's disease. In these cases, the parkinsonian symptoms are resistant to L-dopa therapy.

Another rare condition that may include several parkinsonian features such as akinesia, rigidity, tremor, and postural instability is **corticobasal ganglionic degeneration**. This condition often begins in the sixth decade or later and is relentlessly progressive, ending in death several years later. In addition to parkinsonian features and dystonia, patients show evidence of cortical involvement, including cortical sensory loss, apraxia, alien limb phenomenon, corticospinal tract signs, and a late-appearing dementia. Asymmetry of motor involvement is a consistent feature. Myoclonus and loss of saccadic (particularly vertical) eye movements are also seen. The pathological hallmark of the disease is achromasia (poor staining) and swelling of the neurons accompanied by gliosis within the cortex, substantia nigra, and cerebellar dentate nuclei.

BIBLIOGRAPHY

Agid, Y. Parkinson's disease: pathophysiology. *Lancet* 337:1321–1324, 1991.

Boshes, B. Sinemet and the treatment of parkinsonism. *Ann. Intern. Med.* 94:364–370, 1981.

Burton, K. and Calne, D.B. Pharmacology of Parkinson's disease. *Neurol. Clin.* 2:461–472, 1984.

Carter, J.H. et al. Amount and distribution of dietary protein affects clinical response to levodopa in Parkinson's disease. *Neurology* 39:552–556, 1989.

Cedarbaum, J.M. Pharmacokinetics and pharmacodynamic considerations in management of motor response fluctuations in Parkinson's disease. *Neurol. Clin.* 8:31–49, 1990.

Duvoisin, R. Parkinsonism. *CIBA Clin. Symp.* 29:1–29, 1977.

Duvoisin, R. Parkinson's disease: acquired or inherited? *Can. J. Neurol. Sci.* 11(suppl.): 151–155, 1984.

Fahn, S. Fluctuations of Disability in Parkinson's Disease: Pathophysiology. In C.D. Marsden and S. Fahn (editors). *Movement Disorders*. London: Butterworths, 1982, Pp. 123–145.

Hoehn, M.M. and Yahr, M.D. Parkinsonism: onset, progression and mortality. *Neurology* 17:427–442, 1967.

Hornykiewicz, O. Brain neurotransmitter changes in Parkinson's disease. In C.D. Marsden and S. Fahn (editors). *Movement Disorders*. London: Butterworths, 1982, Pp. 41–58.

Hutton, J.T. and Morris, J.L. Long-acting carbidopa-levodopa in the management of moderate and advanced Parkinson's disease. *Neurology* 42(suppl. 1):51–56, 1992.

Koller, W.C. How accurately can Parkinson's disease be diagnosed? *Neurology* 42(suppl. 1):6–16, 1992.

Langston, J.W. and Ballard, P. Parkinsonism induced by 1-methyl-4-phenyl-1,2,3,6-tetrahydropyridine (MPTP): implications for treatment and the pathogenesis of Parkinson's disease. *Can. J. Neurol. Sci.* 11(suppl.): 160–165, 1984.

Lee, R.G. Physiology of the basal ganglia: an overview. *Can. J. Neurol. Sci.* 11(suppl.): 124–128, 1984.

Lee, R.G. Physiology of the basal ganglia and pathophysiology of Parkinson's disease. *Can. J. Neurol. Sci.* 14:373–380, 1987.

Lesser, R.P., et al. Analysis of the clinical problems in parkinsonism and the complications of long-term levodopa therapy. *Neurology* 29:1253–1260, 1979.

Lieberman, A.N. Parkinson's disease: a clinical review. *Am. J. Med. Sci.* 267:66–80, 1974.

Lieberman, A. Emerging perspectives in Parkinson's disease. *Neurology* 42(suppl. 4):5–7, 1992.

Lieberman, A.N., et al. D-1 and D-2 agonist

in Parkinson's disease. *Can. J. Neurol. Sci.* 14:466–473, 1987.

Marsden, C.D., and Fahn, S. Problems in Parkinson's Disease. In C.D. Marsden and S. Fahn (editors). *Movement Disorders.* London: Butterworths, 1982, Pp. 1–7.

Marsden, C.D., Parkes, J.D., and Quinn, N. Fluctuations of Disability in Parkinson's Disease—Clinical Aspects. In C.D. Marsden and S. Fahn (editors). *Movement Disorders.* London: Butterworths, 1982, Pp. 96–122.

Mayeux, R. Depression and Dementia in Parkinson's Disease. In C.D. Marsden and S. Fahn (editors). *Movement Disorders.* London: Butterworths, 1982, Pp. 75–95.

Moore, R.Y. Catecholamine neuron systems in brain. *Ann. Neurol.* 12:321–327, 1982.

Parkes, J.D. Domperidone and Parkinson's disease. *Clin. Neuropharmacol.* 9:517–532, 1986.

Rajput, A. Epidemiology of Parkinson's disease. *Can. J. Neurol. Sci.* 11(suppl.):156–159, 1984.

Riley, D.E. and Lang, A.E. Cortical-Basal Ganglionic Degeneration. In S. Appel (editor). *Current Neurology.* St. Louis: Mosby–Year Book, 1992, Vol. 12.

Spencer, P.S. Guam ALS/parkinsonism-dementia: a long-latency neurotoxic disorder caused by "slow toxin(s)" in food? *Can. J. Neurol. Sci.* 14:347–357, 1987.

Yahr, M.D. and Duvoisin, R.C. Drug therapy of parkinsonism. *N. Engl. J. Med.* 287:20–24, 1972.

Hyperkinetic Movement Disorders

Several varieties of abnormal involuntary movements have been identified and are generally believed to stem from altered function and possibly neurotransmitter or neuromodulator disturbances in the basal ganglia. The pathological substrates of some of these conditions, such as Huntington's chorea and hemiballism, have been defined, but most are associated with no observable underlying anatomical brain lesions and instead represent disturbances at the biochemical level. The clinical recognition of these syndromes is important because each has its specific causes, prognosis, and potential treatment.

CHOREA AND ATHETOSIS

Chorea or choreiform movements consist of rapid, uncoordinated involuntary jerks that are strong enough to displace a limb or part of a limb. They are multifocal, often distal, and are frequently blended with purposeful movements as if the patient is actively trying to mask them.

For example, a sudden arm jerk may merge into a scratching of the scalp. Choreiform limb movements are also accompanied by grimaces, darting tongue movements, truncal jerks, and irregular respiratory grunts. The gait of affected patients frequently has a bizarre dance-like quality to it, and from this characteristic comes the word *chorea* which is derived from the Greek word for "dance."

Athetosis describes the proximal slow, writhing limb movements that often occur in combination with chorea (choreoathetosis). A particular characteristic of these patients is the hyperpronated position of the forearm with flexion at the wrist and abduction and hyperextension of the fingers when the arms are held outstretched. These are distinguished from dystonic movements mainly by their nonrepetitive nature.

Choreoathetosis and Cerebral Palsy

Birth hypoxia or ischemia may affect the basal ganglia and give rise to athetotic cerebral palsy.

Such patients usually begin to show choreoathetosis around age 2 and severe motor and speech deficits may develop. The caudate and putamen exhibit a marbled appearance due to a disorder of myelination (état marbré). Intelligence is often normal. Kernicterus may also produce athetoid cerebral palsy and affects mainly the globus pallidus.

Huntington's Disease

Huntington's disease, or chorea, is a genetic condition with an autosomal dominant mode of inheritance. Penetrance is complete and spontaneous cases are so rare that, if there is no history of an affected parent, either the diagnosis or the accuracy of the family history must be seriously questioned. The prevalence is 5 per 100,000. The mean age when symptoms appear is around 40, but rare cases can either begin in childhood or in the 7th decade or later.

Pathophysiology and Etiology

The main site of the pathology in Huntington's disease is the caudate nucleus, and it is there that cell loss, particularly of the small Golgi type II interneurons, and gliosis occur (Fig. 13-1). Fibers of passage and afferent axons are relatively spared. The putamen, globus pallidus, and cerebral cortex (especially the frontal and occipital areas) are affected to a lesser degree. Biochemical analysis has revealed a diminution in the content of gamma-aminobutyric acid (GABA), acetylcholine, substance P, and enkephalin in these areas. The dopaminergic systems are preserved and, for unknown reasons, the somatostatin concentration in the caudate is increased. Striatal cholinergic interneurons as well as interneurons containing somatostatin and neuropeptide Y are largely spared.

The pathogenetic mechanism responsible for the neuronal loss is unknown, but an excitotoxic hypothesis has gained some support. Excitatory neurotransmission within the central nervous system (CNS) mainly utilizes the amino acids glutamate and aspartate, which react with four main categories of receptors: N-methyl-D-aspartate, kainate, alpha-amino-3-hydroxy-5-methyl-4-isoxazdepropionic acid, or the metabotropic receptor. The neuropathological and

neurochemical features of kainic acid toxicity in animals somewhat resembles the pattern seen in Huntington's disease. Excessive neuronal excitation by endogenous excitatory amino acids leading to cell death could therefore be involved in the genesis of Huntington's disease. Recent work has demonstrated that the defective gene in Huntington's patients resides on the short arm of chromosome 4. This discovery has made it possible to detect presymptomatic affected individuals for the purposes of genetic counseling.

Clinical Picture and Diagnosis

Juvenile Huntington's (onset earlier than age 20) exhibits atypical features of pronounced rigidity, early severe dementia, a high incidence of seizures, and a more rapid rate of progression. Some patients with late-onset disease may manifest features more reminiscent of parkinsonism than of chorea. Typical cases begin with an insidious personality change, emotional lability, concentration difficulties, and subtle intellectual impairment. Chorea eventually follows (although it may precede any noticeable mental changes) and becomes more and more pronounced, finally interfering significantly with voluntary movement, gait, swallowing, and speech. Rigidity is minimal in most cases. The early impairment of saccadic eye movements can be documented by electrooculography. As the subcortical dementia advances, a patient shows increasing muscle wasting and weakness, and finally becomes bedridden. Death results from malnutrition, sepsis, pneumonia, or pulmonary embolus usually 10 to 20 years following the onset. There is a high incidence of suicide among patients in the early phases of the disease when insight is still preserved.

The typical clinical picture occurring in the context of a history of the disorder in preceding generations confirms the diagnosis. A computed tomographic (CT) scan obtained in the more advanced stages shows fairly characteristic enlargement of the frontal horns due to atrophy of the caudate nuclei. The atrophy can be appreciated best on axial and coronal views of magnetic resonance imaging scans. The electrooculographic demonstration of saccadic gaze

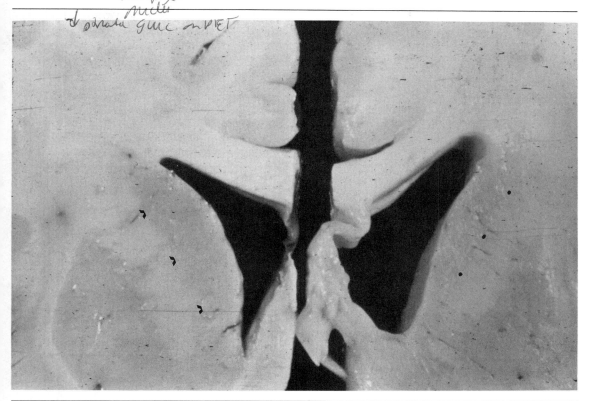

Fig. 13-1. *Coronal section through caudate nucleus of brain in a normal subject (left,* arrowheads*) and in a patient with Huntington's disease (right,* dots*). Note shrinkage of the caudate nucleus and less concavity of the lateral wall of lateral ventricle in the brain affected by Huntington's disease.*

abnormalities may also be helpful in making an early diagnosis. A polymorphic human-linked DNA marker can be used to identify the condition in certain presymptomatic individuals with an approximately 95 percent degree of accuracy. The additional demonstration of reduced striatal glucose metabolism on positron emission tomographic scanning can be further proof of the presence of the disease in presymptomatic individuals.

Management and Prognosis

No known treatment can arrest the progress of the disease or slow or reverse the mental deterioration. The chorea, which is often more disturbing to others than to the patient, can be reduced, if necessary, by administering dopamine-depleting or blocking agents such as haloperidol, reserpine, or tetrabenazine. However, phenothiazines may exacerbate the bradykinesia and tetrabenazine the depression, which are already problems in these patients. High caloric intake to maintain weight and treatment of depression are important measures. Family counseling and psychological support are an important part of the overall management. The identification of presymptomatic individuals with the disease touches on a number of difficult ethical issues, however.

Neuroacanthocytosis

Neuroacanthocytosis is a rare nonfamilial form of chorea that can be misdiagnosed as Huntington's disease. It appears early in life and many patients exhibit rapid ticlike choreic movements in the jaw, tongue, and face. Patients also exhibit dystonia, seizures, and muscle wasting due to a peripheral neuropathy. The dementia in this disease is less marked than the dementia seen in Huntington's disease, but psychiatric disturbances and self-mutilation are common. The diagnostic hallmark of the disease is acanthocytes, which are spiny red blood cells seen with Wright's staining on a thick wet blood film. Letting the blood stand for 12 hours may improve the chances of detecting acanthocytes.

Sydenham's Chorea

One of the major manifestations of rheumatic fever following a beta-hemolytic streptococcal infection in childhood is Sydenham's chorea. This condition used to be the most common cause of chorea in childhood several decades ago, but has now become rare. About one third of these patients also later suffer rheumatic heart disease or migratory polyarthritis. Onset is usually in late childhood and insidious. In addition to the chorea that mainly affects the face and upper extremities, there is emotional lability, listlessness, and generalized hypotonia and weakness. Pathological changes are nonspecific and diffuse, resembling a mild encephalitis with vasculitis affecting the basal ganglia, cortex, and cerebellum. Traditional treatment consists of rest in a darkened room with the administration of minor tranquilizers. Penicillin should also be given. The prognosis is good and the chorea usually disappears within weeks, although recurrences may appear. A rare complication is occlusion of the central retinal artery.

Senile Chorea

Elderly patients may exhibit a nonprogressive form of chorea without dementia and in the absence of a family history. Some of these cases may represent a forme fruste of Huntington's disease.

Paroxysmal and Kinesiogenic Choreoathetoses

The poorly understood entities that make up the paroxysmal and kinesiogenic forms of choreoathetosis include familial (autosomal reces-

sive) and nonfamilial forms of intermittent brief attacks of choreoathetosis (or hemichoreoathetosis) that may, in some instances, be provoked by movement of the involved limbs. Some of these cases may represent a form of basal ganglia epilepsy and respond to treatment with anticonvulsants. Rare cases of the kinesiogenic type have been associated with hypocalcemia stemming from hypoparathyroidism or pseudohypoparathyroidism and basal ganglia calcifications, or associated with thyrotoxicosis.

Other Causes of Chorea

Other causes of chorea include systemic lupus erythematosus, pregnancy (chorea gravidarum), oral contraceptive use, basal ganglia infarction, L-dopa therapy, phenytoin intoxication, Wilson's disease, neurosyphilis, hypoparathyroidism, thyrotoxicosis, and benign familial chorea.

HEMIBALLISM

Hemiballism refers to involuntary, irregular flinging-type movements of a limb around the proximal joint. The movements often appear acutely and commonly arise from a vascular lesion affecting the subthalamic nucleus or its connections. Rarely a metastatic tumor or trauma affecting the same area may be responsible. In some cases, the lesion involves the striatum or thalamus. The movements may evolve from or be replaced by hemichoreic movements. Hemiballism may appear in the context of a hemiplegia or leave a hemiplegia in its wake as it subsides. The movements usually diminish spontaneously within several days of onset. Haloperidol can be used to suppress the movements and thereby prevent patient exhaustion and increase patient comfort.

TREMOR

Tremor refers to a relatively regular, rhythmic, oscillatory movement that may affect the extremities, head, trunk, or voice. It can be characterized as fine or coarse, depending on the amplitude; slow or rapid, depending on the frequency; regular or irregular; or continuous or intermittent. Certain tremors such as primary writing tremor are evoked only by particular movements.

The initial clinical differentiation of tremors is based on whether they occur at rest (but not complete relaxation such as sleep, which will abolish virtually all tremors), with a sustained position (postural tremor), or during movement (action or kinetic tremor). **Tremor at rest** is best illustrated by the 3- to 5-Hz tremor of parkinsonism but is also seen in patients with Wilson's disease or neurosyphilis. **Postural tremor** is frequently accompanied by action tremor and is revealed by having patients hold their hands outstretched with fingers spread or with the index fingers of each hand barely touching. Placing a sheet of paper on the back of the patient's hand will render the tremor more visible. **Action tremor** is easily seen when a patient attempts to drink from a cup.

Intention tremor specifically refers to a type of tremor that increases in amplitude roughly perpendicular to the line of movement as the goal is approached. The finger-nose-finger or heel-knee-shin tests can detect this type of tremor. It is characteristically seen in patients with lesions that affect the main cerebellar efferent pathway—the dentatorubral pathway passing through the superior cerebellar peduncle.

Tremor must be distinguished from other types of involuntary movements. **Asterixis** is a sudden, irregular, flapping-like movement of the hands or feet arising because of a brief lapse of extensor muscle tone. It is best demonstrated by having patients hold their arms outstretched with the wrists extended. This movement disorder is most commonly associated with metabolic disorders such as hepatic, uremic, or pulmonary encephalopathy. It may also occur as the result of drug toxicity (e.g., phenytoin or carbamazepine) or structural lesions (e.g., infarcts) affecting the midbrain, thalamus, or internal capsule, and may be unilateral in these cases.

Rhythmic myoclonus exhibits a slight pause between successive displacements and lacks the to-and-fro quality of tremor. **Fasciculations**, which are spontaneous contractions of muscle motor units, may be frequent and strong enough to displace the fingers and give rise to a pseudotremor. They are recognized by their lack of rhythmicity, the absence of synchrony among fingers, an association with muscle atrophy, and the characteristic electromyographic appearance. Other movements, such as minipolymyoclonus, which appear in some cases of chronic juvenile spinal muscular atrophy, or muscle myokymia (rippling-like muscle movements), may be confused with tremor.

The characteristics of other involuntary movements, which are usually readily distinguished from tremor, are described elsewhere in this chapter. In some cases, tremor may coexist with these other involuntary movements, creating a confusing clinical picture.

Physiological Tremor

Normal physiological tremor has too small an amplitude to be seen, but can be demonstrated by the strong co-contraction of agonist and antagonist muscles in a limb. The normal frequency is 10 to 12 Hz, which tends to decline gradually after the fifth decade. Conditions resulting in catecholamine release such as anxiety, fright, exercise, fatigue, hypoglycemia, thyrotoxicosis, and pheochromocytoma accentuate physiological tremor. Various drugs and toxins can produce tremor, in most cases related to an enhancement of physiological tremor (Table 13-1).

Essential Tremor

Essential tremor is a combined postural and action tremor that occurs in either a sporadic or familial (autosomal dominant) setting and is considered benign because it is generally not associated with other neurological deficits or objective neurological findings. Patients are often referred with a diagnosis of parkinsonism, but essential tremor is usually easily identified on the basis of early-life onset (often childhood), family history, occurrence when the limb is outstretched or moving rather than at rest, greater frequency (6–11 Hz), greater tendency to involve the head, and lack of associated findings such as rigidity, gait disorder, or

Table 13-1. Drugs and Toxins Producing Tremor

Beta-adrenergic agonists
  Epinephrine
  Theophylline
  Isoetharine
  Isoproteronol
  Metaproterenol
  Terbutoline
L-Dopa
Amphetamines
Lithium
Phenothiazines, butyrophenones
Tricyclic antidepressants
Prednisone
Antiepileptics
  Valproic acid
  Carbamazepine
  Xanthines (in coffee and tea)
Heavy metals
  Mercury
  Lead
  Arsenic
  Bismuth

micrographia. In certain patients, the two conditions may occur together, accounting for the postural and resting tremors seen in some parkinsonian patients.

Essential tremor is often relieved by the ingestion of even small amounts of alcohol. The tremor is frequently unilateral at onset, may be asymmetrical, and tends to increase with age. Late-appearing cases are often deemed senile tremor. Interference with fine motor activity or speech may cause some disability. However, the most disabling feature is often the embarrassment it causes, and, because anxiety exacerbates the tremor, a vicious cycle results. Sufferers report that they are frequently mistaken for alcoholics.

Substantial relief is afforded by beta-blocking agents such as propranolol (40 to 160 mg b.i.d.), but this agent is contraindicated in patients with significant congestive heart failure, asthma, hypoglycemic attacks, or insulin-dependent diabetes, and can cause undue bradycardia or hypotension. Side effects of fatigue, impotence, insomnia, constipation, and depression are not uncommon. Other beta-blockers such as metoprolol (preferred in pa-

tients with bronchospastic disease) or timolol can be substituted, and primidone, an antiepileptic barbiturate, has been reported to be effective in some cases.

Other Tremors

Alcohol withdrawal produces a tremor that resembles enhanced physiological tremor. Many alcoholics demonstrate a more persistent postural tremor whose pathogenesis is uncertain. Rubral or midbrain tremor is a fairly coarse, irregular postural tremor seen in conditions such as multiple sclerosis. In severe cases, some relief may be afforded by stereotaxic ventral lateral thalamotomy. Mercury toxicity produces a fine postural tremor in addition to neuropathy.

DYSTONIAS

Dystonia consists of repetitive involuntary and usually twisting movements (i.e., dystonic movements) and postures caused by the co-contraction of agonist and antagonist muscles, with maximal displacement persisting for a second or longer. Typical examples are plantar flexion and inversion (the equinovarus posture) of a foot, an arm flexed behind the back, or hyperextended fingers. In severe cases, patients assume bizarre, fixed dystonic postures with the trunk, neck, and limbs in various twisted and unnatural-appearing positions. Other involuntary movements such as tremor or myoclonus may be combined with dystonia.

Dystonia may occur at rest, at sites distant from movement (overflow dystonia), or only with a specific movement (action dystonia). Although most cases of dystonia are idiopathic and neuropathological examination of the brain yields normal findings, so-called symptomatic cases, due to tumor, infarction, birth anoxia, or Wilson's disease, tend to affect the putamen.

Dystonia that occurs in a hemibody distribution is highly linked to an identifiable etiology. Neurotransmitter disturbances are assumed to be responsible because L-dopa can produce dystonia as a side effect and phenothiazines may give rise to acute dystonic reactions or tardive dystonia. A noradrenergic predominance has been proposed. Rare cases may result from peripheral nerve or root lesions rather than from a CNS pathology. Occasional cases are found to have an hysterical basis and such patients respond to psychotherapy. A classification of dystonia is given in Table 13-2.

Torsion Dystonia (Dystonia Musculorum Deformans)

Torsion dystonia is considered a degenerative condition that may be sporadic or inherited as an autosomal dominant trait exhibiting variable penetrance. Recently the gene was localized to the long arm of chromosome 9 (9q32-q34). An autosomal recessive variety was thought to afflict mainly Ashkenazi Jewish families. This form showed less variation in the age of onset, less involvement of the axial musculature, and a more uniform course. Onset of the autosomal dominant form tends to appear over a wider age range, progresses more slowly, and includes

Table 13-2. Dystonias

Idiopathic torsion dystonia (dystonia musculorum deformans)
    Autosomal dominant
    Autosomal recessive
    Sex-linked
    Sporadic
Symptomatic dystonias
    Tumors, infarcts, trauma affecting the basal ganglia
    Wilson's disease
    Huntington's chorea
    Hallervorden-Spatz disease
    Neuronal ceroid lipofuscinosis
    Chronic GM_1 or GM_2 gangliosidoses
    Drugs (e.g., L-dopa, phenothiazines, metoclopramide)
    Following birth anoxia, kernicterus
    Encephalitis, meningitis
    Parkinsonism
    Progressive supranuclear palsy
    Dopa-responsive dystonia
Special forms of segmental dystonia
    Torticollis
    Writer's cramp and other "occupational" cramps
    Spasmodic dysphonia (laryngeal dystonia)

truncal dystonia and torticollis more frequently and earlier in the course. However, the findings from recent studies have suggested that the Jewish variety may also be mainly autosomal dominant and actually differ little from the non-Jewish variety.

No pathological abnormalities have been discovered in the brains of affected individuals nor have any neurotransmitter disturbances yet been determined. Onset may be gradual and subtle, with incipient manifestations consisting of inturning of a foot while walking, a tendency for the hand to cramp during writing, or dystonic posturing of the upper extremity when reaching out for objects. At the beginning, these abnormalities may appear only during movement or under conditions of emotional excitement. Many of these patients are initially diagnosed as hysterics.

In the late phases, patients may assume fixed dystonic postures leading to severe disability. Childhood-onset cases usually begin between the ages 5 and 12 and are more severe than adult cases.

Treatment is difficult, but high doses of anticholinergic drugs (trihexyphenidyl, gradually increasing to 30–120 mg per day), which are better tolerated by children, may be beneficial. Various other agents, such as benzodiazepines, carbamazepine, baclofen, and tetrabenazine, have been used with some benefit. In some cases, stereotaxic ventrolateral thalamotomy has provided dramatic relief.

Dopa-responsive dystonia (Segawa variant) is a variant of childhood-onset idiopathic torsion dystonia that exhibits an autosomal dominant mode of inheritance, but is seen mainly in non-Jews, as opposed to idiopathic torsion dystonia. The legs and gait are affected earliest but eventually the dystonia becomes generalized. A diurnal fluctuation of symptoms is seen in about three quarters of the cases. Rigidity and late-appearing resting tremor are manifested in some cases, which may make differentiation from child-onset parkinsonism somewhat difficult. The presumed deficit in dopa-responsive dystonia is the decreased central synthesis of dopamine. These patients respond dramatically to even small doses of L-dopa and also do well with anticholinergic agents.

Spasmodic Torticollis

Torticollis refers to an involuntary contraction of the sternocleidomastoid and other nuchal muscles that draws the head to one side and usually rotates it so that the chin points to the opposite side (Fig. 13-2). It may be "spasmodic," imparting a gross tremorlike appearance to the movement. Rare variants are retrocollis, in which the head is pulled backward, or antecollis, in which the head is pulled forward.

Various specific conditions, both congenital and acquired, have been found in some cases: these include cervical muscle deformity or injury, cervical skeletal abnormalities (e.g., C1–C2 subluxation), and posterior fossa tu-

mors. Psychiatric factors have also occasionally been held responsible. However, the vast majority of cases with an adult onset (usually over age 40) are considered to represent a form of segmental dystonia that may progress in some cases and include other dystonic manifestations. As in other forms of dystonia, no underlying neuropathological lesions have been identified in the idiopathic cases.

Characteristically the patient can achieve temporary relief, at least in the early phases, by exerting light counterpressure to the chin—so-called sensory tricks. The condition rarely remits but may do so in some cases. It is usually quite disabling and resistant to most of the treatments that have been tried. Management of secondary psychiatric consequences such as de-

Fig. 13-2. *Patient with spasmodic torticollis.*

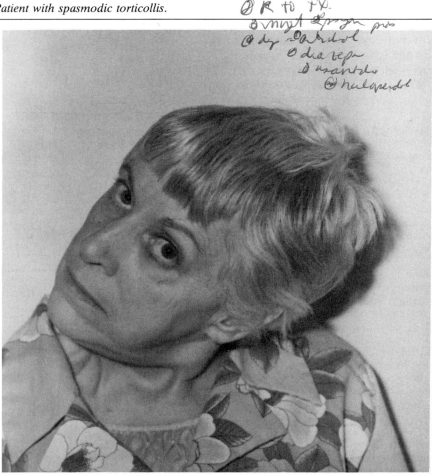

pression is indicated. Drugs such as anticholinergics in high doses, diazepam, amantadine, and haloperidol have provided relief in a limited number of cases. Biofeedback to effect neck muscle relaxation has been claimed successful in certain cases. Some patients require a denervation procedure such as a cervical C1–C6 rhizotomy and section of accessory nerve branches or selective muscle sectioning, but these interventions yield variable results. Botulinum toxin injections into involved muscles have produced significant improvement in some patients, and this has become the treatment of choice (see later discussion).

Blepharospasm

Blepharospasm is an involuntary tendency for the eyes to close, which, in its mildest form, causes increased blinking and, in its most severe form, may qualify as legal blindness. It usually develops gradually and is often preceded by increased blinking frequency, dry eyes, and photophobia. A variety of causes, including ocular disease, psychiatric disturbances, tics, infarcts of the nondominant parietal lobe, parkinsonism (especially postencephalitic), phenothiazine use, and L-dopa therapy have been cited. Severity varies markedly from time to time and symptoms may be reduced in the physician's office, when the patient is concentrating and distracted.

Meige's syndrome is an idiopathic dystonic disorder usually seen in women and combining blepharospasm with oromandibular dystonia. Patients exhibit a variety of lower facial movements, including jaw opening, jaw clenching, tongue twisting and thrusting, grimacing, flaring of the nostrils, and contraction of the platysma (Fig. 13-3). Similar movements may occur in patients with tardive dyskinesia or dystonia following long-term phenothiazine use.

The treatment of this syndrome has been generally disappointing, but localized injections of botulinum A toxin into periorbital muscles has afforded some benefit. The toxin works by binding to presynaptic cholinergic terminals and thereby decreasing the release of acetylcholine. Injections usually have to be given every 3 months, and ptosis, eyelid laxity, and tearing may result.

Writer's Cramp

The commonly seen form of writer's cramp, formerly labeled *occupational neurosis*, is now believed to represent a focal or segmental dystonia. It may become a more generalized dystonia in some cases. The condition is commonly observed in individuals who do a great deal of writing, and usually requires their switching writing hands or learning to keyboard. Typically the neurological findings are negative and the patient has no difficulty performing other fine hand movements. Other allied conditions include typist's cramp and various musician cramps. The condition is more of an inconvenience than a significant disability. Treatment is generally ineffective, although certain writing devices have been employed and the use of botulinum toxin is being investigated. Many patients have to resort to using a handheld word processing device to overcome the problem.

TARDIVE DYSKINESIA

Tardive dyskinesia refers to choreiform movements, most prominently affecting the tongue and mouth, that appear after months or years of treatment with major tranquilizers or other central dopamine-blocking agents (e.g., prochlorperazine and metoclopramide). The movements may appear during ongoing therapy, but more commonly arise following a reduction in dosage or discontinuation of the offending drug. The dyskinetic oral-buccal masticatory movements may be combined with limb chorea, akathisia (motor restlessness), or dystonic movements (tardive dystonia).

All commonly used phenothiazines and butyrophenones can produce this syndrome, although thioridazine and clozapine may be less likely to do so. The disorder is particularly prominent in the elderly, in females, and after prolonged high-dose neuroleptic treatment. Its pathogenesis is believed to relate to postsynaptic basal ganglia dopamine receptor hypersensitivity. Thus, a temporary increase in the dosage

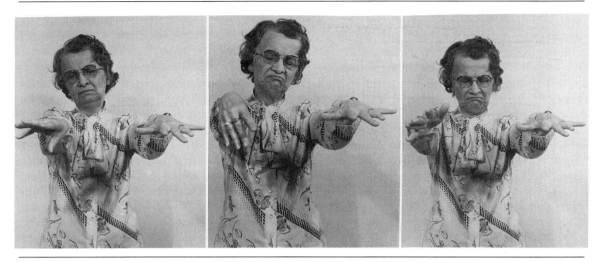

Fig. 13-3. *Patient with Meige's syndrome (blepharospasm and oromandibular dystonia) combined with dystonic arm movements and some athetoid movements. The etiology of this patient's disorder is unknown. Photographs were taken in sequence, from left to right, one second apart.*

of the neuroleptic will suppress the movements but possibly lead to future worsening of the disorder. Tardive dyskinesia must be distinguished from other forms of chorea, such as Huntington's, Meige's syndrome, and various tics and mannerisms.

Many patients tolerate the dyskinesias without distress; others may develop significant swallowing, speaking, and respiratory difficulties. After patients stop taking the offending agent, this frequently leads to remission within several months or a few years. However, some psychotic patients who develop the complication continue to require neuroleptics, in which case they should be given the lowest possible doses and perhaps thioridazine used instead. When the dyskinesias are severe enough to cause discomfort, eating difficulties, muscle tension headache, dysarthria, or respiratory distress, treatment should be attempted.

Once the neuroleptic is discontinued, reserpine, a dopamine-depleting agent, in a dose of 1 to 5 mg per day, frequently brings about improvement. However, side effects of hypotension and depression are common with this agent. Tetrabenazine is one of the most effective agents. Other strategies, though not usually

successful, consist of enhancing central cholinergic activity with purified lecithin, or giving drugs such as clonazepam or baclofen, which may increase central GABAergic tone. Because treatment of this disorder is so ineffectual, clinicians should avoid prescribing neuroleptic agents except when absolutely indicated, use them in the lowest possible doses, and consider withdrawing these agents at the first sign of tardive dyskinesia.

TOURETTE'S SYNDROME

Tics are stereotyped, repetitive movements, such as eye blinking, shoulder shrugging, grimacing, throat clearing, or skipping when walking, that occur at irregular intervals. The underlying cause in the nervous system is not established, but normal voluntary motor pathways do not appear to be involved. Frequently the tics are preceded by a build-up of subjective muscle tension and followed by a feeling of release once expressed. Psychological factors can influence them and they can often be voluntarily suppressed for a period. The tics may resemble chorea, although they tend to be more repetitive and lack the tendency to flow from one body part to another. They also may be difficult to differentiate from myoclonus, which tends to be more rapid and not amenable to voluntary control.

Tics are a common isolated finding in childhood, where they tend to disappear over a few months and are probably psychological in origin. A more persistent, often lifelong idiopathic disorder is the **Tourette's syndrome,** or maladie des tics. This uncommon syndrome is often misdiagnosed as a behavior disorder. It is now generally accepted that it likely originates from an imbalance in basal ganglion neurotransmitters producing a relative dopamine predominance. It is three times more common in males than in females and there is often a familial incidence. Specific criteria for diagnosis include:

1. Onset between ages 2 and 15
2. Multiple motor tics
3. Multiple vocal tics (e.g., involuntary utterances, grunts, and barks)
4. Ability to suppress movements voluntarily for minutes to hours
5. Variations in the intensity of symptoms over weeks and months
6. Duration greater than one year

Patients can also exhibit coprolalia (involuntary swearing), copropraxia (involuntary obscene gesturing), echolalia (involuntary repetition of words or sounds), echopraxia (involuntary imitation of others' movements), palilalia (involuntary repetition of the patient's own words), and self-mutilation tendencies.

The behavior of these patients is so bizarre that, in severe cases, patients frequently suffer ridicule and rejection. The disorder may respond dramatically to haloperidol or pimozide (up to 0.3 mg/kg/day), both of which are central dopamine blockers. Response is less consistent to clonidine or clonazepam, although these agents may be preferred initially to postpone the potential long-term consequences of haloperidol, such as parkinsonism or tardive dyskinesia. Pimozide widens the Q-T interval, and therefore patients taking it should undergo electrocardiographic monitoring.

MYOCLONUS

Myoclonus is a rapid involuntary jerking movement of one or more muscles or parts of muscles arising in the CNS. Its differentiation from tics and chorea, not always easy in the clinical setting, has been discussed earlier in this chapter. Myoclonus may arise from the cerebral cortex (epileptic myoclonus), subcortical levels (e.g., the brainstem reticular formation), or the spinal cord. Pathophysiologically it is related to epilepsy and is often seen concurrently with seizures in many of the same clinical contexts. Epilepsy partialis continua is really a form of repetitive epileptic myoclonus. In myoclonus of cerebral cortical origin, spikes or sharp-wave complexes often appear in the electroencephalogram just prior to the muscle jerks, although computer-averaging techniques may be necessary to separate these discharges from the background recording.

From a clinical perspective, myoclonus can be classified as focal, multifocal, segmental, or generalized. It may also occur in an isolated or repetitive fashion. If repetitive and rhythmic, it may be confused with tremor. It may be spontaneous or induced by various stimuli, such as photic stimulation, startle, or movement of the involved limb. Action myoclonus is a severe form of movement-evoked myoclonus that interferes with limb movement and gait, and is typically seen following recovery from severe generalized cerebral hypoxia or ischemia (e.g., cardiac arrest). **Postanoxic action myoclonus** (the Lance-Adams syndrome) tends to be disabling and permanent. Treatment with clonazepam or 5-hydroxytryptophan plus carbidopa has met with success in some patients. Benzodiazepines or valproic acid are also effective for treating many other forms of myoclonus. An etiological classification of myoclonus is given in Table 13-3.

Palatal myoclonus is a tremorlike rhythmic movement of the soft palate that occurs at a rate of 120 to 140 per minute (range, 40–200 per minute). The larynx, pharynx, floor of the mouth, tongue, diaphragm, intercostal, lower facial, and extraocular muscles may also be involved. In contrast to most other involuntary

Table 13-3. Classification of Myoclonus

Physiological
    Nocturnal myoclonus ("sleep starts")
    Photomyoclonic response to photic
        stimulation
    Hiccoughs

Benign essential myoclonus
    Familial
    Nonfamilial

Myoclonus and epilepsy
    Myoclonus in idiopathic corticoreticular
        epilepsy
    Juvenile myoclonic epilepsy of Janz
    Myoclonic seizures of childhood (e.g., infantile
        spasms of West's syndrome; with Lennox-
        Gastaut syndrome)
    Familial myoclonic epilepsy
        Lipidoses (e.g., Tay-Sachs and Niemann-Pick
            diseases)
        Neuronal ceroid lipofuscinosis
        Lafora's body disease
        Systems degeneration (Unverricht-Lundborg
            disease, Baltic myoclonus, Ramsay Hunt
            disease)
        Myoclonic epilepsy with ragged red fibers and
            other mitochondrial encephalomyopathies
        Cherry-red macular spot myoclonus syndrome
            (type I sialidosis)

Myoclonus due to diffuse central nervous system or
        systemic disease
    Metabolic (uremic, hepatic encephalopathy)
    Infectious (subacute sclerosing panencephalitis,
        Creutzfeldt-Jakob disease, other
        encephalitides)
    Postanoxic action myoclonus (Lance-Adams
        syndrome)
    Alzheimer's disease
    Myoclonus/opsoclonus/ataxia with occult
        neuroblastoma (rarely carcinoma)

Drugs and toxins
    Penicillin
    Tricyclic antidepressants
    Carbamazepine
    L-Dopa
    Methylbromide
    Strychnine

Segmental myoclonus
    Brainstem
        Palatal myoclonus
        Respiratory myoclonus
        ?Opsoclonus
    Spinal cord
        Subacute spinal viral "neuronitis"
        Spinal cord tumors
        Multiple sclerosis

movements, it tends to persist during sleep, and once established, it rarely disappears. Subjectively the patient may experience dysphagia or hear a rhythmical clicking noise due to blockage of the eustachian tube. The syndrome results from a lesion in the so-called triangle of Guillain-Mollaret, consisting of the cerebellar dentate nucleus, contralateral red nucleus in the midbrain, and the inferior olive. The first two structures are connected by the dentatorubral pathway that traverses the superior cerebellar peduncle and the last two, by the central tegmental tract in the brainstem.

BIBLIOGRAPHY

Albin, R.L., et al. Abnormalities of striatal projection neurons and *N*-methyl-D-aspartate receptors in presymptomatic Huntington's disease. *N. Engl. J. Med.* 322:1293–1298, 1990.

Berkovic, S.F., et al. Progressive myoclonus epilepsies: specific causes and diagnosis. *N. Engl. J. Med.* 315:296–305, 1986.

Burke, R.E. Tardive dyskinesia. Current clinical issues. *Neurology* 34:1348–1353, 1984.

Butler, I.J. Tourette's syndrome. Some new concepts. *Neurol. Clin.* 2:571–580, 1984.

Cooper, I. Neurosurgical treatment of dystonia. *Neurology* 20(Part 2):133–148, 1970.

Duvoisin, R.C. Chorea. *Semin. Neurol.* 2:351–358, 1982.

Eldridge, R. The torsion dystonias: literature review and genetic and clinical studies. *Neurology* 20 (Part 2):1–78, 1970.

Fahn, S. The varied clinical expressions of dystonia. *Neurol. Clin.* 2:541–554, 1984.

Fahn, S. Drug treatment of hyperkinetic movement disorders. *Semin. Neurol.* 7:192–210, 1987.

Fahn, S., and Jankovic, J. Practical management of dystonia. *Neurol. Clin.* 2:555–569, 1984.

Fahn, S., Marsden, C.D., and Calne, D.B. Classification and Investigation of Dystonia. In

C.D. Marsden and S. Fahn (editors). *Movement Disorders 2*. London: Butterworths, 1987, Pp. 332–358.

Fahn, S., and Marsden, C.D. The Treatment of Dystonia. In C.D. Marsden and S. Fahn (editors). *Movement Disorders 2*. London: Butterworths, 1987, Pp. 359–382.

Goetz, C.G., and Klawans, H.L. Tardive dyskinesia. *Neurol. Clin.* 2:605–614, 1984.

Greenhouse, A. On chorea, lupus erythematosus, and cerebral arteritis. *Arch. Intern. Med.* 117:389–393, 1966.

Growdon, J.H. and Scheife, R.T. Medical Treatment of Extrapyramidal Diseases. In K.J. Isselbacher, et al. (editors). *Update III: Harrison's Principles of Internal Medicine*. New York: McGraw-Hill, 1982, P. 185.

Hallett, M. Classification and treatment of tremor. *JAMA* 266:1115–1117, 1991.

Harper, P.S. (editor). *Huntington's Disease*. Philadelphia: Saunders, 1991.

Hayden, M.R., et al. The combined use of positron emission tomography and DNA polymorphisms for preclinical detection of Huntington's disease. *Neurology* 37:1441–1447, 1987.

Heathfield, K.W.G. Huntington's chorea: a centenary review. *Postgrad. Med. J.* 49:32–45, 1973.

Herrmann, C. and Brown, J.W. Palatal myoclonus: a reappraisal. *J. Neurol. Sci.* 5:473–492, 1967.

Jankovic, J. Drug-induced and other orofacial-cervical dyskinesias. *Ann. Intern. Med.* 94:788–793, 1981.

Jankovic, J. Blinking and blepharospasm. Mechanism, diagnosis, management. *JAMA* 248:3160–3164, 1982.

Jankovic, J., and Brin, M.F. Therapeutic uses of botulinum toxin. *N. Engl. J. Med.* 324:1186–1194, 1991.

Jankovic, J., and Fahn, S. Physiologic and pathologic tremors. Diagnosis, mechanism, and management. *Ann. Intern. Med.* 93:460–465, 1980.

Jankovic, J., and Pardo, R. Segmental myoclonus: clinical and pharmacologic study. *Arch. Neurol.* 43:1025–1031, 1986.

Klawans, H.L., et al. Treatment and prognosis of hemiballismus. *N. Engl. J. Med.* 295:1348–1350, 1976.

Kurlan, R. Tourette's syndrome: current concepts. *Neurology* 39:1625–1630, 1989.

Lal, S. Pathophysiology and pharmacotherapy of spasmodic torticollis: a review. *Can. J. Neurol. Sci.* 6:427–435, 1979.

Lance, J.W., and Adams, R.D. The syndrome of intention or action myoclonus as a sequel to hypoxic encephalopathy. *Brain* 86:111–136, 1963.

Lou, I.S., and Jankovic, J. Essential tremor: clinical correlates in 350 patients. *Neurology* 41:234–238, 1991.

Marsden, C.D. Blepharospasm-oromandibular dystonia syndrome (Brueghel's syndrome). *J. Neurol. Neurosurg. Psychiatry* 39:1204–1209, 1976.

Marsden, C.D. The pathophysiology of movement disorders. *Neurol. Clin.* 2:435–459, 1984.

Marsden, C.D., Hallett, M., and Fahn, S. The nosology and pathophysiology of myoclonus. In C.D. Marsden and S. Fahn (editors). *Movement Disorders*. London: Butterworths, 1982, Pp. 196–248.

Marsden, C.D., Marion, M.H., and Quinn, N. The treatment of severe dystonia in children and adults. *J. Neurol. Neurosurg. Psychiatry* 47:1166–1173, 1984.

Martin, J.B. Huntington's disease: new approaches to an old problem. *Neurology* 34:1059–1072, 1984.

Myers, R.H., and Martin, J.B. Huntington's disease. *Semin. Neurol.* 2:365–372, 1982.

Nygaard, T.G., Marsden, C.D., and Fahn, S. Dopa-responsive dystonia: long-term treatment response and prognosis. *Neurology* 41:174–181, 1991.

Penney, J.B., Jr., and Young, A.B. Movement

Disorders. In M.V. Johnston, R.L. MacDonald, and A.B. Young (editors). *Principles of Drug Therapy in Neurology*. Philadelphia: Davis, 1992, Pp. 50–86.

Phillips, J.R., and Eldridge, F.L. Respiratory myoclonus (Leeuwenhoek's disease). *N. Engl. J. Med.* 289:1390–1395, 1973.

Scheife, R.T., and Growdon, J.H. Treating tardive dyskinesia. *Semin. Neurol.* 2:305–315, 1982.

Shapiro, A.K., and Shapiro, E. Tourette syndrome: clinical aspects, treatment and etiology. *Semin. Neurol.* 2:373–385, 1982.

Shoulson, I. Huntington's disease. A decade of progress. *Neurol. Clin.* 2:515–526, 1984.

Tahmoush, A.J., Brooks, J.E., and Keltner, J.L. Palatal myoclonus associated with abnormal ocular and extremity movements. *Arch. Neurol.* 27:431–440, 1972.

Weiner, W.J., and Lang, A.E. *Movement Disorders: A Comprehensive Survey*. Mount Kisco, Futura Publishing Company, 1989.

Weakness: Introduction; Motor Neuron and Spinal Cord Disorders

Generalized or localized muscle weakness constitutes one of the most common neurological complaints. Weakness may result from lesions at any level of the central nervous system or peripheral neuromuscular apparatus. Nonneurological problems such as fatigue and lack of energy in depressed patients or conversion reactions in hysterical patients may also masquerade as true muscle weakness. Similarly, systemic illnesses such as cancer, hypothyroidism, or rheumatoid arthritis may give rise to weakness or fatigability with a nonneurological basis. In recent years, the chronic fatigue syndrome, often postviral, has emerged as a relatively common disorder. Patients with this syndrome not only suffer weakness and fatigability but also aches and pains, difficulties with concentration, and a host of other problems. There is an overlap between this syndrome and the fibromyalgia syndrome (fibromyositis), but the organic basis for both remains obscure.

History-taking often provides the initial clues to the localization and etiology of the process responsible for the weakness. Patients with true weakness usually describe their disability in terms of what they can and cannot do. The disabilities thereby mentioned often point to the distribution and degree of the weakness. For example, shoulder girdle weakness leads to difficulty shaving in men, doing up the hair in women, or handling heavy objects at shoulder level or above. Patients with distal upper extremity weakness have trouble holding heavy cooking utensils, opening a car door, turning a key in a lock or unscrewing a jar cap. Patients with proximal lower extremity weakness have difficulty going up or down stairs, assuming a squatting position, or getting up from a low chair or out of the bathtub. Distal lower extremity weakness produces problems standing on tiptoe, pressing on an automobile accelerator pedal, or fitting a foot into a boot or sock.

Other helpful information elicited by the history or examination includes the mode of onset (acute, subacute, or gradual); the fatigability of muscles; any accompanying fasciculations or atrophy; alterations in the deep tendon reflexes and tone; the presence of a Babinski's sign; and accompanying sensory abnormalities. Diagnostic considerations vary depending on whether the weakness exhibits a hemiparetic, quadriparetic, paraparetic (both legs), monoparetic (one limb), segmental (e.g., radicular), mononeuropathic, polyneuropathic, or myopathic pattern. Establishing a clinical diagnosis requires precise delineation of the distribution of the weakness and a knowledge of the segments and nerves supplying individual muscles (Chapter 2). Special tests such as computed tomographic (CT) or magnetic resonance imaging (MRI) scanning, myelography, electromyography and nerve conduction studies, repetitive nerve stimulations and an edrophonium chloride (Tensilon) test, muscle enzyme determinations, or examination of a nerve or muscle biopsy specimen using special techniques are often necessary to identify a specific etiology for the weakness.

FUNCTIONAL ANATOMY OF THE MOTOR SYSTEM

The giant pyramidal (Betz) cells located in layer V of the sensorimotor strip of the cerebral cortex (mainly prerolandic) give rise to axons that cross in the medullary pyramids as they descend to form the corticospinal tracts. These axons pass through the posterior limb of the internal capsule, the midbrain peduncles, and the lower brainstem, to lie mainly in the contralateral lateral funiculus of the spinal cord. They have direct terminations on the anterior horn cells that innervate distal limb muscles and are involved mainly in fine distal skilled limb movements. They are connected to other anterior horn cells by interneurons. A second parallel and somewhat overlapping voluntary motor system, termed the *subcorticospinal system*, includes the reticulospinal, vestibulospinal, tectospinal, and rubrospinal tracts that originate from nuclei in the brainstem. The axons in these tracts terminate bilaterally on anterior horn cells involved with axial, girdle, and proximal limb movements such as locomotion or reaching. The basal ganglia and cerebellum work in conjunction with these voluntary motor systems to ensure that movements are smooth and coordinated.

The neurons lying within the cerebral cortex controlling individual muscles are located in overlapping thin columns that radiate inward from the cortical surface. The rate of firing of cortical motor neurons depends on the magnitude of the force exerted by the particular muscle controlled as well as the rate of change of force. A given pyramidal tract neuron participates primarily in either flexion or extension around a particular joint but may also be involved in other movements as well. The supplementary motor area in the medial frontal cortex plays a role in initiating voluntary motor activities. Positron emission tomographic studies have shown that it tends to be activated along with rolandic areas during voluntary movement.

There is a somatotopic arrangement along the cortical motor strip, such that the top governs the hip and shoulder; the medial surface (supplied by the anterior cerebral artery) controls the leg; and the bottom adjacent to Broca's speech area is responsible for the oropharyngeal structures (Fig. 14-1). The amount of cortex devoted to each body area is proportional to the degree of refinement of movements in that part, with the lips, thumb, and fingers having the greatest representation. This somatotopic arrangement is maintained as the fibers descend to their termination in the spinal cord. The separation between the prerolandic motor cortex and the postrolandic somatosensory cortex is less distinct than was formerly believed, and some fibers in the corticospinal tracts actually originate from postrolandic areas.

Each anterior horn cell (alpha motor neuron) innervates approximately 10 to 1,000 muscle fibers, with the number dictated by the precision of the movements required. An anterior horn cell and its innervated muscle fibers make up a **motor unit**. In addition, smaller gamma motor neurons send their axons to intrafusal muscle fibers lying within muscle spindles. The **muscle spindles** are specially adapted stretch receptors that parallel the main muscle fibers. Specialized sensory endings convey information to the spinal cord concerning the degree of stretch of the muscle spindle. The gamma efferents "set" the spindle sensitivity by providing a specific degree of tension by means of

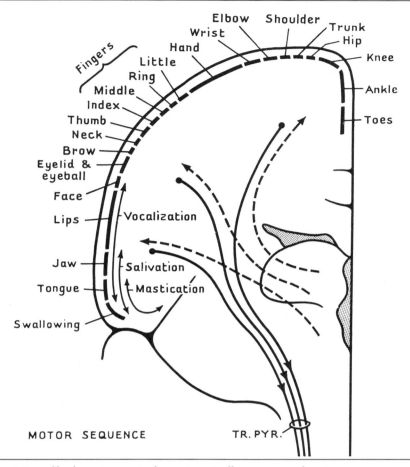

Fig. 14-1. *Representation of body parts arranged somatotopically on a coronal section through the prerolandic motor strip. (TR. PYR. = the pyramidal tract.) (Reprinted with permission from R. Brain,* Clinical Neurology. *London: Oxford University Press, 1960).*

intrafusal muscle fiber contraction. When the main muscle contracts, the muscle spindle tension is unloaded. When the muscle relaxes, the spindle is stretched and alpha motor neurons are excited to increase their firing. Specialized receptors in joints and tendons known as *Golgi tendon organs* also complement the actions of the muscle spindle. This system is helpful, for example, in automatically maintaining posture by keeping muscle tension constant in the lower limbs. The gamma efferent-muscle spindle system furnishes a "servoassistance" function that allows fine adjustments in muscle tension to take place at a reflex spinal level when unex-pected changes in resistance appear during movement.

UPPER AND LOWER MOTOR NEURON LESIONS: SPASTICITY

The first step in localizing the cause of true weakness is to distinguish involvement of the **upper motor neurons** (innervating the anterior horn cell) from that of the **lower motor neurons** or muscle.

In the **upper motor neuron syndrome**, there is weakness in a particular distribution that can best be appreciated by observing a hemiplegic patient several weeks after a stroke. In this setting, the antigravity muscles are particularly affected; these include the shoulder abductors; arm, wrist, and finger extensors; hip flexors and abductors; and foot extensors. The unopposed action of antagonist muscles gives rise to the typical hemiplegic posture and gait seen in such patients, with the arm held against the body flexed at the elbow and wrist, a foot drop, and tendency to drag and circumduct the leg when walking. Fine distal movements are selectively affected in mild cases.

Spasticity is another feature of chronic upper motor neuron involvement, and is best seen in the context of spinal cord lesions. It is a special type of increased muscle tone that exists during passive movement but not at rest. It is also velocity dependent and associated with the clasp-knife phenomenon, which is a sudden release of muscle tone occurring after a gradual increase of tone with muscle stretch, and likely stems from the sudden inhibition of alpha motor neurons as inhibitory input from Golgi tendon organs comes into play with stretch.

The mechanism of spasticity is poorly understood but probably relates to increased excitability of alpha motor neurons due to a reduction in the inhibitory input from the descending corticospinal tract. Afferent segmental input to alpha motor neurons is particularly influenced by gamma aminobutyric (GABA)–ergic interneurons operating under the control of presynaptic inhibition. Mechanisms that have been postulated to account for spasticity include a reduction in segmental GABAergic input, denervation hypersensitivity, or the sprouting of segmental axons to replace the lost suprasegmental inputs to motor neurons. Spasticity may be regarded as a "positive" phenomenon, unlike weakness, which is a "negative" consequence of upper motor neuron lesions. After an acute lesion in upper motor neurons, there is often a variable period of "shock" with muscle flaccidity before spasticity develops. The return of some movement often parallels the development of spasticity.

A symptom that is closely related to spasticity is **flexor spasms**, or involuntary painful flexions of the lower extremities, which are particularly common in the presence of spinal cord lesions. These may be uncomfortable and interfere with sleep. In some patients, tone is most marked in extensor muscles and extensor spasms can occur.

Other components of the upper motor neuron syndrome include hyperactive deep tendon reflexes, clonus, a Babinski's sign, and, less consistently, loss of superficial reflexes (e.g., abdominal and cremasteric).

Treatment of flexor spasms as well as the hyperadducted lower extremity postures in bedridden spastic patients, which may interfere with nursing care, may be accomplished with baclofen, high doses of diazepam, or dantrolene sodium. These agents are most effective in patients with spinal cord lesions and often alleviate spasticity, but at the expense of producing increased weakness or sedation. **Baclofen** is a $GABA_b$ agonist that brings about presynaptic hyperpolarization at the spinal cord interneuron level. It crosses the blood-brain barrier poorly, but attempts to administer it by continuous intrathecal infusion have met with some success. Dantrolene sodium works directly on the muscle membrane and blocks the release of calcium from the sarcoplasmic reticulum that occurs with depolarization. Hepatotoxicity is an occasional side effect. Tizanidine is a newer, potentially effective antispasticity agent that acts as an $alpha_2$-noradrenergic receptor agonist. It reduces the release of excitatory amino acids such as aspartate from interneurons.

Lower motor neuron involvement leads to hypotonia, muscle atrophy (after several weeks), and reduced deep tendon jerks. Fasciculations may also appear, especially if there are anterior horn cell or root lesions.

SOME SPINAL CORD CONDITIONS PRODUCING WEAKNESS

Acute or Subacute Transverse Myelopathy

The rapid development of lower extremity weakness, bladder and bowel impairment, and

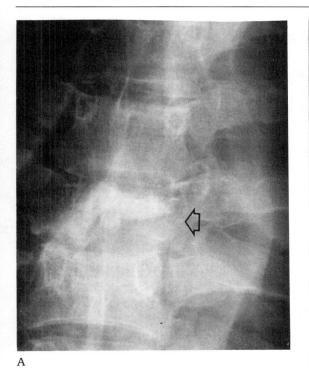

A

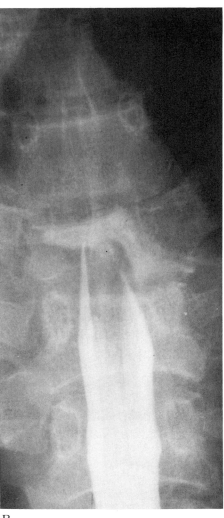

B

Fig. 14-2. *Spinal cord compression due to tuberculous abscess. This 37-year-old man was admitted with paraplegia and urinary retention following a 2-week history of progressive leg weakness and a 6-month history of thoracic back pain, night sweats, fever, and productive cough. He could barely wiggle his toes on examination and there was a T6 sensory level. (A) Plain x-ray study showing collapse of the T6 vertebra with calcification* (arrow). *(B) Myelogram showing complete block at T6.*

ascending sensory loss with a clear-cut level, with or without back pain, are the hallmarks of transverse myelopathy. The lesion may lie at a much higher segmental level than the sensory level or the distribution of weakness indicates. Compression of the spinal cord by an extramedullary lesion and trauma are by far the most common causes. Epidural metastases from a lymphoma or from breast or lung carcinoma, usually in the thoracic region, are common. Pain over the spine at the level of the lesion, vertebral involvement shown by plain spinal x-ray studies, and a positive bone scan of the vertebrae involved often point to the diagnosis (Table 14-1). Epidural abscess (Table 14-2), tuberculous spondylitis (Fig. 14-2), hematomas,

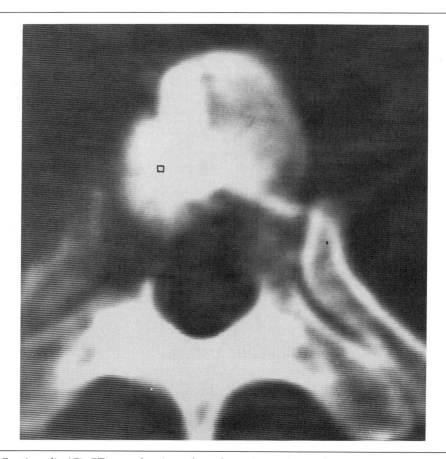

Fig. 14-2 *(Continued). (C) CT scan showing tuberculous abscess* (square).

Table 14-1. Signs and Symptoms of Acute Spinal Cord Compression from Epidural Metastases

Pain
  Present in over 90%
  Over site of lesion with radicular spread:
    Cervical → arms
    Thoracic → trunk
    Lumbar → legs
Paraparesis/paraplegia
  Babinski's signs
Sensory loss
  Especially vibration sense
  Sensory level to pinprick over the trunk
Bladder dysfunction
  Urinary retention

Table 14-2. Features Suggesting Epidural Abscess as a Cause of Spinal Cord Compression

Fever, leukocytosis
Severe root and back pain
Rapid progression of neurological deficit from the time of appearance of root pain
Signs of meningeal irritation (nuchal rigidity, Kernig's sign)
CSF pleocytosis with polymorphonuclear leukocytes

intrinsic tumors of the spinal canal, and rarely thoracic or cervical disc herniations are other causes. The anatomical relationship of various tumors to the spinal cord is depicted in Figure 14-3.

MRI scanning is the best means of identifying the level of the compressive lesion and its location with respect to the spinal cord (Fig. 14-4). CT scanning, performed at the level of the block, can also indicate the nature of the lesion,

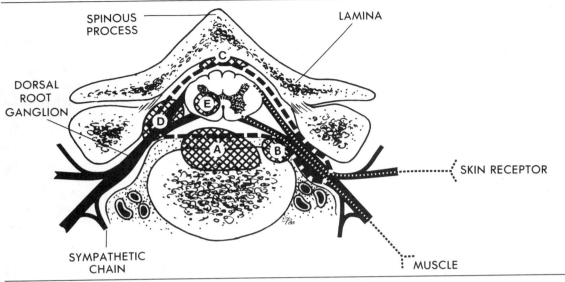

Fig. 14-3. *Cross section of a vertebral body, spinal canal, and spinal cord showing relationship to spinal cord of various tumors causing transverse myelopathy. (A = epidural tumor arising from vertebral body, e.g., lymphoma; B, C = extradural meningioma; D = intradural extramedullary tumor, e.g., schwannoma; E = intramedullary tumor, e.g., astrocytoma, ependymoma, metastatic.)*

but does not provide a full longitudinal view of the cord, as MRI can. It can be combined with myelography, which, done without removing more than a few drops of cerebrospinal fluid (CSF), can also demonstrate the level of the lesion as well as its probable nature (Fig. 14-5). It often reveals a complete or partial spinal block, and a cisternal injection of dye can outline the upper extent. However, unlike CT or MRI, myelography is an invasive procedure and yields less information about the lesion causing the block.

Early diagnosis of this syndrome is essential, before lower extremity paralysis is complete, if surgical decompression is to be beneficial. In certain cases of known neoplastic involvement, management with dexamethasone and localized radiotherapy have proved as effective as surgical decompression.

Transverse myelitis due to intrinsic spinal cord lesions produces a similar syndrome. It may stem from various causes, including multiple sclerosis; following a viral infection, immunization, or vasculitis (e.g., systemic lupus erythematosus); a remote effect of carcinoma; heroin abuse; or exposure to certain toxins. CT and MRI scanning can help differentiate these cases from those due to compressive lesions. A myelogram is usually negative but may show localized widening of the cord. CSF examination may reveal a pleocytosis and raised protein level. Corticosteroids or ACTH are often used in idiopathic cases or those thought to stem from a demyelinating or postviral cause, although their beneficial effect is unproved.

A transverse myelopathy that is acute or subacute in onset may be due to occlusion of the anterior cerebral artery or its main supply vessel (the artery of Adamkiewicz, which enters the spinal canal at a level somewhere between T8 and L4). An infarct of the anterior two thirds of the spinal cord produces paralysis below the level of the lesion as well as sensory loss, mainly to pain and temperature, beginning a few segments below the level of the lesion with vibration sensation preserved. Causes include trauma, vasculitis (e.g., syphilitic aortitis or polyarteritis nodosa), hypotension, atherosclerotic disease of the aorta, cardiac emboli, decompression sickness, and surgery for an aortic aneurysm (see Fig. 19-

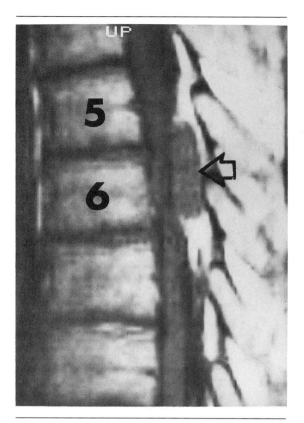

Fig. 14-4. *T₁-weighted MRI scan in a 41-year-old man with a slowly developing spastic paraparesis and sensory level at T8. The arrow points to an extradural meningioma compressing the spinal cord at the T5–T6 level.*

3). Arteriovenous malformations of the spinal cord, which are rare, may precipitate a transverse myelopathy as the result of hemorrhage or venous thrombosis. Arteriovenous malformations usually lie dorsally to the spinal cord and can be visualized by MRI, contrast-enhanced CT scanning, or supine myelography. Spinal arteriography, a time-consuming procedure with a high complication rate, may be necessary in certain cases to identify spinal arteriovenous malformations.

Progressive Spastic Paraparesis or Quadriparesis

A more slowly developing, usually symmetrical, weakness that includes spasticity and other upper motor neuron signs and arising in the lower extremities can be seen in a variety of conditions. In some cases, the upper extremities also become involved. The most common cause is **cervical spondylosis**. Degenerative disease of the cervical spine usually but not always produces prominent neck pain and limitation of movement together with radicular pain and segmental lower motor neuron signs in the upper extremities before gait difficulty and leg weakness supervene. Plain x-ray studies in such patients show degenerative changes in the cervical spine along with disc space narrowing (often at C5–C6 and C6–C7), spondylotic spurs, and bars on the posterior aspect of the vertebral bodies opposite the disc spaces. In compressive cases there is also narrowing of the anteroposterior diameter of the canal to less than approximately 12 mm. CT scans show obvious spinal stenosis with calcified material impinging on the spinal canal (Fig. 14-6), and myelography reveals a partial or complete block and widening of the spinal cord in its lateral dimension that occupies more than two thirds of the width of the spinal canal. In severe cases, management consists of surgical decompression and fusion using an anterior (Cloward) approach to halt progression of the process.

Other conditions such as lesions of the foramen magnum (i.e., developmental abnormalities of the cervicomedullary junction [Fig. 14-7], subluxation of the odontoid, tumors, and cysts), multiple sclerosis, subacute combined degeneration due to vitamin B₁₂ deficiency (see Chapter 19), spinal cord tumors (Table 14-3), and arteriovenous malformations can also produce progressive spastic quadriparesis.

Human T-cell lymphotropic virus type I (HTLV-I) is a retrovirus that produces a progressive myelopathy (tropical spastic paraparesis) among black natives of Africa and the Caribbean with a mean age of onset of 45 years. Epidemiologically, the disease bears many similarities to AIDS. Viral DNA may be detected in the blood cells of these patients using the polymerase chain reaction and there are often oligoclonal bands in the CSF. The spastic paraparesis is slowly progressive and sensory signs are rare.

A progressive myelopathy can occur in patients with hepatic disease who have portal-systemic shunts and also appear months or years

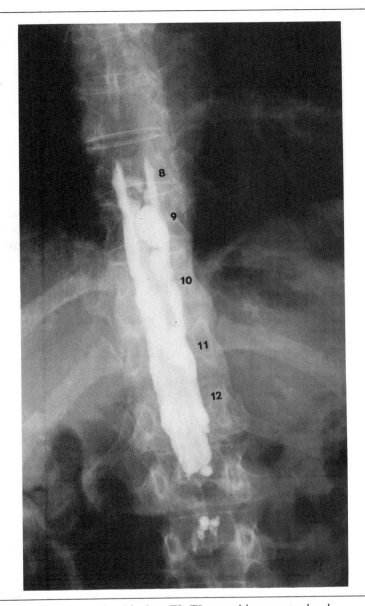

Fig. 14-5. *Myelogram showing a complete block at T8–T9 caused by an extradural multiple myeloma. This 62-year-old woman had a 2-week history of radicular thoracic pain followed by gait ataxia, lower extremity weakness, urinary hesitancy, and a sensory level at T9. Surgical decompression followed by radiotherapy were carried out.*

after irradiation for spinal cord tumors. Furthermore, progressive corticospinal tract lesions as far rostral as the parasagittal region, where meningiomas are particularly common, can be implicated. This means that CT or MRI scanning of the head must be included in the evaluation of every patient with progressive spastic paraparesis. In some cases, full investigation reveals no obvious cause for the syndrome and no other signs are found apart from bilateral corticospinal tract involvement. These cases are classified as a degenerative, often fa-

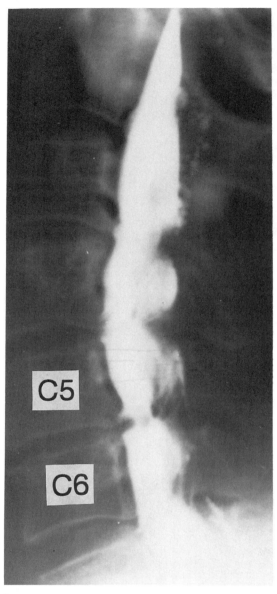

A

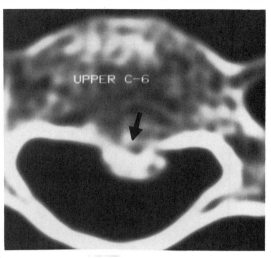

B

Fig. 14-6. *This 49-year-old man had suffered a progressive spastic paraparesis with a stiff, ataxic gait for over 4 years. In addition, he had difficulty with fine coordination in the right hand and deterioration of handwriting, but only minimal neck discomfort. (A) Myelogram shows marked narrowing of the anteroposterior diameter of the spinal canal at C5–C6 as well as posterior impingement from the ligamentum flavum at three levels. (B) CT scan shows a calcified spondylotic midline spur (arrow) projecting backward into the spinal canal. The patient responded well to an anterior decompression and fusion.*

milial form of progressive spastic paraparesis or quadriparesis, and may represent a subvariety of amyotrophic lateral sclerosis (ALS) or be a type of spinocerebellar degeneration.

Amyotrophic Lateral Sclerosis

ALS is the prototype of a group of idiopathic degenerative diseases affecting the motor neurons within the CNS. The age of onset is commonly between 40 and 60, and it shows an incidence of approximately 1 to 2/100,000 per year.

Pathophysiology and Etiology

Pathological changes include the dropout of motor neurons within the motor cortex and brainstem motor cranial nerve nuclei (espe-

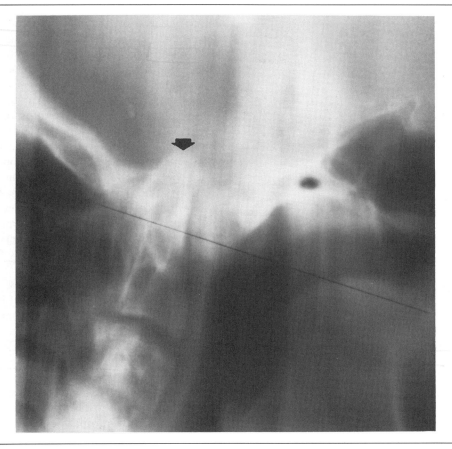

Fig. 14-7. *Compression at the cervicomedullary junction due to basilar impression. This 30-year-old man presented with a mild chronic progressive spastic paraparesis with a right Babinski's sign and loss of pain and temperature sensation below C2, worse on the right. Plain skull x-ray tomograms showed the odontoid* (arrow) *projecting high above the foramen magnum more than 5 mm above McGregor's line (joining the posterior hard palate to the lowermost part of the basis occiput). There was also anterior and posterior fusion of the atlas with the occiput. CT myelography provides a way of viewing the degree of compression of the medulla and cervical cord.*

cially V, VII, IX, and XII) and loss of anterior horn cells. Secondary gliosis occurs in the corticospinal tracts and there is degeneration of ventral spinal roots, motor axons, peripheral nerves, and muscles. About 10 percent of the cases are familial and these cases do not differ appreciably from the sporadic form of ALS, except that rare familial cases have been reported in which patients suffered concurrent dementia or clinically silent posterior column degeneration.

A pathologically distinct variety of ALS-

parkinsonism-dementia (see Chapters 4 and 12) occurs among the Mariana islanders (Chomorros) of the South Pacific and is likely due to a toxin found in the cycad nut flour eaten by these people. A similar disorder is also seen among natives of the Kii peninsula in Japan.

ALS exhibits a clinical spectrum of problems, depending on the degrees of upper motor neuron and lower motor neuron involvement and the amount of brainstem versus spinal involvement. It is termed **progressive bulbar palsy** when the process is confined to the corti-

Table 14-3. Tumors of Spinal Cord and Canal

Intramedullary
  Ependymoma
  Spongioblastoma
  Astrocytoma
  Oligodendroglioma
  Medulloblastoma
  Glioblastoma
  Metastases
Extramedullary–intradural
  Meningioma
  Schwannoma
  Lipoma
  Paraganglioma
  Metastases
Extradural
  Metastases
  Vertebral body tumors
  Lipoma
  Teratoma
  Epidermoid/dermoid

cobulbar tracts and brainstem motor nuclei, producing dysphagia, dysarthria, wasting and weakness of the tongue, facial weakness and wasting, pseudobulbar emotional lability, and a hyperactive jaw jerk. When there is only lower motor neuron spinal involvement, this is considered **progressive spinal muscular atrophy**. Rarely only the corticospinal tracts are involved, producing the picture of progressive spastic paraparesis (see earlier discussion), which is called *primary lateral sclerosis*. Most commonly, however, the full picture of ALS is seen.

Clinical Picture and Diagnosis
Typically the condition begins with gradual asymmetrical weakness, atrophy, and fasciculations that affect one upper extremity. Sensory complaints such as cramps, pain, and vague dysesthesias may be part of the initial picture and forestall accurate diagnosis. As the disease progresses, there is more widespread muscle involvement accompanied by prominent fasciculations. Patients suffer marked weight loss, spasticity, and finally bulbar involvement (e.g., dysphagia, dysarthria, wasting, and fasciculations of the tongue) (Fig. 14-8).

Diagnosis is based on the characteristic clinical picture and the exclusion of other entities that can manifest a combination of upper and lower motor neuron involvement. Characteristically, extraocular movements and bladder function are spared. The presence of objective sensory abnormalities suggests an alternative diagnosis, even though quantitative testing methods have shown subtle sensory deficits in up to 15 percent of the cases. When there is no bulbar involvement, MRI or myelography must be done to rule out the existence of cervical spondylosis or spinal cord tumor. Both of these conditions can produce wasting and fasciculations in the upper extremities and a spastic paraparesis. However, the presence of widespread fasciculations in paraspinal muscles and lower extremities, often seen in ALS, is not encountered in cervical spondylosis. Electromyographic studies frequently reveal marked denervation changes (reduced interference pattern, polyphasic units), giant units (indicating reinnervation of muscle fibers by axonal sprouting from remaining motor units), and increased spontaneous activity in the form of fibrillations and fasciculations. Nerve conduction velocities are usually normal, unlike the finding in many primary neuropathies. Muscle enzymes may be moderately elevated. A muscle biopsy specimen, which is usually not necessary for diagnosis, exhibits neuropathic changes consisting of grouped atrophy, dark-staining angular fibers, and type grouping.

Although some conditions with specific etiologies can mimic ALS, in its fully developed form, ALS is easily recognizable. In rare instances, ALS has been reported as a remote effect of carcinoma, and remission has occurred once the underlying cancer is treated. The subacute motor neuronopathy that constitutes a remote effect of lymphoma, possibly due to viral involvement of anterior horn cells, may also resemble ALS. The motor neuropathy seen with paraproteinemias resulting from an immunological attack on myelin manifests a clinical picture similar to progressive spinal muscular atrophy. Multifocal motor neuropathy with conduction block is a rare idiopathic condition that somewhat superficially resembles motor neuron disease (see Chapter 15). Other possible causes that have occasionally been implicated in the etiology of an ALS-like picture include neurosyphilis, repeated attacks

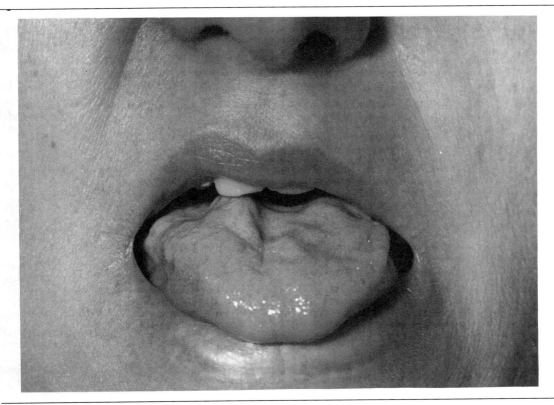

Fig. 14-8. *Marked tongue atrophy in a 32-year-old man with amyoptrophic lateral sclerosis.*

of hypoglycemia, lead intoxication, certain rare inherited gangliosidoses, and thyrotoxicosis. Creutzfeldt-Jakob disease and Pick's disease are also rarely associated with amyotrophy. Because there is no definitive treatment for this nearly uniformly fatal condition, every effort should be made to detect specific etiological factors.

Other forms of progressive motor neuron degeneration that show an autosomal recessive inheritance pattern and pure lower motor neuron involvement appear at an earlier age than does ALS. Werdnig-Hoffman disease is seen at birth and such babies have a "floppy" appearance. They lay in a "froglike" position with marked proximal limb weakness and exhibit a weak suck and cry. The mother may have noticed reduced fetal movements in utero. Pathologically, there is little motor neuron dropout in this disease and muscles tend to show peculiar small rounded, grouped atrophic fibers. The

overwhelming majority of patients do not survive more than a few years. Occasional cases seem to stabilize and patients survive well into adolescence.

This disorder overlaps with what has been termed *juvenile proximal spinal muscular atrophy* (Kugelberg-Welander disease). This autosomal recessive disorder represents a spectrum of spinal motor neuron degeneration that affects proximal muscles but without bulbar or upper motor neuron involvement. These patients may survive for many years, although they are usually wheelchair bound or dependent by the third decade. These conditions are also not clearly distinct from certain hereditary motor neuropathies of the Charcot-Marie-Tooth variety.

Management and Prognosis
Early bulbar involvement is a bad prognostic sign. ALS is almost universally fatal, with a

mean survival of about 3 years. Death occurs as the result of inanition, respiratory failure, and intercurrent infection. Rare cases seem to stabilize and such patients survive for several years. Many patients require the institution of special feeding methods, such as a gastrostomy or a tube inserted through a piriformostomy, as the disease advances. Drugs can provide symptomatic relief for muscle cramps, overflow of saliva, emotional lability, and depression. Rehabilitation methods are recommended that help the patient remain as independent and mobile as possible, and specialized communication devices such as portable computerized and letter display systems should be used to enable patients to communicate once · they are no longer able to speak. One of the most distressing aspects of the illness is that alertness and mental faculties remain unaffected even though the motor capacities relentlessly deteriorate. The decision to provide respiratory support in the terminal stages of the illness is a complex one that must be considered on an individual basis. The issue is best discussed with the patient and family members in the early phases of the illness.

BIBLIOGRAPHY

Adams, R.D., and Salam-Adams, M. Chronic nontraumatic diseases of the spinal cord. *Neurol. Clin.* 9:605–623, 1991.

Aminoff, M.J., and Logue, V. Clinical features of spinal vascular malformations. *Brain* 97:197–210, 1974.

Asanuma, H. Recent developments in the study of the columnar of neurons within the motor cortex. *Physiol. Rev.* 55:143–156, 1975.

Baker, A.S., et al. Spinal epidural abscess. *N. Engl. J. Med.* 293:463–468, 1975.

Berman, M., et al. Acute transverse myelitis: incidence and etiologic considerations. *Neurology* 31:966–971, 1981.

Bobowick, A.R., and Brody, J.A. Epidemiology of motor-neuron disease. *N. Engl. J. Med.* 288:1047–1055, 1973.

Brem, S.S., et al. Spinal subarachnoid hematoma. A hazard of lumbar puncture resulting in reversible paraplegia. *N. Engl. J. Med.* 303:1020–1021, 1981.

Brody, J.A., Hirano, A., and Scott, R.M. Recent neuropathologic observations in amyotrophic lateral sclerosis and parkinsonism-dementia of Guam. *Neurology* 21:528–536, 1971.

Byers, R.K., and Banker, B.Q. Infantile spinal muscular atrophy. *Arch. Neurol.* 5:38–62, 1961.

Byrne, T.N. Spinal cord compression from epidural metastases. *N. Engl. J. Med.* 327:614–619, 1992.

Byrne, T.N., and Waxman, S.G. *Spinal Cord Compression: Diagnosis and Principles of Management.* Philadelphia: Davis, 1990.

Dawson, D.M., and Potts, F. Acute nontraumatic myelopathies. *Neurol. Clin.* 9:585–603, 1991.

Evarts, E.V. Pyramidal tract activity associated with a conditioned hand movement in the monkey. *J. Neurophysiol.* 29:1011–1027, 1966.

Gilbert, R.W., Kim, J., and Posner, J.B. Epidural spinal cord compression from metastatic tumor: diagnosis and treatment. *Ann. Neurol.* 3:40–51, 1978.

Gregorius, F.K., Estrin, T., and Crandall, P.H. Cervical spondylytic radiculopathy and myelopathy: a long-term follow-up. *Arch. Neurol.* 33:618–625, 1976.

Harik, S.I., Raichle, M.E., and Reis, D.J. Spontaneously remitting spinal epidural hematoma in a patient on anticoagulants. *N. Engl. J. Med.* 284:1355–1357, 1971.

Herrick, M.K., and Mills, P.E., Jr. Infarction of spinal cord. Two cases of selective gray matter involvement secondary to asymptomatic aortic disease. *Arch. Neurol.* 24:228–241, 1971.

Hudson, A.J. Amyotrophic lateral sclerosis and its association with dementia, parkinsonism and other neurological disorders: a review. *Brain* 104:217–247, 1981.

Kincaid, J.C., and Dyken, M.L. Myelitis and

Myelopathy. In A.B. Baker and L.H. Baker (editors). *Clinical Neurology*. Philadelphia: Harper & Row, 1984, Pp. 1–32.

Landau, W.M. Spasticity and Rigidity. In F. Plum (editor). *Recent Advances in Neurology*. Philadelphia: Davis, 1969, Pp. 1–32.

Lawrence, D.G., and Kuypers, H.G.J.M. The functional organization of the motor system in the monkey. I. The effects of bilateral pyramidal lesions. *Brain* 91:1–41, 1968.

Lipton, H.L., and Teasdall, R.D. Acute transverse myelopathy in adults. A follow-up study. *Arch. Neurol.* 28:252–257, 1973.

Livingston, K.E., and Perrin, R.G. The neurosurgical management of spinal metastases causing cord and cauda equina compression. *J. Neurosurg.* 49:839–843, 1978.

Logue, V. Angiomas of the spinal cord: review of the pathogenesis, clinical features, and results of surgery. *J. Neurol. Neurosurg. Psychiatry* 42:1–11, 1979.

Lothman, E.W. and Montgomery, E.B., Jr. Control of Motor Activity by the Cerebrum and Cerebellum. In E.D. Frohlich (editor). *Pathophysiology: Altered Regulatory Mechanisms in Disease*, 3rd ed. Philadelphia: Lippincott, 1984, Pp. 741–769.

Mackay, R. Course and prognosis in amyotrophic lateral sclerosis. *Arch. Neurol.* 8:117–127, 1963.

Mcquarrie, I.G. Recovery from paraplegia caused by spontaneous spinal epidural hematoma. *Neurology* 28:224–228, 1978.

Merritt, J.L. Management of spasticity in spinal cord injury. *Mayo Clin. Proc.* 56:614–622, 1981.

Mitsumoto, H., Nanson, M.R., and Chad, D.A. Amyotrophic lateral sclerosis: recent advances in pathogenesis and therapeutic trials. *Arch. Neurol.* 45:189–202, 1988.

Mulder, D.W., and Howard, F.M., Jr. Patient resistance and prognosis in amyotrophic lateral sclerosis. *Mayo Clin. Proc.* 51:537–541, 1978.

Namba, T., Aberfeld, D.C., and Grob, D.

Chronic proximal spinal muscular atrophy. *J. Neurol. Sci.* 11:401–423, 1970.

Palmer, J.J. Radiation myelopathy. *Brain* 95:109–122, 1972.

Phillips, C.G. Laying the ghost of "muscles versus movements." *Can. J. Neurol. Sci.* Aug. 1975, Pp. 209–218.

Phillips, C.G. Motor apparatus of the baboon's hand. *Proc. R. Soc. Br.* 173:141–174, 1969.

Rewcastle, N.B., and Berry, K. Neoplasms of the lower spinal canal. *Neurology* 14:608–615, 1964.

Rosen, A.D. Amyotrophic lateral sclerosis. *Arch. Neurol.* 35:638–642, 1978.

Rowland, L.P. (editor). *Human Motor Neuron Diseases*. New York: Raven, 1982.

Royden Jones, H., Jr. Diseases of the peripheral motor-sensory unit. *CIBA Clin. Symp.* 4:1–32, 1985.

Silver, J.R., and Buxton, P.H. Spinal stroke. *Brain* 97:539–550, 1974.

Sinaki, M., and Mulder, D.W. Rehabilitation techniques for patients with amyotrophic lateral sclerosis. *Mayo Clin. Proc.* 53:173–178, 1975.

Smith, R.A., and Norris, F.H., Jr. Symptomatic care of patients with amyotrophic lateral sclerosis. *JAMA* 234:715–717, 1975.

Tandan, R., and Bradley, W.G. Amyotrophic lateral sclerosis: Part 1. Clinical features, pathology and ethical issues in management. *Ann. Neurol.* 18:271–280, 1985.

Tandan, R., and Bradley, W.G. Amyotrophic lateral sclerosis: Part 2. Etiopathogenesis. *Ann. Neurol.* 18:419–431, 1985.

Tobin, W.D., and Layton, D.D., Jr. The diagnosis and natural history of spinal cord arteriovenous malformations. *Mayo Clin. Proc.* 51:637–646, 1976.

Veron, J.P., et al. Acute necrotic myelopathy. *Eur. Neurol.* 11:83–97, 1974.

Whiteley, A.M., Hauw, J.J., and Escourolle, R. A pathological survey of 41 cases of acute intrinsic spinal cord disease. *J. Neurol. Sci.* 42:229–242, 1979.

Wilkinson, M. *Cervical Spondylosis: Its Early Diagnosis and Treatment.* Philadelphia: Saunders, 1971.

Williams, D.B., and Windebank, A.J. Motor neuron disease (amyotrophic lateral sclerosis). *Mayo Clin. Proc.* 66:54–82, 1991.

Yasuoka, S., et al. Foramen magnum tumors. Analysis of 57 cases of benign extramedullary tumors. *J. Neurosurg.* 49:828–838, 1978.

Young, R.R., and Delwaide, P.J. Spasticity. *N. Engl. J. Med.* 304:28–33; 96–99, 1981.

Weakness: Peripheral Nerve Disorders

Peripheral nerve disorders are among the most common causes of weakness. Although some neuropathies exhibit mainly or exclusively sensory disturbances, they are included in this chapter for the sake of a unified discussion.

FUNCTIONAL ANATOMY OF THE PERIPHERAL NERVOUS SYSTEM

The large peripheral nerves supplying the extremities and trunk are composed of sensory, motor, and autonomic fibers. The motor fibers are the axons of anterior horn cells that leave the spinal dural sheath via the ventral roots. The sensory fibers enter the spinal cord via the dorsal roots, with the cell bodies of the largest fibers residing in the dorsal root ganglia. The mixed peripheral sensory nerve trunk formed by the union of the ventral and dorsal roots begins just at the spinal intervertebral foramen. The larger sensory fibers are myelinated and the smaller ones are unmyelinated or covered by only a thin layer of **myelin**. One Schwann

cell provides the myelin between two **nodes of Ranvier**, which are specialized areas located along the axon that are denuded of myelin where the axon is surrounded only by its basal lamina. Several unmyelinated fibers lie loosely enveloped in the cytoplasm of a single Schwann cell.

Peripheral nerve myelin, which is antigenically and chemically different from central myelin, provides insulation and facilitates more rapid conduction of the nervous impulse (about 60 meters per second). The **action potential** travels by a **saltatory mechanism**, skipping from one node of Ranvier to the next. Another difference between central and peripheral myelinated fibers is that the Schwann cells surrounding the peripheral nerves have the capacity to proliferate and regenerate myelin lost because of damage to the nerve.

Individual nerve fibers, which are enveloped by a connective tissue sheath known as the **endoneurium**, lie in fascicles surrounded by the **perineurium**. The **epineurium** envelopes the whole peripheral nerve. The blood supply to peripheral nerves arises via epineurial arterial branches (the vasa nervorum), which send arterioles through the perineurium. Rarely occlusive disease in the vasa nervorum inflicts ischemic damage to nerves, and this may explain the mild sensory neuropathy frequently seen in peripheral vascular disease.

Besides conducting nervous impulses to and from the periphery, axons also have a transport function. Neurotransmitters, enzymes, nutrients, cellular organelles, and other materials are all transported bidirectionally along the axon through a process known as **axoplasmic flow**. When the nerve is damaged, the previously innervated muscle degenerates due to loss of "trophic" factors arising from the nerve.

DEFINITION AND CLASSIFICATION OF PERIPHERAL NEUROPATHIES

Peripheral neuropathy is a broad term that embraces almost all disorders (except a neoplastic one) that affect peripheral nerves. The term *polyneuropathy* refers to a generalized, usually symmetrical, disorder affecting the peripheral nerves. *Mononeuropathy* refers to a lesion of one individual nerve; *radiculopathy*, to a lesion of one or more spinal roots; and *multiple mononeuropathy*, to a disorder affecting more than one individual nerve.

Neuropathies have been classified into four main groups, based on the pathophysiological mechanisms involved (Fig. 15-1). Each category has relatively specific clinical and electrophysiological features and a limited set of causes. However, in advanced disease there is a great deal of overlap between axonal and demyelinating neuropathies because degeneration of the axon also leads to myelin disruption and an axon denuded of myelin tends to suffer eventual damage.

Myelinopathies

Disorders that affect myelin produce a picture of segmental demyelination. The myelin sheath in certain internodal segments degenerates and may disappear entirely even though adjacent segments may remain well preserved. When the myelin sheath has regenerated in affected segments, it often appears abnormally thin and the internodal distance is shortened. When the cycle of degeneration and regeneration is repeated several times, this causes hypertrophy of the myelin sheath, which presents an "onion bulb" pattern. The pathological attack is waged on the Schwann cell or the myelin itself. Slowed conduction, prolonged terminal latencies, or conduction block are revealed by nerve conduction velocity testing, but electromyography shows no evident denervation affecting the supplied muscles. The muscle or nerve action potential also shows temporal dispersion. Immunological mechanisms are often implicated in these cases. Fairly rapid and complete recovery can be expected in this disorder, except in severe cases that involve secondary axonal damage.

Axonopathies

A picture consisting of an initial degeneration of the terminal portion of axons that progresses proximally ("dying back" phenomenon) is seen when the pathological process attacks either the axon itself or the cell body. Most examples seen clinically are due to toxic or metabolic disorders. The prognosis is poorer for these disorders than for most demyelinating neuropathies and the course may be protracted.

Neuronopathies

The anterior horn cells or dorsal root ganglion cells may be affected directly, and amyotrophic lateral sclerosis and poliomyelitis are examples of such motor neuronopathies. Sensory neuronopathies include herpes zoster, carcinomatous sensory neuropathy, Friedreich's ataxia, and certain toxin-related neuronopathies. A chronic idiopathic sensory neuronopathy can cause severe disabling gait and limb ataxia. Recovery is generally poor in these cases.

Wallerian Degeneration

Wallerian degeneration is the distal axonal and myelin breakdown that occurs in otherwise

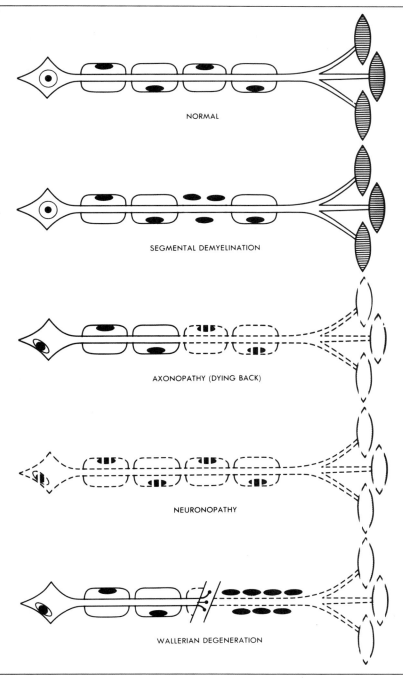

NORMAL

SEGMENTAL DEMYELINATION

AXONOPATHY (DYING BACK)

NEURONOPATHY

WALLERIAN DEGENERATION

Fig. 15-1. *Diagram showing the main sites of damage in the four principal types of polyneuropathy. The cell body of the neuron is shown at the left. An axon with surrounding Schwann cells and myelin is shown joining three muscle fibers. Note that muscle fiber degeneration due to denervation occurs only when the axon is affected.*

healthy nerves following a localized constriction or transection. The degree of recovery depends on the amount of anatomical disruption incurred. If apposition of the distal and proximal segments is maintained and no appreciable mechanical barrier is interposed as the result of hemorrhage and tissue breakdown, the axons will regrow and reinnervate the muscle fibers at a rate of approximately 1 mm per day.

Other Pathologic Features

There are other pathological considerations that pertain to the neuropathies. Some pathological processes are primarily **parenchymal**, attacking the nerve cell, its myelin sheath, or Schwann cells directly; others are mainly **interstitial**, affecting the supporting connective tissue and vasculature. Certain neuropathic processes also have a predilection for neurons of a particular size. **Large-fiber polyneuropathies** tend to produce a distal loss of vibration sense, loss of ankle jerks, ataxia, weakness, and slowed nerve conduction velocities early. **Small-fiber polyneuropathies** produce salient autonomic features, pain and dysesthesias, and a loss of pain sensation with preserved conduction velocities.

POLYNEUROPATHIES

The first step in approaching diagnosis in a patient with a peripheral neuropathy is to differentiate a polyneuropathy from a mononeuropathy or multiple mononeuropathy (discussed later). A polyneuropathy usually presents with fairly symmetrical distal sensory symptoms (paresthesias, loss of sensation, or burning pain) that progress proximally in a stocking-and-glove fashion. In many cases, distal weakness supervenes early in the form of foot drop, hand muscle weakness, and wrist drop. In certain neuropathies, such as Guillain-Barré, porphyria, and thallium poisoning, the weakness may be mainly proximal. Cramping, distal muscle wasting (Fig. 15-2), loss of temperature discrimination, trophic changes in the skin, and uncomfortable dysesthesias are frequently found in these patients. In neuropathies with small-fiber involvement, autonomic symptoms such as orthostatic hypotension, bladder disturbances, impotence, and sweating disturbances may appear (Table 15-1).

Examination in these patients reveals absent or reduced tendon jerks (especially distally); stocking-and-glove loss of sensation to pinprick, temperature, and light touch, and/or a distal loss of posterior column sensation; distal weakness and wasting (in the sensorimotor neuropathies); and trophic skin changes. Palpable or visibly enlarged nerves may be seen in the context of certain hereditary demyelinating neuropathies, leprosy (Fig. 15-3), amyloidosis, or Refsum's disease. Enlarged nerves may be seen best over the dorsum of the foot or at the side of the neck, crossing the sternocleidomastoid muscle. Palpation of the ulnar nerve in the medial upper arm or the common peroneal nerve as it wraps around the fibular neck is most likely to reveal hypertrophy.

The distinction from multiple mononeuropathy may be obscured in two ways. First, when enough individual nerves become involved in multiple mononeuropathy, the clinical picture may resemble a polyneuropathy quite closely. Second, in the presence of a polyneuropathy, individual nerves become more susceptible to compression or entrapment, making superimposed mononeuropathies fairly common.

In a limited number of situations, a nerve biopsy specimen may help clarify the cause of a neuropathy, particularly in patients with multiple mononeuropathy. Polyarteritis nodosa, sarcoidosis, leprosy, infiltrative neuropathy due to carcinoma or lymphoma, amyloidosis, myelomatous demyelinating neuropathy, familial hypertrophic demyelinating neuropathies, and metachromatic leukodystrophy may be specifically diagnosed in this way. The sural nerve above or at the lateral malleolus is the usual site of biopsy, but the superficial branch of the common peroneal nerve or sensory branch of the radial nerve (for neuropathies affecting the upper extremities) can also be used. Occasionally, patients will complain of uncomfortable dysesthesias over the lateral foot and heel, where there is an area of permanent numbness, following a sural nerve biopsy.

Nerve conduction velocity studies are useful

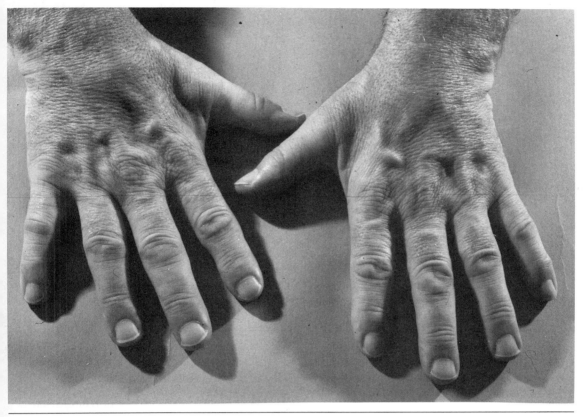

Fig. 15-2. *Atrophy of intrinsic hand muscles ("guttering") in a man with a diabetic sensorimotor polyneuropathy. Note the wasting in the first dorsal interossei bilaterally.*

Table 15-1. Polyneuropathies with Autonomic Involvement

Diabetes mellitus
Guillain-Barré syndrome
Acute pandysautonomia
Riley-Day syndrome
Amyloidosis
Porphyria
Tabes dorsalis

for distinguishing neuropathies from myopathies or anterior horn cell disorders (see Fig. 3-8A). They are also helpful for determining whether a polyneuropathy or multiple confluent mononeuropathies are present, distinguishing sensorimotor from pure motor neuropathies, localizing the site of compression in an entrapment neuropathy, and differentiating axonopathies from myelinopathies (see later discussion).

Acute and Subacute Immune-Mediated Polyneuropathies (Guillain-Barré Syndrome)

Pathophysiology and Etiology

The most common cause of acute or subacute areflexic paralysis is acute inflammatory polyradiculoneuropathy, or the **Guillain-Barré syndrome**, which has an annual incidence of 0.75 to 2 per 100,000. Acute ascending neuropathic paralysis was described by Landry in 1859 and later by Guillain, Barré, and Strohl in 1916. The disorder is a segmental demyelinating neuropathy that is thought to result from an im-

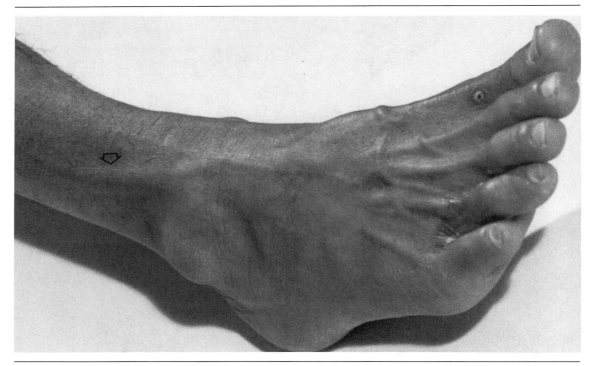

Fig. 15-3. *Marked hypertrophy of the superficial peroneal nerve* (arrow) *in a 32-year-old man with tuberculoid leprosy. Note the skin lesions over the first and fourth toes.*

mune attack on the myelin sheath. An animal model of the disease (experimental allergic neuritis) can be produced by injecting peripheral nerve myelin basic protein (P_2 protein) with Freund's adjuvant into a host animal. This condition can then be passively transferred to other animals by injecting T-lymphocytes from affected animals, suggesting the importance of cell-mediated mechanisms.

An immune pathogenesis is also supported by observations that patients have increased numbers of circulating lymphoblasts and activated T-lymphocytes; humeral factors (presumed antibodies) from patients are toxic to myelin in vitro; and the IgG level may be elevated in serum and cerebrospinal fluid (CSF). In addition, about 50 percent of patients have had a preceding respiratory or gastrointestinal illness or received a vaccination within 4 weeks of the event, and may respond favorably to plasmapheresis.

Pathological studies show that the nerves in these patients are infiltrated, in some cases along their entire length (although the roots are usually most severely affected), by T-lymphocytes, monocytes, and macrophages. There is also deposition of IgM, IgG, IgA, and complement activation products. Segmental demyelination, and, in more severe cases, axonal degeneration are seen.

Whether cell-mediated or humoral autoimmune mechanisms are primarily involved is still not resolved, and both may play a role. Although the analogy to experimental allergic neuritis and some of the pathological features are consistent with a cell-mediated demyelination, circulating complement-fixing IgM antibodies toxic to myelin in vitro have been reported. The specific antigen to which the antibodies react is unknown, but proposed candidates include myelin-associated glycoprotein, a variety of gangliosides including GM_1, and a glycolipid component of myelin that is common to the Forssman antigen found in a variety of infectious agents.

The disorder occurs in all age groups from infancy to the elderly, although it is most common in young adults. Antecedent events that have been associated include viral illnesses (especially infectious mononucleosis, hepatitis, herpes, cytomegalovirus), mycoplasma pneumonia infection, *Campylobacter jejuni* enteritis, vaccination (e.g., swine influenza and smallpox), pregnancy, oral contraceptive use, and underlying carcinoma or lymphoma. HIV infection may also produce an acute neuropathy resembling Guillain-Barré. In recent years, Lyme disease has also been diagnosed in patients with otherwise typical features of Guillain-Barré syndrome (except for CSF pleocytosis).

Clinical Picture and Diagnosis

The disease usually begins with a subacutely developing distal or proximal symmetrical weakness (Table 15-2). Distal paresthesias are often early symptoms, and a possible variant exhibiting a more prominent sensory than motor involvement has been described. Despite this, objective sensory findings are often not conspicuous. Weakness may progress rapidly

Table 15-2. Diagnosis of Guillain-Barré Syndrome

Clinical findings
  Acute/subacute paralysis (usually symmetrical; proximal > distal)
  Areflexia or marked hyporeflexia
  Cranial nerves VII, IX, XII, III, and VI can be involved
  Respiratory muscle involvement in approximately 25 percent
  Autonomic involvement
  Distal sensory involvement (usually mild, mainly subjective paresthesias)
  Muscle pain and tenderness
  Sparing of bladder function and no Babinski responses
  Preceding respiratory or other viral illness in more than 50 percent of the cases
Laboratory findings
  Elevated CSF protein level by the second week with mononuclear pleocytosis <10/mm³ (albuminocytologic dissociation)
  Nerve conduction studies: may be normal early, H and F waves often affected, early conduction block typical
  Electromyogram shows denervation in more severe cases

or over several days in an ascending, descending, or more irregular pattern. Maximum weakness is usually reached within 3 to 4 weeks of onset, and the respiratory muscles are affected in the more severe cases, requiring assisted ventilation in about 20 percent of the patients. Occasional cases exhibit a biphasic, relapsing-remitting, or chronically progressive course.

The cranial nerves are frequently involved. Virtually every nerve except the first two may be affected, and bilateral facial weakness (in one third of the cases), ophthalmoplegia, and dysphagia are particularly common. Bladder involvement is unusual, although there can be transient retention. Other variants of the syndrome include the combination of ophthalmoplegia, ataxia, and areflexia described by Miller-Fisher and possibly a relatively pure pandysautonomic variety.

Examination reveals absent deep tendon reflexes, at least in the areas of weakness, and often in a generalized distribution. Muscles may be painful when squeezed. A very distal mild sensory loss to pinprick sensation on the fingers and toes can usually be demonstrated. By the second week in most cases, the protein level in the CSF is moderately elevated, with fewer than 10 mononuclear cells per cubic millimeter (albuminocytologic dissociation).

The results of nerve conduction velocity studies may be normal early in the course or remain normal throughout in a small number of cases. Special techniques such as H-wave and F-wave measurements often disclose abnormalities in the nerve roots and proximal nerve segments. The most typical finding is conduction block, and this is caused by demyelination. This is revealed by a reduction in the amplitude of the muscle action potential after stimulation of the proximal versus the distal nerve. One predictor of poor prognosis is a marked reduction in the amplitude of the compound motor action potential, which correlates with axonal damage.

Management and Prognosis

Early in the course, the patient's vital signs should be taken at least every 2 hours, especially if weakness is progressing. Bedside indices of respiratory function, including blood gases, vital capacity, and inspiratory forces, should be determined frequently. If the vital capacity falls below approximately 1,000 cc, assisted ventilation should be considered. Weak cough, inability to hold the breath for more than a few seconds, and frequent pauses in conversation due to dyspnea are all signs of deteriorating respiratory function. Management in severe cases requires meticulous respiratory and nursing care in an intensive care unit. Some patients who remain for several months in a ventilator-dependent state experience full recovery.

Tracheostomy is necessary for the administration of prolonged positive-pressure, assisted ventilation, although endotracheal intubation should first be maintained for a week or more because some patients require the respirator for only a short period. Unfortunate tragedies occasionally occur when respirators become disconnected and alarms fail, or when mucous plugs cause tracheal obstruction. It is important for the nursing team to be fully aware that about 80 to 90 percent of these patients should recover completely or nearly so, with only about 10 percent showing severe residual effects.

Other complications that can arise in severe cases and should be anticipated include:

1. Autonomic neuropathy producing wide fluctuations in blood pressure and cardiac arrhythmias. This is one of the most common causes of death in patients with Guillain-Barré syndrome and, for this reason, cardiac monitoring is recommended.
2. Pulmonary embolism. Low-dose subcutaneous prophylactic heparin and the frequent performance of passive limb movements are advisable.
3. Atelectasis, tracheal erosion, respiratory infection, and other complications of assisted ventilation. Attention must be given to proper suctioning, respirator adjustment, tracheostomy care, positioning, and chest physiotherapy. Bronchoscopy may be necessary to clear mucous plugs causing atelectasis.
4. Infection due to urinary catheterization and skin breakdown.
5. Syndrome of inappropriate antidiuretic hor-

mone. The hyponatremia is usually transient and responds to water restriction.
6. Muscle contractures. Preventive therapy consists of passive range of motion exercises, proper positioning, and possibly splinting.
7. Muscle pain is quite frequent and often severe. Carbamazepine, narcotic analgesia, or a single intramuscular injection of methylprednisolone should be tried to ease the pain.
8. Rarely, raised intracranial pressure and papilledema develop, possibly as a result of impaired CSF absorption due to the elevated CSF protein concentration.
9. Finally, the psychological stress resulting from the patient's total paralysis and respirator dependence, physical discomfort, uncertainty about the outcome, and the intensive care unit environment requires a great deal of attention. The patient must be frequently reassured about the usual reversibility of the situation.

Some patients appear to respond dramatically to plasma exchange with albumin or fresh frozen plasma, which is especially recommended for those who are showing rapid progression or developing respiratory failure. It is more likely to be beneficial if started within the first week of the illness. Side effects include hypotension and thrombophlebitis stemming from indwelling catheters inserted into the femoral or subclavian veins. Corticosteroids are not beneficial and are best avoided in acute inflammatory polyradiculoneuropathy. Recently, intravenously administered immune globulin (0.4 gm/kg/day) given over 5 consecutive days has proved to be at least as effective as plasmapheresis and to have fewer side effects.

Other neuropathies that can closely resemble Guillain-Barré syndrome are those caused by porphyria (usually acute intermittent porphyria), diphtheria, thallium or lead intoxication. Poliomyelitis, rarely seen nowadays, except in those who have escaped vaccination, is another cause of acute areflexic paralysis. Features that help distinguish it from Guillain-Barré syndrome are an absence of sensory findings, fever, CSF pleocytosis, preceding gastrointestinal illness, and frequently asymmetrical involvement. In patients with acute spinal cord compression, there is a well-defined sensory level, a high likelihood of urinary retention, possible Babinski's signs, and no cranial nerve involvement. Other causes of acute generalized weakness are listed in Table 15-3.

Chronic Inflammatory Demyelinating Polyradiculoneuropathy

Apart from the course, the clinical, CSF, electrophysiological, and pathological findings in chronic inflammatory demyelinating polyradiculoneuropathy (CIDP) suggest a strong relationship to Guillain-Barré syndrome. Some cases begin with a typical acute polyradiculoneuropathy that continues to progress beyond 2 months after onset. The maximal deficit in usual cases of acute Guillain-Barré syndrome is reached within 4 weeks of onset. Other cases of CIDP have a relapsing-remitting course, rather than the monophasic course typical of acute

Table 15-3. Causes of Acute or Subacute Generalized Weakness

Neuropathies
  Guillain-Barré syndrome (acute inflammatory
    polyradiculoneuropathy)
  Porphyria
  Heavy metal intoxication (lead, thallium)
  Diphtheria
  Buckthorn toxin
  HIV
Anterior horn cells
  Poliomyelitis
  ECHO, Coxsackie viruses
Neuromuscular junction
  Myasthenia gravis
  Botulism
  Anticholinesterase (e.g., insecticide) intoxication
  Tic paralysis
  Mollusk-shellfish consumption
Muscle
  Acute polymyositis
  Periodic paralysis
  Licorice intoxication
  Hypophosphatemia during hyperalimentation
Spinal cord
  Acute compression (e.g., epidural tumor, abscess,
    or hematoma)
  Transverse myelitis
  Spinal cord infarction

Guillain-Barré syndrome, or are unrelentingly progressive from the onset. The nerves may show hypertrophic changes indicative of demyelination and remyelination. About 40 percent of the patients become severely disabled or die from the illness. Intravenous gamma globulin infusions have recently been proved effective in alleviating the disorder. Corticosteroids are frequently beneficial but may produce a steroid-dependent state, such that attempts to taper the dose below a certain level invariably lead to relapse. Other approaches to treatment include repeated plasma exchange or the administration of immunosuppressants such as azathioprine or cyclophosphamide.

A rare distinct chronic neuropathy that is somewhat similar to CIDP but exhibits a neurological picture resembling motor neuron disease has been termed *multifocal motor neuropathy with conduction block*. This condition usually affects young adults and may lead to severe, slowly progressive weakness that spares the cranial nerves. Weak, and in some cases, severely wasted muscles are found within the distribution of specific peripheral nerves with sensory function largely spared. The most striking feature is a conduction block in the motor axons of various nerves demonstrated by electrical studies; this remains stable over time. An autoimmune pathogenesis is assumed and antibodies to GM_1 ganglioside have been observed, although their significance is unclear. Some response to immunosuppression with cyclophosphamide has been reported.

Neuropathies Associated with Plasma Cell Dyscrasias and Neoplastic Disorders

A wide variety of polyneuropathies are seen as a remote effect of carcinoma and lymphoma, most likely stemming from an immune pathogenesis. These are discussed further in Chapter 29. In recent years, investigators have recognized a relatively high association between peripheral neuropathies (often assumed to be idiopathic) and various forms of plasma cell dyscrasias (i.e., monoclonal gammopathy of undetermined significance, osteosclerotic myeloma, multiple myeloma, Waldenström's macroglobulinemia, or gamma–heavy chain disease). These neuropathies are most commonly encountered in older men.

A wide variety of neuropathies accompany the various gammopathies, especially with the overproduction of IgM monoclonal proteins. Some of the neuropathies are distal and mainly sensory but not too disabling. Others are quite disabling because of the severe pain and autonomic or marked motor involvement. The polyneuropathy associated with **osteosclerotic myeloma** is a slowly progressive large-fiber axonopathy causing a secondary demyelinating neuropathy that clinically resembles chronic idiopathic inflammatory demyelinating polyradiculoneuropathy. The neuropathy seen with isolated IgM monoclonal gammopathy is a large-fiber demyelinating neuropathy that likely arises because of the manufacture of antibodies directed against myelin-associated glycoprotein and involves complement fixation. Electron microscopy reveals a characteristic splitting of myelin lamellae. The abnormal immune globulin can be identified in nerve biopsy specimens in some of these cases using immunohistofluorescent techniques. The neuropathy in these patients may abate with treatment of the underlying plasma cell dyscrasia and also with plasmapheresis.

Hereditary Neuropathies

Hereditary Motor and Sensory Neuropathies, Etiology Unknown

Hereditary motor and sensory neuropathy (HMSN) type I corresponds to the classic form of Charcot-Marie-Tooth disease, the usual cause of peroneal muscular atrophy. Demyelination and remyelination occur, causing the formation of hypertrophic nerves with onion bulb patterns that can be observed on microscopical cross sections. Motor nerve conduction velocities are usually markedly slowed (less than 30 meters/sec). An autosomal dominant mode of inheritance is the most common form of transmission, although recessive cases can also present a similar but usually more severe picture. Symptoms usually appear in the first decade and consist of difficulty running and foot deformity (pes cavus). Wasting and weakness

occur predominantly in the distal muscles of the lower extremity (anterior tibial and peroneal), creating the classic "inverted champagne bottle" appearance of the legs. Hypertrophied nerves may be seen over the dorsum of the foot or palpated at the fibular head. Ankle jerks are lost and the deep tendon reflexes are considerably reduced. Vibration sense is typically diminished in the feet. The course is very slowly progressive with the upper extremities becoming involved late. Rarely does severe disability result. The Roussy-Lévy variant of this disorder exhibits additional features of tremor and ataxia.

HMSN type II is the designation now given to the neuronal form of Charcot-Marie-Tooth disease. Because axonal degeneration is the underlying lesion responsible, there is no hypertrophy of nerves and nerve conduction velocities are mildly reduced or normal. In the autosomal dominant form, which is by far the most common, onset is often later and the disability milder than that seen in HMSN type I.

HMSN type III (Dejerine-Sottas disease) is a rare autosomal recessive disorder with onset in infancy. Affected individuals have delayed milestones and are often wheelchair dependent by the end of the first decade. Both hyper- and hypomyelination are seen on nerve biopsy specimens. Conduction velocities in these patients are extremely slow.

There are also several varieties of hereditary pure sensory neuropathies that often occur in combination with autonomic impairment. Because of the loss of pain sensation, many of these patients suffer severe ulcerations of the feet and incur deformities of their digits and joints. The Riley-Day syndrome is discussed further in Chapter 22.

Refsum's Disease

Refsum's disease is a rare autosomal recessive disorder that is of interest because it is caused by the accumulation of excessive amounts of phytanic acid in the peripheral and central nervous system. Because phytanic acid derives entirely from dietary lipid sources, the disease can be partially treated by having patients adhere to a special diet. Besides a chronic, sometimes relapsing-remitting, hypertrophic, demyelinating sensorimotor neuropathy, patients show an atypical form of pigmentary retinal degeneration, sensorineural deafness, ichthyosis (dry, scaly skin), cataracts, and a cardiomyopathy.

Other Hereditary Neuropathies

Neuropathy occurs in the context of certain hereditary diseases involving well-defined metabolic abnormalities. These include Fabry's disease (alpha-galactosidase deficiency), metachromatic leukodystrophy (arylsulfatase deficiency), Krabbe's leukodystrophy (beta-galactosidase deficiency), Tangier disease (hypoalphalipoproteinemia), and the porphyrias. Various other diseases, with less well understood pathogeneses, such as hereditary amyloidosis and ataxia telangiectasia, are also accompanied by neuropathy.

Neuropathies Accompanying Systemic Metabolic, Endocrine, Collagen, and Neoplastic Disorders

These neuropathies, which are extremely common, are discussed in more detail in Chapter 29 and listed in Table 15-4.

Toxic and Nutritional Causes of Neuropathy

An increasing number of industrial toxins, chemicals, and therapeutic agents have been implicated as causes of peripheral neuropathies (Tables 15-4 and 15-5). Vitamin deficiencies with or without alcohol abuse and the recent excess intake of vitamin B_6 can also bring about a painful distal polyneuropathy.

Infectious and Other Causes of Neuropathy

Leprosy is one of the most common causes of neuropathy in the world today. The lepromatous form is mainly responsible for the severe sensory neuropathy that leads to the deformation of distal body parts. The bacillus can be seen on nerve biopsy specimens. Hypertrophied nerves and depigmented anesthetic spots as well as other skin lesions are also characteristic (see Fig. 15-3). Sarcoidosis is another disor-

Table 15-4. Nutritional and Systemic Causes of Neuropathy

Metabolic
  Uremic
  Hepatic
  Porphyria
  Tangier disease
Endocrine
  Diabetes mellitus
  Hypothyroidism
  Acromegaly
Neoplastic, paraproteinemias, dysproteinemias
  Direct infiltrative (metastatic)
  Remote effects (paraneoplastic) of carcinoma or lymphoma
  Associated with plasma cell dyscrasias
  Amyloidosis
  Cryoglobulinemia
Collagen disease
  Polyarteritis nodosa and other necrotizing vasculitides
  Rheumatoid arthritis
  Systemic lupus erythematosus
  Scleroderma
  Sjögren's disease
Infectious and related causes
  Leprosy
  Herpes zoster
  Lyme disease
  HIV
  Sarcoidosis
Nutritional
  Thiamine deficiency
  Vitamin B_{12} deficiency
  Folate deficiency
  Pellagra
  Pantothenic acid deficiency
  Vitamin E deficiency
  Pyridoxine deficiency or excess
Neuropathy of severe systemic illness (ICU neuropathy)

der, likely of immune pathogenesis, that produces peripheral neuropathy, commonly in a multiple mononeuropathy pattern, and can also affect the facial nerves.

Herpes zoster causes a sensory mononeuropathy that is usually confined to one or more dermatomes. Rarely motor impairment occurs in the same distribution. Vesicles appear on the skin in the corresponding dermatome (shingles). In most cases, the process is self-limiting but, in immunosuppressed individuals (e.g., Hodgkins disease), can be particularly severe.

Table 15-5. Drugs, Therapeutic Agents, and Toxins Causing Neuropathy

Drugs and therapeutic agents	
Isoniazid	Vincristine/vinblastine
Phenytoin	*Cis*-platinum
Furadantin	Penicillamine
Hydralazine	Gold
Metronidazole	Tricyclic antidepressants
Sulfamethoxazole	Clioquinalone
Dapsone	Oral contraceptives
Disulfiram	

Industrial chemicals, solvents, and pesticides
Tri-orthocresyl phosphate
Malathion, DDT, lindane
Carbon disulfide
n-Hexane
Acrylamide
Methyl-*n*-butyl-ketone
Chlordecone (Kepone)
Dimethylaminopropionitrile
Heavy metals
Arsenic
Lead
Thallium
Mercury

Postherpetic neuralgia is a frequent consequence in elderly patients, which may persist and be intractable to all forms of treatment. Carbamazepine, tricyclic antidepressants, phenothiazines, transcutaneous nerve stimulation, and more recently capsaicin have been tried in such patients, with a variable degree of success (see Chapters 9 and 24). HIV produces a variety of acute and chronic neuropathies in AIDS patients (see Chapter 24). Cytomegalovirus has also been implicated in a particular form of neuropathy seen in AIDS patients (see Chapter 24).

MONONEUROPATHIES

Mononeuropathies or multiple mononeuropathies are most commonly caused by the compression or entrapment of individual nerves either within narrowly confining anatomical tunnels or at other sites where they are susceptible to repeated trauma against bony prominences (Table 15-6 and Fig. 15-4). Certain occupations (e.g., musicians) that require repetitive limb or finger movements can predispose to damage in particular nerves or branches of nerves.

The pathogenesis of nerve damage in these cases involves the direct physical disruption of the myelin sheath and, in severe cases, the axonal continuity, but may also be partially attributed to ischemia or to interruption of axoplasmic flow. In some cases, there is an underlying familial tendency or a neuronal metabolic disturbance that makes individual nerves susceptible to compression.

Individual nerves are also frequently affected in vasculopathies such as diabetes or collagen disorders and in other vasculitides. Rapid onset, often with pain, and slow recovery over three or four months are characteristic features. When a multiple mononeuropathy becomes extensive, it may be difficult to distinguish it clinically from a more generalized polyneuropathy. When considering the various potential causes of multiple mononeuropathy (Table 15-7), it becomes apparent that peripheral nerve biopsy (providing the nerve biopsied is affected) has a good chance of helping establish a specific diagnosis.

PLEXOPATHIES

Many of the same processes leading to mononeuropathies can also affect the brachial (Fig. 15-5) or lumbosacral plexuses. The involvement of contiguous anatomical sites by the process, CT or MRI findings, and the information yielded by special electrophysiological techniques may point to the existence of a plexopathy. Trauma and neoplastic invasion are common causes of plexus lesions. The thoracic outlet syndrome is discussed along with arm pain in a later chapter.

Brachial Neuritis

The rapid onset of shoulder girdle weakness and pain in conjunction with areflexia and later wasting are the hallmarks of brachial neuritis. The lesion is presumed to consist of inflammation and demyelination as well as axonal damage. Some cases appear after viral infections or immunizations (serum sickness), but most are idiopathic. The weakness may be profound and in

Table 15-6. Common Compression and Entrapment Neuropathies

Nerve	Site of entrapment	Etiology or predisposing factors	Signs and symptoms	Diagnosis
Upper extremity				
Median	Carpal tunnel at the wrist or in the palm	Congenital narrow canal, rheumatoid arthritis, osteoarthritis, excessive wrist flexion movements, pregnancy, gouty tophus, hypothyroidism, diabetes mellitus, acromegaly, amyloidosis	Pain and paresthesias in fingers, especially first 3, at times extending up to the shoulder; awakening at night with symptoms; worsening with wrist flexion movements (e.g., driving); thenar eminence wasting; weakness of thumb abduction and opposition; Tinel's sign at wrist; reduced 250-Hz vibratory sensation in index finger; occasionally objective sensory loss to pinprick in first 3½ fingers and radial two thirds of palm	Reduced or absent sensory potential with stimulation of index finger; increased terminal motor latency with stimulation at wrist and recording over thenar eminence
	Near the elbow: entrapment at ligament of Struthers just above medial epicondyle, at pronator teres muscle, or in forearm at level of anterior interosseus branch	Excessive use of forearm muscles	Paresthesias and pain in hand; tenderness at site of entrapment; variable weakness of pronator teres, flexor carpi radialis, and long flexors of first two fingers	Clinical picture: inability to form an "O" with thumb and index finger; denervation of involved muscles on EMG; nerve conduction abnormalities
Ulnar	Cubital tunnel at elbow	Repeated leaning on elbows; anesthesia; fractures, bony spurs, or deformities at elbow	Paresthesias and sensory loss in 5th finger and medial half of 4th finger and ulnar part of hand below wrist; wasting of interossei ("guttering") and hypothenar eminence; weakness of abductor digiti minimi,	Palpable thickening of ulnar nerve at elbow and excessive nerve movement with elbow flexion; nerve conduction slowing across elbow

Table 15-6 (Continued).

Nerve	Site of entrapment	Etiology or predisposing factors	Signs and symptoms	Diagnosis
	At wrist (canal of Guyon) or deep palmar branch	Arthritis, repeated trauma, ganglion	adductor pollicis, sometimes flexor carpi ulnaris	
			May show wholly motor involvement of hand intrinsics supplied by ulnar; sparing of ulnar sensation over dorsum of hand	EMG and NCVs
Radial	Spiral groove behind humerus in upper arm	"Saturday night palsy" fracture (sleeping with arm hyperabducted over chair after excess alcohol intake; crutches; anesthesia	Wrist drop, finger extensors; brachioradialis weakness; loss of sensation in web space between thumb and first finger (variable)	EMG, NCVs
Long thoracic	Along chest wall	Carrying heavy weight on shoulder or heavy backpack; anesthesia; idiopathic	Serratus anterior weakness (winging of scapula), pain in shoulder	EMG
Suprascapular	Suprascapular notch	Trauma, ganglion	Wasting and weakness of supraspinatus, infraspinatus; shoulder pain	EMG
Brachial plexus	Thoracic outlet	Fibrous band passing between excessively elongated C7 transverse process and first rib; cervical rib; scalenus anticus muscle	Pain, paresthesias in hand, wasting and weakness (especially of ulnar muscles of hand); symptoms increased by carrying or downward traction on arms; BP difference in arms; Adson's maneuver positive	NCVs across Erb's point; CT or MRI scan of thoracic outlet; x-ray study of cervical spine; digital IV subtraction angiography of subclavian artery

Nerve	Site	Causes	Clinical features	Tests
Lower extremity Sciatic	Roots within pelvis, at sciatic notch, at pyriformis muscle, lower nerve behind knee	Obstetrical, bony spur or neoplasm, Baker's cyst	Variable: sciatic pain and tenderness over sciatic notch, hamstring weakness, all muscle groups below knee weak, or just foot drop; sensory loss laterally below knee, over sole of foot, and distal calf	EMG, NCV, x-ray studies of sciatic notch
Femoral	Psoas sheath	Hemophilia, anticoagulation, diabetes, entrapment (rare)	Pain in groin and thigh, weakness of quadriceps; loss of knee jerk; variable sensory loss over anterior thigh and medial leg below knee (saphenous nerve)	EMG, NCV, CT for hemorrhage
Lateral cutaneous nerve of thigh (meralgia paresthetica)	Anterior superior iliac spine or inguinal ligament	Obesity, constricting garments (e.g., girdles), excessive crouching, pregnancy, diabetes	Burning pain, paresthesias and sensory loss in anterolateral thigh ("hip pocket")	Sensory NCV
Obturator	Obturator canal in pelvis	Obturator hernia, fracture, obstetrical, osteitis pubis	Weak thigh adduction; pain and sensory loss in medial thigh	EMG
Common peroneal	Neck of fibula	Excessive crossing of legs, anesthesia, excessive squatting, diabetes, casts, Baker's cyst, ganglion	Foot drop; weakness of toe extension; foot eversion; sensory loss over dorsum of foot (especially space between first and second toes), lateral lower leg, and ankle	NCV, EMG (extensor digitorum brevis)
Superficial peroneal	About 10 cm above lateral malleolus	Entrapment, trauma	Weakness of foot eversion and sensory loss over lateral calf, lateral malleolus, dorsum of foot, and medial 3rd or 4th toes	Sensory nerve action potential, EMG (peroneus longus and brevis)

Table 15-6 (Continued).

Nerve	Site of entrapment	Etiology or predisposing factors	Signs and symptoms	Diagnosis
Deep peroneal	Anterior tarsal tunnel at the ankle	Entrapment	Asymptomatic atrophy of the extensor digitorum brevis and sensory loss in web space between first and second toes	NCV (focal slowing at ankle), EMG (normal above ankle)
Posterior tibial	Tarsal tunnel (medial malleolus), popliteal fossa (rarely)	Arthritis, fracture, ganglion, Baker's cyst	Burning soles of feet especially at night; reduced sensation over heel; weak intrinsic foot muscles	EMG; prolonged terminal latency of motor response recorded from abductor hallucis and reduced sensory action potential recorded over medial plantar nerve with stimulation of big toe

EMG = electromyography; NCV = nerve conduction velocity; BP = blood pressure; CT = computed tomography; MRI = magnetic resonance imaging; IV = intravenous.

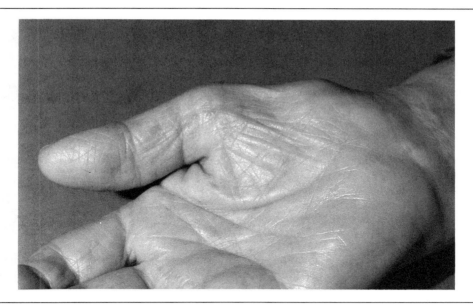

Fig. 15-4. *Carpal tunnel syndrome (bilaterally) in a 74-year-old woman who incurred median nerve compression by using hand crutches improperly.*

Table 15-7. Causes of Multiple Mononeuropathy

Diabetes mellitus
Collagen disease, vasculitis (e.g., polyarteritis
   nodosa)
Sarcoidosis
Leprosy
Herpes zoster
Amyloidosis
Neoplastic infiltration
Multiple compressive neuropathies due to familial
   predilection or underlying polyneuropathy

some cases is bilateral. Major involvement is less commonly distal than proximal. Familial cases with recurrent brachial plexus involvement have been reported. Recovery is the rule but may take 2 or 3 years in severe cases. Steroids may relieve the pain but have not been shown to hasten recovery. A less common analogous syndrome involves the lumbosacral plexus.

Neoplastic Plexus Involvement

Carcinoma of the upper lobe of the lung commonly invades the brachial plexus, giving rise to severe arm pain and motor impairment (Pan-coast's syndrome). The sympathetic chain is frequently involved and this gives rise to a Horner's syndrome. Other infiltrating tumors such as breast carcinoma and lymphoma may also be implicated.

Diagnosis is not usually difficult when a known carcinoma or metastases have been identified near the plexus and there is progressive intractable pain and limb weakness. CT or MRI scanning are often very helpful for demonstrating a soft tissue mass involving the plexus. Surgical exploration may be required to confirm the diagnosis, although negative findings do not rule out plexus invasion and certain cases are only diagnosed during a repeat operation.

In patients who have initially undergone irradiation for cancer in the vicinity of the plexus, late progressive plexus involvement due to the effects of irradiation must be distinguished from recurrent tumor. However, in the event of metastatic plexopathy, the pain tends to be an early and prominent symptom, the lower plexus (C7–T1) is more frequently involved, and Horner's syndrome is more common. Pain is also a prominent feature of lumbosacral plexus metastatic involvement. Radiation plexopathy

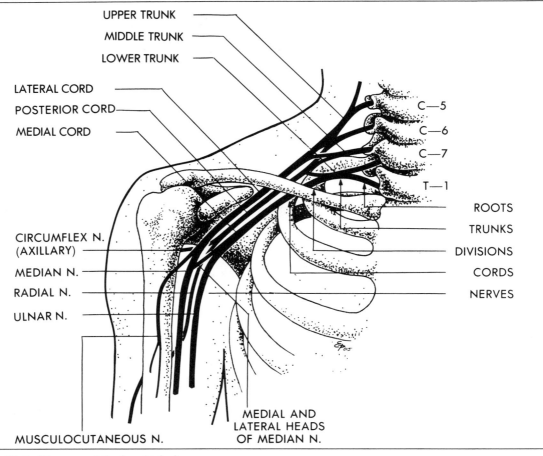

Fig. 15-5. *Diagram of the brachial plexus.*

tends to be confined to patients who have received over 6,000 rads.

BIBLIOGRAPHY

Argov, Z., and Mastaglia, F.L. Drug-induced peripheral neuropathies. *Br. Med. J.* 1:663–666, 1979.

Asbury, A.K., Arnason, B.G., and Adams, R.D. The inflammatory lesion in idiopathic polyneuritis: its role in pathogenesis. *Medicine* 48:173–215, 1969.

Asbury, A.K., and Gibbs, C.J., Jr. (editors). Autoimmune neuropathies: Guillain-Barré syndrome. *Ann. Neurol.* 27(Suppl. 1):S1–S79, 1990.

Asbury, A.K., and Gilliatt, R.W. The Clinical Approach to Neuropathy. In A.K. Asbury and R.W. Gilliatt (editors). *Peripheral Nerve Disorders. A Practical Approach.* London: Butterworths, 1984, Pp. 1–20.

Barohn, R.J., et al. Chronic inflammatory demyelinating polyradiculoneuropathy. *Arch. Neurol.* 46:878–884, 1989.

Brooke, M.H. *A Clinician's View of Neuromuscular Diseases*, 2nd ed. Baltimore: Williams & Wilkins, 1986.

Brown, M.J. Treatable neuropathies. *Adv. Neurol.* 17:235–247, 1977.

Dawson, D.M., Hallett, M., and Millender, L.H. *Entrapment Neuropathies*, 2nd ed. Boston: Little, Brown, 1990.

Downie, A. Peripheral Nerve Compression Syndromes. In W.B. Matthews and G.H. Glaser (editors). *Recent Advances in Clinical Neurology*, No. 3. Edinburgh: Churchill Livingstone, 1982, Pp. 47–66.

Dyck, P.J. (editor). Peripheral neuropathy: new concepts and treatments. *Neurol. Clin. North Am.* 10:601–813, 1992.

Dyck, P.J., et al. Plasma exchange in chronic inflammatory demyelinating polyradiculoneuropathy, *N. Engl. J. Med.* 314:461–465, 1986.

Dyck, P.J., et al. Chronic inflammatory polyradiculoneuropathy. *Mayo Clin. Proc.* 50: 621–637, 1975.

Dyck, P.J., Low, P.A., and Windebank, A.J. Plasma exchange in polyneuropathy associated with monoclonal gammopathy of undetermined significance. *N. Engl. J. Med.* 325:1482–1486, 1991.

Dyck, P.J., Oviatt, K.F., and Lambert, E.H. Intensive evaluation of unclassified neuropathies yields improved diagnosis. *Ann. Neurol.* 10:222–226, 1981.

French Cooperative Group on Plasma Exchange in Guillain-Barré Syndrome. Plasma exchange in Guillain-Barré syndrome: one-year follow-up. *Ann. Neurol.* 32:94–97, 1992.

Gilliatt, R.W., and Harrison, M.J.G. Nerve Compression and Entrapment. In A.K. Asbury and R.W. Gilliatt (editors). *Peripheral Nerve Disorders. A Practical Approach*. London: Butterworths, 1984, Pp. 243–286.

Gosselin, S., Kyle, R.A., and Dyck, P.J. Neuropathy associated with monoclonal gammopathies of undetermined significance. *Ann. Neurol.* 30:54–61, 1991.

Hallett, M., Tandon, P., and Berardelli, A. Treatment of peripheral neuropathies. *J. Neurol. Neurosurg. Psychiatry* 48:1193–1207, 1985.

Harding, A.E., and Thomas, P.K. Genetically determined neuropathies. In A.K. Asbury and R.W. Gilliatt (editors). *Peripheral Nerve Disorders. A Practical Approach*. London: Butterworths, 1984, Pp. 205–242.

Jacob, J.C., Andermann, F., and Robb, J.P.

Heredofamilial neuritis with brachial predilection. *Neurology* 11:1025–1033, 1961.

Kimura, J. Principles and pitfalls of nerve conduction studies. *Ann. Neurol.* 16:413–429, 1984.

Kori, S.H., Foley, K.M., and Posner, J.B. Brachial plexus lesions in patients with cancer: 100 cases. *Neurology* 31:45–50, 1981.

Koski, C.L. Guillain-Barré syndrome. *Neurol. Clin.* 2:355–366, 1984.

Lederman, R.J., and Wilbourn, A.J. Brachial plexopathy: recurrent cancer or radiation? *Neurology* 34:1331–1335, 1984.

Monaco, S., et al. Complement-mediated demyelination in patients with IgM monoclonal gammopathy and polyneuropathy. *N. Engl. J. Med.* 322:649–652, 1990.

Nakano, K.K. The entrapment neuropathies. *Muscle Nerve* 1:264–279, 1978.

Pettigrew, L.C., et al. Diagnosis and treatment of lumbosacral plexopathies in patients with cancer. *Arch. Neurol.* 41:1282–1285, 1984.

Ropper, A.H. The Guillain-Barré syndrome. *N. Engl. J. Med.* 326:1130–1136, 1992.

Ropper, A.H., and Shahani, B.T. Diagnosis and management of acute areflexic paralysis with emphasis on Guillain-Barré syndrome. In A.K. Asbury and R.W. Gilliatt (editors). *Peripheral Nerve Disorders. A Practical Approach*. London: Butterworths, 1984, Pp. 21–45.

Ropper, A.H., Wijdicks, E.F.M., and Truax, B.T. *The Guillain-Barré Syndrome*. Philadelphia: Davis, 1992.

Schaumburg, H.H., Berger, A.R., and Thomas, P.K. *Disorders of Peripheral Nerves*, 2nd ed. Philadelphia: Davis, 1992.

Sibley, W.A. Polyneuritis. *Med. Clin. North Am.* 56:1299–1319, 1972.

Steck, A.J., et al. Peripheral neuropathy associated with monoclonal IgM autoantibody. *Ann. Neurol.* 22:768–770, 1987.

Sterman, A.B., Schaumburg, H.H., and Asbury, A.K. The acute sensory neuronopathy syndrome: a distinct clinical entity. *Ann. Neurol.* 7:354–358, 1980.

Stewart, J.D., and Bray, G.M. Peripheral neuropathy. *Curr. Neurol.* 5:201–228, 1984.

Thomas, P.K. Inherited neuropathies. *Mayo Clin. Proc.* 58:476–480, 1983.

Warmolts, J.R. Electrodiagnosis in neuromuscular disorders. *Ann. Intern. Med.* 95:599–608, 1981.

Windebank, A.J., et al. The syndrome of acute sensory neuropathy: clinical features and electrophysiologic and pathologic changes. *Neurology* 40:584–591, 1990.

Young, R.R., et al. Pure pandysautonomia with recovery—description and discussion of diagnostic criteria. *Brain* 98:613–636, 1975.

Weakness: Disorders of Muscle

The contraction of muscles in response to nervous signals translates into the movement of body parts and the performance of work. In the adult, the muscle cell, or **fiber,** is cylindrical or fusiform with a diameter of 30 to 60 μm and length of 2 to 15 cm. Its outer membrane, or **sarcolemma,** consists of a plasma membrane and basement membrane with multiple nuclei lying directly beneath it. Muscle fibers are organized into bundles or fascicles, each surrounded by connective tissue (perimysium) through which small arterioles pass. Around each muscle fiber is a small amount of areolar tissue (endomysium).

Each muscle fiber is innervated by a terminal axonal branch located at a specialized region near its midpoint known as the **motor endplate.** This is where acetylcholine is released by the nerve terminals in response to an action potential and diffuses across the synaptic cleft to make contact with special receptors located on numerous subsysnaptic infoldings of the muscle membrane. A localized depolarization of the muscle fiber membrane is then conducted along the fiber from this site and also into the interior of the muscle fiber through a series of transverse tubules known as the **T system.**

A longitudinally oriented series of **myofibrils** (Fig. 16-1), the actual contractile elements, lie within the muscle fiber. Still smaller **myofilaments** are located within the myofibrils. Thinner filaments contain the protein molecule **actin,** which is attached to either side of dark-appearing transverse lines (the Z discs). These interdigitate with and partially overlap thicker filaments containing the molecule **myosin.** The fibrils are aligned so that, on light and electron microscopy, they appear as a regular pattern of alternating light and dark areas along the whole length of the fiber (see Fig. 16-1). The repeating unit consists of a 2-μm segment situated between two Z discs, known as a **sarcomere.** A light area, the I band, is located on either side of the Z discs. In the center of the sarcomere are darker areas, the A bands, where myosin and actin overlap. A lighter area (the H zone), with a dark line at its center (the M line), is seen at the midpoint of the sarcomere, and this

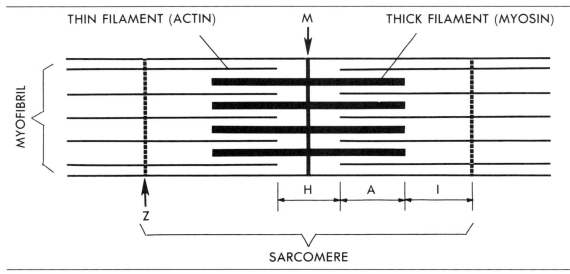

Fig. 16-1. *The arrangement of myosin and actin filaments within striated muscle. This regular arrangement gives the muscle a regular, striated appearance on histological sections. Note the Z and M lines and alternating A (anisotropic) and I (isotropic) bands. The I band becomes smaller with contraction of the fiber as actin and myosin filaments slide over each other.*

is where myosin filaments are not overlapped by actin. The fibrils are enveloped by a system of cisternae and this forms the **sarcoplasmic reticulum.** The T tubules are intimately related to the sarcoplasmic reticulum and, at the level of the junction between the A and I bands, form structures known as **triads**:—two terminal cisternae flanking a single T tubule.

Excitation-contraction coupling is the process whereby depolarization of the axon terminals is transformed into the mechanical energy necessary for contraction. The release of calcium from the sarcoplasmic reticulum into the cytoplasm brought about by depolarization, which is then conducted through the T system, constitutes the critical initiating event for contraction. The actual contractile process involves the splitting of ATP by myosin ATPase and the rapid formation and breaking of cross-links between actin and myosin so that the actin filaments at opposite ends of each sarcomere slide toward each other. This process involves the interaction between calcium and a troponin-tropomyosin complex, which is bound to actin. Normally, this complex prevents the attachment of myosin and actin but, in the presence of calcium, this inhibition is lost and cross-links are formed.

The muscle relaxation following contraction is accomplished through the re-uptake of calcium by the cisternae.

The muscle cell requires a relatively large amount of energy for the restoration of ionic equilibrium of membranes, protein synthesis, and especially contraction. Energy is stored in muscle in the form of phosphocreatine, glycogen, and lipids. The enzyme **creatine kinase** (CK) catalyzes the transphosphorylation reaction, whereby ATP, the immediate source of energy for contraction, is regenerated from ADP by the formation of creatine from phosphocreatine. Several enzymes are involved in the breakdown of glycogen to glucose, with phosphorylase as the rate-limiting step. The conversion of glucose from glycogen, which is stored in muscle, and glucose circulating in the serum are the major energy sources for short bursts of high-intensity work and for the early stages of more prolonged strenuous exercise.

Under anaerobic conditions, lactate is produced via the glycolytic pathway. Under aerobic conditions, much more energy is generated through the tricarboxylic acid cycle and electron transport chain within the mitochondria. The pyruvate dehydrogenase enzyme complex is involved in the oxidative decarboxylation of pyruvate to acetyl–coenzyme A (CoA). Free fatty acids (especially long-chain fatty acids) from the blood or from triglycerides stored within the muscle are an important energy substrate at rest or under conditions of prolonged submaximal exercise. Long-chain fatty acyl-CoA is transported into the mitochondrion for oxidation by a carrier system utilizing **carnitine** (L-3-hydroxy-4-trimethyl-aminobutyrate) and two enzymes, carnitine palmitoyl transferase 1 and 2. Under certain conditions, branched-chain amino acids can also serve as an energy substrate.

Two main types of muscle fibers have been identified on the basis of their histochemical properties (Table 16-1). Utilizing myofibrillar ATPase at a pH of 9.4, light-staining (type I) and dark-staining (type II) fibers can be seen (Fig. 16-2). Normally the two fiber types are intermixed in a checkerboard-like pattern. The fiber type is determined by the anterior horn cell innervating the fiber, and all the fibers of a particular motor unit are of one type. There is also a rough correlation between the histochemical fiber type and certain physiological properties of the fiber.

SIGNS OF MUSCLE DISEASE

Weakness, either unvarying or episodic, is the major sign of muscle disease. True fatigability, or a marked reduction in strength during the performance of a particular action, is more consistent with a neuromuscular junction deficit than with intrinsic muscle disease. However, certain types of muscle weakness may be provoked by exercise, such as that due to familial periodic paralysis or metabolic myopathies.

The differentiation of myopathic from neuropathic weakness is a common clinical problem (Table 16-2), but the distribution of the weakness is frequently helpful in making this distinction, because myopathic disorders tend to produce proximal, symmetrical involvement as well as neck flexion weakness and, in certain cases, ptosis, facial weakness, dysphagia, and rarely neck extension weakness ("head-lolling"). Conversely, neuropathies usually produce more distal weakness. However, certain myopathic disorders such as myotonic dystrophy and Gowers' distal myopathy may also produce mainly distal weakness. Guillain-Barré syndrome (acute inflammatory polyradiculoneuropathy) is also an exception, but the diagnosis is often evident on other grounds (see Chapter 15). When sensory abnormalities are present, the deep tendon reflexes are depressed disproportionately to the weakness, and fasciculations are prominent, neuropathic illness is more likely than myopathic disease.

Myopathies are less easily differentiated from the slowly progressive proximal spinal muscular atrophies caused by anterior horn cell degeneration. Electrical studies and muscle biopsy are often needed to distinguish these cases from myopathy, but even these tests may reveal the presence of "myopathic" changes in advanced stages of spinal muscular atrophy. Asymmetrical involvement and preserved strength in the muscles adjacent to affected muscles indicate spinal muscular atrophy. Some other helpful clues to specific myopathies are pseudohypertrophy of muscle (e.g., in muscular dystrophy), sparing of the extensor digitorum brevis bulge

Table 16-1. Muscle Fiber Types

Features	Type I	Type II
Myofibrillar ATPase	Lower (light-staining)	Higher (dark-staining)
Metabolism	Oxidative, more neutral lipid storage	Better equipped for glycogenolysis and anaerobic glycolysis
Mitochondria	Fewer	More stored glycogen
Function	Sustained contraction (slow twitch)	"Fight or flight" (fast twitch)
Blood supply	Greater capillarity	—
Color	Red (rich in myoglobin)	White

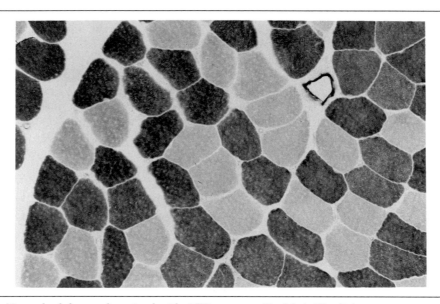

Fig. 16-2. *Normal adult muscle stained with ATPase at a pH of 9.4. The light-staining fibers are type I and dark-staining fibers are type II. Note the fairly even distribution of fiber types arranged in a checkerboard pattern.*

Table 16-2. Neuropathic Versus Myopathic Weakness

	Neuropathic	Myopathic
Distribution of weakness	Usually distal, may be asymmetrical	Usually proximal, symmetrical
Cranial nerves	Often involved	Often ptosis, facial weakness, neck flexion weakness, dysphagia
Atrophy	Early and disproportionate to weakness	Late and proportionate to weakness
Deep tendon reflexes	Lost early	Lost late
Sensory findings	Frequent	Absent
Creatine kinase level	May be moderately elevated	Often very high
Muscle biopsy	Denervation changes	Often specific findings
Nerve conduction velocities	Often reduced	Normal
Electromyographic findings	Neuropathy	Myopathy

on the lateral dorsum of the foot in myopathic scapuloperoneal syndromes, percussion or grip myotonia (e.g., in myotonic dystrophy), and skin findings characteristic of dermatomyositis.

Various other complaints besides weakness may point to the existence of muscle disease. Muscle aches and pains, cramps, and stiffness may be features of various inflammatory muscle diseases such as polymyositis, polymyalgia rheumatica, or viral myositis. Some patients with a prolonged postviral chronic fatigue syndrome may complain of intolerable muscle discomfort and fatigue as well as mental "fogginess" following attempts at even minimal exercise.

The myofascial pain syndrome and fibromyalgia are two ill-defined rheumatological syndromes that are commonly encountered in patients with persistent and often effort-related muscle pain and trigger points that can be detected by palpation. Muscles may be enlarged in either a generalized or localized manner in disorders such as hypothyroid myopathy, Pompe's disease, sarcoidosis, and other inflammatory myopathies. Another sign of muscle disease is intermittent myoglobinuria, due to rhabdomyolysis, that is often exercise-related. This may be severe enough to cause renal failure. Various inherited metabolic myopathies as well as toxic and infectious agents may also produce this picture (Table 16-3).

There are also syndromes involving the excessive or even continuous contraction of muscle, some neuropathic and some due to an intrinsic abnormality of muscle membranes. These disorders produce muscle cramps and stiffness and may be associated with other features such as excessive sweating. They include Isaac's syndrome (neuromyotonia), the stiff-person syndrome, and the Schwartz-Jampel syndrome.

Table 16-3. Causes of Myoglobinuria and Rhabdomyolysis

Inherited metabolic myopathies
  McArdle's disease
  Phosphofructokinase deficiency
  Carnitine palmitoyl transferase deficiency
  Malignant hyperthermia
Trauma
  Crush injury
  Excessive exercise
  Prolonged coma
  Status epilepticus
Toxins
  Alcohol
  Heroin
  Amphetamine
  Phencyclidine
  Snake venoms
Inflammatory myopathies
  Polymyositis/dermatomyositis
  Viral myositis (e.g., influenza A/B)
Electrolyte disturbances
  Hypernatremia
  Hyponatremia
  Hypokalemia
  Hyophosphatemia
Disturbances of body temperature
  Extreme hypothermia
  Heat injury

The **stiff-person syndrome** is a rare, chronic disorder occurring in adulthood that is associated with stiffness and rigidity of the axial muscles and intermittent painful spasms which are provoked by movement. The primary abnormality likely does not reside in the muscles but in the central nervous system. Antibodies to the intraneuronal enzyme glutamic acid decarboxylase have been found in the serum and cerebrospinal fluid (CSF) of some patients and this may lead to a reduction in central gamma-aminobutyric acid–ergic inhibition. High doses of benzodiazepines are effective in reducing the excessive muscle tone in affected patients, and recently prednisone treatment has also been claimed beneficial.

Malignant hyperthermia is a sporadic or autosomal dominant inherited, sometimes fatal, metabolic disorder of muscle. It is manifested as an extreme generalized muscular rigidity that includes the masseters, and patients also exhibit rhabdomyolysis (producing very high serum CK values) and a very high fever. The disorder is precipitated by the administration of inhalational anesthetics such as halothane or by succinylcholine. Treatment with cooling measures, diazepam, and dantrolene sodium may be lifesaving in these individuals. The in vitro testing of muscle fibers with the application of halothane or caffeine has been used to identify susceptible individuals. A genetic locus for malignant hyperthermia has been identified on chromosome 19q and it is now possible to use DNA probes to identify affected individuals from families at risk. Phenothiazines and other neuroleptics have also provoked a similar although less acute syndrome (the malignant neuroleptic syndrome) in susceptible individuals.

INVESTIGATION OF MUSCLE DISEASE

Muscle Enzymes

Serum levels of CK are substantially elevated in early Duchenne's muscular dystrophy, acute rhabdomyolysis due to various causes, and some inflammatory myopathies. More moderate elevations are observed in other myopathic

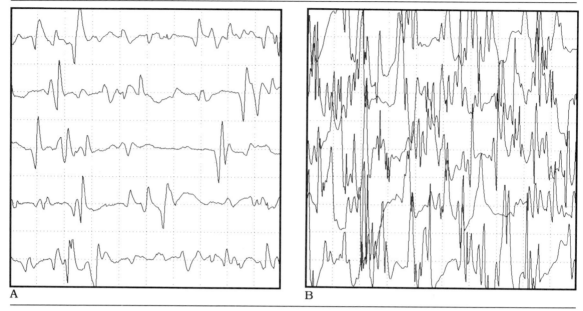

Fig. 16-3. *Electromyographic findings in myopathic and neuropathic disorders. (A) Normal motor units during the minimal voluntary muscle contraction. (B) A full interference pattern during strong contraction in a normal patient. Note that the individual motor units are obscured.*

disorders and in some neuropathic disorders such as progressive spinal muscular atrophy and chronic neuropathies. An elevated CK level may also be seen in patients with hypothyroidism or following heavy exercise, epileptic seizures, intramuscular injections, muscle injury, or heavy alcohol ingestion. Myocardial infarction and cerebral infarction may also cause an elevation in the levels of mainly the MB-CK and BB-CK isoenzymes, respectively, which can be differentiated from the MM subtype found in skeletal muscle. However, skeletal muscle contains significant amounts of the MB subtype, especially in immature regenerating muscle. Therefore, in a myopathic disorder such as polymyositis, an elevation in the level of MB-CK does not necessarily point to cardiac involvement. CK elevation is not only a useful indicator of possible muscle disease but may serve as an index to the activity, regression, or response to therapy of disorders such as polymyositis. The levels of other muscle enzymes, including aldolase, lactic dehydrogenase, and aspartate aminotransferase, are also frequently elevated in the presence of muscle disease, but these are less sensitive indicators than CK.

Electromyography

Standard needle electromyography (EMG) may help distinguish neuropathic from myopathic disease, may better define the distribution of muscle involvement, and aid in the identification of specific myopathic disorders that exhibit characteristic EMG features (Fig. 16-3). However, the technique is uncomfortable, relies on patient cooperation, and may yield false-negative findings in cases with patchy involvement. Muscles that are to be used later for muscle biopsy should not be needled because this may produce artifacts in the muscle specimens. Typical myopathic features include low-voltage polyphasic units, the over-rapid recruitment of motor units with minimal effort, and an excessively "spiky" interference pattern. Although the presence of abnormal spontaneous activity in resting muscle, such as positive sharp waves and even fibrillations, can

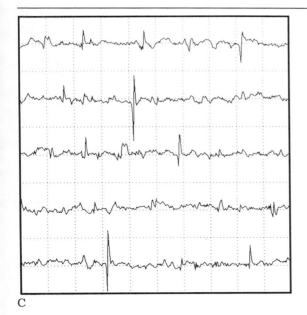

C

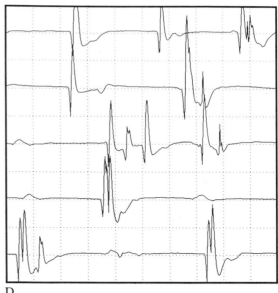

D

Fig. 16-3. *(C) Spontaneous activity at rest (fibrillations) in a patient with denervation. At least three separate muscle fiber potentials are shown. (D) Typical motor units seen with denervation. Note the polyphasic, high-amplitude units with prolonged duration. (E) Myopathic motor units recorded from the deltoid in a patient with dermatomyositis. Note that the units are polyphasic, of low amplitude, and short duration. There is also an over-rapid recruitment of units despite a minimal voluntary contraction. All tracings were done with a sweep speed of 10 msec per division and a gain of 0.5 mV per division except in A, where gain was increased to 0.2 mV per division, and D, where it was decreased to 2.0 mV per division.*

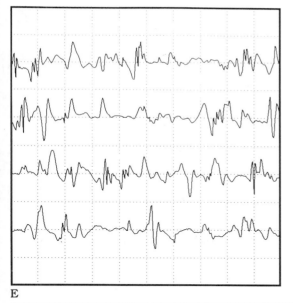

E

be seen in polymyositis, spontaneous discharges are more typical of denervation. Bizarre high-frequency discharges are typical of polymyositis. Myotonic discharges, waxing and waning high-frequency firing of units provoked by needle insertion, and contraction on percussion of muscle are seen in disorders such as myotonic dystrophy and myotonia congenita.

Muscle Biopsy

A moderately affected proximal muscle such as the deltoid or quadriceps is commonly chosen as the biopsy site in the investigation of myopathic disorders. The biopsy is done with the patient under local anesthesia and special techniques must be used in the handling of specimens to avoid artifacts and allow for proper histochemical staining and electron microscopic examination, if required.

In muscular dystrophy, fibers show evidence of excessive variation in size, areas of necrosis, regeneration (basophilia), and central nuclei, and muscle is replaced by connective tissue and fat (Fig. 16-4). In myotonic dystrophy, there are subsarcolemmal masses, nuclear chains, and ring fibers. Muscle specimens from patients with inflammatory muscle disease exhibit cellular infiltration around intramuscular arterioles, at times perifascicular atrophy (in dermatomyositis), and fiber necrosis (Fig. 16-5). Histochemical staining techniques and electron microscopic examination reveal the presence of distinctive features in numerous congenital myopathies (see later discussion). Special staining techniques also allow the demonstration of excessive amounts of stored glycogen or lipid or a lack of specific enzymes characteristic of metabolic myopathies. Swollen vacuoles are seen in the muscle fibers of patients with hypokalemic myopathy or periodic paralysis. Amy-loid, granulomas typical of sarcoidosis, and parasites are other specific findings obtainable by muscle biopsy.

With denervation, muscles show group atrophy, type grouping (with reinnervation), small angular fibers, and target fibers (Fig. 16-6). Type I or II fibers may be selectively involved in the myopathic disorders (e.g., type II atrophy in steroid myopathy and type I atrophy in myotonic dystrophy), but both fiber types tend to be affected in the neuropathic disorders. Disuse leads mainly to type II atrophy.

Other Tests

Computed tomographic (CT) scanning of muscle has been used to define the extent and degree of muscle atrophy and may also detect specific findings in muscle, such as calcification. Magnetic resonance imaging (MRI) and magnetic resonance spectroscopy (MRS) of muscle represent promising techniques for the studying of energy metabolism in certain hereditary and

Fig. 16-4. *Muscle biopsy section stained with hematoxylin-eosin from a 4-year-old boy who was seen because of a delayed onset of walking, progressive weakness of hip-girdle muscles, pseudohypertrophy of the calf muscles, and a markedly elevated creatine kinase level of 7,000 units/liter. The diagnosis was Duchenne type muscular dystrophy. Note the variation in fiber size and their rounded appearance, plus the smallness of many fibers and the marked increase in the connective tissue between fibers.*

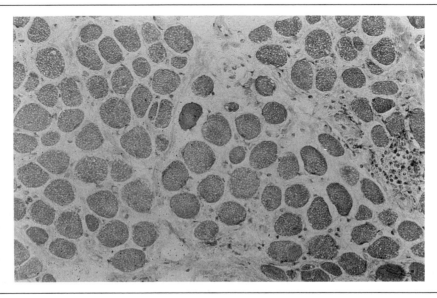

acquired metabolic myopathies such as the mitochondrial encephalomyopathies.

In McArdle's disease or phosphofructokinase deficiency, an ischemic forearm exercise test shows no rise in the lactate level of venous blood following exercise performed with a tourniquet around the arm. In addition, phosphorus MRS shows a characteristic lack of shift of the phosphorus peak following exercise. Serum carnitine levels are reduced in the presence of systemic carnitine deficiency. In hypokalemic periodic paralysis, attacks can be induced by the administration of glucose and insulin, or following exercise and a high carbohydrate meal. Potassium loading can be used to induce muscle weakness in patients with clinically suspected hyperkalemic periodic paralysis.

MUSCULAR DYSTROPHIES

The muscular dystrophies are a group of hereditary disorders in which patients suffer progressive muscular weakness due to necrosis of muscle fibers with gradual replacement by connective tissue and fat. The different varieties (Table 16-4) are distinguished on the basis of the mode of inheritance, distribution of weakness, and rate of progression. The pathogenesis is based on an inherited defect in the muscle cell membrane, which has also been observed in the red blood cells of dystrophic patients. The membrane defect permits the leakage of the intracellular enzyme CK and also, through unknown mechanisms, leads to early cell death.

Duchenne and Becker Muscular Dystrophy

Pathophysiology and Etiology
Unraveling the pathogenesis of the Duchenne and Becker types of muscular dystrophy was one of the early triumphs to come from the application of reverse molecular genetics techniques to the study of human illness (see Chapter 26). The abnormal gene responsible for both the Duchenne and Becker types of dystrophy resides on the short arm of the X chromosome (Xp21) and is extremely large and complex,

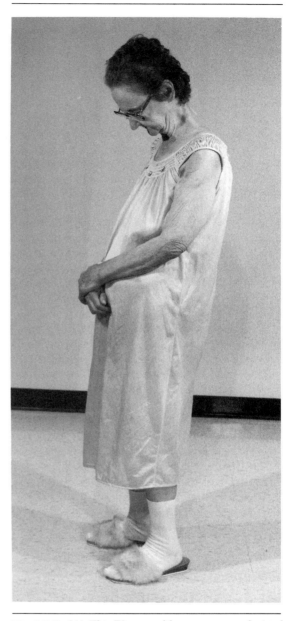

Fig. 16-5. *(A) This 70-year-old woman was admitted following a 2-month history of progressive proximal leg and arm weakness as well as neck extension weakness. She also exhibited dysphagia and decreased voice volume and had a 6-month history of a skin rash, especially over the extensor surfaces of the hands, a 20-lb (9-kg) weight loss, and Raynaud's phenomenon. This photo shows her marked neck extension weakness (head-lolling) and increased lumbar lordosis, indicating hip-girdle weakness. Her creatine kinase level was elevated and EMG showed the irritative phenomena typical of inflammatory myopathies.*

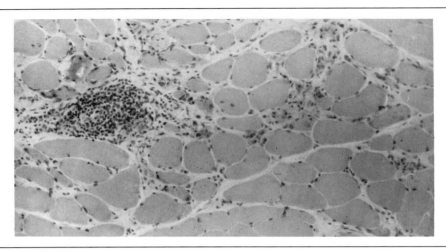

Fig. 16-5 *(Continued). (B) Muscle biopsy (deltoid) confirmed the diagnosis of dermatomyositis. Note the marked inflammatory perivascular changes and some shrunken, necrotic fibers seen on hematoxylin-eosin staining. Despite initial improvement on prednisone (80 mg/day), she died 3 weeks following admission from respiratory arrest due to progressive weakness of respiratory muscles.*

with approximately 2.5 Mb of DNA. In 70 percent of the cases of Duchenne's dystrophy, deletions or duplications are found at the Xp21 locus. Cloning and sequencing have shown that it codes for a 4.7-kD protein known as **dystrophin.** Dystrophin is found in skeletal, cardiac, and smooth muscle and is a cytoskeletal protein contained in the subsarcolemmal membrane region. It interacts with actin at its N terminal to bind to the intracellular cytoskeletal network and is attached to the surface membrane near its 3′ terminal via a transmembrane glycoprotein complex.

One theory for how muscle fibers become damaged in Duchenne's dystrophy proposes that, without dystrophin, there is less redundancy and strength in the membrane, making it susceptible to tears and mechanical disruption during contraction. In Duchenne's dystrophy, the stores of dystrophin are severely reduced to less than 3 percent of their normal amounts. In Becker's dystrophy, a truncated form of dystrophin is present in moderately reduced amounts.

Epidemiology
The Duchenne type of muscular dystrophy is the most common and best-defined of the mus-

cular dystrophies. It occurs in 1 of 4,000 live male births and has a prevalence of 3 per 100,000. Although it exclusively affects boys, girls with Turner's syndrome (XO) may be affected.

Clinical Picture and Diagnosis
The disease becomes evident clinically around the time that walking begins, and about half the patients do not walk until after 18 months of age. The gait is clumsy, falls are frequent, and running is difficult. Between the ages of 3 to 5, patients experience proximal lower extremity, hip, and truncal weakness, which is manifested by a waddling gait, difficulty in climbing stairs, and a hyperlordotic posture. Toe-walking may occur and there may be an equinovarus foot deformity.

Patients use the classic Gowers' maneuver to rise from the floor: first they turn to a prone position, support themselves on both their legs and hands (the "tripod" position), and then use their hands to "walk" gradually up the legs to assume the upright position. Initially the weakness is mainly confined to the lower extremities, but gradually becomes more generalized. By the age of 9 to 12, the affected boy becomes wheelchair bound and

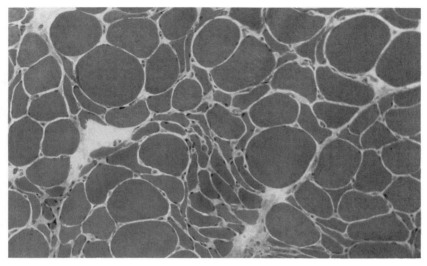

A

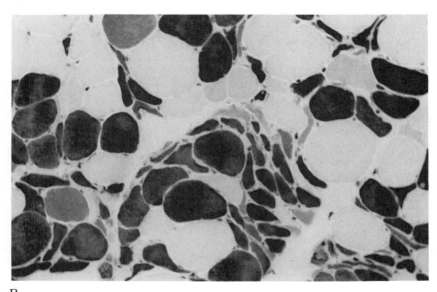

B

Fig. 16-6. *(A) Muscle tissue stained with hematoxylin-eosin from a patient with amyotrophic lateral sclerosis showing a typical denervation pattern. Note the small angular atrophic fibers occurring mainly in groups (group atrophy). (B) Specimen stained with ATPase (pH 9.4) obtained from the same muscle block, showing that most of the atrophic fibers in this region are type II.*

a gradually progressive kyphoscoliosis and contractures of the calf muscles, hips, elbows, and wrists occur. Respiratory insufficiency results from thoracic deformity and muscle weakness, and patients die (usually due to pneumonia) most often before the age of 20.

Other features of the disease include pseudo-hypertrophy of the calves and other muscles (e.g., vastus lateralis, deltoids, and forearm extensors), cardiac hypertrophy and electrocardiographic changes, and, in about one quarter of the cases, mental retardation.

Table 16-4. Classification of Muscular Dystrophies

Type	Heredity	Age of onset of symptoms	Specific features	Course
Duchenne/Becker	X-linked (Xp21 dystrophin gene)	Infancy	Pseudohypertrophy, M.R. 30%, CK $\uparrow\uparrow$ early	Nonambulatory by 12 years
Emery-Dreifuss	X-linked (Xq28)	Late teens	Early contractures of elbows and Achilles tendon, cardiac conduction abnormalities	Slow progression
Limb-girdle	Autosomal recessive, autosomal dominant (rare), sporadic	Teens, young adult	May have scapuloperoneal distribution, heterogeneous group	Slow progression, longevity
Facioscapulohumeral	Autosomal dominant, autosomal recessive (rare)	Childhood or teens	May have inflammatory features on biopsy	Slow progression, longevity
Oculopharyngeal	Autosomal dominant	Adult	Often French Canadian, ptosis and dysphagia (rarely limb weakness)	Slow progression, longevity
Distal	Autosomal dominant	Adult	Scandinavian	Slow progression
Myotonic [a]	Autosomal dominant (unstable gene fragment with triplet repeats on chromosome 19)	Variable, may be present at birth	Weakness mainly distal, myotonia, M.R. common, cataracts, frontal baldness, testicular atrophy, cardiac involvement	Slow progression

[a]Not strictly speaking a dystrophy but included by tradition.
M.R. = mental retardation; CK = creatine kinase.

The Becker type of dystrophy resembles the Duchenne type in its inheritance pattern, distribution of weakness, calf pseudohypertrophy, and very high CK levels. However, the onset is usually in the second decade and the progression is much slower, with only a slightly reduced life expectancy.

Diagnosis is based on the clinical picture as well as myopathic findings on EMG and very high levels of serum CK (50–400 times normal). The CK level is high by the age of 1 year but falls steadily toward normal as the disease progresses and greater numbers of muscle fibers degenerate. Lactic dehydrogenase and aldolase levels are also elevated. A muscle biopsy should be done to confirm the diagnosis (especially if only one family member is affected), and specimens show an increased variation in fiber size with hypertrophied fibers, segmental necrosis of fibers, rounded opaque fibers, grouped basophilic fibers, forking or branching of fibers representing attempts at regeneration, and increased amounts of connective tissue and fat. In the end stages, specific features are not easily recognized.

Management and Prognosis

No specific treatment is available to halt the inexorable downhill course of the disease, but management consists of attempting to maintain mobility and prevent muscle contractures and kyphoscoliosis. Proper wheelchair fitting, bracing, exercises, and chest physiotherapy are important. Fetal myoblasts have been transplanted into the muscle tissue of affected patients in an attempt to restore the dystrophin level. The technique is still experimental, however, and has not yet been shown to improve strength. The possibility of gene therapy is now being discussed. Adenovirus vectors are theoretically capable of delivering the dystrophin gene to affected muscle fibers.

Genetic counseling must be provided for families with an affected individual. Because up to one third of cases represent spontaneous mutations, every effort must be made to determine the carrier status of the mother and sisters of the patient. A mother who either has two affected sons or one son and a male relative affected with the disease almost certainly carries

the gene. In other cases, special methods should be used to determine carrier status. In 45 to 70 percent of cases, carriers have been found to have an elevated CK level. The CK level should be determined on three separate occasions, because elevated levels may return to normal during pregnancy or with advancing age. Female carriers may exhibit mild proximal weakness (5–10%), calf hypertrophy, or minor changes on EMG or muscle biopsy (70%), including an increased proportion of type I fibers.

Special techniques can now be employed for the definitive diagnosis of the Duchenne and Becker types of muscular dystrophy. Dystrophin assay of muscle tissue using immunohistochemical methods permits the differentiation of the two forms of dystrophy and allows the distinction of Becker's dystrophy from conditions such as limb-girdle dystrophy, which resemble it clinically. Dystrophin assay may be useful in detecting carriers of Duchenne type dystrophy, who often show a mosaic pattern, in that some muscle fibers contain near normal amounts of dystrophin and other fibers, virtually none.

Genetic analysis is a much more specific and sensitive way of detecting carriers or performing antenatal diagnosis (on a chorionic villus biopsy sample or cells obtained by amniocentesis). The usual method is to analyze restriction-fragment-length polymorphisms using several DNA probes to cover the span of the dystrophin gene. White blood cells can be used for DNA analysis. The participation of several family members, both affected and unaffected, is necessary for this type of linkage analysis and errors may occur as the result of recombination. Genomic probes that can detect deletions directly are applicable in some cases.

Emery-Dreifuss Muscular Dystrophy

Emery-Dreifuss muscular dystrophy is a rare X-linked (abnormal gene at Xq28) form of the disorder that begins in adolescence and runs a chronic course, with only a mild shortening of the patient's life span. Patients exhibit a slowly progressive wasting and weakness, mainly in a humeroperoneal distribution. One of the hallmarks is early contractures of the elbows, Achilles tendon, and posterior cervical muscles. The CK level is only moderately elevated. Cardiac involvement is a common problem, with a predisposition to sudden fatal arrhythmias, and, for this reason, prophylactic pacemaker insertion is recommended. Carrier detection is important because carriers must be screened for cardiac abnormalities.

Facioscapulohumeral Muscular Dystrophy

Facioscapulohumeral muscular dystrophy is an autosomal dominant disorder in which patients exhibit a variable degree of weakness but rarely significant disability. Onset is in adolescence or adult life. Patients may notice winging of the scapula or proximal arm wasting and weakness, but rarely may be seen in consultation because they cannot smile properly or their lips are everted (Fig. 16-7). Often the degree of involvement within a family varies markedly. Some patients also have mild weakness of their peroneal muscles, and these cases overlap with the myopathic scapuloperoneal syndromes. Neurogenic scapuloperoneal syndromes have also been described. A muscle biopsy specimen may show few abnormalities and, occasionally, inflammatory changes.

Limb-Girdle Dystrophy

Limb-girdle dystrophy embraces a heterogeneous group of adult-onset slowly progressive proximal myopathies associated with moderately elevated CK levels and dystrophic features on biopsy specimens. Some patients have been found to be carriers of Duchenne's muscular dystrophy. Similar clinical pictures are manifested by the proximal spinal muscular atrophies, endocrine myopathies, polymyositis, and certain benign congenital, histologically distinct myopathies (see later discussion).

Oculopharyngeal Dystrophy

Oculopharyngeal dystrophy is an autosomal dominant, adult-onset disorder that has been observed mainly in French-Canadian families. Affected patients suffer progressive ptosis and dysphagia, but there is only mild limb involvement.

Gowers' Distal Myopathy

Gowers' distal dystrophy is rare except in Sweden, where it occurs as an autosomal dominant disorder. Typically patients suffer onset in adulthood and the disease is slowly progressive. It must be distinguished from Charcot-Marie-Tooth hereditary sensorimotor neuropathy.

MYOTONIA AND MYOTONIC DYSTROPHY

Myotonia is due to a defect in the electrical properties of the muscle membrane that leads to repetitive firing, prolonged involuntary contraction, and delayed relaxation that can be elicited by electrical or mechanical stimuli such as percussion. When severe, myotonia may be symptomatic, producing generalized muscle stiffness or localized "cramps" or "spasms" that, for example, make it impossible for a patient to relax a handgrip for several seconds. Percussion of the thenar eminence, brachioradialis muscle, or tongue (using a tongue blade placed underneath) can demonstrate the abnormally prolonged muscle contraction. In mild cases, the myotonia can best be revealed by EMG. Movement of the needle, percussion of the muscle, or voluntary contraction will provoke high-frequency waxing and waning discharges that give off a "dive bomber" sound.

Myotonic Dystrophy (Steinert's Disease)

Pathophysiology and Etiology

Although traditionally classified with the muscular dystrophies, myotonic dystrophy is a distinct entity that shows atrophic rather than dystrophic changes on muscle biopsy specimens. The fundamental abnormality responsible is an inherited defect in the muscle membranes that leads to a lowered resting membrane potential and increased excitability with a tendency toward repetitive firing. It has a prevalence of 5 per 100,000.

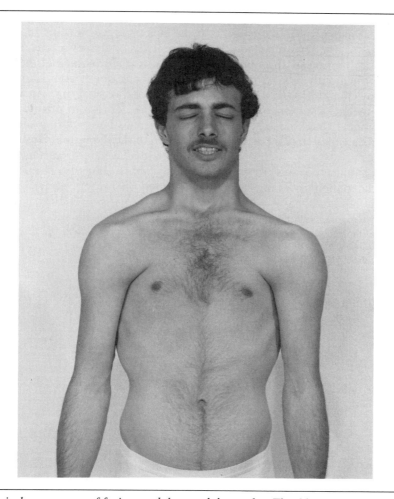

Fig. 16-7. *Typical appearance of facioscapulohumeral dystrophy. This 20-year-old man complained of a 4-year history of mild shoulder girdle weakness with difficulty lifting heavy objects. He was unaware of any muscle problems in the family but family members were not examined. Note the inability to bury his eyelashes or turn the corners of his mouth upward as he tried to smile and close his eyes maximally. Also note the low shoulders, horizontal position of his clavicles, high-riding winged scapulae (apparent as a bulge above the trapezius on the right), axillary creases, pectoral atrophy, and well-developed deltoids compared to his biceps.*

The disorder is inherited as an autosomal dominant trait and there is a large variation in the expressivity within a family. The gene for myotonic dystrophy has recently been localized to chromosome 19 and found to contain an unstable fragment with a variable number of triplet (cytosine-thymidine-guanidine) repeats. The number of repeats determines the severity of the phenotypic expression. This variable genetic abnormality accounts for the wide range in the expressivity associated with the disease. It also may explain the phenomenon of anticipation seen in this illness, whereby the phenotypic features appear earlier and with greater severity in successive generations of family members.

Clinical Picture and Diagnosis
Besides both skeletal and smooth muscle involvement, multiple other organs are also affected, leading to a characteristic constellation

of findings. Diagnosis is often possible on the basis of the facial appearance with frontal balding; temporalis, masseter, and sternocleidomastoid atrophy; ptosis; tenting of the upper lip with a tendency for the mouth to hang open; and cataract formation (Fig. 16-8). The cataracts, which may be detected by slit-lamp examination in asymptomatic individuals, are typically posterior subcapsular and exhibit a "stardust" appearance.

Cramping due to myotonia is rarely a presenting complaint in these patients. Some seek medical attention because of the progressive distal weakness and wasting that often become apparent by adolescence. In others, the presenting complaint is mental dullness, which is a relatively frequent complaint, especially in the childhood-onset form. An undue susceptibility to the depressant effects of barbiturates and other anesthetics during surgery may draw attention to the diagnosis. Obstetrical difficulties, with increased fetal wastage and prolonged difficult labors, may also suggest the diagnosis in affected offspring.

Fig. 16-8. *This 38-year-old woman with myotonic dystrophy shows facial features that are relatively subtle compared to those seen in more severe cases. The face is rather expressionless; she has cataracts (indicated by the eyeglasses), bilateral atrophy of the temporalis muscle, a fairly high hairline frontally, and a somewhat thin neck.*

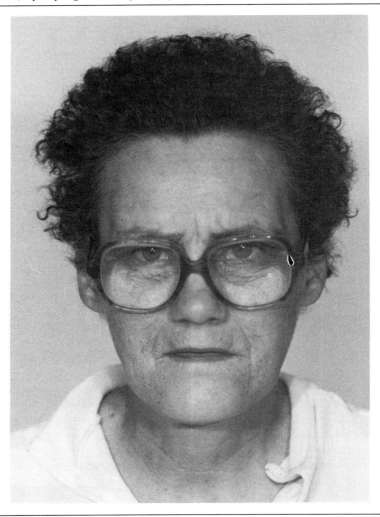

Other features, in addition to the muscle weakness, include dysphagia, megacolon or diarrhea due to smooth muscle involvement; testicular atrophy and infertility in males; abnormal glucose tolerance with insulin resistance and high levels of circulating insulin; hypercatabolism; and lowered serum levels of IgG. Cardiac conduction defects producing a prolonged A-V interval may cause syncope or even sudden death.

The EMG can be helpful in confirming the diagnosis. A muscle biopsy specimen shows typical features of atrophic fibers (especially type I), central nuclear chains, ring fibers, and subsarcolemmal masses. The CK level is often moderately elevated.

By utilizing linked polymorphic markers on chromosome 19, it is now possible for genetic testing to identify, with a high degree of certainty, presymptomatic carriers of the gene. Using genetic analysis, approximately 8 to 9 percent of the asymptomatic patients whose results from supplementary tests were negative (i.e., EMG and slit-lamp examination), but who had a 50 percent risk of carrying the gene, were actually found to have inherited the gene.

The identification of carriers is important so that they can be observed for the development of cataracts and cardiac abnormalities. This also allows for the anticipation of risks during anesthesia and makes possible genetic counseling.

Congenital myotonic dystrophy is virtually always transmitted by the mother. Affected infants exhibit a floppy appearance, poor suck and swallowing, facial diplegia, a characteristic inverted U appearance of the mouth, and talipes equinovarus. Mental retardation and significant weakness, which may abate somewhat, are the rule. It is now possible to identify affected fetuses with the abnormal gene in utero.

Management and Prognosis

Most patients become gradually weaker over the course of several years. Myotonia, if symptomatic, may be relieved by procainamide, phenytoin, or carbamazepine. Patients may require pacemaker insertion because of symptomatic cardiac arrhythmias.

Myotonia Congenita (Thomsen's Disease)

Myotonia producing muscle stiffness and diffuse muscle hypertrophy with onset in early childhood are the main features of myotonia congenita. There is an autosomal dominant and a more severe autosomal recessive variety, both more frequent in men. Rest worsens the muscle stiffness and exercise relieves it.

Paramyotonia Congenita (Eulenburg's Disease)

Paramyotonia congenita is a rare autosomal dominant disorder. Affected patients manifest myotonia and stiffness, mainly in facial, forearm, and hand muscles, which is worsened by exposure to cold as well as exercise. The distinction from the myotonia (especially affecting eyelids) with attacks of weakness that are seen in patients with hyperkalemic periodic paralysis is not clear.

INFLAMMATORY MYOPATHIES

Polymyositis/Dermatomyositis

Bohan and Peter have classified the idiopathic group of inflammatory myopathies into the following clinical categories: adult polymyositis, adult dermatomyositis, polymyositis/dermatomyositis (PM/DM) associated with neoplasm, childhood PM/DM, and PM/DM associated with the overlap syndrome. Inclusion-body myositis (see later discussion) can be added to this classification.

Polymyositis is a relatively uncommon disorder, but serves as the prototype for the idiopathic inflammatory myopathies. It is thought to be due to an autoimmune, mainly cytotoxic T-cell–mediated, attack on muscle, perhaps triggered by a virus. The disorder afflicts females twice as frequently as males and tends to occur in the middle age groups.

Clinical Picture and Diagnosis

The usual presenting picture is a proximal, usually symmetrical, painless progressive weakness that affects the shoulder and hip girdles and neck flexion. In rare cases, patients suffer asymmetrical weakness affecting one limb, a fulminant onset of weakness affecting respiratory muscles, or an acute rhabdomyolysis with myoglobinuria. Dysphagia, which is a poor prognostic sign, may be seen and stems from the involvement of upper esophageal striated muscle. Facial weakness and ptosis are not uncommonly seen, but extraocular muscles are usually spared. Head-lolling may occur because of neck extensor weakness (see Fig. 16-5). Myalgias, although uncommon, may be prominent in some patients. Raynaud's phenomenon and positive antinuclear factors appear in some cases, supporting the link between idiopathic PM/DM and the group of collagen diseases. Interstitial lung disease, cardiac involvement, and focal glomerulonephritis are other rarer features.

Diagnosis is supported by the presence of elevated CK and other muscle enzyme levels, although serum enzyme levels are normal in a small proportion of patients (Table 16-5). EMG typically shows small-amplitude, short-duration, polyphasic "myopathic" units; increased

Table 16-5. Diagnosis of Polymyositis/Dermatomyositis

Clinical findings
  Progressive weakness of:
    Proximal limbs
    Neck flexion/extension
    ± Respiratory, eyelid, facial, pharyngeal muscles
  ± Muscle pain and tenderness
  May be associated with collagen disease
  Dermatomyositis: heliotrope rash of eyelids, Gottron's papules over knuckles, periungual telangiectasias
  Occult malignancy in 15–25% of cases of adult dermatomyositis
Laboratory findings
  Elevated serum creatine kinase level in vast majority
  Electromyography: myopathic features, fibrillations, positive sharp waves, bizarre high-frequency potentials
Muscle biopsy
  Fiber necrosis, perivascular mononuclear infiltrates
  Childhood dermatomyositis: vasculitis, perifascicular atrophy
  May be normal (patchy lesions)

---

spontaneous activity (fibrillations) and evidence of increased muscle irritability upon needle insertion; positive sharp waves; and bizarre, high-frequency repetitive discharges. Muscle biopsy specimens, most commonly obtained from the quadriceps or deltoid, show evidence of fiber degeneration and regeneration affecting both fiber types, fiber necrosis, increased endomysial fibrosis, and round-cell infiltrates around vessels. In the childhood form of dermatomyositis, there is also evidence of vasculitis and often perifascicular atrophy (i.e., a degeneration of the muscle fibers at the periphery of the fascicle) due to ischemia. However, the biopsy findings may be normal because of the patchy inflammatory involvement of muscles.

Patients with dermatomyositis, besides the myopathy, exhibit certain characteristic skin changes. These include the "heliotrope" rash, which is a violaceous to erythematous edematous rash of the eyelids; Gottron's atrophic papules or plaques over the knuckles; periungual telangiectasias; a poikilodermatous rash over exposed areas; and a photosensitive "butterfly" rash similar to that seen with lupus erythematosus. Adult dermatomyositis may be associated with an underlying malignancy in 15 to 25 percent of the cases, especially in older patients. Patients with underlying malignancy may be more resistant to treatment.

Childhood dermatomyositis has several features that distinguish it from the usual PM/DM and appears to represent a form of systemic vasculitis in which there is a very early involvement of muscle capillaries mediated by the complement C5b–9 membranolytic attack complex. Unlike polymyositis, a primarily humeral mechanism is postulated. Bowel infarction and retinal vasculitis are other potential signs of a widespread vasculitis in this disorder. Calcinosis of subcutaneous tissues and muscles is another distinguishing feature, which may contribute to the overall disability. Children with the disease also have a greater tendency to suffer contractures, and toe-walking may be a presenting sign.

Cases of polymyositis due to the overlap syndrome are most frequently seen with mixed connective tissue disease and progressive systemic sclerosis (scleroderma). Joint involvement is a feature that should suggest an overlap syndrome in a patient with PM/DM. The prognosis in these cases is often determined by the extent of the underlying collagen disease.

Management and Prognosis

The overall prognosis in patients with PM/DM is variable and unpredictable, with exacerbations and remissions and a significant mortality. In many patients, the disease either burns itself out or remains at a smouldering level after the initial few years. Childhood dermatomyositis tends to run a more monophasic course than the other varieties. Treatment consists of an initial course of high-dose steroids (e.g., prednisone 60 to 100 mg per day) for at least 4 weeks, slowly tapering to an alternate-day regimen over the next 10 weeks so that the weakness can be treated. It is important to assess the weakness as objectively as possible (e.g., by timing how long one leg can be held at 45 degrees in the supine position) to gauge the efficacy of therapy. Serum enzyme levels typically return toward normal 4 to 6 weeks before clinical improvement commences and often increase several weeks before an exacerbation. Only after the patient's condition has been stable for several weeks should the gradual tapering of steroids (e.g., 5 mg per week) be attempted.

Many practitioners advocate keeping the patient on low-dose prednisone (e.g., 10–30 mg per day) for up to 2 years. Immunosuppressants such as azathioprine, cyclophosphamide, or methotrexate have been used for steroid-resistant cases or because of their steroid-sparing properties. Complications of steroid therapy, such as osteoporosis, growth retardation in children, and steroid myopathy, have led to the increasing popularity of alternative treatments, although none of these approaches has yet proved to arrest the disorder satisfactorily. Recently high-dose intravenous immunoglobulin treatment, although expensive, has shown promise. Physiotherapy, avoiding overly vigorous exercise, which could provoke muscle necrosis, and a high-protein diet are other common recommendations in the treatment of this disorder.

Other Types of Inflammatory Myositis

Inclusion-body myositis is a histologically distinct form of inflammatory myopathy that usually has a later onset and exhibits a more chronic course than polymyositis. Dysphagia is rarely seen, weakness is often pronounced distally as well as proximally, and serum muscle enzyme levels are only mildly elevated. Weakness is most prominent in finger and wrist flexors, foot extensors, and the quadriceps, leading to falls and absent patellar jerks. Muscle biopsy specimens exhibit marked fiber atrophy, fiber necrosis and regeneration, and a variable mononuclear infiltrate. Electron microscopy reveals the existence of intracytoplasmic vacuoles containing characteristic 14- to 18-nm filaments. This appears to be due to an attack of cytotoxic T lymphocytes on muscle, similar to what takes place in polymyositis. These patients do not respond to steroid therapy and no adequate treatment has been discovered.

Sarcoidosis may produce a slowly progressive proximal myopathy. Granulomatous changes are also seen in muscle biopsy specimens from patients with sarcoidosis in whom there is no symptomatic muscle involvement.

Eosinophilic polymyositis is a rare inflammatory myopathy that occurs as part of the idiopathic hypereosinophilic syndrome. The muscle weakness in affected patients may be quite severe and include the heart. There is a peripheral blood eosinophilia and the muscles are invaded by eosinophils. Several identifiable infectious agents have been implicated in the genesis of inflammatory myopathies, usually through the direct invasion of muscles, including influenza A and B, parainfluenza, coxsackie B5, ECHO 9, and herpesvirus. Some severe cases have been associated with acute rhabdomyolysis. Toxoplasmosis, Lyme disease, and HIV infection can also produce a polymyositis-like myopathy.

Drugs such as clofibrate, cimetidine, *d*-penicillamine, and azidothymidine (AZT) can produce a myopathy with inflammatory features, but only the latter two agents cause an endomysial inflammatory response similar to that found in idiopathic polymyositis. Ragged red fibers are also found in AZT-induced myositis.

METABOLIC MYOPATHIES

An increasing number of defined hereditary and acquired metabolic abnormalities of muscle are being characterized (Table 16-6). These disorders usually present as a slowly progressive weakness mimicking muscular dystrophy, severe congenital weakness (floppy infant syndrome) with short survival, or recurrent bouts of exercise-related muscle cramps with myoglobinuria. Some of these disorders exhibit distinct histological and histochemical features on muscle biopsy specimens and may involve other organs besides muscle, including the brain.

Carbohydrate Metabolism Disorders

A variety of enzymatic deficiencies affecting the breakdown of glycogen and glycolysis have been described. **McArdle's disease,** which is a muscle phosphorylase deficiency that is inherited as an autosomal recessive trait, is the proto-

Table 16-6. Acquired Endocrine, Metabolic, and Drug-induced Myopathies

Endocrine
  Hypothyroidism
  Hyperthyroidism
  Hyperparathyroidism
  Osteomalacia
  Cushing's disease
  Acromegaly
Electrolyte disturbances
  Hypokalemia
  Hyperkalemia
  Hypophosphatemia
  Hypomagnesemia
Toxic
  Alcohol
  Drugs
    Chloroquine
    Clofibrate
    Lovastatin
    Steroids
    Emetine
    Heroin
    Cimetidine
    Drugs causing hypokalemia
    Cytotoxic agents
    Azidothymidine
    Ipecac

type of this group of disorders. Normally muscle phosphorylase cleaves terminal 1,4–linked glucose units of glycogen to produce glucose-1-phosphate. Muscle energy metabolism which relies mainly on glycolysis is impaired. The clinical manifestations are often delayed until adolescence when painful muscle cramps and at times myoglobinuria may become apparent with exercise. The disorder may also present as an adult-onset progressive generalized weakness. The cramps (contractures) are electrically silent on EMGs. Muscle biopsy specimens show the existence of subsarcolemmal vacuoles containing glycogen.

The ischemic forearm exercise test is used to aid in diagnosis. In a standard task, a blood pressure cuff is placed around the patient's upper arm and venous blood samples are obtained at 0, 2, 5, 10, and 20 minutes after exercise to determine the lactate levels. There is no increase in the lactate levels in patients with the disease. Should pain occur before the standard 2 minutes is reached, the test must be aborted because muscle necrosis can occur. Many patients are unable to complete more than 1 minute of ischemic exercise without experiencing painful contractures. Muscle biopsy specimens from affected patients usually show no histochemical reaction for phosphorylase, but are not usually helpful in cases of partial enzyme deficiency. P^{31}-MRS can be used to confirm the diagnosis when the findings from muscle biopsy are nondiagnostic. The avoidance of strenuous exercise is the most important aspect of management, but recently a high-protein diet has been suggested to improve endurance.

Phosphofructokinase deficiency, an autosomal recessive disorder that involves defective glycolysis, bears many clinical similarities to McArdle's.

Acid maltase deficiency is a lysosomal storage disease that involves the accumulation of excess glycogen in muscles. It includes an infantile form (Pompe's), which is fatal in the first year due to cardiac involvement, a childhood onset form with a much slower progression of muscle weakness, and an adult form. The adult form presents in the third or fourth decade and may resemble limb-girdle dystrophy.

Mitochondrial Myopathies

A bewildering variety of rare, and sometimes clinically disparate, syndromes that involve abnormal mitochondrial function are increasingly being recognized. When both cerebral function and muscle are involved, the disorder is called a *mitochondrial encephalomyopathy*. In some, histological examination of muscle tissue using a modification of the Gomori's trichrome stain shows the existence of abnormal mitochondria—ragged red fibers. However, these are not found in every case and are not specific to the mitochondrial encephalomyopathies. In many of these disorders, the mitochondria are abnormal on electron microscopic studies, displaying abnormal shapes, an abnormal internal structure, or various inclusions. Maternal inheritance is common in these illnesses, as mitochondrial DNA is inherited through the mother. A number of specific defects in the respiratory chain enzyme complex, which resides on the inner surface of the mitochondrial membrane, have been identified in these disorders. The fact that only certain cell lines may carry the genetic defect may explain the marked clinical heterogeneity of these disorders.

Three of the better-defined clinical syndromes in this category are the Kearns-Sayre syndrome (which is discussed in Chapter 11), the myoclonus epilepsy with ragged red fibers syndrome (MERRF), and the mitochondrial myopathy, encephalopathy, lactic acidosis, and strokelike episodes syndrome (MELAS).

MELAS involves muscle and brain and is caused by a point mutation in mitochondrial DNA leading to a complex I deficiency in the electron transport chain. The disease may appear in children or adults, and includes a variable combination of signs and symptoms, including classic migraine-like episodes, occipital infarcts, seizures (e.g., epilepsy partialis continua), cortical blindness, deafness, dementia, muscle weakness, short stature, cardiomyopathy, ragged red fibers on muscle biopsy specimens, and episodes of lactic acidosis. The strokelike episodes are likely related to the increased number of abnormal mitochondria in the smooth muscle cells around small and medium-sized brain arteries. Diagnosis is based on the clinical features, muscle biopsy findings, elevated lactate levels following exercise (not invariably present), MRS, and mitochondrial enzyme assays.

MERRF is due to a different point mutation of mitochondrial DNA but its features broadly overlap those of MELAS. Reduced cytochrome oxidase may be the main enzyme affected. Action myoclonus, generalized tonic-clonic or myoclonic seizures, cerebellar ataxia, dementia, neurosensory hearing loss, short stature, muscle weakness, ragged red fibers, optic atrophy, and lipomas are some of the features of this disorder. The age of onset and clinical features are extremely variable.

Other rare abnormalities of muscle intramitochondrial energy metabolism involving defects either in oxidation and phosphorylation coupling or in the respiratory chain have also been described. One of the better-studied members of this group of disorders is cytochrome C oxidase deficiency, which has been implicated in various childhood encephalomyopathies, including Menkes' disease (trichopoliodystrophy), Leigh disease (subacute necrotizing encephalomyelopathy), and Alpers' disease (progressive sclerosing poliodystrophy). Leigh disease is discussed further in Chapter 27. Leber's hereditary optic atrophy is another member of this group of disorders, but does not produce a myopathy (see Chapter 11).

Defects in the utilization of long-chain fatty acids as a substrate for muscle have now been well described. In **carnitine palmitoyl transferase deficiency,** an autosomal recessive disorder mainly affecting males, fasting or exercise leads to myoglobinuria. Affected patients benefit from a frequent dietary intake of carbohydrate. **Muscle carnitine deficiency,** a probable autosomal recessive disorder, causes a progressive and usually early-onset proximal myopathy with lipid droplet accumulation in muscles. Some success has been obtained with oral carnitine or steroid treatment. **Systemic carnitine deficiency** is a much more severe disorder that presents mainly as recurrent attacks of hepatic encephalopathy in childhood.

Periodic Paralysis

Both hypo- and hyperkalemic forms of familial (usually autosomal dominant) periodic paralysis have been documented. The former is usually more severe, and attacks of total weakness (sparing the extraocular muscles) may last for up to 24 hours. Respiratory muscles may also be affected. The age of onset is usually earlier in the hyperkalemic form, beginning early in the first decade. Myotonic phenomena are common in the hyperkalemic form and there may be an overlap with paramyotonia congenita. In both forms, attacks tend to occur upon awakening and during rest following exercise. High carbohydrate or sodium intake may precipitate an attack in patients with the hypokalemic form, while fasting may provoke an attack in patients with the hyperkalemic form. During the acute attack, the serum potassium level may decrease enough to precipitate cardiac arrhythmias in the hypokalemic variety. To provoke attacks for diagnostic purposes, glucose and insulin can be administered to produce hypokalemia or oral potassium taken to elevate serum potassium levels.

The weakness encountered in hypokalemic periodic paralysis is treated by the oral administration of potassium. In the hyperkalemic form, the serum potassium level may actually be normal during an attack. Acetazolamide may prevent attacks in both forms, but thiazides may be preferable and glucose administration may abort an attack in the hyperkalemic variety. A fixed myopathic weakness may eventually develop in patients with periodic paralysis. Muscle biopsy specimens obtained during an attack show vacuoles containing glycogen. This finding tends to persist when a fixed myopathy occurs.

Another form of hypokalemic periodic paralysis, affecting mainly Oriental males, occurs in the presence of thyrotoxicosis. Many other acquired disorders that cause hypokalemia or hyperkalemia may lead to episodic weakness.

Acquired Metabolic and Toxic Myopathies

Myopathic weakness is part of the clinical picture in a variety of acquired metabolic, endocrine, and toxic conditions (see Table 16-6).

HISTOLOGICALLY DISTINCT CONGENITAL MYOPATHIES

Although the histologically distinct congenital myopathies usually present in the neonatal period or early infancy as congenital hypotonia (floppy infant syndrome), the prognosis is much more benign than that in patients with many other conditions affecting the central nervous system, anterior horn cells, or peripheral nerves, which cause a similar clinical picture. Most of these syndromes are nonfamilial, although both dominant and recessive inheritance patterns occur. Skeletal deformities and a high-arched palate are sometimes associated findings, and facial and neck flexion weakness as well as ptosis is common. The best-defined of these disorders are nemaline myopathy, central core disease, centronuclear myopathy, and congenital fiber–type disproportion, although several others have been reported. These conditions are diagnosed on the basis of distinct histological features on muscle biopsy specimens. Although they are rare, precise diagnosis is essential because most but not all cases carry a relatively benign prognosis.

BIBLIOGRAPHY

Armstrong, R. M., and Appel, S. H. Neuromuscular Disorders. In S. H. Appel (editor). *Current Neurology*. New York: Wiley, 1982, Vol. 4, Pp. 1–16.

Armstrong, R. M., and Armstrong, D. L. Congenital and Mitochondrial Myopathies. In S. H. Appel (editor). *Current Neurology*. New York: Wiley, 1984, Vol. 5, Pp. 163–200.

Auger, R. G., et al. Hereditary form of sustained muscle activity of peripheral nerve origin causing generalized myokymia and muscle stiffness. *Ann. Neurol.* 15:13–21, 1984.

Bohan, A., and Peter, J. B. Polymyositis and dermatomyositis: Parts I and II. *N. Engl. J. Med.* 292:344–347;403–407, 1975.

Braun, S. R., et al. Intermittent negative pressure ventilation in the treatment of respiratory failure in progressive neuromuscular disease. *Neurology* 37:1874–1875, 1987.

Brooke, M. H. *A Clinician's View of Neuro-muscular Disease,* 2nd ed. Baltimore: Williams & Wilkins, 1986.

Burke, R. E., and Tsairis, P. The correlation of the physiological properties with histochemical characteristics in single motor units. *Ann. NY Acad. Sci.* 228:145–159, 1974.

Callen, J. P. Dermatomyositis. *Int. J. Dermatol.* 18:423–433, 1979.

Carpenter, S., and Karpati, G. *Pathology of Skeletal Muscle.* New York: Churchill Livingstone, 1984.

Carroll, J. E., and Brooke, M. H. Muscle. In A. L. Pearlman and R. C. Collins (editors). *Neurological Pathophysiology,* 3rd ed. New York: Oxford University Press, 1984, Pp. 56–73.

Chad, D., Munsat, T. L., and Adelman, L. S. Diseases of Muscle. In R. N. Rosenberg (editor). *The Clinical Neurosciences.* New York: Churchill Livingstone, 1983, Vol. 1, Pp. 569–608.

Clemens, P. R., and Caskey CT. Duchenne muscular dystrophy. In S. H. Appel (editor). *Current Neurology.* St. Louis: Mosby–Year Book, 1992, Vol. 12, Pp. 1–22.

Dalakas, M. C. Polymyositis, dermatomyositis, and inclusion-body myositis. *N. Engl. J. Med.* 325:1487–1498, 1992.

Danon, M. J., et al. Inclusion body myositis. A corticosteroid-resistant idiopathic inflammatory myopathy. *Arch. Neurol.* 39:760–764, 1982.

DiMauro, S., et al. Mitochondrial encephalo-myopathies. *Neurol. Clin.* 8:483–506, 1990.

Downey, G. P., et al. Neuroleptic malignant syndrome. Patient with unique clinical and physiologic features. *Am. J. Med.* 77:338–340, 1984.

Dubowitz, V. Carrier detection and genetic counselling in Duchenne dystrophy. *Dev. Med. Child. Neurol.* 17:352–356, 1975.

Dubowitz, V., and Brooke, M. H. *Muscle Biopsy: A Modern Approach.* Philadelphia: Saunders, 1973.

Emery, A. E. H. Emery-Dreifuss muscular dystrophy and other related disorders. *Br. Med. Bull.* 45:772–787, 1989.

Furukawa, T., and Peter, J. B. The muscular dystrophies and related disorders. I. The muscular dystrophies. *JAMA* 239:1537–1542, 1978.

Furukawa, T., and Peter, J. B. The muscular dystrophies and related disorders. II. Diseases simulating muscular dystrophies. *JAMA* 239:1654–1659, 1978.

Gardner-Medwin, D. Clinical features and classification of the muscular dystrophies. *Br. Med. Bull.* 36:109–115, 1980.

Griggs, R. C., and Karpati, G. The pathogenesis of dermatomyositis. *Arch. Neurol.* 48:21–22, 1991.

Griggs, R. C., and Moxley, R. T. (editor). Metabolic myopathies. *Semin. Neurol.* 3:225–318, 1983.

Gutmann, D. H., and Fischbeck, K. H. Molecular biology of Duchenne and Becker's muscular dystrophy: clinical applications. *Ann. Neurol.* 26:189–194, 1989.

Harding, A. E., and Holt, I. J. Mitochondrial myopathies. *Br. Med. Bull.* 45:760–771, 1989.

Harper, P. S. *Myotonic Dystrophy.* Philadelphia: Saunders, 1979.

Hodgson, S. V., and Bobrow, M. Carrier detection and prenatal diagnosis in Duchenne and Becker muscular dystrophy. *Br. Med. Bull.* 45:719–744, 1989.

Hoffman, E. P., et al. Improved diagnosis of Becker muscular dystrophy by dystrophin testing. *Neurology* 39:1011–1017, 1989.

Holden, D. J., Brownell, A. K. W., and Fritzler, M. J. Clinical and serologic features of patients with polymyositis and dermatomyositis. *Can. Med. Assoc. J.* 132:649–653, 1985.

Holt, I. J., et al. Mitochondrial myopathies: clinical and biochemical features of 30 patients with major deletions of muscle mitochondrial DNA. *Arch. Neurol.* 26:699–708, 1989.

Jog, M. S. Lambert, C. D., and Lang, A. E. Stiff-person syndrome. *Can. J. Neurol. Sci.* 19:383–388, 1992.

Karpati, G. Recent developments in the biology of dystrophin and related molecules. *Curr. Opin. Neurol. Neurosurg.* 5:615–621, 1992.

Kissel, J. T., et al. The relationship of complement-mediated microvasculopathy to the histologic features and clinical duration of disease in dermatomyositis. *Arch. Neurol.* 48:26–30, 1991.

Kunkel, L. M., and Hoffman, E. P. Duchenne/ Becker muscular dystrophy: a short overview of the gene, the protein, and current diagnostics. *Br. Med. Bull.* 45:630–643, 1989.

Lane, R. J. M., and Mastaglia, F. L. Drug-induced myopathies in man. *Lancet* 2:562–566, 1978.

Layzer, R. B. McArdle's disease in the 1980's (editorial). *N. Engl. J. Med.* 312:370–371, 1985.

Lorish, T. R., Thorsteinsson, G., and Howard, F. M., Jr. Stiff-man syndrome updated. *Mayo Clin. Proc.* 64:629–634, 1989.

Mastaglia, F. L., and Ojeda, V. J. Inflammatory myopathies. Parts I and II. *Ann. Neurol.* 17:215–227;317–323, 1985.

Moorman, J. R., et al. Cardiac involvement in myotonic muscular dystrophy. *Medicine* 64:371–387, 1985.

Morgan-Hughes, J. A., et al. Mitochondrial encephalomyopathies. Biochemical studies in two cases revealing defects in the respiratory chain. *Brain* 105:553–582, 1982.

Munsat, T. Creatine phosphokinase alterations in neuromuscular diseases. *Isr. J. Med. Sci.* 13:93–97, 1977.

Nonaka, I. Mitochondrial diseases. *Curr. Opin. Neurol. Neurosurg.* 5:622–632, 1992.

Pascuzzi, R. M. (editor). Stiff muscle syndrome. *Semin. Neurol.* 11:197–294, 1991.

Plotz, P. H. (moderator). Current concepts in the idiopathic inflammatory myopathies: polymyositis, dermatomyositis and related disorders. *Ann. Intern. Med.* 111:143–157, 1989.

Reardon, W., and Harper, P. S. Advances in myotonic dystrophy: a clinical and genetic perspective. *Curr. Opin. Neurol. Neurosurg.* 5:605–609, 1992.

Riggs, J. E. (editor). Muscle disease. *Neurol. Clin.* 6:429–648, 1988.

Rowland, L. Myoglobinuria, 1984. *Can. J. Neurol. Sci.* 11:1–13, 1984.

Rowland, L. Cramps, spasms and muscle stiffness. *Rev. Neurol.* (Paris) 141:261–273, 1985.

Sigurgeirsson, B., et al. Risk of cancer in patients with dermatomyositis or polymyositis: a population-based study. *N. Engl. J. Med.* 326:363–367, 1992.

Simpson, J. A. Muscle. In M. Critchley, J. O'Leary, and B. Jennett (editors). *Scientific Foundations of Neurology,* Philadelphia: Davis, 1972, Pp. 44–58.

Smith, P. E. M., et al. Practical problems in the respiratory care of patients with muscular dystrophy. *N. Engl. J. Med.* 316:1197–1204, 1987.

Warmolts, J. R. Electrodiagnosis in neuromuscular disorders. *Ann. Intern. Med.* 95:599–608, 1981.

Woodward, J. B., and Ringel, S. P. Neuromuscular diseases. In W. J. Weiner, C. G. Goetz (editors). *Neurology for the Non-Neurologist.* Philadelphia: Harper & Row, 1981, Pp. 284–317.

Zeviani, M., et al. Deletions of mitochondrial DNA in Kearns-Sayre syndrome. *Neurology* 38:1339–1346, 1988.

Weakness: Myasthenia Gravis and Other Disorders of the Neuromuscular Junction

MYASTHENIA GRAVIS

Myasthenia gravis is the prototype and most common of the disorders affecting neuromuscular transmission. Myasthenia gravis exhibits a spectrum of clinical manifestations, but all cases share the common feature of muscle fatigability, either generalized or localized. Thanks to recent advances in our understanding of the pathogenesis of this disorder, effective treatment is now available in most cases.

Pathophysiology and Etiology

Myasthenia gravis is an autoimmune disorder in which antibodies to the acetylcholine (ACh) receptor protein at the postsynaptic site interfere with neuromuscular transmission and eventually cause an alteration in the morphological characteristics of the subsynaptic region with simplification of membranous infoldings. The antibodies bind to the alpha subunit of the receptor, which changes the configuration of the receptor and decreases the likelihood of acetylcholine binding.

Various animal models duplicating many of the clinical and electrical features of myasthenia gravis have been developed. A snake toxin, alpha-bungarotoxin, can bind selectively to ACh receptors, thus allowing both the isolation and quantification of the receptors. Using this technique, it has been possible to show that fewer ACh receptor sites are available in myasthenic muscle than in normals. Administration of this substance or alpha-cobra toxin to animals (e.g., rats) has also reproduced a good model of myasthenia gravis. When antibodies to purified eel ACh receptor protein are produced in rabbits, a syndrome almost identical to myasthenia gravis results. Immunofluorescent techniques have been used to localize the antibodies to the postsynaptic ACh receptor.

The major antibody measured for clinical purposes is the ACh receptor binding antibody. Blocking or modulating antibodies, or both, exist in a small percentage of patients whose levels of binding antibody are not elevated. In humans, circulating anti–ACh receptor IgG antibodies are found in 90 percent of patients with generalized myasthenia gravis but are often not found in patients with pure ocular myasthenia gravis. The antibody level does not correlate well with the severity or activity of the disease, but sequential studies of antibody levels are useful for monitoring the response to therapy. Sero-negative patients generally respond less well to therapy than do those with detectable antibodies.

Other features of myasthenia gravis that suggest an autoimmune pathogenesis have been known for some time. About 15 percent of patients with myasthenia gravis have an underlying thymoma. Most other patients exhibit thymic hyperplasia in the form of germinal centers located in the medulla of the thymus. Because thymic myoid cells and muscle share certain common antigens (including ACh receptor antigens), the abnormal autoimmune response may originate from a breakdown of immune tolerance at the thymic level. An autoimmune or viral "thymitis" has therefore been postulated as an initiating event in myasthenia gravis. The improvement that often follows thymectomy lends further support to the role of the thymus gland in the pathogenesis of myasthenia gravis.

There is also an abnormally high incidence (and familial incidence) of other autoimmune diseases in patients with myasthenia gravis, including Hashimoto's thyroiditis, pernicious anemia, and collagen vascular diseases. Anti–muscle antibodies that bind to the cross striations are also found in the sera of 25 percent of patients with myasthenia gravis (75% of patients with thymoma).

HLA typing has revealed some association between generalized myasthenia and HLA-B8 and DRW3. Penicillamine, which is used to treat rheumatoid arthritis, may produce a fairly typical, although reversible, myasthenia gravis syndrome by affecting the ACh receptor.

Clinical Picture and Diagnosis

Myasthenia gravis affects all age groups, but there is a peak incidence in females in the second and third decades and in males in the sixth and seventh decades. Females are affected twice as often as males. The onset is usually insidious, with fluctuating weakness that tends to be worse at the end of the day or following exercise. Most commonly the bulbar muscles are involved early, with diplopia, ptosis and/or difficulty chewing, and dysphagia constituting the most common presenting symptoms. As the disease advances, limb and neck muscles and eventually respiratory muscles become involved. In occasional cases, there is an acute fulminant onset with the rapid development of respiratory failure.

Weakness may be provoked or worsened by specific factors such as intercurrent infection, hypokalemia, hypocalcemia, or the administration of drugs affecting neuromuscular transmission, such as quinine or quinidine, beta-blockers, procainamide, phenytoin, chlorpromazine, and antibodies (streptomycin, neomycin, colistin, kanamycin, gentamicin, polymyxins, tobramycin, and amikacin). Other nonspecific exacerbating factors include surgery and pregnancy.

On examination, a degree of fixed weakness may be detected along with obvious fatigability following the sustained use of the involved muscles. A useful test is to have the patient maintain maximum up-gaze for a minute or more, which often produces objective worsening of the ptosis. The extraocular muscle weakness does not correspond to the involvement of a particular cranial nerve and pupils are spared. Weakness of eye closure and other facial muscles as well as neck flexion is also a common finding. A lid-twitch sign may be seen and elicited by having the patient maintain down-gaze then look upward quickly. If present, the upper lid will elevate and then immediately descend, appearing to twitch. Deep tendon reflexes are preserved and at times even hyperactive.

The differential diagnosis includes other disorders that present with diplopia (at times intermittent), such as thyroid ophthalmopathy and lesions of the brainstem; the myasthenic syndrome of Eaton-Lambert (see later discussion), motor neuron disease (especially progressive bulbar palsy), which may exhibit certain "myasthenic features," including some response to anticholinesterase agents (see later discussion);

oculopharyngeal dystrophy; and neurasthenia, which is a subjective sense of fatigability of psychogenic origin. This last disorder may be particularly difficult to differentiate from early cases of myasthenia gravis.

The diagnosis of myasthenia gravis is based on the clinical picture, electrodiagnostic features, and the patient's response to anticholinesterase agents (Table 17-1). When objective signs of weakness, such as ptosis, limb weakness, low voice volume, or diminished vital capacity, are present, a Tensilon (edrophonium) test can be performed to establish the diagnosis (Fig. 17-1). In this test, the patient is first given an intravenous control injection of saline or calcium chloride, which may provoke some subjective sensation of flushing. Following this, 2 mg of Tensilon is administered and, if no undue hypotension or hypersensitivity is observed, 8 mg is then given over 1 minute. If objectively the weakness abates within the next 1 or 2 minutes, this constitutes a positive result and a diagnosis of myasthenia gravis is highly likely. Occasional patients respond better to 1.5 mg of prostigmine given intramuscularly (along with 0.5 mg of atropine to counter the muscarinic side effects). The more prolonged duration of action allows a longer assessment time of the response, which is particularly useful in children. In some patients, especially those who

Table 17-1. Diagnostic Features of Myasthenia Gravis

Clinical findings
    Muscle fatigability (especially extraocular, levator palpebrae, and bulbar)
    Lid-twitch sign
    Normal deep tendon reflexes and sensory findings
    Concurrent autoimmune disease
Laboratory findings
    Positive edrophonium (Tensilon) or neostigmine test
    Electromyography
        Decremental response to supramaximal repetitive stimulation reversed by edrophonium
        Posttetanic potentiation and exhaustion
        Increased jitter on single-fiber recordings
    Acetylcholine receptor antibodies
    Chest x-ray study or mediastinal CT scan (thymoma in 15%)
    Edrophonium tonometry

are already on anticholinesterase agents, certain muscles may improve in strength following Tensilon administration, but others may weaken. Side effects due to cholinergic excess, such as muscle twitching, salivation, and bradycardia, are common and may require the administration of atropine.

Electrical nerve stimulation studies are useful for demonstrating the characteristic electrical phenomena of myasthenia gravis, but the procedure is quite painful. The ulnar nerve is often chosen as the site for stimulation, with recording done over the abductor digiti minimi, and trains of supramaximal stimuli are given at frequencies ranging from 2 to 50 Hz. At low rates of stimulation, the amplitude of the muscle action potential in myasthenics declines by at least 12 percent by the third or fourth stimulus, with some mild subsequent recovery (Fig. 17-2). Exercise for 1 to 2 minutes may be necessary to bring out this decremental response. The phenomena of posttetanic potentiation, transient augmentation of muscle potential amplitude following a conditioning tetanus, and posttetanic exhaustion, which is an exaggeration in the decrement 2 to 4 minutes following a tetanus, are all characteristic findings. These electrical phenomena are usually partially reversible by Tensilon administration.

Increased "jitter" can be demonstrated on single-fiber electromyographic studies, reflecting a greater than normal variability in delay of neuromuscular transmission from fiber to fiber. The regional curare test is used in patients with apparently isolated ocular myasthenia to uncover the presence of subclinical spinal muscular involvement. In this test, a tourniquet is placed on the patient's arm and a low dose of curare is administered intravenously. This dose is too small to produce noticeable effects in normal subjects but may provoke weakness and a decremental electrical response in the hand muscles of myasthenics.

All patients with myasthenia gravis should have their thyroid function evaluated and undergo chest x-ray study (anteroposterior and oblique views), tomography, or computed tomography of the mediastinum to search for a thymoma. Measurement of the serum anti–ACh receptor antibody levels may also aid

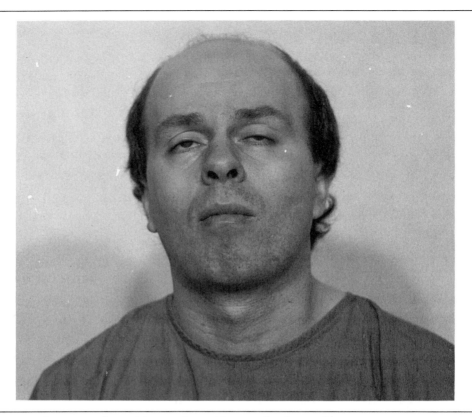

Fig. 17-1. *Tensilon test performed in a patient with generalized myasthenia gravis. The patient is requested to look up and smile. (A) Before intravenous administration of 10 mg of Tensilon.*

in confirming diagnosis. Despite extensive testing, the diagnosis may be uncertain in some patients. Trial treatment with anticholinesterase agents may help clarify the picture in these patients.

Management and Prognosis

The long-term prognosis in patients with myasthenia gravis is variable but is unfavorable in about 10 percent. In some individuals the disease seems to burn itself out, but in others, the course is unrelenting and leads to significant disability and recurrent bouts of life-threatening bulbar and respiratory weakness, often associated with intercurrent illness. The course appears to be particularly treacherous in elderly males. However, with modern management and intensive care facilities, death from the disease itself is extremely rare.

Patients with pure ocular myasthenia may require nothing more than anticholinesterase treatment or intermittent eye-patching to eliminate the bothersome diplopia, with prednisone reserved for the more severe cases. However, nearly 90 percent of the cases with ocular myasthenia become generalized within 3 to 4 years.

In most cases, anticholinesterase agents constitute the initial treatment (Table 17-2). They act by prolonging the action of ACh at the synapse. Pyridostigmine (60 mg, 1–3 tablets every 4–6 hours) and a long-acting preparation (180 mg) taken at bedtime are commonly prescribed. Supplemental doses of the shorter-acting preparation, neostigmine (15 mg), can be taken before excessive physical activity is performed or before meals. Symptoms of muscarinic cholinergic excess, such as increased bronchial secretions, bronchospasm, diarrhea, miosis, ab-

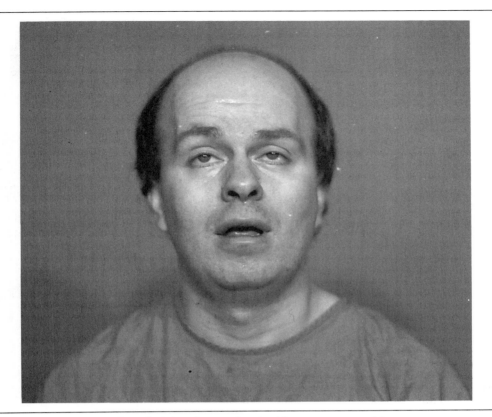

Fig. 17-1. *(B) One minute after administration, patient is able to open eyes wider and retract mouth better.*

dominal cramps, bradycardia, and nicotinic effects of increased weakness, may limit therapy. Loperamide is a useful anticholinergic agent that can counteract the diarrhea. The absorption of anticholinesterase compounds is somewhat variable and bioavailability is low.

In many, especially younger, patients, early thymectomy via the suprasternal or sternal-splitting approach is advocated. The latter approach is often preferred because it offers a better chance of identifying and removing all thymic tissue. Thymectomy likely works in part by reducing the number of cells producing the ACh receptor antibody. In addition, antigenic material that is triggering the abnormal immune response may be removed.

About 80 percent of the patients show improvement postoperatively, although sometimes response is delayed for up to 2 or more years. In some unresponsive cases, repeat oper-ation to search for residual or ectopic thymic tissue is worthwhile. Thymectomy appears to work best in young women with mild disease and high antibody titers, especially if done early in the illness.

Before thymectomy, patients are taken off anticholinesterase agent and, if necessary, placed on respiratory support, which is often continued for several days postoperatively depending on the severity of the disease. Anticholinesterases are restarted 24 hours postoperatively at one half the previous dose.

All patients with thymoma should undergo thymectomy. In uncommon cases in which the tumor is malignant, cobalt irradiation is carried out postoperatively. Occasionally thymomas may arise from an ectopic cervical thymus and present as a mass in the neck.

Prednisone is very effective in 80 to 90 percent of the patients with severe involvement.

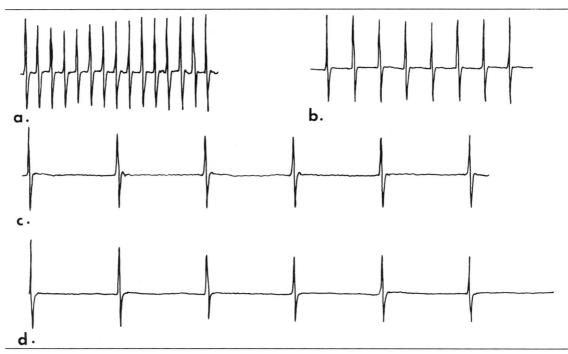

Fig. 17-2. *Supramaximal stimulation of ulnar nerve at the wrist, recorded over the hypothenar eminence in a 60-year-old woman with mild, treated myasthenia gravis. (A) Stimulation at 20/sec produces an 18 percent decrement in the amplitude of the response at the fourth stimulus. (B) Stimulation at 10/sec produces a 15 percent decrement. (C) Stimulation at 3/sec produces a 16 percent decrement, but, at 2 minutes after exercise (D), a 20 percent decrement.*

Table 17-2. Treatment of Myasthenia Gravis

Anticholinesterases
    Pyridostigmine
    Pyridostigmine (slow-release form)
    Neostigmine
Prednisone
Immunosuppressants
Plasmapheresis
Thymectomy
Intravenous gamma globulin

In the initial phases of treatment, the weakness may worsen transiently, requiring temporary respiratory support, but a gradual increase in the prednisone dosage may prevent this complication. Frequently treatment must be maintained for several months, leading to a high incidence of steroid-related side effects such as gastrointestinal bleeding, cushingoid appear-ance, hypertension, diabetes mellitus, osteoporosis with vertebral fractures, aseptic necrosis of the hip, and steroid-induced myopathy. For this reason, alternate-day therapy is often instituted after a few months, once the patient's condition is stabilized. Immunosuppressants such as azathioprine and cyclophosphamide are also being used increasingly to take advantage of their steroid-sparing effects. Severe blood dyscrasias and hepatotoxicity are potential rare side effects of azathioprine use.

Another mode of treatment that has been used as a temporary measure for managing acute exacerbations or in preparation for thymectomy is plasmapheresis or plasma exchange. The exact mechanism responsible for its efficacy is unknown, since improvement does not correlate very well with a reduction in the anti–ACh receptor antibody titers. The role of intermittent courses of plasmapheresis in the long-term management is still unknown but, in any event, often proves impractical. Recently, a 5-day course of high-dose immunoglobulin given intravenously has been reported to provide therapeutic benefit, at least in the short term.

Other nonspecific measures consist of having patients avoid certain substances and drugs (mentioned previously) that would further impair neuromuscular transmission, treating respiratory infections aggressively, and instituting chest physiotherapy when respiratory complications intervene.

Patients who present in "crisis" with acutely reduced respiratory reserve and generalized weakness represent worsening of myasthenia in the vast majority of cases. In rare cases, an excessive anticholinesterase dosage can precipitate a cholinergic crisis with increased weakness. The most prudent way of managing such a crisis initially is to institute respiratory support and stop anticholinesterase agents. Rapid recovery of strength in the presence of initial systemic signs of acetylcholine excess (e.g., muscle twitching, bradycardia, myosis, and sweating) suggests that the problem was a cholinergic crisis.

NEONATAL AND CONGENITAL MYASTHENIA

The occurrence of transient neonatal myasthenia in the offspring of 12 to 16 percent of mothers with myasthenia gravis is likely due to the transplacental transfer of maternal circulating anti–ACh receptor antibody, which is not present in every case, however. Affected infants exhibit muscle weakness, ptosis, poor cry and suck, and may require the temporary administration of anticholinesterase agents. The syndrome disappears within 6 weeks, at which time anti–ACh receptor antibodies are no longer detectable.

Rare familial or sporadic forms of congenital myasthenia that do not have an immunological basis have recently been described. The pathogenesis in these patients involves a lack of acetylcholinesterase or specific deficits in the interaction of acetylcholine with its receptor.

EATON-LAMBERT "MYASTHENIC" SYNDROME

The Eaton-Lambert syndrome has a strong male predominance, a later mean age of onset than myasthenia gravis, and is associated with underlying oat-cell carcinoma of the lung in 70 percent of the cases (Table 17-3; see Chapter 29). The proximal lower extremities are particularly affected, with sparing of the bulbar and ocular muscles. The deep tendon reflexes are depressed, patients experience autonomic symptoms such as dry mouth, and the CSF protein level is usually elevated. The syndrome may occur in conjunction with other remote effects of the carcinoma on the nervous system, such as cerebellar degeneration. The administration of Tensilon may bring about a transient improvement in strength but the response to anticholinesterases is usually only partial.

An unusual feature of the disease is that patients show initial fatigability but their strength improves with continuing effort, which can also be demonstrated electrically. The defect responsible is presynaptic and involves the impairment of acetylcholine release due to the binding of antibodies to voltage-dependent calcium channels. There is a proliferation of postsynaptic infoldings at the muscle endplate, unlike the simplification seen with myasthenia gravis. It has recently been suggested that antibody which is cross-reacting with tumor antigen binds to the presynaptic site. Treatment of the underlying carcinoma may yield some improvement. Specific agents that enhance presynaptic acetylcholine release such as guanidine have also been tried, but with limited success.

BOTULISM

Clostridium botulinum, an anaerobic spore-forming bacteria, may proliferate and produce its deadly toxin in improperly canned foods. To kill the spores, food must be heated in a pressure cooker to 120°C. The organism also occasionally grows in contaminated wounds or the gastrointestinal tract (especially in infants). In a recent survey of food-borne botulism in adults,

Table 17-3. Characteristics of Eaton-Lambert "Myasthenic" Syndrome Versus Myasthenia Gravis

Characteristics	Eaton-Lambert syndrome	Myasthenia gravis
Age of onset (yr)	Mean, 55	Mean, 20; all ages
Male–female	10:1	1:2 (1:4.5, adolescents)
Muscles affected	Proximal and distal limb >> bulbar	Extraocular and bulbar >> limbs
Effect of exercise once weakness occurs	Improvement in strength	Increasing weakness
Remissions	No	Yes
Deep tendon reflexes	Diminished	Normal
Autonomic features (e.g., dry mouth)	Yes	No
Associated tumor	Oat-cell carcinoma of lung (70%)	Thymoma (15%)
Association with other nonmetastatic neurological syndromes	Yes	No
Circulating antibodies	To presynaptic calcium channels	Acetylcholine receptor
Electromyography	Decremental response at stimuli <10/sec; incremental response at stimuli >10/sec	Decremental response, posttetanic exhaustion
Response to anticholinesterases	Minimal	Yes
Defect	Presynaptic impairment of acetylcholine release	Postsynaptic acetylcholine receptor defect

most cases were found to be due to the consumption of raw, "parboiled," or fermented meats from marine animals. Types A, B, E, and G are all known to cause human botulism, but types A and B are the most common.

The toxin impairs presynaptic ACh release by affecting the calcium channels and, once taken in, causes the acute onset of diplopia and bulbar weakness, dry mouth, and gastrointestinal upset as well as respiratory paralysis that can last for months. Patients typically have dilated, fixed pupils, which indicates autonomic involvement.

Symptoms usually appear 12 to 72 hours after the ingestion of the contaminated food, and the more rapid the onset, the worse the prognosis. Progression may occur in the first 3 to 4 weeks after onset. Detection of the toxin in food and body fluids establishes the diagnosis.

Botulin trivalent antitoxin (A, B, and E) is used initially in the management, although it only acts on circulating antitoxin. Cathartics and enemas, if used early enough, may help remove the toxin from the gut. Guanidine hydrochloride may be tried to augment the pre-synaptic release of ACh. Antibiotics (penicillin) may kill live organisms such as those in contaminated wounds, but are contraindicated in infants with botulism because the toxin can be released into the gastrointestinal tract by the dead organisms. Treatment is generally supportive and includes prolonged tracheostomy and ventilation in severe cases. Despite these measures, recovery is often prolonged and the mortality rate is approximately 15 percent.

BIBLIOGRAPHY

Argov, Z., and Mastaglia, F. L. Disorders of neuromuscular transmission caused by drugs. *N. Engl. J. Med.* 301:409–413, 1979.

Drachman, D. B. Myasthenia gravis. *N. Engl. J. Med.* 298:136–142;186-193, 1978.

Engel, A. G. Myasthenia gravis and myasthenia syndromes. *Ann. Neurol.* 16:519–534, 1984.

Foldes, F. F., and Glaser, G. H. Diagnostic tests in myasthenia gravis: an overview. *Ann. NY Acad. Sci.* 183:275–286, 1971.

Glaser, G. H. Crisis, precrisis and drug resistance in myasthenia gravis. *Ann. NY Acad. Sci.* 135:335–349, 1966.

Johns, T. R. (editor). Myasthenia gravis. *Semin. Neurol.* 2:194–302, 1982.

Johns, T. R. Treatment of myasthenia gravis: long-term administration of corticosteroids with remarks on thymectomy. *Adv. Neurol.* 17:99–122, 1977.

Lambert, E. H., and Elmqvist, D. Quantal components of end-plate potentials in the myasthenic syndrome. *Ann. NY Acad. Sci.* 183:183–199, 1977.

Linton, D. M., and Philcox, D. Myasthenia gravis. *Disease-a-Month* November, 1990, Pp. 597–637.

Lisak, R. P., and Barchi, R. L. *Myasthenia Gravis* (Vol. 11, Major Problems in Neurology). Philadelphia: Saunders, 1982.

Namba, T., Brown, S. B., and Grob, D. Neonatal myasthenia gravis: report of two cases and review of the literature. *Pediatrics* 45:488–504, 1970.

Newson-Davis, J. Myasthenia. In W. B. Matthews and G. H. Glaser (editors). *Recent Advances in Clinical Neurology—4.* Edinburgh: Churchill Livingstone, 1984, Pp. 1–18.

Oosterhuis, H. J. G. H. *Myasthenia Gravis.* New York: Churchill Livingstone, 1984, P. 269.

Oosterhuis, H. J. G. H., and Kuks, J. B. M. Myasthenia gravis and myasthenic syndromes. *Curr. Opin. Neurol. Neurosurg.* 5:638–644, 1992.

Papatestas, A. E., et al. Studies in myasthenia gravis: effects of thymectomy. Results in 185 patients with nonthymomatous and thymomatous myasthenia gravis; 1941–1969. *Am. J. Med.* 50:465–474, 1971.

Patten, B. M. Myasthenia gravis: review of diagnosis and management. *Muscle Nerve* 1:190–205, 1978.

Pearlman, A. Neuromuscular Junction. In A. L. Pearlman and R.C. Collins (editors). *Neurological Pathophysiology.* New York: Oxford University Press, 1984, Pp. 41–55.

Penn, A. S. Neuromuscular junction. In E. D. Frohlich (editor). *Pathophysiology. Altered Regulatory Mechanisms in Disease,* 3rd ed. Philadelphia: Lippincott, 1984, Pp. 789–804.

Schwab, R., and Perlo, V. P. Syndromes simulating myasthenia gravis. *Ann. NY Acad. Sci.* 135:350–365, 1966.

Verma, P., and Oger, J. Treatment of acquired autoimmune myasthenia gravis: a topic review. *Can. J. Neurol. Sci.* 19:360–375, 1992.

Witte, A. S., et al. Azathioprine in the treatment of myasthenia gravis. *Ann. Neurol.* 15:602–605, 1984.

18

Ataxia and Cerebellar Disorders

Ataxia, which is an incoordination of movement, may affect gait, or it may involve the limbs individually, together, or bilaterally, the lower extremities only, or various combinations of the preceding. Discussion in this chapter concentrates mainly on derangements that involve the cerebellum and its connections as a cause for ataxia. Disturbances of proprioception (sensory ataxia), vestibular input, and weakness may also produce ataxia, and have been discussed in previous chapters. The various causes of recurrent falling attacks without apparent loss of consciousness are listed in Table 18-1.

THE CEREBELLUM

The cerebellum is concerned with regulating the timing, coordination, and integration of movements, including extraocular movements and speech. It functions closely with the motor cortex, basal ganglia, vestibular system, and spinal motor system.

Table 18-1. Causes of Recurrent Falling Attacks Without Apparent Loss of Consciousness

---

Gait ataxia due to cerebellar, vestibular, or proprioceptive disorders

Atonic seizures

Cataplexy

Basal ganglia disorders
  Parkinson's disease
  Progressive supranuclear palsy

Vertebrobasilar insufficiency

Spinal cord compression at foramen magnum level (e.g., subluxation of odontoid, basilar impression)

Orthopedic disorders (e.g., patellar subluxation, arthritis of hip joints)

Normal-pressure hydrocephalus

Idiopathic falling attacks (especially affecting middle-aged women)

Anatomy

The cerebellum occupies most of the infratentorial compartment and is connected to the brainstem by three bundles of white matter (peduncles): the superior (brachium conjunctivum), middle (brachium pontis), and inferior (restiform body). The middle peduncle contains only afferent fibers but the other two are composed of both afferent and efferent projections.

The cerebellar cortex consists of infoldings of gray matter known as *folia*. From an anatomical perspective, the cerebellum can be divided in the sagittal plane into the midline vermis and lateral hemispheres and in the coronal plane into the anterior, posterior, and flocculonodular lobes. There are numerous identifiable lobules within these divisions. Beneath the gray matter lie white matter fiber projections in which are embedded gray matter masses known as the *deep nuclei*. In functional terms, there are three longitudinal zones on each side, distinguished according to their major afferent and efferent connections: (1) a midline zone consisting of vermian and paravermian cortical areas projecting to the fastigial nucleus; (2) an intermediate zone sending fibers to the globose and emboliform nuclei (nuclei interpositi); and (3) a lateral zone providing efferents to the dentate nucleus. The flocculonodular lobe constitutes a fourth functional division; its cortical cells send axons directly to the vestibular nuclei, which can be thought of as homologues of the cerebellar deep nuclei.

The histological organization of the cerebellum is quite uniform and closely linked to its physiological functioning (Fig. 18-1). A Purkinje cell monolayer furnishes the main cerebellar outflow, largely by way of projections to the deep nuclear cells. Excitatory inputs to Purkinje cells arrive via two principal fiber systems. The **parallel fiber system** consists of bifurcating axons originating from the deep granular cell layer, each traveling a lengthy distance and contacting hundreds of Purkinje cells. Some afferents arrive directly on Purkinje cells via **climbing fibers** that arise principally from the contralateral inferior olivary nucleus. Most of the afferent input to the cerebellum, which arises from spinocerebellar, vestibulocerebellar, and pontocerebellar pathways, is carried by **mossy fibers** that terminate on granular cells in a complex fashion to form **glomeruli**. Golgi II inhibitory cells also contact granular cells.

The molecular layer lies over the Purkinje cell layer and contains parallel fibers, branching Purkinje cell dendrites, and inhibitory basket and stellate cells. These two cell types serve to limit the duration and spread of Purkinje cell discharges, thereby confining the zone of excitation to a narrow band.

Physiology

Purkinje cells normally fire at a relatively constant rate of about 50 to 100 per second, which increases or decreases according to excitatory-inhibitory interplay. Parallel fibers terminate on the dendritic spines of Purkinje cells and produce a strong excitatory response known as the *simple spike*. Climbing fibers contact one or very few Purkinje cells near the soma or proximal dendrites and produce a so-called complex-spike response. The Purkinje cell itself has an inhibitory influence on deep and vestibular nuclei. Specific neurotransmitters have been postulated to exist at various sites: glutamic acid for the granular cell–Purkinje cell (parallel fiber) synapse, gamma-aminobutyric acid at the Purkinje cell–nuclear synapse, aspartic acid in the climbing fibers from the inferior olive, and noradrenergic fibers from the locus ceruleus.

The functional organization of the cerebellum can also be viewed in phylogenetic or evolutionary terms. The **archicerebellum** corresponds to the flocculonodular lobe and has strong vestibular connections. The **paleocerebellum** comprises mainly the vermis and parafloccular areas and principally influences spinal mechanisms involved in gait and posture. The **neocerebellum** consists of the more lateral cortical areas, a small midvermal area, and the dentate nucleus, which has strong interconnections with the cerebral cortex. There is also a somatotopic arrangement of projections to various cerebellar functional areas as well as to the deep nuclei. Caudal body parts are represented in the anterior lobe.

The cerebellum is essentially involved in four major reverberating circuits: (1) vestibulocerebellar-vestibular, whereby information is conveyed regarding head and eye move-

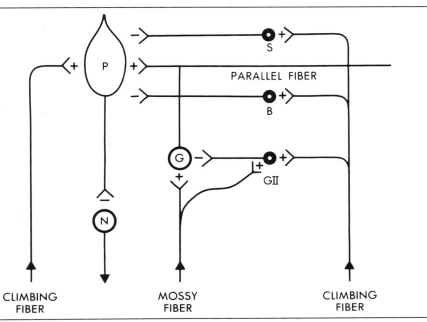

Fig.18-1. *Simplified diagram of cerebellar circuitry. Afferent input arrives via climbing fibers (mainly from contralateral inferior olive) and mossy fibers (mainly from spinocerebellar, pontocerebellar, and vestibulocerebellar pathways). Granular cells (G) provide parallel fibers excitatory to Purkinje cells (P). Purkinje cell output is inhibitory on nuclear cells (N), which provide main cerebellar efferents. Inhibitory interneurons are black. (S = stellate cell; B = basket cell; GII = Golgi II cell.)*

ments; (2) reticulocerebellar-reticular influences; (3) spinocerebellar-spinal, in which proprioceptive information is communicated to the cerebellum via spinocerebellar pathways and both alpha and gamma motor cells receive information via vestibulospinal, rubrospinal, and reticulospinal routes, thus promoting appropriate timing, force, and speed of movement (spinal influences from cerebellum are mainly ipsilateral); (4) cerebrocerebellar-cerebral connections, principally arriving by corticopontine fibers projecting via pontine nuclei to the contralateral cerebellum and reaching the contralateral cerebral cortex via dentatorubral-thalamic (VL nucleus) connections as well as projections from the fastigial and interpositi nuclei. Cerebral interconnections play a role in both the initiation of voluntary movements and the appropriate modification of speed and

direction of motor responses as they are being carried out.

Pathophysiology

It is not always possible to predict the clinical consequences of cerebellar lesions or identify precise anatomoclinical correlations, for several reasons. First, common disorders such as degenerations, tumors, or vascular lesions frequently also affect brainstem structures, either primarily or secondarily, as the result of raised intracranial pressure and distortion. Second, the system possesses a great capacity to adapt to the presence of cerebellar lesions, and therefore the chronicity and timing of the lesion may greatly determine the clinical manifestations. Third, lesions that affect cerebellar connections, such as the peduncles, or the areas contacted, such as the vestibular nuclei or even cerebral cortex, may produce signs that resemble those seen when the cerebellum is directly involved. Finally, despite the generalizations that can be made concerning the precise functions of the various cerebellar zones, there is actually a great deal of overlap in this regard.

In general, cerebellar impairment in humans may produce combinations of the following symptoms: ataxia, postural instability, dysmetria (i.e., a disturbance of the trajectory or placement of a body part during active movement), decomposition of movement, some slowness of movement, dysdiadochokinesia (difficulty performing rapid alternating movements), mild delay in initiating or terminating movements, overshoot, rebound, hypotonia, dysarthria, tremor (3–5 per second postural tremor), pendular deep tendon reflexes, eye movement disorders (e.g., rebound nystagmus, gaze-evoked direction-changing nystagmus, ipsilateral gaze palsy, ocular dysmetria, flutter, and square-wave jerks), and head or truncal titubation. Many of these signs may stem from more fundamental disturbances in the regulation of timing and force of movements.

In humans there is a **midline vermian and anterior lobe syndrome** (e.g., alcohol cerebellar degeneration) that displays features mainly of gait, truncal, and at times lower extremity ataxia and possibly nystagmus. In a similar **flocculonodular syndrome,** patients exhibit gait and postural instability and nystagmus, but limb movements are normal when they are recumbent. Lateral cerebellar lesions affecting the cortex, dentate nucleus, or its projections produce limb ataxia and dysmetria as well as hypotonia and intention tremor, mainly affecting skilled learned movements. Dysarthria occurs most frequently in the presence of left-sided lateral cerebellar lesions, but can also be seen with lesions of other areas. Eye movement disturbances are less precisely localized. A **pancerebellar syndrome,** which combines many of the features already mentioned, also appears in the context of such conditions as postanoxia, phenytoin toxicity, multiple sclerosis, and viral or postviral disorders affecting the cerebellum.

SPINOCEREBELLAR AND OLIVOPONTOCEREBELLAR DEGENERATIONS

Hereditary ataxias have long been considered part of the systems degeneration disorders, but classification has been difficult and controversial. Some practitioners favor grouping cases with clinically similar characteristics, even though there may be minor variations on a central theme. The thinking underlying this approach is that affected members within a family (especially in dominantly inherited cases) may themselves show variable clinical features. Others prefer to classify each new clinical variant separately. Further confusion arises from the fact that the phenotypic patterns can be similar despite a variable heredity, and all may occur sporadically. Besides gait ataxia, limb ataxia, and dysarthria, patients with spinocerebellar (SCD) or olivopontocerebellar (OPCD) degenerations may show varying combinations of peripheral neuropathy, peroneal muscular atrophy, corticospinal tract degeneration, myoclonus, epilepsy, dementia, optic atrophy, pigmentary retinal degeneration, autonomic disorders, deafness, extrapyramidal signs such as parkinsonism or tremor, slow eye movements, or pes cavus. The recent elaboration of the specific biochemical defects responsible for some of these disorders has sparked hope for the eventual formulation of a more rational basis for classification.

Despite the reigning confusion in this area, however, some recurrent clinical themes and specific syndromes can be distinguished. A simplified classification of the hereditary SCDs and other ataxias is shown in Table 18-2. More detailed classifications have been proposed by Harding (1983) and Currier (1984). The investigation of these patients should include a detailed family history and first-hand observation of family members, computed tomography (CT) or magnetic resonance imaging (MRI), and, in certain cases, electrooculography, CSF examination for oligoclonal banding, and measurement of brainstem auditory evoked potentials, peripheral nerve conduction velocities,

Table 18-2. Simplified Classification of Hereditary Progressive Ataxias

Spinocerebellar degenerations
    Spinal (usual onset: before age 20; usual heredity: recessive)
        Hyporeflexic (including Friedreich's ataxia)
        Spastic
    Cerebellar (usual onset: mid–adult life; usual heredity: dominant)
        Cerebellar (or cerebelloolivary) atrophies (Holmes)
        Cerebellar + brainstem (olivopontocerebellar degenerations)
            Dominant types
            Sporadic types or recessive: With glutamate dehydrogenase deficiency; Joseph disease
Other hereditary progressive ataxias (usual childhood onset)
    Bassen-Kornzweig syndrome (abetalipoproteinemia and vitamin E deficiency)
    Refsum disease (phytanic acid–alpha hydroxylase deficiency)
    Wilson's disease (copper excess)
    Hexosaminidase A and/or B deficiency
    Biotinidase deficiency
    Cerebrotendinous xanthomatosis (cholestanol deposition in the nervous system)
    Ataxia telangiectasia

glutamate dehydrogenase activity, or lysosomal enzyme levels.

Friedreich's Ataxia

Friedreich's ataxia is an uncommon autosomal recessive or sporadic form of SCD that serves as the prototype for the spinal forms of the disorder. Barbeau and his group have formulated the following criteria for diagnosis in typical cases: onset of symptoms before the end of puberty, early lower extremity and gait ataxia accompanied by weakness and eventually affecting all four limbs, early dysarthria, absent vibration and joint position sense in the lower extremities, absent deep tendon reflexes in the lower extremities, progressive pes cavus (high-arched feet with claw toe and equinovarus deformity) and kyphoscoliosis within 2 years of onset, absent sensory nerve action potentials in the lower extremities and reduced sensory conduction velocities in the upper extremities, and progressive (usually hypertrophic) cardiomyopathy. In addition, many patients exhibit corticospinal tract signs such as upgoing toes and tend to have hyperactive jaw jerks, even when other deep tendon reflexes are depressed.

About 40 percent of the patients are glucose intolerant and half of these are insulin-dependent diabetics. Most patients are wheelchair bound by the age of 25 and die in their 40s from progressive muscle wasting and respiratory or cardiac failure.

The pathological findings in patients with Friedreich's ataxia consist of degenerative changes with demyelination, fiber breakdown, and gliosis affecting the posterior columns and spinocerebellar tracts of the spinal cord. In some cases, there is also degeneration of the cells within Clarke's column of the spinal cord and corticospinal tract involvement. The cerebellum is only mildly affected and CT scans may show nothing more than mild atrophy of the anterior-superior vermis. Loss of dorsal root ganglion cells, optic nerve atrophy, and retinal ganglion cell loss are also frequently noted. Patients can suffer a dying-back axonopathy that principally affects large-diameter sensory fibers.

An extensive search has been conducted for the basic underlying biochemical deficit responsible for this disorder. Results from the Quebec study suggested that an energy deprivation state existed in the mitochondria. Other researchers have identified a mitochondrial malic enzyme deficiency in some cases.

Management consists of vigorous rehabilitation, early correction of the scoliosis with a brace or, when severe, surgery, treatment of the congestive heart failure and arrhythmias, and psychological counseling.

Familial Progressive Spastic Paraplegias

The familial progressive spastic paraplegias exhibit a variable inheritance pattern, and, on the basis of their clinical and pathological characteristics, they overlap with familial motor neuron disease (see Chapter 14). Features of spasticity may dominate the clinical picture. Some patients also show ataxia, optic atrophy, deafness, or dementia.

Olivopontocerebellar Degenerations

The clinical diversity of the OPCDs has been more clearly defined by Duvoisin and Plaitakis. Classically an OPCD is inherited as a dominant trait, but recessive and sporadic forms are frequent. Onset is usually in mid or late life and progression is relatively slow. Whether "pure" late-onset cerebellar degeneration, which may show pathological signs of olivary degeneration, should be included in this group is unclear.

The OPCDs represent a true systems degeneration commonly consisting of a progressive late-onset cerebellar ataxia in combination with dysarthria and extrapyramidal features such as parkinsonism or dystonia. The CT scan usually shows striking cerebellar (especially vermian) and brainstem atrophy and, in certain cases, also enlargement of the third ventricle and cerebral cortical atrophy. Additional features, such as spasticity, bulbar involvement, sphincter disturbances, amyotrophy, severe postural vertigo, sleep apnea, and dementia may be seen. Prominent autonomic involvement is seen in one subgroup of the disorder, which is mainly sporadic in occurrence. In another subvariety, patients have very slow eye movements with virtually absent saccades and peripheral neuropathy. Some patients with recessive OPCD suffer from glutamate dehydrogenase deficiency, although a fair amount of phenotypic variability is observed in this group.

Joseph disease is a dominantly inherited multisystem degeneration of the nervous system that is exclusively encountered in Portuguese inhabitants of the Azores and their descendants. Rosenberg has studied a very large pedigree with the disorder dating back several generations. Three clinical subtypes have been defined, with marked phenotypic variation exhibited within the same family: type I, onset in the second or third decades with mainly pyramidal and extrapyramidal features; type II, onset in the fourth decade with pyramidal, extrapyramidal, and cerebellar findings; and type III, onset from the fifth to seventh decades with cerebellar ataxia and peripheral neuropathy. In addition, lid retraction, ophthalmoparesis, loss of saccadic eye movements, and facial and lingual fasciculations without atrophy may be seen. Although this disorder resembles other cases of OPCD, postmortem studies have revealed that the inferior olive is not involved and there is often striatonigral degeneration, in addition to the spinal, brainstem, and cerebellar involvement.

Ramsay Hunt Syndrome

Patients with Ramsay Hunt syndrome (dyssynergia cerebellaris myoclonia and dyssynergia cerebellaris progressiva) show signs of progressive cerebellar degeneration that is accompanied by myoclonus, severe intention tremor, and epilepsy. Its pathological features overlap those of Friedreich's ataxia and, in fact, it probably does not represent a distinct entity. Some cases appear to have distinct mitochondrial abnormalities with ragged red fibers on muscle specimens obtained by biopsy. Similar cases have been termed *dentatorubral atrophy* because of the predominant degeneration within the dentate nucleus and dentatorubral outflow pathway. A similar clinical picture, but usually with earlier onset and added features of marked mental deterioration, may occur in Lafora's disease, some of the sphingolipidoses, or neuronal ceroid lipofuscinosis.

Ataxia Telangiectasia

Ataxia telangiectasia is an autosomal recessive, multisystem disorder affecting the nervous system, immune system, and skin. Neurological symptoms, consisting of head tremors and gait instability, appear in infancy or early childhood. Limb tremors and ataxia, nystagmus, abnormal extraocular movements, ocular apraxia (inability to refixate voluntarily), and dysarthria are other features. The patient's motor performance continues to deteriorate throughout childhood, with dystonic posturing, choreoathetosis, myoclonus, and dementia supervening. There are often signs of posterior column and peripheral nerve involvement.

Telangiectasias can be seen from an early stage, especially on the bulbar conjunctiva, earlobes, chest, and antecubital areas. Patients suffer characteristic cellular (T-cell impairment) and humoral (IgA and IgE deficiency) immune deficits that predispose them to recurrent infections as well as early death stemming from lymphoreticular and other malignancies. Glucose intolerance is also common. Defective repair of DNA may represent the fundamental disturbance in this disorder.

OTHER CAUSES OF PROGRESSIVE OR CHRONIC ATAXIA

Congenital Disorders

An ataxic form of **cerebral palsy** may result from anoxic cerebellar damage incurred at birth, since the Purkinje cells are relatively susceptible to hypoxia. Developmental anomalies of the cerebellum may be clinically silent or lead to chronic and at times recurrent bouts of ataxia.

The **Dandy-Walker syndrome** consists of a cystic dilatation of the fourth ventricle with dysgenesis of the cerebellar vermis and frequently atresia of the foramina of Luschka and Magendie, which normally allow egress of cerebrospinal fluid (CSF) from the fourth ventricle. It is the hydrocephalus, which frequently accompanies this anomaly, and not the cerebellar dysfunction that brings the child to medical attention. Frequently the child has other brain anomalies as well.

A type II Chiari or **Arnold-Chiari malformation** includes distortion and anomalous development of the cerebellum, but usually patients are seen because of signs of hydrocephalus or spasticity, rather than because of ataxia. **Midline subarachnoid cysts** may occur in the posterior fossa, usually in association with a hypoplastic cerebellar vermis. The cysts may or may not communicate with the fourth ventricle. They may be asymptomatic, give rise to intermittent or progressive symptoms of raised intracranial pressure due to hydrocephalus, or be manifested by symptoms of gait ataxia, which may be intermittent.

Diagnosis is readily accomplished by CT or MRI scanning, and the communication with the fourth ventricle can be ascertained by intrathecal radionuclide injection and posterior fossa scanning.

Alcoholic Cerebellar Degeneration

One of the more common effects of chronic excessive alcohol intake, or an accompanying aspect of nutritional deficiency, is anterior-superior vermian atrophy. Clinical manifestations may be minimal, or patients may exhibit a progressively ataxic wide-based gait, inability to perform tandem walking, unstable posture, and, at times, titubation of the head and trunk and lower limb ataxia when supine. The postural tremor of the hands, which is frequently seen in alcoholics, has also been attributed to cerebellar degeneration.

At autopsy, all layers of the midline cerebellum are noted to be atrophied with marked loss of Purkinje cells (see Chapter 29). CT scanning reveals diffuse cerebellar atrophy that is most marked in the vermian area. In some cases, symptoms may appear subacutely or intermittently, but not necessarily linked to alcohol intake, which suggests that other causative factors are superimposed on a preexisting cerebellar degeneration. With adequate nutrition and abstinence from alcohol, the gait ataxia may somewhat abate in these patients.

Other Toxic, Metabolic, and Endocrine Disorders

Exposure to DDT or lindane and 5-fluorouracil and long-term phenytoin use may lead to permanent cerebellar impairment. In long-standing epileptic patients on phenytoin therapy, there may be additional factors that contribute to the process. These include repeated bouts of

anoxia or head trauma, which are a consequence of the seizures. Long-term sedative
overdosing may produce a reversible ataxic syndrome. Repeated bouts of hypoxia or hypotension, or both, due to pulmonary disease or
cardiac arrhythmias, repeated bouts of hypoglycemia, and heat stroke may also cause Purkinje
cell damage and bring about a cerebellar syndrome. Patients with hypothyroidism may occasionally present with gait ataxia, which is
reversible with thyroid replacement.

Neoplasms

Patients with primary or secondary cerebellar
neoplasms may present with a progressive cerebellar syndrome, often accompanied by signs
of elevated intracranial pressure. The location
of the tumor in the cerebellum and whether
there is fourth ventricular obstruction or secondary brainstem involvement are the most important determinants of the clinical picture. A
wide variety of tumor types can affect the cerebellum, including gliomas, lymphomas, sarco-
mas, meningiomas, hemangioblastomas (e.g.,
with von Hippel–Lindau disease), schwannomas, and metastatic tumors. Medulloblastomas, which are most common in children,
mainly affect midline structures and commonly
cause progressive gait and truncal ataxia, vomiting, nystagmus, and head tilt. Cerebellar
astrocytomas in childhood tend to be located
in the cerebellar hemispheres and produce both
limb and gait ataxia. Metastatic tumors figure
most prominently among the cerebellar tumors
that afflict older age groups.

Infectious Conditions

The cerebellum is a particularly common intracranial site for abscess formation, and a high
proportion of intracranial tuberculomas, especially in children, are found there. Cerebellar
abscesses most commonly give rise to headache
and signs of an expanding posterior fossa mass
lesion, besides the cerebellar signs. Certain
slow viral infections such as Creutzfeldt-Jacob
disease, kuru, and progressive rubella panencephalitis can present with or produce prominent cerebellar signs.

Remote Effects of Carcinoma

Subacute or chronic gait ataxia, frequently accompanied by dysarthria and limb ataxia, can
develop insidiously or subacutely as a remote
effect of carcinoma (see Chapter 29). The syndrome may also occur in conjunction with other
neurological nonmetastatic manifestations such
as peripheral neuropathy or the Eaton-Lambert
myasthenic syndrome. Among the underlying
primary tumors responsible for the syndrome,
which include lung, breast, and uterine tumors,
ovarian carcinoma has been particularly prominent. Pathological examination in patients with
a nonmetastatic cause shows a loss of Purkinje
cells and granule cells as well as inflammatory
perivascular infiltrate. The syndrome may precede the clinical appearance of the carcinoma
and persist despite treatment of the malignancy.
Anti–Purkinje cell antibodies are found in the
serum of a high proportion of affected patients.

Multiple Sclerosis

Multiple sclerosis frequently attacks cerebellar
white matter but usually in conjunction with
other areas of the central nervous system. In
many patients, MRI or autopsy reveals the unexpected presence of widespread plaques in the
cerebellum. Patients with advanced disease frequently show the characteristic Charcot's triad
of nystagmus, intention tremor, and scanning
speech. Although approximately 15 percent of
the cases of multiple sclerosis are familial, these
may be distinguished from the SCDs or OPCDs
by their relapsing and remitting course, absence
of peripheral nerve involvement, frequent asymmetrical involvement of the optic nerves, the appearance of plaques on CT or MRI scans, and
the presence of oligoclonal bands in the CSF.

ACUTE OR SUBACUTE ATAXIA

Infectious and Parainfectious Causes

Several viruses, including Epstein-Barr,
ECHO, coxsackie, herpes simplex, herpes zoster, and poliomyelitis, may cause cerebellitis,
and aseptic meningitis may occur concomitantly

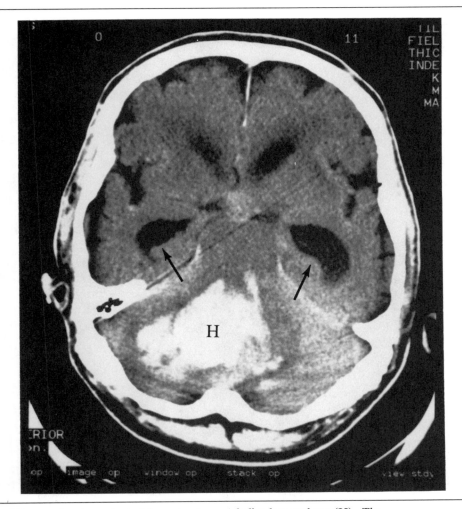

Fig. 18-2. *CT scan showing a typical hypertensive cerebellar hemorrhage* (H). *The patient presented with sudden severe ataxia, inability to stand, and vomiting, followed rapidly by coma. The arrows indicate the dilated temporal horns of the lateral ventricles resulting from obstructive hydrocephalus due to compression of the fourth ventricle.*

in these cases. *Mycoplasma* pneumonia may produce a similar syndrome. Rarely patients with bacterial or fungal meningitis manifest prominent and early signs of ataxia. In children, ataxia may also occur acutely after an exanthematous condition, such as measles, mumps, rubella, and especially varicella, or following immunization. Fisher's syndrome consists of acute cerebellar ataxia, ophthalmoplegia, and areflexia that frequently appears after an upper respiratory infection. This syndrome appears to be a variant of Guillain-Barré inflammatory

polyradiculoneuropathy and there has never been proof that the ataxia stems from direct cerebellar involvement.

Vascular Causes

Vertebrobasilar insufficiency, cerebellar or brainstem infarction, and cerebellar hemorrhage (Fig. 18-2) can produce ataxia, frequently in combination with other neurological symptoms. These vascular conditions are discussed further in Chapter 23. Vertebrobasilar mi-

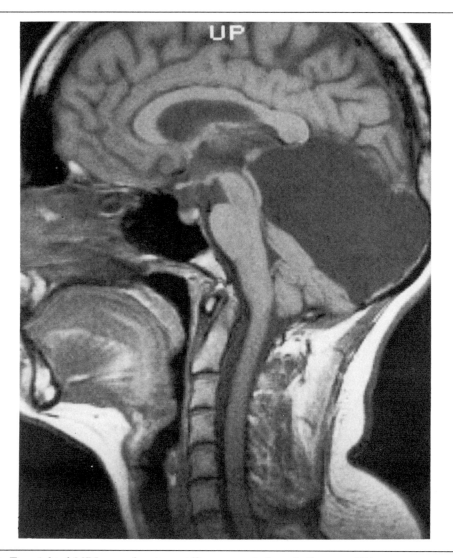

Fig. 18-3. T_1-weighted MRI scan showing midline congenital cerebellar cyst. This patient exhibited no abnormal neurological findings.

graine, especially in children, can cause recurrent bouts of ataxia and vomiting, often accompanied by headache and visual disturbances.

Toxic Disorders

The drugs mentioned in the preceding section on chronic ataxias, as well as heavy metals such as lead, mercury, and thallium, various chemicals and solvents, plus tick toxin, have been implicated as causes of acute or subacute ataxia.

Posterior Fossa Mass Lesions

Previously silent neoplasms, abscesses, and cysts may abruptly become symptomatic, perhaps because of sudden vascular compromise or rapid expansion beyond a critical volume (Fig. 18-3).

Metabolic Disorders

Recurrent bouts of ataxia, nausea, and vomiting, and perhaps stupor, in association with infection or "metabolic stresses," occur in several unusual inherited metabolic conditions. Hartnup disease, the intermittent form of maple syrup urine disease, pyruvate decarboxylase deficiency, urea cycle abnormalities, and Leigh disease all fall into this category.

Special Syndromes of Childhood

Acute Idiopathic Ataxia of Childhood

Acute idiopathic ataxia of childhood appears most frequently between the ages of 1 and 4 years and may arise after a nonspecific upper respiratory or gastrointestinal infection. Patients experience the rapid development of truncal and gait ataxia and a milder limb ataxia, especially in the lower extremities. Hypotonia, tremor, and ocular dysmetria are frequent accompaniments, and nystagmus, opsoclonus, lethargy, or delirium is less common. CSF may show a mild mononuclear pleocytosis, but findings are usually normal. Most patients recover rapidly over one to several weeks, but up to one third of the patients may be left with prolonged or permanent ataxic deficits, or less commonly intellectual deterioration.

Opsoclonus-Myoclonus Ataxia Syndrome with Underlying Neuroblastoma

Acute ataxia accompanied by myoclonus and chaotic multidirectional conjugate eye movements (opsoclonus) may occur in infants or children and even occasionally in adults. The disorder may run a relapsing and remitting course, with each bout triggered by an infectious illness. In children, the syndrome is highly linked to an underlying neuroblastoma and represents virtually the only well-defined remote effect of malignancy in childhood. Therefore, when it is encountered, a search for occult neuroblastoma should be undertaken that includes radiographs and CT scans of the chest and abdomen, skeletal survey, intravenous pyelography or ultrasound of the kidneys, bone marrow examination, and measurement of urinary vanillylmandelic acid and other catecholamine metabolite levels. Symptoms may regress spontaneously or with ACTH treatment. Whether a similar syndrome can occur as a parainfectious

complication without an underlying neuroblastoma is currently unclear.

Miscellaneous

Conditions that have already been discussed, such as multiple sclerosis, global hypoxia or ischemia, hypoglycemia, epilepsy, and alcoholic cerebellar degeneration, may present in a relatively acute manner in the form of ataxia. In addition, head trauma, particularly a blow to the occiput or contrecoup injury to the cerebellum, may cause a temporary ataxic syndrome.

BIBLIOGRAPHY

Barbeau, A. Pathophysiology of Friedreich's Ataxia. In W. B. Matthews and G. H. Glaser (editors). *Recent Advances in Clinical Neurology—3.* Edinburgh: Churchill Livingstone, 1982, Pp. 125–145.

Blass, J. P. The Hereditary Ataxias. In S. Appel (editor). *Current Neurology.* New York: Wiley, 1981, Vol. 3, Pp. 66–91.

Brown, J. R. Diseases of the Cerebellum. In A. B. Baker and R. J. Joynt (editors). *Clinical Neurology.* Philadelphia: Harper & Row, 1985, Vol. 3, Pp. 1–43.

Currier, R. D. A Classification of Ataxia. In R. C. Duvoisin and A. Plaitakis (editors). *The Olivopontocerebellar Atrophies.* New York: Raven, 1984.

Duvoisin, R. C., and Plaitakis, A. (editors). *The Olivopontocerebellar Atrophies* (Advances in Neurology, Vol. 41). New York: Raven, 1984.

Gilman, S., Bloedel, J. R., and Lechtenberg, R. *Disorders of the Cerebellum.* Philadelphia: Davis, 1981.

Harding, A. E. Classification of the hereditary ataxias and paraplegias. *Lancet* 1:1151–1155, 1983.

Lothman, E. W., and Montgomery, E. B., Jr. Control of Motor Activity of the Cerebrum and Cerebellum. In E. D. Frohlich (editor). *Patho-*

physiology: Altered Regulatory Mechanisms in Disease, 3rd ed. Philadelphia: Lippincott, 1984, Pp. 741–770.

Netsky, M. Degeneration of the Cerebellum and Its Pathways. In J. Minckler (editor). *Pathology of the Nervous System.* New York: McGraw-Hill, 1968, Pp. 1163–1184.

Nyberg-Hansen, R., and Horn, J. Functional aspects of cerebellar signs in clinical neurology. *Acta Neurol. Scand.* 48(Suppl. 58):219–245, 1972.

Plaitakis, A., and Gudesblatt, M. The hereditary ataxias. In S. H. Appel (editor). *Current Neurology.* New York: Wiley, 1984, Vol. 5, Pp. 471–509.

Rosenberg, R. N. Joseph disease: An autosomal dominant motor system degeneration. In R.C. Duvoisin and A. Plaitakis (editors). *The Olivopontocerebellar Atrophies.* New York: Raven, 1984.

Stumpf, D. A. The inherited ataxias. *Neurol. Clin.* 2:47–57, 1985.

Thach, W. T., Jr., and Montgomery, E. B., Jr. Motor system. In A. L. Pearlman and R. C. Collins (editors). *Neurological Pathophysiology,* 3rd ed. New York: Oxford University Press, 1984, Pp. 151–178.

Victor, M., Adams, R. D., and Mancall, E. L. A restricted form of cerebellar cortical degeneration occurring in alcoholic patients. *Arch. Neurol* 1:579–588, 1959.

Weiss, S., and Guberman, A. Acute cerebellar ataxia in infectious disease. In P. J. Vinken and G. W. Bruyn (editors). *Infections of the Nervous System* (Handbook of Clinical Neurology, Vol. 34). Amsterdam: North-Holland, 1978, Pp. 619–639.

Ziter, F. A., Bray, P. F., and Cancilla, P. A. Neuropathologic findings in a patient with neuroblastoma and myoclonic encephalopathy. *Arch. Neurol.* 36:51, 1979.

Zoghbi, H. The Spinocerebellar Degenerations. In S. H. Appel (editor). *Current Neurology.* St. Louis: Mosby–Year Book, Vol. 11, 1991.

Disorders with Prominent Sensory Complaints and Pain

ANATOMY OF THE SOMATOSENSORY SYSTEM

Primary somatic sensation, including light touch, deep pressure, position and movement, vibration, pain, and temperature, is conveyed to the brain by relatively modality-specific pathways. Histologically specialized peripheral skin, subcutaneous, tendon, and joint receptors, which serve as transducers, impart a degree of specificity to the initial sensory receptive process, though many of the receptors are potentially multimodal. Pain reception is primarily associated with free nerve endings. Localization of the stimulus is accomplished by a somatotopic arrangement of fibers, which is more or less maintained at higher central levels. This is less true for pain, and its precise localization partially depends on information received from parallel fiber systems mediating touch and pressure. The intensity of the stimulus is coded in terms of the frequency of firing in afferent

pathways and the size of the receptor population activated.

Primary afferent peripheral nerve fibers, which are mainly bipolar neurons with their cell bodies located in the dorsal root ganglia, enter the dorsal root of the spinal cord as two distinct populations. Those lying more dorsomedially are larger myelinated fibers that convey vibration, joint position, and pressure sensation. These fibers generally ascend ipsilaterally in the posterior columns and synapse in the nuclei gracilis and cuneatus of the medulla. Fibers entering the dorsal columns from higher levels are located more laterally. The somatotopic arrangement within the main sensory and motor tracts of the spinal cord is shown in Figure 19-1. The second-order medullary neurons then cross (internal arcuate fibers) to form the medial lemniscus and then ascend in the brainstem to terminate in the ventroposterolateral thalamic nucleus (VPL). Sensory fibers from the trigeminal and glossopharyngeal cranial nerves originating from the facial and pharyngeal regions join the medial lemniscus.

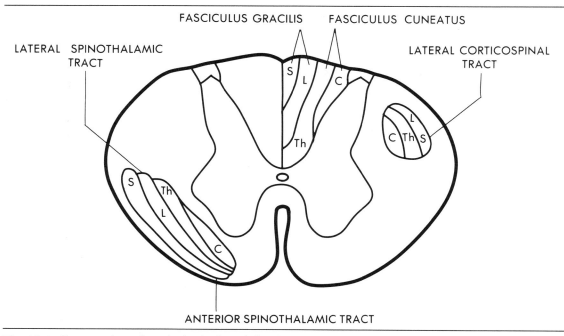

Fig. 19-1. *Cross section of cervical spinal cord showing somatotopic arrangement of fibers in the corticospinal tract and the principal ascending sensory tracts. (S = sacral; L = lumbar; Th = thoracic; C = cervical.)*

Smaller unmyelinated C or sparsely myelinated A-delta fibers that convey pain enter the dorsal horn more ventromedially. These fibers largely terminate in the dorsal root entry zone on second-order neurons in laminae I or V of Rexed or on interneurons in lamina II (the substantia gelatinosa). Some of the entering fibers are distributed to higher or lower segments via the dorsolateral fasciculus (Lissauer's tract).

The vast majority of fibers carrying pain and temperature sensation cross over within one or two segments of their entry to form the ascending anterolateral spinothalamic tract. The fibers entering most caudally end up more superficially as fibers from higher segments are incorporated. In the lower brainstem, the spinothalamic tract lies dorsolaterally, quite separate from the medial lemniscus. However, the two successively merge above the pontine level and, in fact, terminate somatotopically on the same VPL nucleus of the thalamus. Most of the spinothalamic pain fibers nevertheless actually terminate in the brainstem reticular formation or the periaqueductal gray area.

Thalamocortical projections that traverse the posterior limb of the internal capsule and terminate mainly on the postcentral primary somatosensory receiving area are responsible for the conscious perception of most somatic sensations. Pain seems to be perceived mainly at the thalamic level, although frontal and limbic areas may furnish the emotional coloring and "suffering" that so frequently accompany pain. Somatosensory evoked potentials can be recorded from sensory cortex when pure pain fibers are stimulated. Whether localized loss of pain can occur secondary to a purely cortical lesion is still a matter of controversy.

Derangements in sensation may occur in the form of sensory loss or anesthesia; paresthesias, which can be thought of as unprovoked positive primitive sensory phenomena (e.g., "numbness," "tingling," "pins and needles," "crawling sensations"); or dysesthesias, which are aberrant or distorted sensations experienced in response to a stimulus (e.g., a tingling sensation when touched). Paresthesias may occur in the presence of lesions affecting virtually any portion of the sensory pathways. **Hyperalgesia** indicates an abnormal hypersensitivity to pain stimuli, whereas **hyperpathia** (which is seen with lesions of the thalamus or spinothalamic tract) constitutes an excessively strong pain response experienced once an initial abnormally high pain threshold is exceeded.

PAIN

Physiology

The principal pain pathways have already been discussed. Only in recent years have the complex phenomena of pain become better understood and the many observed clinical aspects of pain been explained in physiological terms.

Pain Fibers and Pathways

There appear to be two distinct types of pain, each possessing its own system of afferents. Sharp, superficial, well-localized, acute pain is conducted mainly by the faster A-delta fibers (average, 19 m/sec) and ascends in a somatotopically arranged fashion in the spinothalamic tract to the VPL of the thalamus. A duller, more distressing, longer-lasting, and less well-localized form of pain signaling ongoing tissue damage is conducted more slowly along unmyelinated C fibers (1 m/sec), which terminate mainly in lamina V of the spinal cord. The rostral projections of these neurons are more diffuse and polysynaptic, and provide input mainly to the brainstem reticular formation, nonspecific thalamic nuclei, and eventually limbic system and cerebral cortex.

Two common features of many of the peripheral stimuli causing pain are that they produce tissue damage and trigger the release of certain vasoactive and pain-promoting substances, such as bradykinin, serotonin, histamine, substance P, or prostaglandins. These substances may stimulate receptors or nerve endings either directly or indirectly by modulating their sensitivity to mechanical or other stimuli. Receptors responsive to chemical stimulation (which are also multimodal) have been particularly linked with C fibers, whereas mechanical and heat stimuli producing pain are linked more to A-delta transmission.

The central integration of pain transmission initially takes place in the dorsal horn, especially in lamina II, the substantia gelatinosa, where C-fiber terminations predominate. Suprasegmental, especially brainstem inhibitory, influences occur at this level. In the "gate" theory of Melzack and Wall, interneurons at this level were theorized to have a gate function. This consisted of a tendency to prevent the entrance of C and A-delta fiber impulses to neurons forming the spinothalamic tract by inhibiting them presynaptically. Although newer physiological data have contradicted the theory, it is still a useful way of thinking about certain clinical pain phenomena. Large-fiber inputs were thought to "close the gate" and reduce pain, which explained how rubbing or applying either vibration or electrical stimulation to a painful area could reduce the pain. Smaller-fiber (C-fiber) input was believed to "open the gate" through the inhibition of interneurons in the substantia gelatinosa, thereby accounting for such phenomena as postherpetic neuralgia, in which larger dorsal root ganglion neurons are selectively lost.

Recent investigations have shown that there are strong inhibitory influences originating from serotonin-containing neurons that arise from the nucleus raphe magnus of the medulla, whose fibers descend in Lissauer's tract and terminate in laminae I, II, and V of the dorsal horn. The periaqueductal gray area of the midbrain sends neurons to this and other brainstem nuclei involved with pain modulation and, when stimulated experimentally, produces analgesia.

The Endorphins

A system of endogenous neuropeptides with opiate properties has been discovered. These substances, known as *endorphins,* function as neuromodulators or neurotransmitters, and are concentrated in the periaqueductal gray area as well as in laminae I, II, and V (mainly interneurons) of the spinal dorsal horn. They not only serve an endogenous analgesic function but are also widely distributed throughout the brain, including the limbic system, striatum, and hypothalamus, and likely influence several aspects of nervous function. Specific receptors for these substances account for the analgesic as well as other actions of morphine and like narcotic agents.

One class of endorphins consists of the **enkephalins,** two pentapeptides, one with methionine (met-enkephalin) and the other with leucine (leu-enkephalin) on its terminal. These substances are found in the brain, the dorsal horn of the spinal cord, autonomic nerves, and the adrenal medulla. It is postulated that the release of these substances from interneurons inhibits incoming pain-conducting fibers, thus reducing their release of the neurotransmitter substance P. A larger endorphin substance (31 amino acids), known as *beta-endorphin,* is found in the brain and pituitary gland. **Dynorphins,** a third class of endorphins, are found in the posterior pituitary and gastrointestinal tract, but probably play no endogenous role in modulating pain. A precursor molecule with a molecular weight of 31,000, known as *proopiomelanocortin,* is found in the anterior pituitary and contains ACTH, beta-lipotropin, beta-endorphin, and melanocyte-stimulating hormone within its structure.

The administration of endorphins or endorphin analogues into the CSF in humans provides potent and long-lasting analgesia, and this may eventually find a clinical application. The discovery of these endogenous opioid substances also brought to light possible explanations for many of the observed clinical phenomena relating to pain and its control, including the documented effects of placebos in certain individuals, the ability of the person's mental "set" to modify the response to pain, the effects of tricyclic antidepressants (which increase the central availability of serotonin and norepinephrine), and the effects of acupuncture.

Other Pain Regulatory Factors

Two other aspects of pain regulation require mention. First, pain is a subjective phenomenon and, as such, is variably influenced by factors such as cultural background, prior experience with pain, the potential impact of the pain and accompanying injury on the patient's life, and secondary gain. Second, the peripheral sympathetic nervous system appears to have some influence on peripheral pain trans-

mission. Many painful neuropathies involving small fibers such as amyloidosis and diabetes mellitus also have a marked autonomic component. In certain chronic painful conditions, such as reflex sympathetic dystrophy or causalgia, in which there are also autonomic and trophic changes in the limb, sympathectomy may prove successful in reducing or eliminating the pain.

Types of Pain

Referred Pain

Visceral pain arising from intrathoracic, intraabdominal, and intrapelvic structures is conducted along sympathetic and parasympathetic afferents. This type of pain is often poorly localized and may be referred to specific surface areas supplied by the same spinal segments (e.g., the pain from cholecystitis felt in the right shoulder or the pain from ischemic heart disease referred to left arm). The convergence of afferent input from visceral and somatic areas on the same dorsal horn nociceptive cells is thought to be the mechanism responsible.

Central Pain

An infarct of the thalamus in the territory of the thalamogeniculate artery may give rise to the syndrome first described by Déjerine and Roussy. The syndrome may include a contralateral transient hemiparesis, choreoathetoid movements of the opposite hand, an ipsilateral Horner's syndrome, or a contralateral reduction of pain sensation with hyperpathia or allodynia. Hyperpathia refers to a delay and overreaction to pain-producing, especially repetitive, stimuli ("recruitment"). Patients with allodynia experience a painful response to normally nonpainful stimuli such as light touch or scratching. Other nonvascular lesions in the thalamus or affecting spinothalamic pathways may produce this persistent pain state, which can be very difficult to treat. Treatment with antiepileptic drugs such as carbamazepine may be of benefit in some cases.

Postherpetic Neuralgia

At a variable interval following an attack of cutaneous herpes zoster, a severe disabling persistent neuralgic pain may appear in the involved areas, even when sensation may otherwise be lost within these areas. The V1 dermatome in the face and the midthoracic dermatomes are the most frequently involved and this complication most commonly afflicts the elderly. Depression is a frequent component. In many patients, the disorder resolves spontaneously after several months. The underlying pathology appears to be the selective loss of larger dorsal root ganglion cells that allows the establishment of chronic reverberating circuits at the dorsal root entry zone. Treatment has been largely unsuccessful, but conservative measures such as regular gentle rubbing of the involved area with a rough towel, the application of a hand vibrator, transcutaneous electrical nerve stimulation, the application of ethylchloride spray, or the use of carbamazepine or tricyclic antidepressants, or both, are occasionally helpful. Capsaicin, the active component in hot chili peppers, can be applied topically four to five times a day for 4 weeks, although burning of the skin upon application is an unpleasant side effect. It is thought to act by releasing and eventually depleting the store of substance P, a pain-modulating substance, from presynaptic terminals. Initial treatment of the herpetic condition with steroids lessens the likelihood of postherpetic neuralgia. Surgical destruction of the dorsal root entry zone by creating a radiofrequency lesion or using a laser has been successful in some cases.

Causalgia

Causalgia, a spontaneous burning pain, which is usually intense and persistent, occurs in a small proportion of patients after injury to a nerve trunk or plexus. The sciatic and median nerves are most commonly involved and the nerve is usually not completely transected. High-velocity missile injuries, such as those incurred under combat conditions, are the most common source of the problem, but stab wounds, surgery, and misplaced intramuscular injections have also been implicated. Typically symptoms begin at a variable interval following injury and may be delayed for months. Patients experience extreme hyperpathia and allodynia, often finding the slightest touch unbearable. There can be sympathetic alterations in the limb, such as discoloration, coolness, and trophic skin changes, but these are more common in the related state of **reflex sympathetic dystrophy,** which is not necessarily a result of nerve injury. Emotional distress is an almost inevitable accompaniment and many patients are mistakenly diagnosed as having psychogenic pain. Treatment consists of a trial of transcutaneous nerve stimulation and tricyclic antidepressants. Sympathetic blocks followed by sympathectomy can be used if the condition does not remit.

Phantom Limb Pain

Persistent pain in the stump following amputation, often appearing to arise from the missing limb, is common in amputees. Only rarely does this stem from neuroma formation at the stump. It is believed to be caused by an alteration in the peripheral input which changes the configuration of central pain integration. Treatment is ineffective in most cases, but measures such as transcutaneous nerve stimulation or tricyclic antidepressants may bring about some improvement.

Chronic Pain

Besides the conditions already mentioned, there exists a variety of other chronic pain states that may be very resistant to treatment. Low back pain (see later discussion), pain due to cancer, and the persistent, intractable, incapacitating myalgia and muscle tenderness known as fibromyalgia, or myofascial pain syndrome, are examples. This last condition is a poorly understood pain syndrome that is usually seen by rheumatologists, and is usually diagnosed in patients with diffuse musculoskeletal pain once other disorders such as osteoporosis, myositis, arthritis, metastatic bone disease, and polymyalgia rheumatica have been excluded. Typically these patients, who are usually women, have various sensitive trigger points that are elicited by palpation of the muscles. In addition, affected patients are usually depressed and find virtually any physical activity exacerbates their symptoms. Pain and stiffness are mainly confined to the neck, shoulders, and upper back. Sleep is usually disturbed and symptoms are worse upon awakening in the morning.

Treatment should be attempted with nonsteroidal antiinflammatory medication, physiotherapy (e.g., heat, ultrasound, and mild exercise), massage, tricyclic antidepressants, and perhaps low-dose steroids. Patients require intensive rehabilitation that also focuses on contributing psychological and social factors that may be prolonging the disability.

New medical and surgical approaches are being tried in patients with intractable pain due to malignancy or injury. The intrathecal infusion of narcotics is one such approach. Neuroaugmentation procedures, which involve the implantation of stimulators in the brainstem, thalamus, or other areas, have been used in certain cases. Localized ablative procedures, such as cordotomy or midbrain tractotomy, often fail or afford only temporary relief because of the complex central circuitry involved in mediating pain. As a last resort, prefrontal leukotomy or anterior cingulectomy has been carried out to relieve the suffering in these unfortunate individuals.

Congenital Insensitivity to Pain

A diverse group of patients with congenital hyporesponsivity, insensitivity, or "indifference" to pain has been recognized, and this represents a rare disorder. Some of these patients have hereditary sensory and autonomic neuropathies such as the Riley-Day syndrome. Others appear to lack the small C fibers that mediate pain. In still others, the pathogenesis remains obscure and may stem from central biochemical alterations that affect pain regulatory systems, perhaps involving the endorphins. These patients suffer frequent trauma, burns, skin ulcers, and severe degeneration of joints because they lack the normal protective reflexes.

PATTERNS OF SENSORY LOSS IN SPINAL CORD DISEASE

The distribution of sensory loss or alteration is often a valuable clue to the location of lesions within the peripheral and central nervous systems (Fig. 19-2). Sensory loss associated with lesions of the cutaneous nerves, plexuses, or roots has been dealt with previously.

Brown-Séquard (Hemicord) Syndrome

A transverse lesion that affects only half of the spinal cord is rare, except in cases of trauma. In this setting, posterior column sensation on the same side as the lesion below the involved level and contralateral pain and temperature sensation up to a few segments below the lesion are impaired. Touch sensation is much less affected. There is also ipsilateral weakness below the lesion due to corticospinal tract involvement.

Anterior Spinal Artery Syndrome

The anterior spinal artery supplying the ventral two thirds of the spinal cord is the most frequently involved vessel in vascular disease affecting the cord, especially around the T6 watershed area where anastomoses are most tenuous. The etiology may be trauma, hypotension, embolization, vasculitis, or surgery on the aorta. The characteristic syndrome includes paraplegia and a well-defined sensory level to pain and temperature, which are lost up to a few segments below the lesion. The posterior columns are usually spared, and therefore vibration, joint position sense, and pressure sensation are preserved. MRI scanning may readily demonstrate a spinal cord infarct (Fig. 19-3).

Sacral Sparing

Intramedullary expanding lesions such as tumors may produce a sensory level that characteristically leaves sacral segments intact, because afferent fibers from those areas lie most superficially in the spinothalamic tracts.

Subacute Combined Degeneration of the Spinal Cord

Subacute combined degeneration of the spinal cord constitutes the classic neurological manifestation of vitamin B_{12} deficiency secondary to pernicious anemia. Pernicious anemia is a genetic autoimmune condition in which a deficit in the production of gastric intrinsic factor resulting from gastric parietal cell atrophy leads to defective vitamin B_{12} absorption. The disease is most prevalent in Northern Europeans (e.g., Scandinavians) of fair coloring, and patients typically exhibit other features such as vitiligo, a red "beefy" tongue, achlorhydria (lack of gastric acid), and a high incidence of concurrent autoimmune disorders. Both patients and their relatives also carry a relatively high risk for developing gastric cancer. The diagnosis may be suspected on the basis of the hematological picture, consisting of a megaloblastic anemia (which may be severe), hypersegmented neutrophils in the peripheral blood, or, in mild cases, intermediate megaloblastic changes in the bone marrow. The serum vitamin B_{12} level is very low in these patients. A Schilling test, done to establish diagnosis, demonstrates an increase in B_{12} absorption when intrinsic factor is provided.

Other causes of vitamin B_{12} deficiency, such as strict vegetarianism, gastrectomy, intestinal tapeworm, and severe malabsorption, are much less frequent. Normally the body stores of vitamin B_{12} are adequate for several years, and only severe prolonged dietary deficiency can provoke symptoms. It is well known that the neurological complications of B_{12} deficiency can occasionally occur in the absence of any hematological changes. Besides subacute combined degeneration, patients may suffer a distal sensory neuropathy, an optic neuropathy, and a mild dementia.

The subacute combined degeneration selectively affects the corticospinal tracts and posterior columns. In this disorder the involved tracts in the spinal cord exhibit a spongy degenerated appearance that affects both myelin and axons and there is also gliosis. The patient frequently complains of uncomfortable truncal and limb paresthesias, and progressive gait difficulty is the usual presenting feature. Spasticity of the lower extremities and Babinski's signs occur, but deep tendon reflexes may be depressed rather than increased. A similar clinical picture with loss of vibration and joint position sense and paraparesis may be encountered in patients with spinal cord compression caused by tumor or cervical spondylosis and in the vacuolar myelopathy seen with AIDS. Treatment with monthly vitamin B_{12} injections can bring about improvement in all patients but those with well-advanced disease, who may show some minimal improvement after several months.

Syringomyelia

The term *syringomyelia* derives from the Greek word *syrinx*, meaning a tube or pipe, and refers to a progressive cavitation within the central part of the spinal cord. However, when the cavity is linked to the central spinal canal, and is lined by ependymal cells and filled with normal cerebrospinal fluid (CSF), *hydromyelia* is probably a more appropriate designation for the disorder.

Pathophysiology and Etiology

There has been much debate concerning the pathogenesis of the disorder, but the work of Gardner has revealed that many cases of syringomyelia and hydromyelia are associated with congenital or acquired abnormalities in the posterior fossa such as the Arnold-Chiari malformation or arachnoiditis. Scarring and distortion of the anatomy in the posterior fossa (e.g., herniation of the cerebellar tonsils through the foramen magnum) are believed to prevent the egress of CSF from the fourth ventricle, and also impede the normal flow of CSF from basal cisterns to the spinal canal. The pressure exerted by normal choroid plexus pulsations and from other sources is then transmitted by the CSF from the fourth ventricle down the central spinal canal, causing it to dilate progressively. Eventually a cavity forms within the substance of the spinal cord. This variety of syringomyelia is termed *communicating*, because the central canal and syrinx communicate with the fourth ventricle. In other cases, however, there is no communication between the syrinx and the fourth ventricle or even with the central canal.

Not all cases are associated with anomalies of the posterior fossa. Syringomyelia may also arise as a late sequela in paraplegics who have sustained spinal trauma. It can also occur in conjunction with spinal cord tumors (particularly intramedullary). In these instances, the

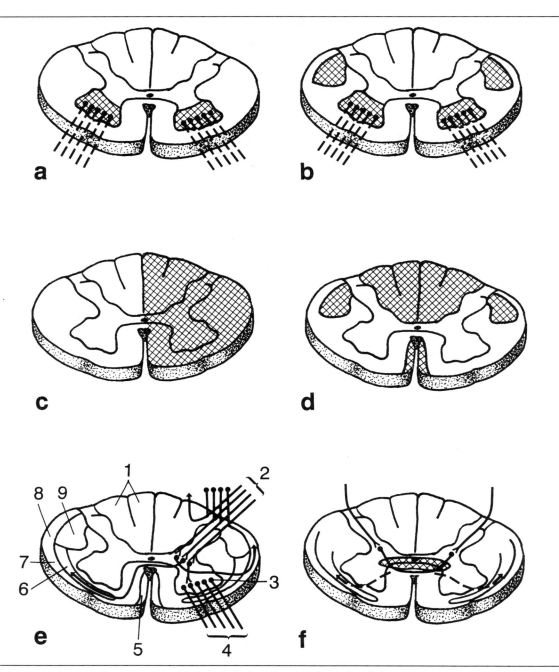

Fig. 19-2. *Lesions* (cross hatching) *in various disorders affecting the spinal cord. Interrupted lines indicate degenerated fibers in the nerve roots. (1 = posterior columns; 2 = posterior (sensory) nerve root; 3 = anterior horn cells; 4 = anterior (motor) nerve root; 5 = anterior corticospinal tract; 6 = spinothalamic tract; 7 = anterior spinocerebellar tract; 8 = posterior spinocerebellar tract; 9 = lateral corticospinal tract.) (A) Acute poliomyelitis and progressive spinal muscular atrophy. (B) Amyotrophic lateral sclerosis. (C) Brown-Séquard syndrome. (D) Subacute combined degeneration. (E) Normal spinal cord. (F) Syringomyelia.*

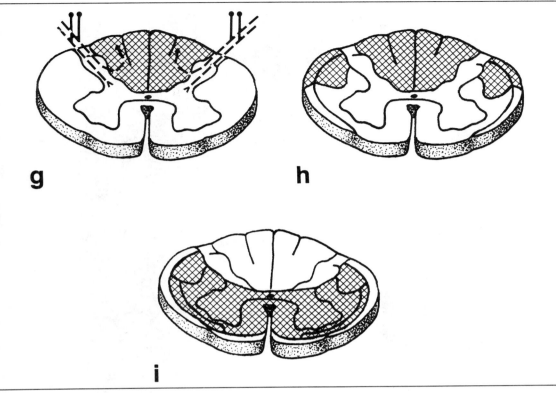

Fig. 19-2 *(Continued). (G) Tabes dorsalis. (H) Friedreich's ataxia. (I) Anterior spinal artery syndrome. (Adapted from W. Blackwood, T. C. Dodds, and J. C. Sommerville,* Atlas of Neuropathology, *2nd ed. Edinburgh; E & S Livingstone, 1964.)*

fluid in the syrinx is often yellowish and has a high protein content. Some cases of syringomyelia may arise as an isolated congenital developmental abnormality of the spinal cord.

Clinical Picture and Diagnosis

Symptoms may first appear in childhood or late adult life, but, in one large series, the mean age of onset was around 30 years. Symptoms may also appear following neck or back trauma. Because the cavity most commonly forms in the lower cervical area, affected patients typically exhibit a clinical picture consisting of sensory loss and segmental wasting, weakness and fasciculations in the arms and hands, and paraparesis and upper motor neuron findings in the legs. Deep tendon reflexes are often absent in the upper extremities, which also show trophic changes. A "dissociated" sensory loss with absent pain and temperature and preserved touch

and posterior column sensation almost confirms the diagnosis. The sensory findings may occur over the arms and trunk or over the trunk and shoulders in a "suspended cape" or "hemicape" distribution.

The sensory findings are explained by the fact that the crossing pain fibers from the dorsal horn cells projecting to the spinothalamic tracts travel just anterior to the central spinal canal and are affected early by the dilating syrinx. With progression, anterior horn cells, corticospinal tracts, and finally posterior columns may become involved. Ultimately only a thin ribbon of spinal cord may remain intact around an irregular large syrinx with surrounding gliosis.

Other features observed in the disorder include Horner's syndrome, the preservation of sphincter function until late, and scoliosis. There may be severe degeneration of the joints (Charcot's joints), especially in the elbow and

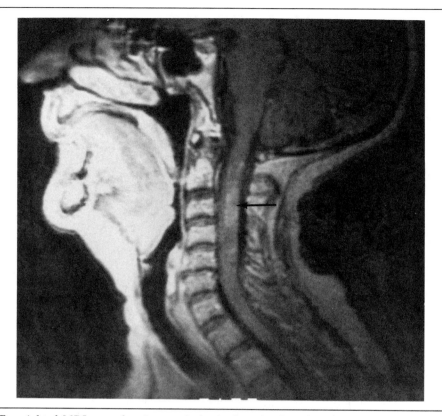

Fig. 19-3. *T₁-weighted MRI scan showing cervical spinal cord infarct* (arrow).

shoulder, resulting from the loss of pain and normal protective reflexes. Likewise, painless burn wounds are often seen on the hands. Patients may also show developmental anomalies such as a short neck, an asymmetrical thorax, sternal depression or prominence, cervical ribs, or unequal breast development.

Diagnosis is based on the clinical picture and the radiological findings. Plain x-ray studies may reveal anomalies at the cervical cranial junction such as atlantooccipital fusion or basilar impression. Rarely, the cervical spinal canal may be widened in its anteroposterior diameter. Myelography frequently demonstrates descent of the cervical tonsils, a widened cervical canal, or failure of the dye to enter the posterior fossa. High-resolution CT scanning of the spine, using metrizamide or other water-soluble agents, may reveal delayed uptake of the contrast material into

the central canal. Magnetic resonance imaging (MRI) scanning is now the method of choice for delineating the syrinx (Fig. 19-4). Longitudinal images of the spinal canal, without the interference of bone, can precisely define the extent of the cavity and readily differentiate a syrinx from an intramedullary tumor, with which it is sometimes associated.

Syringobulbia, which may occur either in isolation or together with syringomyelia, usually affects the lower brainstem at characteristic sites. In this disorder, slitlike cavities appear in the dorsal midline. These can affect the medial longitudinal fasciculus; extend ventrolaterally from the fourth ventricle and interrupt the descending root of the fifth nerve, the tractus solitarius, and the ninth and tenth nerves; or extend between the olive and pyramid, thus compromising the twelfth nerve. Symptoms include

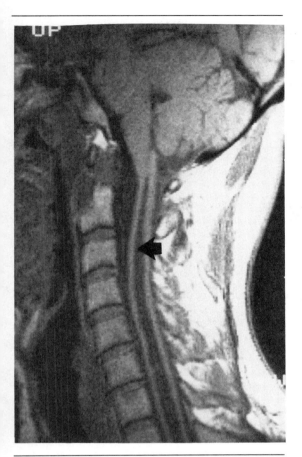

Fig. 19-4. *T_1-weighted MRI scan showing syringomyelia (arrow). This 40-year-old woman presented following a 10-year history of neck and shoulder pain, progressive numbness and weakness of the right arm, and mild gait difficulty. The syrinx extended from the medulla to the lumbar region.*

stridor in the newborn, dysphagia and nasal speech, and facial paresthesias. Rarely symptoms may appear acutely.

Management

The treatment of syringomyelia is controversial. When symptoms are progressive and disabling, surgical intervention should be attempted. Some advocate a posterior fossa approach, even if a clear-cut pathology is not demonstrated in advance. Decompression and allowing the egress of CSF from the fourth ventricle and into the spinal canal are the objectives. Posterior fossa surgery has a relatively high morbidity and

mortality, however. Patients with concurrent hydrocephalus should have a ventricular shunt installed. A shunt placed from the syrinx into the subarachnoid space has also been tried, as has section of the filum terminale, to allow drainage of CSF from the central canal. No method of treatment has yet provided a sure means of halting the progression of the disorder.

"Hysterical" Sensory Loss

Patients suffering from hysteria, a conversion reaction, or malingering may exhibit bizarre, anatomically inconsistent, and fluctuating sensory findings. A stocking-and-glove sensory loss to all modalities over the extremity with a very sharp border constitutes a classic hysterical pattern. Hemisensory loss with a sharp border exactly in the midline or several inches past the midline are other typical patterns. Hysterical patients may claim they cannot detect displacement about a joint yet other tests of proprioception, such as the Romberg test or having the patient touch his or her fingers together with eyes closed, may be performed perfectly. Patients who have "functional" hemisensory loss to pinprick and touch may also claim they cannot feel a vibrating tuning fork on only half of the sternum or forehead. Because vibration is transmitted throughout these bones, this is usually a clue to hysteria or malingering. The presence of abdominal cutaneous reflexes or a withdrawal response to nose tickle is also incompatible with a claimed sensory loss in these areas.

PAIN IN THE NECK AND UPPER EXTREMITY

One of the most common problems faced by neurologists, rheumatologists, and orthopedists is pain localized to the neck, shoulder, or arm. Despite extensive investigation, many of these patients remain without a precise diagnosis, although some respond well to symptomatic treatment. The major conditions to be considered in the differential diagnosis are listed in Table 19-1. Some of these conditions, such as

Table 19-1. Major Causes of Neck, Shoulder, and Arm Pain

Musculoskeletal causes
    Cervical muscle or ligament strain (e.g., whiplash injury)
    Calcific tendonitis of shoulder
    Bursitis, tendonitis (e.g., subacromial or olecranon bursitis, tennis elbow)
    Arthritis
        Cervical spondylosis/osteoarthritis
        Rheumatoid
        Ankylosing spondylitis
        Diffuse idiopathic skeletal hyperostosis (Forestier's disease)
    Subluxation of the odontoid
    Myofascial pain syndrome
Neurologic causes
    Root compression due to disc protrusion or foramen encroachment from spondylosis
    Root involvement from other causes (e.g., herpes zoster, malignancy, schwannoma)
    Brachial plexus involvement
        Pancoast's tumor of lung
        Brachial neuritis
        Thoracic outlet compression
        Hyperabduction syndrome
    Compression/entrapment neuropathies in arm (e.g., carpal tunnel, cubital tunnel)
Referred pain (e.g., from cardiac source)

carpal tunnel syndrome and fibrositis, have already been discussed.

Cervical Root Compression Due to Cervical Disc Disease or Cervical Spondylosis

Pathophysiology and Etiology

Cervical spondylosis is an extremely common degenerative condition that affects the vertebrae, discs, and ligaments of the cervical spine. The changes commonly responsible include hypertrophic bony overgrowth and spurs that form at the anterior and posterior edges of the vertebral bodies (especially adjacent to disc spaces), hypertrophy of the ligamentum flavum running posterior to the spinal cord between the laminae of adjacent vertebrae, articular facet hypertrophy, and encroachment of bony material on the root exit foramina.

Intervertebral discs degenerate with age and undergo chemical changes that cause them to lose their elasticity. This produces distortion of the normal anatomy and alters the dynamics of neck movements. These changes, along with excessive wear and tear and other unknown factors, predispose individuals to cervical spondylosis in later life. Ischemic factors stemming from radicular and anterior spinal artery compression may also contribute to the pathogenesis of spinal cord involvement.

Clinical Picture and Diagnosis

Typically patients experience gradually progressive paraparesis and posterior column sensory loss. Many patients complain of nuchal pain and stiffness, occipital (and sometimes frontal) muscle tension headache, and trapezius and shoulder pain—all exacerbated by neck movements. Many cases are symptomatic, but some patients may have only minor neck complaints, even though neck x-ray studies show severe changes. Narrowing of the anteroposterior diameter of the cervical canal to 12 mm or less (measuring from a posterior osteophyte to the anterior portion of the vertebral spinous process) indicates a high likelihood of spinal cord compression leading to myelopathy.

When spondylosis or intervertebral disc protrusion causes foraminal narrowing, symptoms of individual root compression appear. In acute cases of disc herniation, in which the nucleus pulposus is extruded through the annulus fibrosus into the spinal canal, patients experience severe acute neck and arm pain with muscle spasm in the neck and paresthesias in the arm.

Coughing, sneezing, or straining frequently exacerbates the symptoms and precipitates a shooting pain down the arm that is typical of root irritation. In the early phases of cervical root compromise, pain may be felt in the scapular area, which constitutes a useful differentiating feature from arm pain due to more distal nerve entrapment. The distribution of pain and paresthesias and the existence of certain objective neurological signs in the arm can accurately point to the root involved in about 90 percent of cases (Table 19-2). The C7 root is by far the most frequent root affected by disc disease, with C6, C8, and C5 succeeding in that order. Men are more commonly affected than women. Besides the usual neurological examination that looks for weakness, fasciculations, tendon reflex changes, and sensory loss, various foraminal compression tests can be employed that reproduce the pain and paresthesias for diagnostic purposes. A most useful maneuver is to have the patient extend the neck and laterally flex it to the side of involvement in an attempt to provoke symptoms.

Plain cervical spine x-ray studies, including oblique views which permit visualization of the foramina, are indicated in all cases. Cervical myelography (Fig. 19-5) and computed tomographic (CT) scanning with metrizamide enhancement can accurately identify the level of root compromise and differentiate disc disease from a tumoral cause in most cases. The CSF protein level is frequently elevated in patients with disc herniation or spondylosis.

Thoracic disc disease, which is uncommon, tends to occur at the lower thoracic levels and produces localized back pain as well as radicular pain in the trunk. Spinal cord compression is a relatively frequent component of this condition. It may be missed on myelography and is probably best diagnosed either by CT scanning with metrizamide enhancement or by MRI scanning.

Management

Management of acute cervical-brachial pain due to root compression initially consists of immobilizing the neck with a soft cervical collar worn night and day, the application of cold (and later heat) to relieve neck muscle spasm, analgesia, and gentle cervical traction performed by a physiotherapist. Diathermy and ultrasound treatment to the neck may also be of benefit.

Surgical therapy may be indicated in patients with intractable pain or progressive neurological deficits, although surgery may be difficult if there are multiple levels of involvement and the spondylosis is severe. An anterior approach is being used increasingly because it allows direct access to the protruded disc or spondylotic bars and permits the easy fusion of vertebrae when necessary.

Thoracic Outlet Syndromes

The neurovascular bundle passing through the thoracic outlet superior to the first rib and underneath the clavicle may be compromised at this level. A cervical rib, the anterior scalene muscle, or fibrous bands coming off an elongated C7 transverse process and attaching to the first rib can all compress the brachial plexus and have all been implicated in the etiology of this condition. Female patients with poor muscle tone and low-hanging shoulders who use their arms extensively seem to be particularly prone to this problem.

Thoracic outlet syndrome is overdiagnosed and the sole presence of a cervical rib should not automatically be construed to indicate the condition. Most commonly, patients complain of pain and paresthesias in the ulnar distribution of the hand and medial forearm when carrying heavy objects (e.g., luggage or grocery bags) or when using the arm for prolonged periods above the shoulder level. Most patients exhibit few objective neurological signs, although there may be weakness and wasting of the muscles supplied by C8 and T1 as well as sensory loss in the medial hand. In more severe cases, there is a vascular compromise, which may be manifested by Raynaud's phenomenon in the hand, a radial pulse delay on the involved side, a supraclavicular bruit, or blood pressure difference in the two arms. A helpful diagnostic sign is the ability to elicit symptoms by exerting downward traction on the arms or forced abduction of the arm. Obliteration of the radial pulse with the patient's arm abducted and forced

Table 19-2. Subjective and Objective Findings in Cervical Root Syndromes

Root	Pain	Paresthesias	Weakness or fasciculations	Reduced tendon reflex
C5	Shoulder, lateral upper arm to elbow	Shoulder	Deltoid, infraspinatus	Biceps, brachioradialis
C6	Shoulder, scapula, biceps area, radial aspect forearm	First two fingers	Biceps, brachioradialis	Biceps, brachioradialis
C7	Shoulder, scapula, posterolateral arm, posterior and anterior forearm	2nd, 3rd fingers	Triceps	Triceps
C8	Scapula, posterior arm and medial forearm	4th, 5th fingers	Intrinsic hand muscles	Triceps occasionally

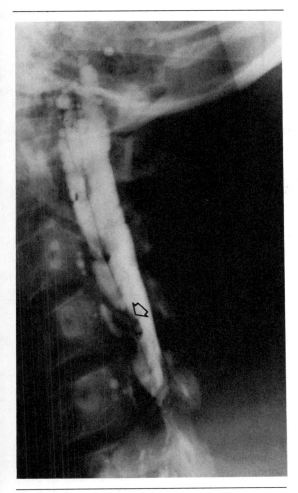

Fig. 19-5. *The patient was a 45-year-old woman who had experienced neck and bilateral arm pain for several months followed by gait ataxia and a sense of "heaviness" in the lower extremities. On examination she exhibited a mild spastic quadriparesis, worse on the left, and a partial sensory loss below C3 on the left. Myelogram showed a large central disc protrusion at C5–C6 (arrow)* that was compressing the spinal cord and causing a partial block.

backward while the head is turned in the opposite direction with the chin elevated is not very helpful diagnostically, because it is also a relatively common finding in normal subjects.

When thoracic outlet syndrome is suspected, plain neck x-ray studies should be obtained that look specifically for signs of spondylotic

or disc disease, a cervical rib, or elongated C7 transverse process. Nerve conduction studies performed across the clavicle (Erb's point) may occasionally demonstrate slowing, but are technically difficult and painful to carry out. Subclavian Doppler studies or angiography may be helpful in patients with symptoms of vascular compromise.

Initial management is directed toward having the patient avoid activities or postures that produce the symptoms and perform a series of exercises designed to improve shoulder posture by strengthening shoulder and neck muscles. In cases with a clear-cut diagnosis, removal of a portion of the first rib by a transaxillary approach, excision of a cervical rib if present, or section of constricting fibrous bands or the anterior scalene muscle may be successful.

LOW BACK PAIN

Pain in the lumbosacral region is one of the most common ailments afflicting mankind and is the major cause of work-related disability. One study found 18 percent of the population between the ages of 18 and 68 suffers from low back pain. Patients with chronic low back pain are typically those who suffer persistent pain following a lumbar spinal operation and who have often been referred from one physician to another, frequently ending up in a pain management or special rehabilitation center. Newer neuroimaging techniques, such as high-resolution CT and MRI, are contributing to our knowledge of the pathoanatomical basis of back pain syndromes. Figures 19-6 and 19-7 show a cross-sectional view of a vertebral body and the relationship of spinal segments to the vertebral bodies. It is important to keep these anatomical relationships in mind when evaluating syndromes of root or cord compression.

Differential Diagnosis

Major causes of back pain are listed in Table 19-3. So-called mechanical low back pain, resulting from improper lifting or twisting the spine while bending over, accounts for the vast

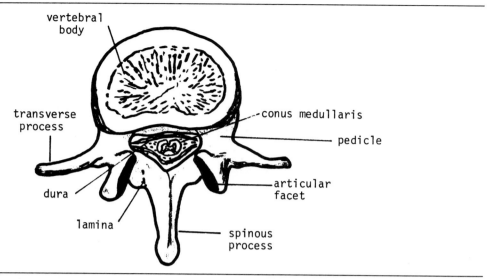

Fig. 19-6. *Schematic cross section of a lumbar vertebral body.*

majority of patients. Poor abdominal muscle tone and obesity, which produce a hyperlordotic posture, as well as congenital bony anomalies, such as partial lumbarization of the S1 vertebra or facet tropism, all predispose to this problem by creating unusual strains and forces in the lower spinal column. Low back pain may be chronic, acute, recurrent acute, or a combination of these temporal patterns.

Pain that is unremitting and progressively worsens over several weeks always suggests the possibility of a neoplastic etiology. A thorough physical examination that searches for vertebral tenderness and lymphadenopathy, and that includes abdominal palpation, pelvic and breast examination in women, and rectal examination with prostate palpation in men, should be performed in all cases. When a neoplastic etiology is suspected, plain spinal x-ray studies followed by bone and CT scans of the painful areas as well as a chest x-ray study plus serum protein electrophoresis may yield information that can confirm the diagnosis. The discussion in this chapter will concentrate on those causes of low back pain that are likely to be the source of problems in patients referred to the neurologist or neurosurgeon.

Herniation of Lumbar Discs

Adjacent vertebrae are separated by a fibrocartilaginous structure, the disc, which serves as a shock absorber. With age and use, the proteoglycan composition of the central portion of the disc (nucleus pulposus) becomes altered; its collagen content also increases and water is lost, thereby reducing the disc's force-absorption capacity. Hyaline degeneration, neovascularization, and tears also develop in the surrounding annulus fibrosus, which allows the protrusion or bulging of the nucleus pulposus posteriorly where the annulus fibrosus is the thinnest. As the process advances, prolapse may occur, causing the displacement of nuclear material backward into the vertebral canal. Nuclear material may later be extruded as the posterior annular fibers rupture and, if the posterior longitudinal ligament is breached, the disc material may become sequestered and lie free within the vertebral canal.

The neurological consequences that may develop depend on several factors: (1) the level of the disc herniation (Table 19-4), with each disc tending to compress the root corresponding to the level of the vertebra below it; (2) whether

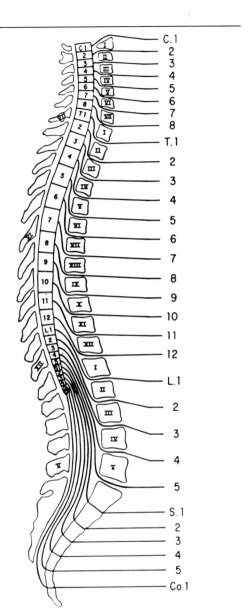

C.1
2
3
4
5
6
7
8
T.1
2
3
4
5
6
7
8
9
10
11
12
L.1
2
3
4
5
S.1
2
3
4
5
Co.1

Fig. 19-7. *Longitudinal section showing relationship of spinal segments and roots to the vertebral column. Note that the spinal cord ends at L1–L2 with the cauda equina below that level, and that almost all lumbar and sacral segments are located opposite T12 and L1 vertebrae. (Adapted from J. Favill, Outline of the Spinal Nerves. Springfield, IL: Thomas, 1946.)*

Table 19-3. Causes of Low Back Pain (With or Without Sciatica)

Lumbosacral strain due to, e.g., poor posture, trauma, obesity, pregnancy
Neoplastic or infectious disease of vertebrae or adjacent structures
  Multiple myeloma
  Metastases (e.g., breast, lung, lymphoma, prostate)
  Tuberculosis (e.g., Pott's disease)
  Pyogenic disc space infection
Degenerative disc disease
  With root compression causing sciatica
  Without root compression
Lumbar spondylosis
  With root compression causing sciatica
  Without root compression
Osteoarthritis of facet joints
Spinal stenosis
  Congenital
  Acquired (i.e., degeneration)
Spondylolisthesis
  With spondylolysis
  Without
Arthritides
  Rheumatoid
  Ankylosing spondylitis
  Other
Intraabdominal and intrapelvic disorders
  Severe uterine fibroids
  Aortic aneurysm
  Retroperitoneal neoplasms
Psychogenic back pain (including malingering)
Other
  Compression fracture
  Osteoporosis
  Osteoid osteoma of vertebra
  Paget's disease

the herniation is in the midline (cauda equina compression or no symptoms may occur), lateral, or extremely lateral (root compression likely); (3) the amount of herniated disc material; and (4) whether there is accompanying spinal stenosis (see later discussion).

Patients with degenerative disc disease often cite a history of recurrent bouts of back pain occurring over several years, which usually abates after a few days of bed rest. At one point, perhaps after minor trauma, unaccustomed exercise, or heavy lifting, there is an acute (at times incapacitating) onset of back pain that tends to radiate down the buttock, posterior thigh, and leg (sciatica) as the disc prolapses or extrudes. Sciatica, which is due to root irritation and inflammation, is worsened by

Table 19-4. Subjective and Objective Findings in Lumbosacral Root Syndromes

Root	Pain	Paresthesias	Weakness or fasciculations	Reduced tendon reflex
L4	Posterolateral hip, anterior thigh and knee	Anterior thigh, knee, medial leg	Quadriceps	Knee jerk
L5	Posterolateral thigh, lateral leg, dorsum of foot	Lateral calf, dorsum of foot, first three toes	Foot and first toe extensors, foot inversion, foot eversion, hamstrings, gluteus medius	Internal hamstring or posterior tibial (inconsistent)
S1	Posterior thigh, calf, heel	Posterior calf, heel, lateral side of foot	Gastrocnemius, hamstrings, gluteus maximus, foot eversion	Ankle jerk

coughing, straining, or performing maneuvers that stretch the involved root, such as bending laterally toward or away from the involved side. In acute cases, paravertebral muscle spasm is severe, scoliosis may be apparent, and the patient walks with a list. Standing and especially sitting may be extremely uncomfortable, and the patient may choose to lie supine or on his or her side on a firm surface with the knees partially flexed.

Over 90 percent of these degenerative discs occur at the L4–L5 and L5–S1 levels, and only about 7 percent at L3–L4. The neurological signs present usually reflect root involvement at these levels (see Table 19-4). In addition, sciatica and back pain are typically elicited or worsened by certain maneuvers. Passive raising of the involved leg, which is held straight while the patient lies supine, may be severely limited. Similarly, extending the knee while the patient lies supine with the hip flexed may be impossible (Lasègue's sign). The "crossed-leg" sign, in which symptoms are reproduced when the opposite leg is held straight and raised by the examiner, is very suggestive of disc herniation. The "bowstring" sign is elicited by having the patient lie supine and place the involved extended leg on the examiner's shoulder, who presses down on the knee to produce the pain. The femoral nerve stretch test is used for detecting upper lumbar root involvement (L2–L4). To perform it, the patient lies prone with his or her leg flexed at the knee while the examiner attempts to reproduce the radicular pain by hyperextending the patient's leg at the hip. There is also loss of the usual lumbar lordosis when patients are in the relaxed standing position and back movements are greatly limited.

Plain x-ray studies of the spine may reveal the existence of disc space narrowing or additional spondylotic changes at the appropriate level, but can be normal, even in cases of massive disc protrusion. Oblique (foraminal) views are mandatory to search for bony impingement on the foramina that may be the source of radicular symptoms. High-resolution axial CT scanning carried out at clinically indicated levels is increasingly replacing conventional myelography as a definitive, safe, and comfortable diagnostic tool (Fig. 19-8). When there is a straightforward clinical picture that correlates well with the CT findings, no other preoperative test may be required. CT, performed with intrathecally administered water-soluble contrast material, is useful for detecting neoplastic lesions in the spinal cord or canal. However, conventional myelography may prove superior in some cases, especially when multiple levels or concurrent severe spinal stenosis are involved. An extreme lateral disc extrusion may be missed entirely by conventional myelography, and therefore CT must also be done in patients with a clinically likely disc herniation or protrusion but negative myelogram (Fig. 19-9). MRI scanning provides a longitudinal view of several vertebral levels and can furnish direct evidence of disc protrusion or herniation.

Other possibilities must be considered in patients with sciatica when no radiological evidence of disc is found. Spinal stenosis (see later discussion) or spondylolisthesis (one vertebra displaced forward on the vertebra below) should be apparent radiologically. Tumors of the roots (e.g., neurofibroma or a metastatic growth) can usually be visualized by CT scanning with or without the intrathecal instillation of water-soluble contrast material. Lesions of the lumbosacral plexus such as metastatic tumors may pose diagnostic difficulties, but there is usually clinical and electromyographic evidence of the involvement of several roots, and these growths may also be visualized by plain or contrast-enhanced CT. Lesions of the sciatic nerve itself can present with pain in the sciatic distribution. Entrapment at the piriform muscle can be difficult to diagnose but abnormalities may be detected by specialized electrophysiological tests. A bony spur at the sciatic notch, which can be visualized on an x-ray film, is a rare cause of sciatica. A sciatic mononeuropathy due to diabetes or vasculitis may mimic certain features of a herniated disc. Neurofibrosarcomas, neurofibromas, and neurilemomas are tumors that can involve the sciatic nerve and affected patients typically present with foot and leg pain (especially nocturnal) and dysesthesias. The tumor may be palpable along the course of the nerve. CT scanning of the pelvis and thighs is the diagnostic procedure of choice. In most patients,

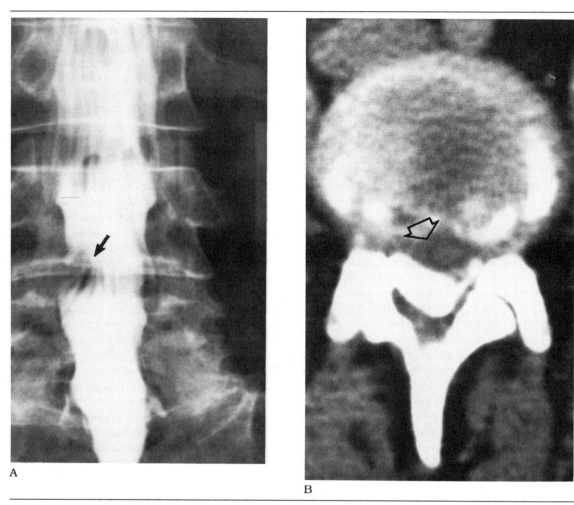

A

B

Fig. 19-8. *Typical appearance of lumbar disc herniation* (arrows) *on myelogram (A) and CT scan (B). Note the indentation of the dye column on the CT scan.*

a combination of back pain and spasm in conjunction with signs and symptoms attributable to a single root distribution readily distinguish a herniated disc from a sciatic nerve lesion.

Spinal Stenosis

Spinal stenosis in its broadest sense represents narrowing of the spinal canal in its transverse or sagittal dimension. Central lumbar spinal stenosis is diagnosed when an axial CT scan shows the anteroposterior diameter of the spinal canal to be less than 11.5 mm. Lateral recess stenosis is diagnosed when the anteroposterior diameter of the lateral recess is less than 3 mm. Spinal stenosis, especially affecting the posterior half of the spinal canal, may be congenital. Much more commonly it is acquired and results from degenerative changes. Osteoarthritis of the facet joints may lead to hypertrophy and subluxation, which tends to impinge on the lateral recesses forming the intervertebral nerve root canals. Ligamentum flavum hypertrophy, marginal osteophytes projecting posteriorly from vertebral bodies, and protruding intervertebral discs frequently contribute to the evolution of spinal stenosis. The most commonly involved levels are L2 through L4.

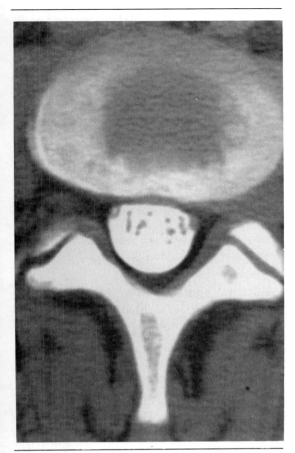

Fig. 19-9. *Far lateral L3–L4 disc herniation* (arrow) *seen on CT scan. This patient's myelogram was normal.*

Neurogenic intermittent claudication is the most common symptom of spinal stenosis, which is described by patients as pain, numbness, or weakness usually affecting both lower extremities. Symptoms appear in the upright position while walking or other positions requiring lumbar extension. Extension causes further narrowing of the already compromised spinal canal. Unlike patients with true intermittent claudication in the lower extremities due to vascular insufficiency, these patients may become symptomatic with prolonged standing. In addition, patients must bend forward or lie down for symptoms to remit, symptoms are often referred to the whole limb rather than just the calf, low back pain is common, and the periph-

eral pulses are generally intact. Sciatica is uncommon in this group and the result of the straight-leg raising test is usually negative. The condition may be treated surgically by doing multilevel laminectomies with or without foraminotomies.

Management of Acute Back Pain

The initial management of acute back pain or sciatica due to a herniated disc, lumbar strain, and most other causes consists first and foremost of bed rest for up to 3 weeks. The application of ice, massage, and ultrasound, and the administration of analgesics, antiinflammatory agents, and muscle relaxants may all promote comfort and healing. Rest on a firm surface such as a special orthopedic mattress placed on a bed board or the floor is essential. As soon as the pain has subsided, the patient should undertake a series of graded specialized back flexion exercises. Once the pain is resolved and the patient mobile, attention should be directed toward preventive measures to lessen the likelihood of further exacerbations. Weight loss, abdominal strengthening, hamstring stretching, postural correction, correct sitting postures, and not sitting in low soft chairs and not lifting while bent over at the waist should all be stressed. Active, early back rehabilitation with strengthening and flexibility exercises is being increasingly recommended. This approach allows the best chance for early functional recovery.

The indications for surgery in the treatment of disc disease are somewhat controversial. In general, surgery should be considered in patients with intractable recurrent back pain or sciatica that does not respond to conservative measures or in those with neurological deficits such as a foot drop or significant sensory loss. Radiological confirmation of the diagnosis must be obtained by CT, MRI, or myelography. Cauda equina compression is an indication for urgent surgery. The approaches to disc surgery vary, although the standard method involves laminectomy or hemilaminectomy and removal of disc material.

If operation does not relieve the symptoms or symptoms recur (failed disc syndrome), this may be due to several factors. Most commonly the initial diagnosis was wrong or a concurrent condition such as lateral recess stenosis was overlooked. Rarely the wrong level is operated on. A sequestered disc fragment may have been missed. In addition, patients may also suffer instability of the back with spondylolisthesis or disc herniation at a new level.

In patients with chronic incapacitating back pain, psychological management is an important part of the treatment. The goal of treatment should be functional rehabilitation and not necessarily full pain relief. A team approach involving psychologists, psychiatrists, rehabilitation specialists, pain experts, counselors, and physiotherapists offers the best chance of helping these difficult cases. In many patients, the resolution of any legal actions related to work-related injury or the awarding of compensation has a markedly positive therapeutic effect.

BIBLIOGRAPHY

Pain

Basbaum, A. I., and Fields, H. L. Endogenous pain control mechanisms: review and hypothesis. *Ann. Neurol.* 4:451–462, 1978.

Bonica, J. J (editor). Causalgia and Other Reflex Sympathetic Dystrophies. *Adv. Pain Res. Ther.* 3:141–166, 1979.

Clement-Jones, V., and Besser, G. M. Clinical perspectives in opioid peptides. *Br. Med. Bull.* 39:95–100, 1983.

Clifford, D. B. The Somatosensory System and Pain. In A. L. Pearlman and R. C. Collins (editors). *Neurological Pathophysiology,* 3rd ed. New York: Oxford University Press, 1984, Pp. 74–85.

Fields, H. L. Pain: II. New approaches to management. *Ann. Neurol.* 9:101–106, 1981.

Goodman, C. E. Pathophysiology of pain. *Arch. Intern. Med.* 143:527–530, 1983.

Horowitz, S. Iatrogenic causalgia. Classification, clinical findings, and legal ramifications. *Arch. Neurol.* 41:821–824, 1984.

Kosterlitz, H. W., and McKnight, A. T. *Endorphins and Enkephalins* (Advances in Internal Medicine). Chicago: Mosby–Year Book, 1980, Pp. 1–36.

Melzack, R., and Wall, P. D. Pain mechanisms: a new theory. *Science* 150:971–979, 1965.

Morley, G. K., Erickson, D. L., and Morley, J. E. The neurology of pain. In A. B. Baker and R. J. Joynt (editors). *Clinical Neurology,* Philadelphia: Harper & Row, 1985, Vol. 2, Pp. 1–81.

Nathan, P. Pain. In W. B. Matthews and G. H. Glaser (editors). *Recent Advances in Clinical Neurology,* 3. Edinburgh: Churchill Livingstone, 1982, Pp. 83–94.

Payne, R., and Pasternak, G. W. Pain. In M. V. Johnston, R. L. Macdonald, and A. B. Young (editors). *Principles of Drug Therapy in Neurology.* Philadelphia: Davis, 1992, Pp. 268–301.

Portenoy, R. K. (editor). Pain: mechanisms and syndromes. *Neurol. Clin.* 7:183–445, 1989.

Richards, R. L. Causalgia: a centennial review. *Arch. Neurol.* 16:339–350, 1967.

Tuttle, C. B. Drug management of pain in cancer patients. *Can. Med. Assoc. J.* 132:121–134, 1985.

Yiannikas, C., and Shahani, B. T. Painful sequelae of injuries to peripheral nerves. *Am. J. Phys. Med.* 63:53–83, 1984.

Arm and Neck Pain

Bennett, R. M. (editor). The fibrositis/fibromyalgia syndrome. Current issues and perspectives. *Am. J. Med.* 81(3A):1–115, 1986.

Corbin, K. B. Common neurological brachial pain problem. *Med. Clin. North Am.* 52:773–779, 1968.

Dawson, D. M., Hallett, M., and Millender, L. H. Thoracic outlet syndromes. In D. M. Dawson, M. Hallett, and L. H. Millender (editor). *Entrapment Neuropathies.* Boston: Little, Brown, 1983, Pp. 169–183.

Fam, A. G., and Smythe, H. A. Musculoskeletal chest wall pain. *Can. Med. Assoc. J.* 133:379–389, 1985.

Fields, W. S. Neurovascular syndromes of the neck and shoulders. *Semin. Neurol.* 1:301–309, 1981.

Friction, J. R. Myofascial pain syndrome. *Neurol. Clin.* 7:413–427, 1989.

McNaughton, F. L. Neurological aspects of shoulder lesions. In H. F. Moseley (editor). *Shoulder Lesions*. Edinburgh: Churchill Livingstone, 1969, Pp. 260–281.

Smythe, H. A. Fibrositis and other diffuse musculoskeletal syndromes. In W. N. Kelly, E. D. Harris, and S. Ruddy (editors). *Textbook of Rheumatology*. Philadelphia: Saunders, 1981.

Yoss, R. E., et al. Significance of symptoms and signs in localization of involved root in cervical disk protrusion. *Neurology* 7:673–683, 1957.

Subacute Combined Degeneration

Castle, W. B. Current concepts of pernicious anemia. *Am. J. Med.* 48:541–548, 1970.

Victor, M., and Lear, A. A. Subacute combined degeneration of the spinal cord. Current concepts of the disease process. Value of serum vitamin B12 determinations in clarifying some of the common clinical problems. *Am. J. Med.* 20:896–911, 1956.

Syringomyelia

Barnett, H. M. F., Foster, J. B., and Hudgson, P. *Syringomyelia*. Philadelphia: Saunders, 1973.

Bonafé, A., et al. High resolution computed tomography in cervical syringomyelia. *J. Comput. Assist. Tomogr.* 4:42–47, 1980.

Duffy, P. E. Syringomyelia and syringobulbia. In E. S. Goldensohn and S. H. Appel (editors). *Scientific Approaches to Neurology*. Philadelphia: Lea & Febiger, 1977, Pp. 589–603.

Gardner, W. J. Hydrodynamic mechanism of syringomyelia: its relationship to myelocele. *J. Neurol. Neurosurg. Psychiatry* 28:247–259, 1965.

Klawans, H. L., Jr. Delayed traumatic syringomyelia. *Dis. Nerv. Syst.* 29:525–528, 1968.

McIllroy, W. J., and Richardson, J. C. Syringomyelia: a clinical review of 75 cases. *Can. Med. Assoc. J.* 93:731–734, 1965.

McRae, D. L., and Standen, J. Roentgenologic findings in syringomyelia and hydromyelia. *Am. J. Roentgenol.* 98:695, 1966.

Rhoton, A. L., Jr. Syringomyelia. In C. B. Wilson and J. T. Hoff (editors). *Current Surgical Management of Neurological Disease*. Edinburgh: Churchill Livingstone, 1980.

Schlesinger, E. B., et al. Hydromyelia: clinical presentation and comparison of modalities of treatment. *Neurosurgery* 9:356–365, 1981.

Williams, B. A critical appraisal of posterior fossa surgery for communicating syringomyelia. *Brain* 101:223–250, 1978.

Low Back Pain

Abdullah, A. F., et al. Extreme-lateral lumbar disc herniations. Clinical syndrome and special problems of diagnosis. *J. Neurosurg.* 41:229–234, 1974.

Bogduk, N. The anatomy of the lumbar intervertebral disc syndrome. *Med. J. Aust.* 1:878–881, 1976.

Ciric, I., and Mikhael, M. A. Lumbar spinal-lateral recess stenosis. *Neurol. Clin.* 3:417–423, 1985.

Dorwart, R. H., and Genant, H. K. Anatomy of the lumbosacral spine. *Radiol. Clin. North Am.* 21:201–220, 1983.

Dorwart, R. H., Vogler, J. B. III, and Helms, C. A. Spinal stenosis. *Radiol. Clin. North Am.* 21:301–325, 1983.

Elliot, F. A., and Schutta, H. S. The differential diagnosis of sciatica. *Orthop. Clin. North Am.* 2:477–484, 1971.

Hall, S., et al. Lumbar spinal stenosis. Clinical

features, diagnostic procedures and results of surgical treatment in 68 patients. *Ann. Intern. Med.* 103:271–275, 1985.

Keim, H. A., and Kirkaldy-Willis, W. H. Low back pain. *CIBA Clin. Symp.* 32:1–35, 1980.

Kranzler, L. I., Schaffer, L., and Sigueira, E. B. Recent advances in the treatment of ruptured lumbar intervertebral disks. *Neurol. Clin.* 3:405–416, 1985.

Rothman, R. H. The clinical syndrome of lumbar disc disease. *Orthop. Clin. North Am.* 2:463–475, 1971.

Sander, J. E., and Sharp, F. R. Lumbosacral plexus neuritis. *Neurology* 31:470–473, 1981.

Schellinger, D. The low back pain syndrome. Diagnostic impact of high-resolution computed tomography. *Med. Clin. North Am.* 68:1631–1646, 1984.

Teplick, J. G., and Haskin, M. E. CT and lumbar disc herniation. *Radiol. Clin. North Am.* 21:259–288, 1983.

Thomas, J. E., et al. Neurogenic tumors of the sciatic nerve. A clinicopathologic study of 35 cases. *Mayo Clin. Proc.* 58:640–647, 1983.

Waddell, G. A new clinical model for the treatment of low-back pain. *Spine* 12:632–644, 1987.

Wier, B., and de Leo, R. Lumbar spinal stenosis: analysis of factors affecting outcome in 81 surgical cases. *Can. J. Neurol. Sci.* 8:295–298, 1981.

Wilkinson, H. A. Failed disk syndrome. *Am. Fam. Physician* 617:86–94, 1978.

Williams, A. L. CT diagnosis of degenerative disc disease. The bulging annulus. *Radiol. Clin. North Am.* 21:289–300, 1983.

Wilson, C. B. Significance of the small lumbar spinal canal: cauda equina compression syndromes due to spondylosis. Part 3: Intermittent claudication. *J. Neurosurg.* 31:499–506, 1969.

Wiltse, L. L., Newman, P. H., and McNab, I. Classification of spondylolysis and spondylolisthesis. *Clin. Orthop.* 117:23–29, 1976.

Raised Intracranial Pressure, Hydrocephalus, and Brain Tumors

RAISED INTRACRANIAL PRESSURE

Physiology of the Intracranial Compartment

In the adult, the cranium consists of a relatively rigid closed box with an outlet to the spinal canal at the foramen magnum. The intracranial contents comprise three components: brain tissue (about 1,500 ml), CSF (about 75 ml), and blood (about 100 ml, mostly located within the venous sinuses) (Fig. 20-1). Any increase in volume of one of these compartments must be countered by an equal reduction in volume elsewhere within the intracranial cavity, or else the intracranial pressure (ICP) will rise.

The brain itself is relatively noncompliant and the main buffering of volume is accomplished either by the downward movement of CSF into the spinal subarachnoid space or by increased resorption into the venous sinuses. A reduction in the intracranial blood volume is somewhat lim-ited because there is a constant critical need for a minimal cerebral blood flow (CBF). A theoretical curve that plots the ICP versus volume takes a hyperbolic shape, in that there is an initial compensated phase in which pressure rises only slightly with added volume, followed by a transitional phase of increasing slope, and finally an arm of the curve where even small volume changes result in marked pressure elevation. Such curves are governed by a number of other variables that affect the ICP, one of the most important being the time factor.

The brain accommodates itself much better to gradual increases of intracranial volume than to sudden catastrophic rises. Normal ICP is less than 15 mm Hg (200 mm H_2O). There are transient, well-tolerated rises to much higher levels during such maneuvers as straining, coughing, and standing on one's head. There are also minor fluctuations in the baseline pressure due to pulse pressure and respirations. When the intracranial compartment is tight and compliance is reduced, however, these normal fluctuations are no longer tolerated but become

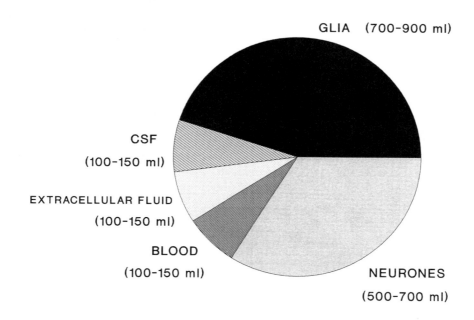

Fig. 20-1. *Components of the intracranial compartment.*

exaggerated, so that even minimal further volume changes may spawn dramatic rises in the ICP.

Cerebral Blood Flow and Autoregulation

Cerebral function depends on constant blood flow to supply glucose and oxygen, the main substrates for energy metabolism. Within about 10 seconds after global ischemia occurs, consciousness is lost and cerebral energy supplies start to diminish. If cerebral perfusion is not restored within approximately 3 minutes, the neurons and capillaries incur irreversible cellular damage.

CBF depends on both the cerebral perfusion pressure (CPP) and the cerebral vascular resis-

tance (CVR). Under normal circumstances, a system of **autoregulation** operates that maintains a fairly constant CBF in the face of changing CPP between limits of 60 to 160 mm Hg (Fig. 20-2). This constancy of CBF is maintained by the dilatation of cerebral arterioles to reduce resistance when CPP falls and constriction when CPP rises. The main factor that governs autoregulation is the pH of the extracellular fluid which bathes the brain arterioles. When the pH falls, these vessels dilate.

The most potent determinants of extracellular fluid pH are the arterial partial pressure of carbon dioxide (P_{CO_2}) and the rate of metabolism of brain cells that produce carbon dioxide and lactate as metabolic end products under aerobic and anaerobic conditions, respectively. Through this mechanism of pH dependence, arteriolar caliber (i.e., regional CBF) is linked

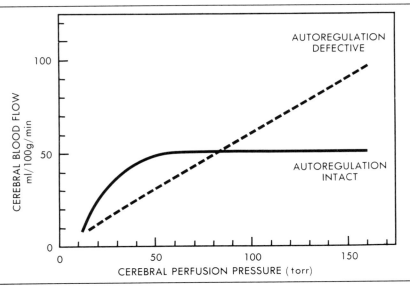

Fig. 20-2. *Relationship between cerebral blood flow and cerebral perfusion pressure. With intact autoregulation, cerebral blood flow is kept constant over a wide range of perfusion pressures.*

to regional metabolic demand. Myogenic reflexes intrinsic to arteriolar smooth muscle play a lesser role in the automatic adjustment of lumen caliber. Blood viscosity is another factor affecting CBF, but actually remains relatively constant under most circumstances. The normal resting average CBF for the whole brain is about 750 ml per minute, or 55 ml/100 gm/min. Flow is three to four times greater in the gray matter than in the white matter, reflecting a greater metabolic demand in the former.

The CPP is generally equal to the mean systemic arterial pressure minus the ICP, which in turn, is closely approximated by the intraventricular CSF pressure. It is clear from all these considerations that one of the main consequences of elevated ICP is a reduced CPP, and, as the limits of compensation are exceeded, a reduced CBF. The global cerebral ischemia that ensues becomes evident when the CPP drops below 50 mm Hg; CBF ceases altogether as the ICP approaches the mean systemic arterial pressure (normally about 100 mm Hg). These ischemic changes cause further brain swelling and edema, which compound the already elevated ICP and its effects plus those of the attendant brain distortions on central vasomotor control centers, with resultant impairment of cardiac and systemic vasoregulatory function.

Cerebral Edema

One of the most common causes of raised ICP seen clinically is cerebral edema, and therefore management is often directed toward its reduction. The precise effects of edema on brain function are uncertain, but it is clear that brain edema is a frequent contributor to increased ICP and abnormal brain shifts. Cerebral edema is defined as an increase in brain water content leading to brain swelling. Brain extracellular fluid that is in intimate contact with CSF normally constitutes about 15 percent of the total brain volume. Normally there is a very effective **blood-brain barrier** interposed between the brain extracellular space and the intravascular compartment (Fig. 20-3). Histologically this barrier consists of tight junctions of brain capillaries, which are also specialized by their lack of fenestrations. Astrocytic foot processes are in close contact with about 80 percent of the outside surface of brain capillaries and may

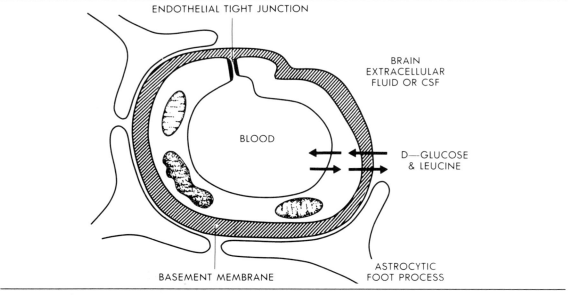

Fig. 20-3. *Schematic representation of a cerebral capillary showing the histological components of the blood-brain barrier.*

serve some additional role in the functioning of the blood-brain barrier. Edema normally preferentially accumulates and spreads within the white matter, probably because of intrinsic tissue characteristics that foster this.

Two major types of edema have been identified, **vasogenic** and **cytotoxic**. Vasogenic edema is due mainly to a disruption of the blood-brain barrier and is the most common form seen clinically. It occurs in the context of tumors, head injury, infarcts, hemorrhages, abscesses, meningitis, and lead encephalopathy. The edema fluid, which is a plasma ultrafiltrate possessing a relatively high protein content, accumulates in the extracellular space with a particular predilection for white matter. Cytotoxic edema is due to the accumulation of water and sodium within neurons, glial cells, and endothelial cells. This form of edema may be seen in the presence of acute cerebral hypoxia, water intoxication or sodium depletion, and the osmotic dysequilibrium syndromes associated with hemodialysis or diabetic ketoacidosis. Stupor and diffuse encephalopathic changes are seen with this type of edema. A third type of edema, **interstitial edema,** is seen most commonly in patients with

obstructive hydrocephalus. In this condition, periventricular white matter contains increased amounts of water and sodium, which can be seen as periventricular low-density areas on computed tomographic (CT) scans.

Causes and Consequences of Raised ICP

Raised ICP may be caused by head injury, mass lesions (e.g., tumors, hematomas, and abscesses), various metabolic and toxic disorders (e.g., Reye's syndrome and lead encephalopathy), encephalitis and meningitis, subarachnoid hemorrhage, cerebrovascular engorgement (e.g., venous sinus or jugular venous obstruction), hydrocephalus (see later discussion), or pseudotumor cerebri (discussed later). Cerebral edema constitutes a significant element of most of these entities.

One of the major consequences of raised ICP is that the CPP may be continuously or transiently impaired. Two factors contribute to this, even when the baseline ICP is only moderately elevated. First, the fundamental cause of the elevated ICP may also impair cerebral autoregulation. Under these circumstances, CBF becomes totally dependent on CPP and is very susceptible to minor changes in such variables as the systemic blood pressure and the positioning of the patient. Secondly, **plateau waves** appear. These are recurrent, sudden rises in ICP lasting 5 to 20 minutes and occurring several times per hour. Suctioning, anesthesia, hypoxia, pain, rapid eye movement sleep, and other factors can trigger their appearance. During the plateau waves, neurological function can deteriorate and lead to symptoms of blindness, decerebrate "spasms," deepening stupor or coma, respiratory irregularities, and dilated pupils. The appearance of these waves is considered an indication that the patient is on the verge of decompensation (i.e., the steep slope of the compliance curve), and therapeutic measures to reduce ICP are required urgently in this setting. Spontaneous resolution of each plateau wave may coincide with spontaneous hyperventilation of the patient.

Elevated ICP may either be generalized throughout the intracranial cavity, as occurs in lead encephalopathy and Reye's syndrome, or it may be prominent in one of the intracranial compartments, as in the region of a tumor or hematoma. When the ICP elevation originates in a particular region within the cranium, such as one cerebral hemisphere, brain tissue can be displaced, which can then lead to various brain herniations (Fig. 20-4). Herniation of the cingulate gyrus under the falx cerebri, which is relatively rigid and fixed, may occur in the presence of large unilateral anterior cerebral hemispheric lesions. One or both anterior cerebral arteries may be secondarily occluded, leading to infarction in the mesial frontal areas. More commonly, herniation of the uncus and parahippocampal gyrus of the mesial temporal lobe occurs through the tentorial notch. The third nerve is compromised early in this form of herniation, producing an ipsilateral dilated pupil, and a contralateral hemiparesis commonly occurs when the ipsilateral midbrain peduncle is also compressed by the herniating uncus and parahippocampus. The midbrain, which lies at the level of the tentorial notch, may also be shifted laterally, thereby compressing the opposite cerebral peduncle against the

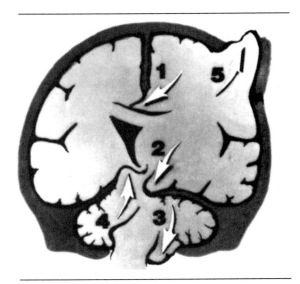

Fig. 20-4. *Schematic representation of the various forms of brain herniation. (1 = cingulate gyrus; 2 = uncal (temporal lobe); 3 = cerebellar tonsillar; 4 = upward cerebellar; 5 = transcalvarial.)* (Reprinted with permission from R. A. Fishman, Cerebrospinal Fluid in Diseases of the Nervous System. *Philadelphia: Saunders, 1980.)*

rigid tentorium with a resultant ipsilateral hemiparesis. The sylvian aqueduct, which is also at the level of the tentorial notch, is easily obstructed, causing hydrocephalus and compounding the elevated pressure in the supratentorial compartment. The deepening coma, which is a sign of this form of herniation, is largely due to compromise of the midbrain reticular activating system.

The syndrome of rostral-caudal deterioration, which may occur with either transtentorial or central herniation of the brainstem, is described in Chapter 5. A possible secondary vascular consequence of transtentorial herniation is occlusion of the posterior cerebral artery. Downward displacement of the brainstem may also lead to tearing of brainstem penetrating arteries, causing the socalled Duret's hemorrhages in the pons and midbrain. Downward herniation of the cerebellar tonsils through the foramen magnum, often seen with posterior fossa mass lesions, exerts pressure effects on the medulla and may lead to rapid vasomotor collapse and apnea. Occasional upward herniation of the cerebellum through the tentorial notch evokes signs similar to those of uncal herniation.

Diagnosis of Elevated ICP

The classic clinical triad of a deteriorating level of consciousness, bradycardia, and increased systolic blood pressure may not appear even though intracranial hypertension is significant. The most reliable signs are deepening stupor and papilledema, but even papilledema may be absent in patients with raised ICP. A sixth nerve palsy may constitute a nonlocalizing sign of elevated ICP. A CT scan that shows brain shifts or significant edema is a good indicator of elevated ICP, but CT findings may be normal despite a high ICP. The only sure way of diagnosing elevated ICP is through actual measurement. This can be accomplished by a variety of methods, such as recording pressures from the epidural space by special transducers (e.g., Ladd monitor) or by directly measuring the ventricular CSF pressure by an indwelling ventricular catheter. Although an advantage of the latter method is that it permits the withdrawal of CSF to reduce pressure, the risk of infection during long-term ICP recording is much greater than that with epidural transducers.

The level of ICP per se is not the most important consideration in patients who may be on the verge of decompensation. If sudden deterioration is to be prevented, intracranial compliance should ideally be determined. Attempts have been made to do this by rapidly infusing or removing fixed amounts of saline (1 ml) via an intraventricular catheter and measuring the attendant effects on the ICP.

Management of Elevated ICP

Attempts should be made to keep the ICP within the range of 15 to 20 mm Hg using both conservative and surgical means. The strategies for reducing ICP are fourfold (Table 20-1):

1. Neurosurgical removal of the intracranial mass lesion (e.g., subdural hematoma or cerebellar infarction)
2. Reduction of the cerebral edema

Table 20-1. Management of Elevated Intracranial Pressure

Medical approaches
  Reduce cerebral edema
    Hyperventilation
    Osmotic agents (mannitol)
    Corticosteroids (dexamethasone)
  Reduce fluid intake
  Keep patient in head-up position
  Prevent hypertension and seizures
  Sedation and analgesia when necessary
  Hypothermia (avoid fever)
  Adequate ventilation
Surgical treatment
  Remove the cause (e.g., tumor, subdural
    hematoma)
  Ventriculostomy or shunt to treat hydrocephalus
  Subtemporal decompression and removal of
    necrotic brain tissue in certain cases

3. Reduction of intracranial blood volume by hyperventilation
4. Withdrawal of fluid from the cerebral ventricles and shunt installation when hydrocephalus is present

In extreme cases of intractable brain swelling, bone has been removed to permit subtemporal decompression.

When possible, the primary cause of the elevated ICP should be treated neurosurgically. Unfortunately, this is not always immediately practical because many cases of elevated ICP are not due to discrete operable brain lesions. Additionally, operating on a patient who is deeply comatose and possibly in a poor general state poses a high risk. A craniotomy can be performed but brain displacement and swelling may continue in the face of severe cerebral edema.

Osmotic agents such as mannitol are given in the acute stages to reduce cerebral edema and the extracellular fluid volume. They are very effective in reducing ICP and the effects may be witnessed within minutes. The initial dose is 0.25 gm per kilogram of body weight given rapidly intravenously through a large-bore needle in a 25% solution, with a urinary catheter in place. The aim is to elevate the serum osmolality to between 305 and 315 mOsm/L but at the same time to avoid severe dehydration. This dose may be repeated every 2 to 3 hours as needed, to a total dose of 2 gm/kg/day. Efficacy may be diminished following several doses, and a rebound effect may rarely occur. Furosemide is less effective but is often given in addition to the mannitol. Steroids are less effective and take 8 to 12 hours to begin working. However, dexamethasone (10 mg intravenously in the acute phase followed by 4 mg every 6 hours) may help control cerebral edema in patients suffering from a tumor or head trauma. A very effective temporary measure that can often sustain a patient until more definitive therapy is implemented is intubation and hyperventilation to achieve an arterial P_{CO_2} of 25 to 30 mm Hg. This lowers ICP by causing vasoconstriction and hence reduces the intracranial blood volume.

Attention to general measures that influence ICP is also an important part of management. The head should be elevated, usually to 15 to 30 degrees, and neck twisting or manipulation avoided. Hyperthermia, which elevates ICP through increased CBF, should be reduced. Normal fluid volume and electrolyte balance should be maintained. Dehydration should be prevented because it can diminish the general circulatory volume and cardiac output. Seizures should be treated or prophylactic therapy instituted if they pose a significant threat. Hypoxia with levels of P_{O_2} below 50 mm Hg can also worsen raised ICP. It is especially important to prevent hypotension because CPP is often barely adequate in these cases.

ABNORMALITIES OF CSF FLOW AND PRODUCTION

Physiology of CSF

The CSF serves as a "sink" for brain extracellular fluid, which helps maintain the chemical homeostasis of the brain. It also serves as a buffer to help regulate ICP, as discussed earlier. The CSF may also furnish mechanical support for the brain, maintain a constant brain temperature, and serve as a substitute lymphatic system. Seventy percent of the CSF is manufactured by the choroid plexus within the lateral, third, and fourth ventricles, and 30 percent by transependymal and possibly transpial production. The capillaries of the choroid plexus bear many similarities to those of the glomeruli of the kidney. CSF is formed as an ultrafiltrate of blood as well as by active secretion. Its rate of formation of 0.35 ml per minute is remarkably constant even when CSF pressure is high. The total CSF volume of 150 ml (100 ml, intracranial; 50 ml, spinal) is turned over three to four times per day.

After formation, CSF exits the ventricular system via the two lateral foramina of Luschka and the midline foramen of Magendie of the fourth ventricle. Some CSF descends into the spinal subarachnoid spaces but, after entering the basal cisterns, most ascends over the cerebral convexity to the arachnoid villae, where absorption occurs. The arachnoid villae are specialized structures possessing a postulated valvelike mechanism that empty into the sagittal venous sinus. CSF is absorbed by bulk flow, with resorption normally starting at an outflow pressure of about 70 mm H_2O. With further increases in CSF pressure, absorption increases linearly to a level of four to six times the baseline values. This capacity to augment absorption, partially by the increased use of other absorption sites (e.g., transependymally or via subarachnoid spaces around spinal roots) is a possible compensatory mechanism that operates in hydrocephalus.

Hydrocephalus

Hydrocephalus represents a condition of increased CSF volume within enlarged ventricular spaces, usually under increased pressure. When ventricles enlarge secondary to cerebral atrophy, this is termed *hydrocephalus ex vacuo*. There are two main groups of hydrocephalus: **noncommunicating (obstructive)**, in which the CSF flow is blocked within the ventricular system or at the outlet foramina, and **communicating**, in which the CSF flow is impaired in the subarachnoid spaces or at the actual site of absorption (e.g., normal-pressure hydrocephalus). Very rare cases are possibly due to an

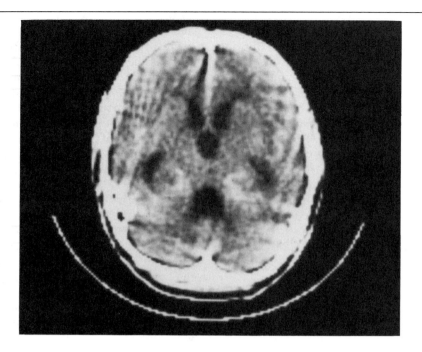

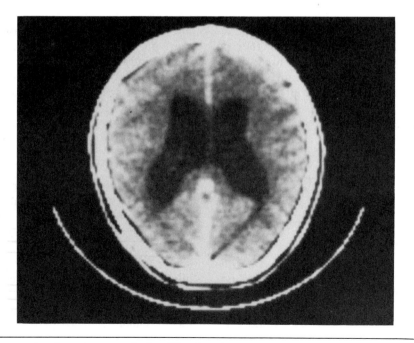

Fig. 20-5. *CT scans showing acute ventricular dilatation due to communicating hydrocephalus. Note dilatation of temporal horns and fourth ventricle. Patient had Arnold-Chiari malformation.*

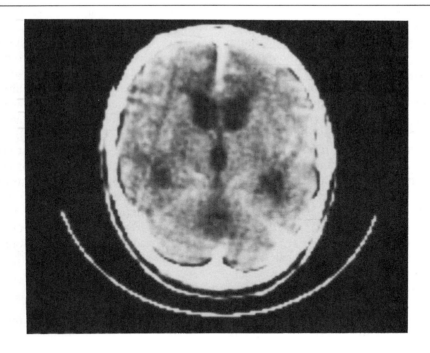

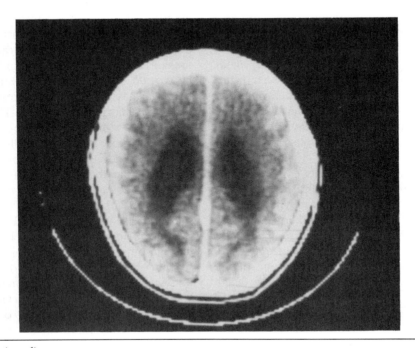

Fig. 20-5 *(Continued)*.

increase in CSF production (e.g., papilloma of the choroid plexus).

Most cases of hydrocephalus are congenital and fall into two major categories: those associated with spina bifida cystica or the Arnold-Chiari malformation, and those due to congenital lesions of the sylvian aqueduct (aqueductal stenosis). The Chiari type II (Arnold-Chiari) malformation consists of herniation of the cerebellar vermis and fourth ventricle into the upper cervical canal, often in conjunction with spina bifida cystica and bony anomalies at the craniocervical junction area. The hydrocephalus associated with this disorder is usually due to aqueductal stenosis but may also be of the communicating variety (Fig. 20-5).

Congenital aqueductal stenosis has an unknown etiology, but could stem from developmental abnormalities or an intrauterine viral infection that affected the ependymal cells. A sex-linked inherited variety has been described.

Another developmental abnormality producing hydrocephalus and a largely dilated cystic fourth ventricle is the **Dandy-Walker malformation,** which is due to atresia of the foramina of Luschka and Magendie. Other conditions associated with hydrocephalus in children and adults are intraventricular tumors (e.g., colloid cyst of the third ventricle and ependymoma); paraventricular tumors; cysts and other mass lesions of the posterior fossa; aneurysms of the vein of Galen and other vascular malformations in children; and previous meningitis, head injuries, or ependymitis. Communicating (normal-pressure) hydrocephalus is discussed in Chapter 4.

Patients with hydrocephalus exhibit a progressive picture of elevated ICP or an acute picture of suddenly decompensated intracranial hypertension. Gradual abnormal head enlargement is often the presenting feature in children because the cranial sutures are not yet fused and permit expansion. There is disproportional growth of the cranium compared to the facial bones, frontal bossing of the skull, thinning of the cranial vault, dilatation of scalp veins, difficulty with vertical gaze ("sunset eyes" in extreme cases), intellectual deterioration, and gait difficulty with spasticity in the legs. Adult patients may present with headache, papilledema, intellectual deterioration, and gait difficulties.

In certain cases, hydrocephalus arrests spontaneously and, when the neurological picture has been stable for a number of years, treatment is not indicated. Hydrocephalus is usually readily apparent on CT scans, which may also indicate the site of the blockage in cases of obstruction. In certain cases, dynamic CT scanning with water-soluble contrast material or radionuclide cisternography helps determine the site of obstruction. Many patients require diversionary procedures, such as ventriculoatrial or ventriculoperitoneal shunts. Unfortunately, many children with shunts suffer repeated shunt infections and other complications that require multiple shunt revisions.

Pseudotumor Cerebri

Pseudotumor cerebri (benign intracranial hypertension) is an uncommon syndrome with a diverse etiology. In this disorder, brain extracellular water content is increased, which leads to an elevated ICP without hydrocephalus. Patients show diffuse brain swelling and frequently small slitlike ventricles. Despite a significantly elevated ICP, brain herniation does not occur because the intracranial hypertension is generalized. Lumbar puncture can be carried out safely in this setting, once CT scanning has ruled out the presence of brain shifts or enlarged ventricles. The usual presenting symptom is headache, at times with vomiting. There is usually papilledema and perhaps a sixth nerve palsy. Neurological signs are otherwise lacking and patients are alert and quite well, considering what would be expected in patients with comparable CSF pressure due to an intracranial mass lesion. The CSF in these patients is normal, apart from low protein values in some. Most patients are obese young women who manifest evidence of some endocrinological disturbance such as menstrual irregularities or pregnancy. Hypervitaminosis A, tetracycline ingestion, steroid or oral contraceptive use, Cushing's syndrome, and hypoparathyroidism are some other identifiable causes.

The majority of cases remit spontaneously

within about 6 months. Weight loss should be encouraged. Repeated lumbar punctures should be done every few weeks to lower the CSF pressure to within the normal range, or when the patient becomes symptomatic. The most pressing concern in these patients is the threat of visual loss, which can occur suddenly but is usually preceded by a stepwise deterioration or obscurations, consisting of very brief bouts of blindness due to papilledema. Visual fields should be defined by perimetry and acuity should be charted on a regular basis. If vision appears to be deteriorating and the ICP cannot be controlled, the installation of a lumboperitoneal shunt or operative slitting of the optic nerve sheath should be considered. Agents such as glycerol, which is poorly tolerated and high in calories, and steroids, which themselves can cause this syndrome, as well as acetazolamide or furosemide are frequently used in the management of this disorder.

BRAIN TUMORS

Pathophysiology and Etiology

The etiology of primary brain tumors is unknown, but some evidence suggests that viruses (e.g., papovaviruses), irradiation, and exposure to certain petrochemicals may be responsible in some patients, as is the case for cancer in general. The most common histological tumor types in adults are glioma (especially glioblastoma, the most malignant form of primary brain tumor, which comprises about 30% of all the cases of primary brain tumors), meningioma, pituitary adenoma, and acoustic neuroma. In children, medulloblastoma, cystic astrocytoma, ependymoma, and pontine glioma are the most common tumors, all of which tend to be located infratentorially. Table 20-2 summarizes the main features of the most common brain tumors.

Most tumors arise from glial and supporting elements of the nervous system and only rarely do they originate from neural elements (e.g., a ganglioglioma). The histological makeup of the tumor is the most important factor dictating the growth pattern and malignancy, but the location of the tumor is also an important determinant of morbidity as well as accessibility to treatment. Certain tumors, although histologically benign, by virtue of their proximity to vital neural structures and growth within a confined space deep in the brain may produce disproportionately high morbidity. For example, meningiomas, pinealomas, and craniopharyngiomas behave in this manner. Many malignant brain tumors invade normal brain tissue in a diffuse and widespread manner, and therefore cannot be easily extirpated at operation. The tumor cells in gliomas tend to spread along white matter tracts and may invade the contralateral hemisphere across the corpus callosum. Other tumors such as acoustic neuromas and meningiomas tend to be primarily extraaxial, although they may compress and even invade adjacent brain tissue. Tumors such as medulloblastomas, ependymomas, and glioblastomas produce widespread seeding throughout intracranial and spinal subarachnoid spaces. These same tumors may also rarely produce distant metastases to such sites as the lymph nodes and bone, especially following operation.

Epidemiology

The approximate incidence of primary and secondary (metastatic) brain tumors is about 8 per 100,000 population. Primary brain tumors exhibit a minor peak in incidence in children, and are second only to leukemia as a cause of cancer in this age group. There is a steadily rising incidence throughout adulthood, which peaks in the sixth and seventh decades. Certain tumors such as meningiomas and pituitary adenomas show a higher incidence in females. A familial tendency toward the formation of CNS neoplasms, especially gliomas, is a rare occurrence. Certain inherited neuroectodermal developmental syndromes are linked with intracranial neoplasms. For example, neurofibromatosis is associated with an increased incidence of optic gliomas, thalamic gliomas, meningiomas, and bilateral acoustic neuromas. Cerebellar hemangioblastoma occurs in von Hippel–Lindau syndrome. Medulloblastoma can be associated with the multiple basal-cell nevus syndrome.

Table 20-2. Characteristics of Most Common Brain Tumors

Tumor	Age occurrence and incidence	Location	Symptoms	Therapy	Prognosis	Special features
Astrocytoma (low-grade)	Adults	Cerebral hemispheres, thalamus	Seizures, neurological deficit	Biopsy, radical excision where possible, possibly RTx	Survival many years	May transform to glioblastoma
Cerebellar astrocytoma of childhood	Children, rarely adults	Midline cerebellum, cerebellar hemispheres	Limb ataxia, ↑ICP, HA	Drain cyst, excise tumor nodule, RTx	Excellent, cure possible	Essentially benign in childhood cases
Brainstem glioma	Children, young adults	Pons	Multiple bilateral cranial nerve palsies, facial myokymia, gait difficulty	RTx, shunt as needed	Survival several years	Expansion of brainstem, rarely causes hydrocephalus, may mimic multiple sclerosis
Astrocytoma (malignant or glioblastoma multiforme)	Adults	Cerebral hemispheres	HA, ↑ICP, seizures, neurological and behavioral deficits	Radical excision, RTx, CTx	Survival 6–30 months	Hemorrhages common, rarely metastasizes outside CNS, may seed in subarachnoid spaces
Oligodendro-glioma	Adults	Cerebral hemispheres	Seizures, HA, neurological deficits	Excision, RTx	Fairly good	Calcifications common, may present as intracerebral hemorrhage, symptoms may go back for several years

Tumor	Age	Location	Clinical features	Treatment	Prognosis	Comments
Medullo-blastoma	Two thirds, 5–9 yr; one third, 15–35 yr	Midline cerebellum, lateral cerebellum (especially adults)	Head tilt, wide-based ataxic gait, HA, V, and ↑ICP	Excision, RTx including spinal and CNS axis, CTx, shunt	Survival many years	Tends to seed spinal canal and may metastasize outside CNS via circulation or shunt
Ependymoma	Children, adults	Intraventricular 4th ventricle, cerebral hemisphere (intraventricular)	↑ICP, HA, cranial nerve palsies	Excision, RTx, shunt	Fair	May seed spinal canal
CNS lymphoma	Adults	Variable, hemispheres, deep midline, diffuse	Behavioral changes, seizures, hydrocephalus	RTx, CTx	Survival for many years possible	Well seen on contrast-enhanced CT scan, associated with AIDS
Meningioma	Adults, especially middle-aged women	Cerebral convexity parasagittal, sphenoid wing, intraventricular, base of brain, posterior fossa	Seizures, headaches, TIA-like symptoms, neurological deficits	Excision, RTx	Good, cure possible but regrowth common if not completely excised	May be multiple (e.g., in neurofibromatosis) and may recur, often calcified, supplied mainly by external carotid artery, tends to erode bone, occasionally malignant features, rapid growth during pregnancy
Acoustic neuroma	Adults	Cerebello-pontine angle	Hearing loss, vertigo, Vth and VIIth nerve involvement, ataxia, rarely hydrocephalus	Excision by posterior fossa or translabyrinthine approach	Excellent	Bilateral in neurofibromatosis-2

Table 20-2 (Continued).

Tumor	Age occurrence and incidence	Location	Symptoms	Therapy	Prognosis	Special features
Optic glioma	Children (16 mo–16 yr)	Optic nerve, chiasm, tract	Headache, optic atrophy, visual loss, field changes, proptosis, hypothalamic involvement, hydrocephalus	Excision if possible and progressing, RTx, CTx, shunt as needed	Good, long survival	Associated with neurofibromatosis in about 40%, may show calcifications, cysts
Hemangio-blastoma	Adults	Cerebellum, rarely elsewhere	HA, vomiting, ataxia, ↑ICP	Excision	Excellent	Associated with von Hippel–Lindau syndrome (plus retinal angiomas), associated with polycythemia, may be cystic
Pinealoma	Children, young adults	Pineal, rarely elsewhere	Parinaud's syndrome, hydro-cephalus, personality changes, precocious or delayed puberty	Excision, RTx, shunt	Good	Various degrees of malignancy, may metastasize outside CNS
Cranio-pharyngioma	Children, young adults, adults	Suprasellar	Behavioral changes, visual loss, HA, hypothalamic and endocrine disturbances, hydro-cephalus, growth retardation	Excision, RTx	Good	Tends to be calcified in children, surgery may be difficult due to adherence to carotid arteries and hypothalamus

Tumor	Age	Location	Clinical features	Treatment	Prognosis	Comments
Pituitary adenoma	Adults, children	Sellar, may extend suprasellar	Visual loss (superior quadrantanopia, optic atrophy), amenorrhea and galactorrhea, Cushing's disease, hypopituitarism, acromegaly, growth failure	Transsphenoidal surgery for microadenoma, transsphenoidal biopsy and RTx, transfrontal excision, proton beam RTx, bromocriptine	Good	Microadenoma most common, especially prolactinoma; may bleed
Metastatic	Adults, occasionally children; most common intracranial tumor	Superficial gray matter, subcortical, cerebellum	Seizures, HA, ↑ICP, neurological deficits	Excision when single, RTx depending on sensitivity, dexamethasone for edema	Poor, depends mainly on primary tumor	May be multiple even if not visualized, ring enhancement with surrounding edema on CT, may bleed, most common primaries: lung, breast, melanoma, renal carcinoma, GI, choriocarcinoma

HA = headache; CTx = chemotherapy; RTx = radiotherapy; V = vomiting; ↑ICP = raised intracranial pressure; TIA = transient ischemic attack; GI = gastrointestinal.

Clinical Picture and Diagnosis

Brain tumors tend to produce symptoms by one of the following mechanisms:

1. Elevation of ICP and production of brain shifts through mass effect, edema, and obstruction of CSF pathways
2. Irritation of gray matter, which produces seizures
3. Destruction of localized areas of brain tissue, either directly or through effects on vasculature
4. Bleeding, which leads to intracranial hemorrhage (most commonly glioblastoma, oligodendroglioma, or metastases from melanoma, renal cell carcinoma, or choriocarcinoma)
5. Affecting hormone levels, either the overproduction or underproduction (pituitary and other parasellar tumors)
6. Affecting adjacent bony structures, which causes erosion or thickening of bone (e.g., meningiomas)

With the foregoing in mind, it is easy to understand why the major presenting features of brain tumors are headache, vomiting, behavior and personality changes, increasing stupor, visual symptoms such as diplopia, seizures, and focal neurological deficits such as aphasia, hemiparesis, or visual field defects. Certain tumors such as meningiomas may give rise to transient focal neurological deficits resembling transient ischemic attacks.

Some tumors grow in relatively silent areas of the brain such as the nondominant (right) frontal or temporal areas, where they may reach substantial size before symptoms such as seizures occur. Some tumors are discovered incidentally by neuroimaging studies done for unrelated reasons.

The electroencephalogram characteristically shows slowing with polymorphic delta waves that are often intermixed with sharp waves in the area of the tumor, which may spread to involve the whole hemisphere in the case of malignant invasive tumors (Fig. 20-6). Plain skull x-ray studies can reveal evidence of ele-

Fig. 20-6. *EEG from an 82-year-old man with a left frontoparietal glioblastoma. Note the absence of normal background, widespread polymorphic delta activity, and sharp waves over the left hemisphere.*

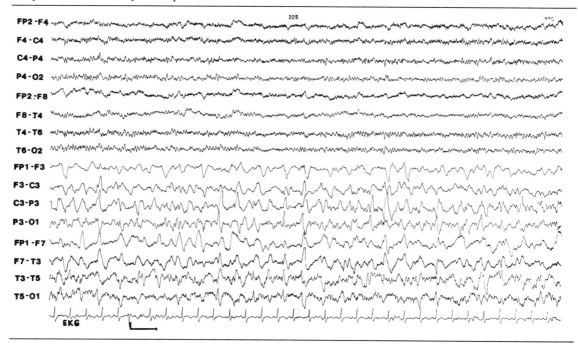

vated ICP such as erosion of the posterior clinoids (Fig. 20-7), shift of the pineal gland, calcifications within the tumor, increased vascular markings (with meningioma), or enlargement of the sella turcica (with pituitary neoplasms) (Fig. 20-8).

Angiography, which may be important for preoperative planning, is frequently helpful in defining the blood supply of the tumor and often depicts a capillary blush in the area of primary brain tumors that is produced by tumor vessels, especially in the case of malignant gliomas. In addition, the mass effect of the tumor gives rise to stretching, bowing, and displacement of various vessels. For investigational purposes, CT or MRI scanning is the method of choice (Figs. 20-9 to 20-17). Many vascular tumors exhibit contrast enhancement. Glioblastomas frequently appear as a serpiginous contrast-enhanced ring surrounding an area of low density (necrosis) with edema encompassing the tumor. MRI scanning has the potential to detect early low-grade gliomas and also to demonstrate small gliomas in the posterior fossa. CT scanning can also fairly accurately portray the extent of ventricular distortion and hydrocephalus. Frequently studies in the coronal plane are advantageous for the demonstration of small pituitary neoplasms. In many cases, a presumptive preoperative diagnosis can be made on the basis of CT, MRI, and angiographic findings. However, for definitive diagnosis and treatment planning, a histological diagnosis should be obtained, either using tissue acquired at the time of tumor removal or, in the case of inaccessible tumors, by stereotaxic CT-guided needle biopsy.

Management and Prognosis

Advances in neurosurgical technique such as the operating microscope, ultrasonic aspirator, and laser coagulation now permit the more complete removal of brain tumors with less morbidity than witnessed in the past. Whenever possible, a brain tumor should be surgically excised to the maximal degree allowable, without producing undue additional neurological disability. Although cure cannot be achieved in patients with primary malignant brain tumors, mere debulk-

Fig. 20-7. *Plain skull x-ray study showing erosion of the dorsum sellae* (arrow) *due to raised intracranial pressure.*

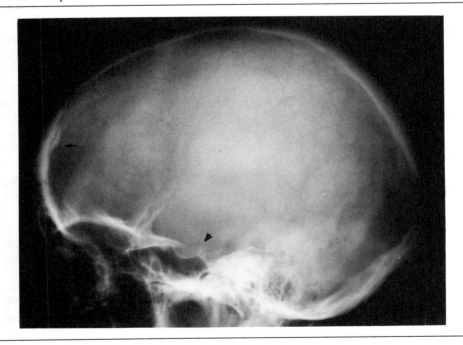

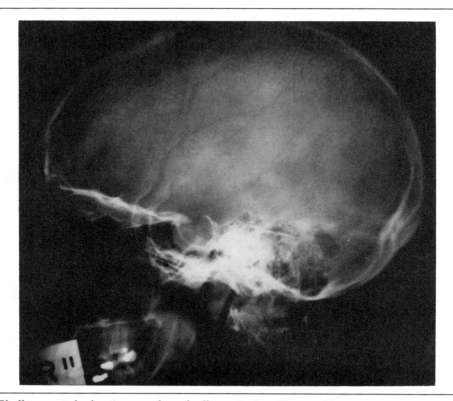

Fig. 20-8. *Skull x-ray study showing an enlarged sella turcica in a 28-year-old woman with a pituitary adenoma (prolactinoma).*

ing of the tumor can provide symptomatic relief from the pressure effects plus additional weeks of useful life, and also allow time for other modes of therapy to take effect. Reoperation may be necessary once the tumor regrows.

Whether surgery is advocated for single or multiple metastases to the brain depends on considerations such as the location of the tumor, or tumors, the age and overall condition of the patient, the prognosis for the primary cancer, and the degree of the tumor's radiosensitivity. The findings from a recent randomized trial have shown that surgical removal of single brain metastases followed by radiotherapy translates into longer survival, fewer recurrences, and a better quality of life, compared to the course seen in patients treated by radiotherapy alone.

In certain cases, irradiation to the tumor and other areas of the neuraxis using fractionated doses of up to 6,000 rads remains the most frequently used adjunctive therapy in patients with malignant brain tumors. However, this treatment carries the risk of inducing brain necrosis, which may appear several months afterwards and be difficult to distinguish from recurrent tumor. PET or SPECT scanning may, however, be useful in this regard. A very uncommon risk of radiotherapy in long-term survivors is the induction of a second primary brain neoplasm.

Chemotherapy, particularly using nitrosourea agents such as carmustine (BCNU) or methotrexate, is being used increasingly. A currently popular regimen includes procarbazine, vincristine, and lomustine (CCNU). Methods that enhance the delivery of drugs to the tumor, such as intracarotid injection, are being adopted, as are other modes of treatment such as immunotherapy and hyperthermia. Utilizing various combinations of these treatments, survival has been increased from 6 months to up to 2½ years or longer in a significant number of patients with glioblastoma. Unfortunately long-

Fig. 20-9. *Enhanced CT scan showing a massive bifrontal meningioma in a 55-year-old woman with a 1-year history of vague headaches, personality changes, memory problems, and vertigo.*

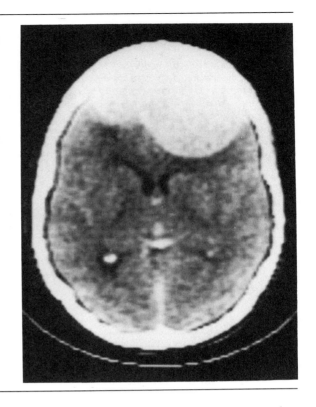

Fig. 20-10. *Coronal enhanced CT image showing a suprasellar calcified lesion with some surrounding edema in a 56-year-old woman with a 6-month history of change in personality, hyperphagia, hypersomnia, loss of libido, headache, and hypothyroidism. The patient had a craniopharyngioma. Also note the enlarged lateral ventricles (hydrocephalus).*

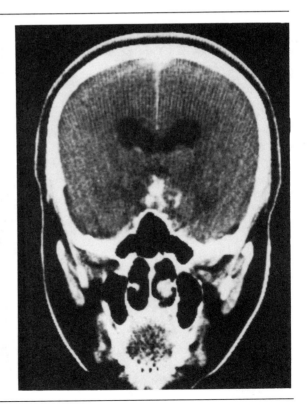

Fig. 20-11. *Coronal enhanced CT image showing intrasellar chromophobe adenoma extending slightly above the sella* (arrow) *This 54-year-old woman presented with a 3-month history of right-sided retroorbital headache, decreased balance, anorexia, increased thirst, loss of libido, bitemporal visual field defects, a prolactin level of 44 μgm/L, and mild diminution of growth hormone and follicle stimulating hormone–luteinizing hormone reserve on stimulation testing. The tumor was removed by a transsphenoidal approach.*

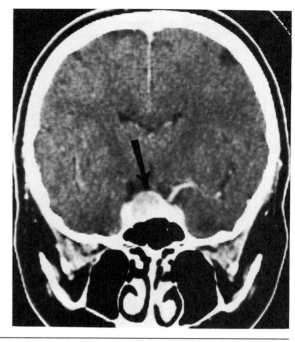

Fig. 20-12. *Enhanced CT image of a left temporal glioblastoma. Note contrast enhancement* (arrowhead), *extensive edema, hemorrhagic areas in the tumor, marked ventricular compression, midline shift, and hydrocephalus.*

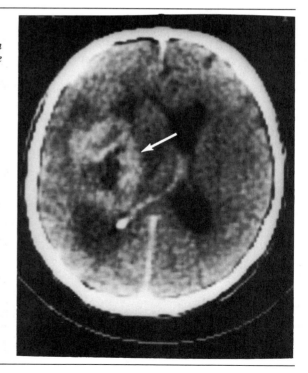

Fig. 20-13. *Enhanced CT scan showing typical ring-enhancing appearance with marked surrounding white matter edema in a patient with left parietal metastatic lung carcinoma.*

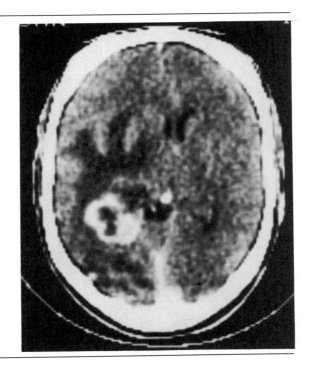

Fig. 20-14. *Enhanced CT image showing bilateral acoustic neuromas* (arrows), *more prominent on the left, in a patient with neurofibromatosis-2. The patient was a 35-year-old woman with a 3-month history of headaches, but normal hearing and balance. She had two café-au-lait spots. Audiograms were normal but brainstem auditory evoked potentials were abnormal.*

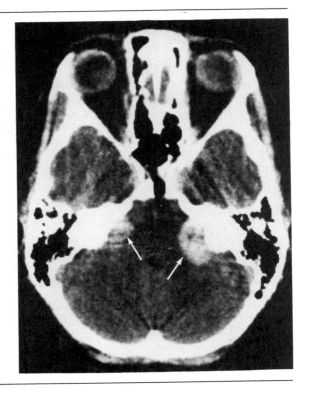

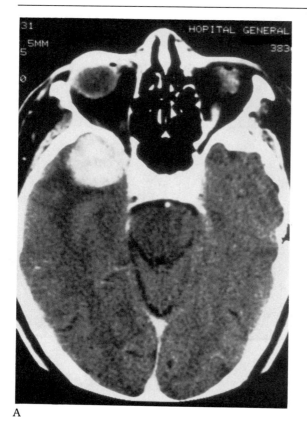

A

Fig. 20-15. *(A) Enhanced CT scan in a 68-year-old woman with a right sphenoid wing meningioma. The patient presented with a spell, which was initially thought to be transient global amnesia, followed the next day by a generalized tonic-clonic seizure. (B) Hematoxylin-eosin–stained histological section from the meningioma showing a typical psammoma body. The dark area represents calcium. (Original magnification ×25.)*

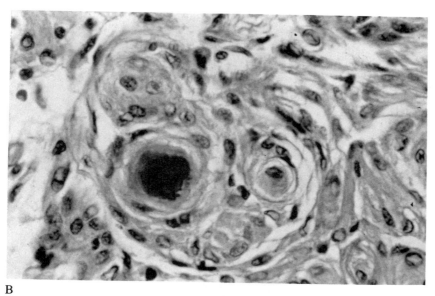

B

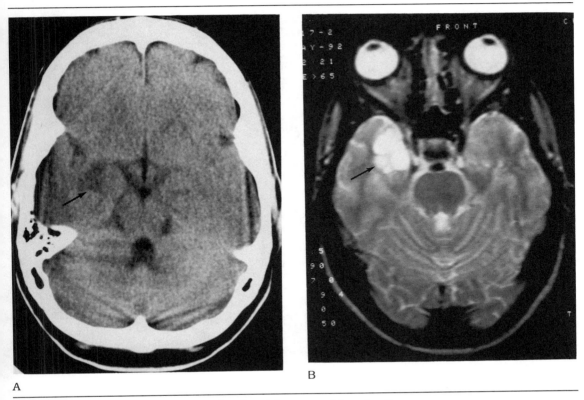

Fig. 20-16. *(A) Unenhanced CT scan showing right temporal low-density area* (arrow) *in a patient with temporal lobe epilepsy. (B) T₂-weighted MRI scan from the same patient clearly showing an area of increased signal* (arrow), *representing a low-grade glioma.*

term survivors frequently suffer neurobehavioral side effects secondary to the treatment proper.

Palliative measures are also an important part of the protocol. Dexamethasone (4 to 20 mg taken orally every 6 hours) is used to reduce cerebral edema. Anticonvulsants are prescribed in patients with seizures and as prophylaxis. In certain cases, ventricular shunting must be performed to relieve hydrocephalus, but carries the risk of providing an additional pathway for tumor metastases to occur. The overall prognosis in patients with primary malignant brain tumors is poor. Many untreated patients with such tumors die within 3 months after symptoms first appear. Elderly patients with a significant neurological disability prior to treatment have the poorest prognosis.

Meningeal Carcinomatosis

Primary cancers of the breast, lung, kidney, melanomas, and lymphomas are among those that may spread diffusely to the meninges. Typically, patients are gravely ill with severe headache, meningeal signs, stupor, papilledema, and focal cranial nerve findings. CT scans may reveal the existence of enlarged ventricles and diffuse meningeal enhancement. The CSF is characteristically under high pressure with an elevated protein level and a low glucose concentration. Several lumbar punctures may be necessary before CSF specimens are obtained that yield tumor cells on cytological studies. Treatment with dexamethasone, radiotherapy to the spinal axis, and intrathecal chemotherapy may extend survival for a short period.

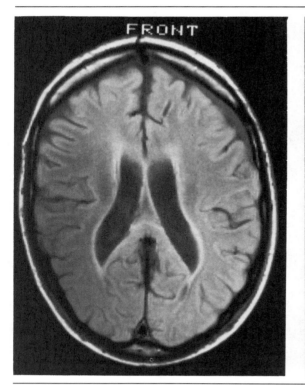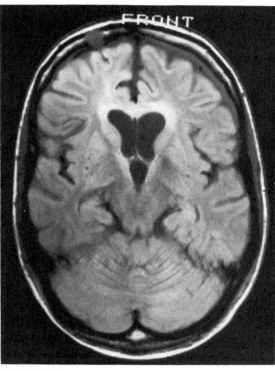

Fig. 20-17. *Proton-density MRI cuts showing increased signal around enlarged ventricles, including the third. The patient was a 24-year-old man with a 5-month history of intractable vomiting with minimal nausea, weight loss from 120 to 70 pounds (54 to 31.5 kg), apathy, intermittent ataxia, and a left visual field defect. His condition suddenly deteriorated with coma and decerebration. Stereotaxic biopsy of the periventricular tumor revealed a dysgerminoma that responded very well to radiotherapy.*

BIBLIOGRAPHY

Raised Intracranial Pressure and Hydrocephalus

Ahlskog, J. E. Pseudotumor cerebri. *Ann. Intern. Med.* 97:249–256, 1982.

Bruce, D. A. The pathophysiology of increased intracranial pressure. In *Current Concepts*. Kalamazoo, MI: Upjohn Company, 1978, Pp. 3–51.

De Meyer, W. Megalencephaly in children. *Neurology* 22:634–643, 1972.

Fishman, R. A. Brain edema. *N. Engl. J. Med.* 293:706–711, 1975.

Fishman, R. A. The pathophysiology and treatment of brain edema. In W. B. Matthews and G. H. Glaser (editors). *Recent Advances in Clinical Neurology*, No. 2. Edinburgh: Churchill Livingstone, 1978, Pp. 119–127.

Fishman, R. A. *Cerebrospinal Fluid in Diseases of the Nervous System*. Philadelphia: Saunders, 1980.

Forrest, D. M., and Cooper, D. G. W. Complications of ventriculo-atrial shunts: a review of 455 cases. *J. Neurosurg.* 29:506–512, 1968.

Goldstein, G. W. Pathogenesis of brain edema and hemorrhage: role of the brain capillary. *Pediatrics* 64:357–360, 1979.

Ignelzi, R. J. Cerebral edema: present perspectives. *Neurosurgery* 4:338–342, 1979.

McDermott, M. W., and Wilson, C. B. Management of primary brain tumors. In V. C. Hachinski (editor). *Challenges in Neurology.* Philadelphia: Davis, 1992, Pp. 215–255.

Milhorat, T. H. Hydrocephalus. In T. H. Milhorat. *Pediatric Neurosurgery.* Philadelphia: Davis, 1978, Pp. 91–135.

Miller, D., and Adams, H. Physiopathology and management of increased intracranial pressure. In M. C. Mitckley, J. L. O'Leary, and B. Jennett (editors). *Scientific Foundations of Neurology.* Philadelphia: Davis, 1972, Pp. 308–324.

Miller, J. D. The management of cerebral oedema. *Br. J. Hosp. Med.* Feb. 1979, Pp. 152–164.

Rockoff, M. A., and Ropper, A. H. Treatment of intracranial hypertension. In A. H. Ropper, S. K. Kennedy, and N. T. Zervas (editors). *Neurological and Neurosurgical Intensive Care.* Baltimore: University Park Press, 1983, Pp. 21–38.

Rogers, M. C., and Traystman, R.J. An overview of the intracranial vault. Physiology and philosophy. *Crit. Care Clin.* 1:195–204, 1985.

Ropper, A. H. Raised intracranial pressure in neurologic disease. *Semin. Neurol.* 4:397–407, 1984.

Sklar, F. H., et al. Cerebrospinal fluid dynamics in patients with pseudotumor cerebri. *Neurosurgery* 5:208–216, 1979.

Weisberg, L. A. Benign intracranial hypertension. *Medicine* 54:197–207, 1975.

Brain Tumors

Ausman, J. I., French, L A., and Baker, A. B. Intracranial neoplasms. In A. B. Baker and L. H. Baker (editors). *Clinical Neurology,* revised edition. Philadelphia: Harper & Row, 1984.

Brown, R. C., Gunderson, L., and Plenk, H. P. Medulloblastoma. A review of the LDS hospital experience. *Cancer* 40:56–60, 1977.

Coxe, W. S. Intracranial tumors. In S. G. Eliasson, A. L. Prensky, and W. B. Hardin, Jr. *Neurological Pathophysiology,* 2nd ed. New York: Oxford University Press, 1978, Pp. 305–320.

Daly, D. D., Svien, H. J., and Yoss, R. E. Intermittent cerebral symptoms with meningiomas. *Arch. Neurol.* 5:287–293, 1961.

Kahn, E. A., et al. Forty-five years experience with craniopharyngiomas. *Surg. Neurol.* 1:5–12, 1973.

Little, J. R., et al. Brain hemorrhage from intracranial tumor. *Stroke* 10:283–288, 1979.

Menezes, A. H., Bell, W. E., and Perret, G. E. Hypothalamic tumors in children. Their diagnosis and management. *Child Brain* 3:265–280, 1977.

Patchell, R. A., et al. A randomized trial of surgery in the treatment of single metastases to the brain. *N. Engl. J. Med.* 322:494–500, 1990.

Raimondi, A. J., and Gutierrez, F. A. Diagnosis and surgical treatment of choroid plexus papillomas. *Child Brain* 1:81–115, 1975.

Ransohoff, J. Surgical management of metastatic tumors. *Semin. Oncol.* 2:21–27, 1975.

Rubinstein, L. *Tumors of the Central Nervous System.* Washington: Armed Forces Institute of Pathology, 1972.

Salomon, M. The morbidity and mortality of brain tumors. A perspective on recent advances in therapy. *Neurol. Clin.* 3:229–257, 1985.

Schaumburg, H. H., Plank, C. R., and Adams, R. D. The reticulum cell sarcoma-microglioma group of brain tumours. A consideration of their clinical features and therapy. *Brain* 95:199–212, 1972.

Walker, A. E., Robins, M., and Weinfeld, F. D. Epidemiology of brain tumors: the national survey of intracranial neoplasms. *Neurology* 35:219–226, 1985.

Walker, M. D., et al. Randomized comparisons of radiotherapy and nitrosylureas for the treatment of malignant glioma after surgery. *N. Engl. J. Med.* 303:1323–1329, 1980.

Walker, R. W., and Posner, J. B. Central nervous system neoplasms. In S. H. Appel (editor). *Current Neurology.* New York: Wiley, 1984, Vol. 5, Pp. 285–322.

Weir, B. W., and Elvidge, A. R. Oligodendrogliomas. An analysis of 63 cases. *J. Neurosurg.* 20:500–505, 1968.

Yasuoka, S., et al. Foramen magnum tumors. Analysis of 57 cases of benign extramedullary tumors. *J. Neurosurg.* 49:828–838, 1978.

Cranial Nerve Disorders

Syndromes affecting the third, fourth, sixth, and eight cranial nerves as well as trigeminal neuralgia have already been discussed. Other disorders that involve one or more cranial nerves are described here.

TRIGEMINAL SENSORY NEUROPATHY AND FACIAL NUMBNESS

There is a unilateral form of facial numbness, with a postviral or idiopathic etiology, that usually remits over several weeks. The lower face is mainly affected and the condition is usually painless. Although the pathogenesis is unknown, this disorder may represent a sensory equivalent of Bell's palsy. Isolated facial numbness may also occur as the result of trigeminal neuropathy secondary to herpes zoster, collagen diseases such as scleroderma, metastatic carcinoma or lymphoreticular malignancy affecting the base of the skull or meninges, diabetes, acoustic or fifth nerve neuroma, tortuous

vertebral arteries or lesions of the brainstem including multiple sclerosis, pontine infarction or glioma, syringobulbia, or an Arnold-Chiari malformation.

FACIAL NERVE PALSY

Bell's Palsy [acute or subacute idiopathic fac nerve weakness]

Bell's palsy consists of an acute or subacute idiopathic facial nerve weakness (Fig. 21-1). Because some patients also experience subjective (and occasionally objective) sensory symptoms over the face and may show evidence of vestibular nerve involvement, the condition may actually represent a multiple cranial mononeuropathy.

Pathophysiology and Etiology [unknown]

The etiology of Bell's palsy is unknown. A certain proportion of cases occur after a nonspecific viral infection, suggesting an immune-mediated demyelination of the facial nerve in these

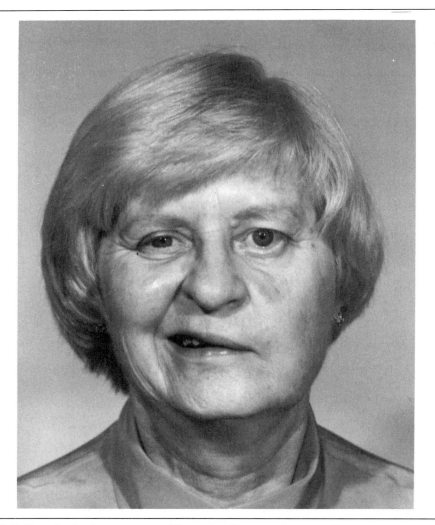

Fig. 21-1. *Left Bell's palsy in the acute stage. The patient is attempting to smile. Note overflow of tears (epiphora).*

instances. In some patients who undergo surgical decompression, the nerve is found to be edematous and hemorrhagic. These findings, along with the anatomical containment of the nerve within the bony facial canal and the success of decompressive surgery in some instances, imply that swelling of the nerve and ischemia play a role in the pathogenesis. The association of a small percentage of cases with diabetes mellitus, hypertension, pregnancy, and pseudotumor cerebri in children lends further credence to this hypothesis.

Epidemiology

There is an incidence of about 20 cases of Bell's palsy per 100,000 population per year, and this rises from a low in the first decade to a maximum in the fourth decade, although it may afflict all age groups. There is a family history of the disorder in about 10 percent of the patients.

Clinical Picture and Diagnosis

Most patients experience pain in the retroauricular area or deep within the ear, either prior to or at the onset of facial weakness. Facial weakness may be first evident upon awakening in the morning. Paralysis is usually maximal within 4 to 7 days of onset, but rarely weakness may progress for up to 2 weeks. Patients also commonly complain of an overflow of tears, food getting caught in the cheek, and biting the inner cheek when eating. Taste is impaired subjectively in about 60 percent of the cases and occasionally patients complain of hyperacusis on the involved side.

Fibrillations on needle electromyographic studies of the facial muscles do not appear until about 10 days after the onset of palsy. Nerve excitability studies, which measure the amount of current required to produce a visible facial twitch with stimulation over the mastoid area, are often conducted about 5 to 7 days after onset. Latency, amplitude, and the form of muscle evoked potentials with nerve stimulation may also be measured. If the amplitude of the evoked muscle response is less than half that on the normal side, denervation is likely. The blink reflexes are also abnormal in patients with Bell's palsy.

More refined tests such as electrogustometry (measurement of the current thresholds required to produce a metallic taste on each side of the tongue) and cannulation of the sublingual ducts to measure salivary output have also been attempted in an effort to identify patients who are at greater risk for incomplete recovery. Unfortunately, the correlation between these test results and the occurrence of denervation remains to be clarified. Furthermore, once denervation is actually detected, treatment is not likely to influence the course of the disease.

In any case of seventh nerve palsy, the etiological factors must be sought (Table 21-1). In the Ramsay Hunt syndrome, a cutaneous vesicular eruption due to herpes zoster occurs over the ear in conjunction with a seventh nerve palsy that stems from herpetic invasion of the geniculate ganglion. In children with facial palsy, additional considerations are birth injury, Möbius' syndrome (congenital absence of the sixth and seventh nerve nuclei), mumps, histiocytosis X, pseudotumor cerebri, and a postimmunization condition. In cases of bilateral facial palsy, the main etiologies are sarcoidosis, Guillain-Barré syndrome, leprosy,

Table 21-1. Causes of Unilateral or Bilateral Facial Palsy

Idiopathic Bell's palsy
Ramsay-Hunt syndrome (herpes zoster of geniculate ganglion)
Lyme disease
Sarcoidosis
Diabetes mellitus
Collagen vascular disease
Hematoma of facial nerve canal (e.g., in blood dyscrasias)
Fracture of the temporal bone
Guillain-Barré syndrome
Cerebellopontine angle tumors
Multiple sclerosis
Pontine infarction (Millard-Gubler syndrome, Foville's syndrome)
Pontine glioma
Parotid gland tumors

meningitis, pontine glioma, and ethylene glycol intoxication. Bilateral facial weakness also occurs in the context of motor neuron disease, myasthenia gravis, and various congenital and acquired myopathies.

Management and Prognosis

Attempts have been made to formulate specific prognostic criteria that would identify poor-risk patients who might benefit from early medical or surgical intervention intended to prevent denervation. Based on the clinical experience, the following factors have been found to be associated with a more unfavorable outcome: age over 60; the development of complete paralysis; loss of taste, hyperacusis, markedly diminished lacrimation (all implying a proximal lesion of the nerve); recovery delayed for over 2 months; and associated hypertension or diabetes. The absence of electrical signs of denervation is not often a useful indicator of prognosis, because they may not be manifested for several days, even though axonal damage has already occurred in the proximal nerve.

The first consideration in treatment is protecting the patient's eye from abrasion and infection when eyelid closure is incomplete. The patient should apply a lubricating ointment and patch the eye closed at night. Massage and the application of a vibrator to the paralyzed facial muscles may help maintain muscle tone but their benefit is unproved.

The results of two controlled trials, in which patients took a total of 60 mg of prednisone per day beginning within the first week of onset, indicate this regimen is mildly beneficial in reducing the incidence of autonomic synkinesias and incomplete recovery. Steroid treatment also effectively lessens the accompanying pain. Unroofing of the facial canal is sometimes advocated by otolaryngologists, especially if recovery is delayed for more than 2 months. Surgery is of unproved value and theoretically would not be helpful once denervation has taken place or if the facial nerve is involved more proximally.

About 80 percent of patients experience an excellent recovery within 2 to several weeks. Some patients, however, are left with minor synkinesias such as twitching of the mouth when blinking. More bothersome autonomic synkinesias such as "crocodile tears" (tearing when eating) and gustatory sweating (facial sweating when eating) are rare. These synkinesias are due to denervation and subsequent aberrant reinnervation. Incomplete recovery or facial contracture produces cosmetic problems in rare instances.

Other Conditions Affecting the Facial Nerve or Face

Hemifacial Spasm
Spontaneous, brief clonic contractions of the facial muscles on one side often begin in the orbicularis oculi with only eye twitching, but progress over time to involve the hemiface and ultimately produce brief eye closure and drawing back of the mouth. Eventually persistent mild facial weakness may also occur. The frequent spasms may be quite bothersome and interfere with sleep. These movements are different from facial tics, which have a less stereotyped character and are closely linked to emotional stress. Partial seizures involving the face exhibit a more rhythmic quality and may be accompanied by electroencephalographic abnormalities.

The pathogenesis of the disorder appears to be varied. Tumors in the cerebellopontine angle as well as aberrant arterial loops in the posterior fossa (from the anterior inferior cerebellar artery, posterior inferior cerebellar artery, or vertebral arteries) can compress and irritate the nerve, causing partial demyelination and possible short circuiting of nervous impulses (ephaptic transmission).

Angiography seldom demonstrates abnormal arterial loops, even though at surgery they may often be readily seen as they cross-compress the root of the nerve. Separation of the compressing artery from the nerve can eradicate the condition. Rarely patients with Paget's disease present a triad of findings, consisting of basilar impression, trigeminal neuralgia, and hemifacial spasm.

Some patients with hemifacial spasm may respond to carbamazepine for a while, and localized injections of botulinum toxin have proved successful in some cases.

Facial Myokymia
Facial myokymia consists of fine, continuous, undulating, involuntary movements of the face on one side, of which the patient is not usually aware. The most common causes of the disorder are intrinsic pontine lesions such as multiple sclerosis or glioma that affect the facial nerve nucleus or adjacent areas.

Facial Contracture
A progressive continuous "spastic" contracture of the facial muscles on one side (Fig. 21-2) can be associated with pontine glioma as well as multiple sclerosis.

Hemifacial Atrophy
Progressive hemifacial atrophy of unknown cause usually begins in the first or second decade and worsens over the ensuing few years before it finally arrests. Skin, subcutaneous tissue, and even bone may be affected. Sympathetic changes may also occur on the involved side and the disorder has been hypothesized to resemble the reflex sympathetic dystrophies of the hand. Restorative plastic surgery can be used to treat the deformity.

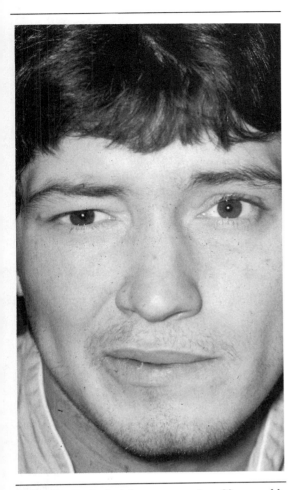

Fig. 21-2. *Right facial contracture in a 22-year-old man with a pontine glioma. The patient is at rest. Notice the continuously contracted right face with narrowing of the right palpebral fissure.*

DISORDERS OF SMELL AND TASTE

Anatomy and Physiology

The chemical senses, olfaction and gustation, serve to alert one to the presence of toxic substances in the environment or ingested material or to the threat of fire. They also impart flavor to food, give pleasure to certain activities such as sniffing a flower, and, possibly, in the case of olfaction, play a sexual role. Strong connections between olfactory pathways and the limbic system endow olfactory experiences and memo-

ries with a special emotional coloring. Disorders of smell and taste are relatively common and must not be trivialized because they can cause significant distress.

Olfaction

The nasal olfactory epithelium is a 2 to 5 cm^2, specialized area in the nasal cavity situated along the superior-posterior nasal septum and lateral wall. The specialized bipolar receptor cells possess a knoblike projection at their tip from which extend cilia that contain the actual olfactory receptors. Various odorant molecules fit into these receptors in a lock-and-key sort of arrangement, and particular odors are then identified according to the pattern of receptor excitation.

Unmyelinated axons from the receptor cells traverse the cribriform plate (where they are susceptible to traumatic damage) to enter the olfactory bulb lying on the floor of the anterior cranial fossa. The synapse at the olfactory bulb level forms a complex structure known as a *glomerulus*. Several other cell types are found in the olfactory bulb and some processing of information takes place at this level. The axons of the olfactory bulb cells proceed posteriorly as the olfactory tract, which divides into median and lateral olfactory stria. There is some decussation of fibers in the anterior commissure. The primary olfactory cortex lies in the piriform part of the temporal lobe (uncus and surrounding cortex). Fibers also pass to the amygdaloid nucleus, septal nuclei, and hypothalamus.

Gustation

The sense of taste is strongly dependent on olfaction, and therefore anosmic patients complain of food tasting bland. Taste buds, the structures that contain the taste receptor cells, are widely distributed over the tongue, palate, and pharynx. Taste sensation is conveyed principally by the facial nerve (anterior two thirds of the tongue and palate) through the chorda tympani, but also through the glossopharyngeal (posterior third of the tongue) and vagus nerves. The axons conveying taste descend in the brainstem via the solitary tract and synapse in the solitary nucleus of the medulla. Second-order neurons ascend to the ipsilateral ventroposteromedial nucleus of the thalamus and from there to the ipsilateral parainsular portion of the parietal operculum, which is the primary cortical receiving area. There are also projections from the solitary nucleus to the hypothalamus and amygdala.

Pathophysiology and Etiology

Anosmia, or the total loss of smell, may affect either all or only certain odors. **Hyposmia** represents a decreased sensitivity or raised threshold to odors. In some patients smell is distorted, usually with an unpleasant smell substituted for a normally pleasant one, and this is known as **dysosmia.** Patients with epileptic seizures arising from the uncal portion of the temporal lobe can experience olfactory hallucinations, which are usually unpleasant ("something rotten or burning"). Such "uncinate fits" have a strong association with primary brain tumors.

The most common benign cause of anosmia, usually temporary, is intranasal disease such as allergic or atrophic rhinitis, sinusitis, the common cold, or intranasal polyps. Tumors represent another, obviously more serious, cause. Head trauma can tear the fibers passing through the cribriform plate or damage the olfactory bulbs or tracts. Several endocrine and nutritional disorders can be associated with anosmia or hyposmia, including Addison's disease, Cushing's syndrome, diabetes mellitus, pseudohypoparathyroidism, vitamin B_{12} deficiency, and Korsakoff's psychosis. A diverse group of neurological conditions can also involve disorders of smell, including Alzheimer's disease, Huntington's disease, Parkinson's disease, multiple sclerosis, herpes simplex encephalitis, anterior communicating aneurysms, meningiomas of the floor of the anterior cranial fossa, and frontal lobe gliomas. The Foster Kennedy syndrome, which is due to a meningioma in the olfactory groove or sphenoid wing, consists of ipsilateral anosmia, ipsilateral optic atrophy (resulting from pressure on the optic nerve), and papilledema.

The first consideration in evaluating a complaint of loss of taste (ageusia) or decreased taste (hypogeusia) is to test olfactory sensation since a reduction in smell will be accompanied by a diminution of taste. Disorders of the oral cavity and tongue, including excessive dryness, infection, and tumor infiltration of the tongue, can cause reduced or distorted taste. Bell's palsy or other lesions of the seventh cranial nerve located proximal to the takeoff of the chorda tympani (and especially proximal to the emergence of the greater superficial petrosal nerve) give rise to a loss of taste on the ipsilateral two thirds of the tongue. Loss of taste has also been documented as being consequent to lesions of the central gustatory pathways at the level of the solitary nucleus or tract of the medulla, the ventroposteromedial nucleus of the thalamus, or the parainsular parietal cortex near the area where tongue sensation is represented. A variety of other conditions, such as vitamin A deficiency, zinc deficiency, chronic renal failure, hypothyroidism, depression, and penicillamine administration, have been associated with taste disturbances.

Diagnosis

Smell can be tested qualitatively at the bedside using odoriferous nonirritating substances that can be prepared in small bottles at various dilutions in mineral oil. Standardized tests are available, such as the University of Pennsylvania Smell Identification Test (UPSIT), which makes use of "scratch 'n sniff" microencapsulated odors.

Testing of the four principal tastes, sweet, sour, salt, and bitter, requires special techniques that are outlined in Chapter 2.

MULTIPLE LOWER CRANIAL NERVE PALSIES

Lesions affecting various combinations of the upper cranial nerves, such as orbital tumors, Gradenigo's syndrome, nasopharyngeal tumors, chordomas, and aneurysms, have already been discussed (see Chapter 11). Some classic patterns of multiple lower cranial nerve involvement and some specific causes of these and related syndromes are briefly described here.

Localizing Syndromes

Cerebellopontine Angle Syndrome
The eighth, seventh, and, later on, fifth nerves are involved in the cerebellopontine angle syndrome. Acoustic neuromas (schwannomas), meningiomas, metastatic tumors, cysts, tuberculomas, and tortuous arteries are the most common causes. If the tumor becomes large enough, cranial nerves VI, IX, X, and XI may also become involved. However, by that time, cerebellar signs and raised intracranial pressure are also prominent.

Jugular Foramen Syndrome
In the jugular foramen syndrome, the ninth, tenth, and eleventh nerves are affected. Various causes include basilar skull fractures, tumors (especially glomus jugulare and metastatic tumors), abscesses, arachnoiditis, osteitis, and basilar impression (Fig. 21-3).

Jugular Foramen and Hypoglossal Canal (Collet-Sicard) Syndrome
The ninth, tenth, eleventh, and twelfth nerves are compromised in the Collet-Sicard syndrome. Patients may also exhibit a Horner's syndrome. The lesions responsible are similar to those that cause the jugular foramen syndrome alone.

Tapia's Syndrome
Tapia's syndrome consists of a twelfth nerve lesion, producing tongue hemiatrophy, in combination with a tenth nerve lesion, producing ipsilateral vocal cord paralysis. Trauma and rarely tumors can be the cause.

Hemibase Syndrome (Bertolotti-Garcin Syndrome)
In patients with hemibase syndrome, all of the cranial nerves on one side may be affected, but frequently the first four are spared. Progressive neoplastic invasion of the base of the skull and meninges is the usual cause.

Specific Causes

Malignant Otitis Externa
Invasive or "malignant" otitis externa is a very aggressive form of *Pseudomonas* infection that

Fig. 21-3. *A 73-year-old woman who presented with a 1-year history of right shoulder pain, dysphagia, decreased voice volume, spasms of the right face on two occasions, decreased hearing and tinnitus in the right ear, vertigo, and gait ataxia. Examination revealed impairment of cranial nerves VIII to XII on the right. The right jugular foramen was enlarged on the skull x-ray study. CT revealed a mass in the region of the right jugular foramen, which was invading the petrous and mastoid areas. Angiography showed a vascular glomus jugulare tumor that responded very well to irradiation. Note wasting of the right trapezius and sternocleidomastoid muscles.*

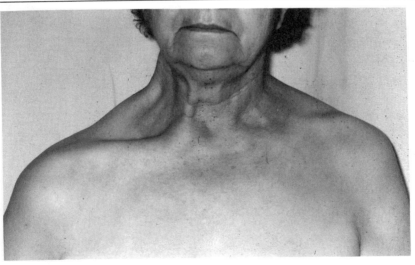

begins in the external ear canal, almost always in elderly patients with long-standing diabetes mellitus. Subcutaneous tissues become involved and the infectious process penetrates into the middle ear and base of the skull, where osteomyelitis may occur. Pain in the ear, discharge from the ear, and palsies of the seventh or eighth cranial nerves are the usual presenting features. Despite the severity of the infection, patients do not manifest systemic signs such as fever. *Pseudomonas* may be cultured from the external auditory canal, and radiological studies such as tomograms or computed tomography (CT) may reveal the presence of erosion at the base of the skull. Several lower cranial nerves may become involved and lateral sinus thrombosis may also occur. In patients who exhibit either cranial nerve findings or other signs of central nervous system involvement, the mortality is as high as 50 percent. Treatment should consist of intravenously administered aminoglycosides and semisynthetic penicillin antibiotics effective against *Pseudomonas*. Surgical intervention may be necessary to treat the basal osteomyelitis in patients who do not respond to antibiotics alone.

Tortuous Vertebral or Basilar Arteries

Dilated, elongated, and tortuous vertebral, basilar, or posterior inferior cerebellar arteries may compress one or more cranial nerves in the posterior fossa. The fifth, seventh, eighth, and ninth nerves are the ones most typically

Fig. 21-4. *This patient was a 72-year-old man with metastatic carcinoma of the prostate who presented with the subacute onset of diplopia due to a left sixth nerve palsy, bilateral headache, and mild sensory loss in the left face. (A) CT scan shows erosion of the clivus caused by a metastatic tumor* (arrow).

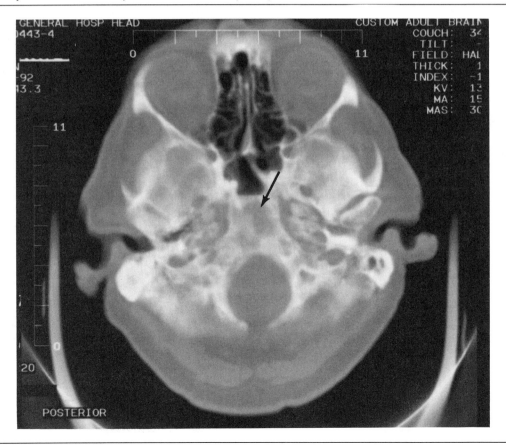

involved. Angiography reveals the aberrant vessels well in most cases, and they also may appear as contrast-enhancing lesions that resemble berry aneurysms on CT scans. Treatment in these cases is difficult because surgical attempts to relieve the compression often inflict ischemic damage on neural structures.

Idiopathic Multiple Cranial Mononeuropathy

Some view the rare entity of idiopathic multiple cranial mononeuropathy as a restricted form of Guillain-Barré syndrome. Some cases are recurrent and involve different combinations of the cranial nerves at different times and may be precipitated by upper respiratory infections. The seventh nerve is most commonly involved, along with the upper cranial nerves.

Other Causes of Multiple Lower Cranial Nerve Involvement

Patients with Hodgkin's disease as well as histiocytic lymphomas may rarely present with signs and symptoms of selective multiple cranial nerve involvement. Basilar impression, cholesteatomas, glomus jugulare tumors, sarcoidosis, metastases to the base of the skull (Fig. 21-4), and carcinomatous meningitis are other causes. Bilateral seventh, eighth, and ninth nerve involvement rarely occurs as a sequela of ethylene glycol intoxication. Meningitis due to *Listeria monocytogenes* may seldom produce multiple upper and lower cranial nerve findings resulting from brainstem involvement. Motor neuron disease, multiple sclerosis, and pontine gliomas represent intrinsic diseases of the pons that may compromise multiple lower cranial

Fig. 21-4. *(B) T_1-weighted MRI scan shows replacement of fat in the sphenoid bone by tumor, giving a bright signal* (arrow). *The tumor was invading the cavernous sinus.*

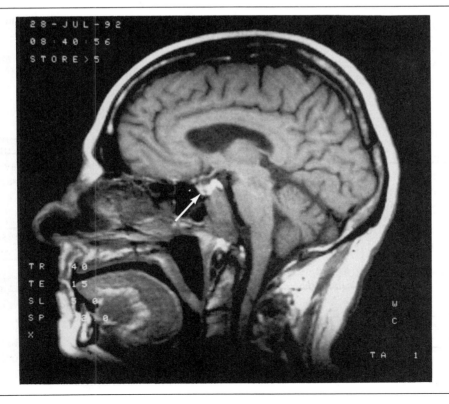

nerves, rarely in the absence of other findings. Myasthenia gravis must be suspected in any case in which the multiple lower cranial nerves controlling bulbar motor function appear to be affected.

BIBLIOGRAPHY

Abbasy, M., et al. Etiology and definitive microsurgical treatment of hemifacial spasm. Operative techniques and results in 47 patients. *J. Neurosurg.* 47:321–328, 1977.

Adour, K. K. Diagnosis and management of facial paralysis. *N. Engl. J. Med.* 307:348–351, 1982.

Adour, K. K., and Wingerd, J. Idiopathic facial paralysis (Bell's palsy): factors affecting severity and outcome in 446 patients. *Neurology* 24:1112–1116, 1974.

Adour, K. K., et al. Predinsone treatment for idiopathic facial paralysis (Bell's palsy). *N. Engl. J. Med.* 287:1268–1272, 1972.

Aminoff, M. J. Bell's palsy and its treatment. *Postgrad. Med. J.* 49:46–51, 1973.

Andermann, F., et al. Facial myokymia in multiple sclerosis. *Brain* 81:31–44, 1961.

Blau, J. N., Harris, M., and Kennett, S. Trigeminal sensory neuropathy. *N. Engl. J. Med.* 281:873–876, 1969.

Boghen, D., Filiatrault, R., and Descarries, L. Myokymia and facial contracture in brainstem tuberculoma. *Neurology* 27:270–272, 1977.

Brackmann, D. E. Bell's palsy: incidence, etiology, and results of medical treatment. *Otolaryngol. Clin. North Am.* 7:357–367, 1974.

Crabtree, J. A. Herpes zoster oticus and facial paralysis. *Otolaryngol. Clin. North Am.* 7:369–373, 1974.

Dedo, D. D. Hemifacial atrophy. A review of an unusual craniofacial deformity with a report of a case. *Arch. Otolaryngol.* 104:538–541, 1978.

Doroghazi, R. M., et al. Invasive external otitis. Report of 21 cases and review of the literature. *Am. J. Med.* 71:603–614, 1981.

Hauser, W. A., et al. Incidence and prognosis of Bell's palsy in the population of Rochester, Minnesota. *Mayo Clin. Proc.* 46:258–264, 1971.

Horowitz, S. H. Isolated facial numbness. Clinical significance and relation to trigeminal neuropathy. *Ann. Intern. Med.* 80:49–53, 1974.

Manning, J. J., and Adour, K. K. Etiology of facial palsy in children. *Pediatrics* 49:102–109, 1972.

Matthews, W. B. The treatment of Bell's palsy. In W. B. Matthews and G. H. Glaser (editors). *Recent Advances in Clinical Neurology.* Edinburgh: Churchill Livingstone, 1982, Vol. 3, Pp. 239–248.

May, M., et al. Natural history of Bell's palsy: the salivary flow test and other prognostic indications. *Laryngoscope* 86:704–712, 1976.

May, M., et al. The use of steroids in Bell's palsy: a prospective controlled study. *Laryngoscope* 86:1111–1112, 1976.

Nelson, J. R. Facial paralysis of central nervous system origin. *Otolaryngol. Clin. North Am.* 7:411–424, 1974.

Sadé, J. Pathology of Bell's palsy. *Arch. Otolaryngol.* 95:406–414, 1972.

Steele, J. C., and Vasuvat, A. Recurrent multiple cranial nerve palsies: a distinctive syndrome of cranial polyneuropathy. *J. Neurol. Neurosurg. Psychiatry* 33:828–832, 1970.

Teoh, R., Barnard, R. O., and Gautier-Smith, P. C. Polyneuritis cranialis as a presentation of malignant lymphoma. *J. Neurol. Sci.* 48:399–412, 1980.

Van Allen, M. W., and Blodi, F. C. Neurologic aspects of Möbius syndrome. *Otolaryngol. Clin. North Am.* 7:411–424, 1974.

Wolf, S. M., et al. Treatment of Bell palsy with prednisone: a prospective, randomized study. *Neurology* 28:158–161, 1978.

Disorders of the Autonomic Nervous System

The autonomic nervous system (ANS) is concerned with the regulation of visceral and vital functions, the maintenance of internal homeostasis, and the preparation of the body to deal with stress or emergency situations. It operates in close conjunction with the endocrine system. Although it is mainly governed by reflex or involuntary mechanisms, some voluntary influence over the system is possible. It is largely an efferent system that controls smooth muscle, cardiac muscle, and glands, but afferent fibers from the heart, gastrointestinal tract, and bladder are also involved. Clinical autonomic disorders may occur in an isolated fashion but are usually part of a more widespread systems degeneration disorder or a peripheral neuropathy.

ANATOMY AND PHYSIOLOGY

The autonomic outflow of the central nervous system arises principally from the hypothalamus, which furnishes a close link between autonomic and neuroendocrine functions. The prefrontal cortex, paracentral lobule, and limbic structures are believed to influence hypothalamic autonomic output. The anterior hypothalamus is thought to be more involved with the parasympathetic division of the ANS, and the posterior more with the sympathetic. Descending influences are carried via reticulospinal pathways. Autonomic disturbances stemming from central suprasegmental lesions, except Horner's syndrome, are relatively rare.

The peripheral ANS is divided into two distinct divisions, usually operating in an antagonistic fashion; these are the sympathetic and parasympathetic systems (Table 22-1). The **sympathetic system** serves to prepare the organism for quick action in the face of stress (the "fight or flight" response) and, when stimulated, increases blood pressure, heart rate, cardiac output, and blood flow to muscle, as well as triggering bronchodilation, sweating, pupillary dilation, quieting of bowel function, and increased output of the adrenal medullary hormones epinephrine and norepinephrine. Its peripheral fibers arise from cells lying in the

Table 22-1. Innervation and Function of Autonomic Effectors

	Preganglionic neuron	Postganglionic neuron	Function
HEAD STRUCTURES			
Eye: pupillary and ciliary muscles			
Sympathetic	Cord segments T1 to T2	Superior cervical ganglion	Pupillary dilation (mydriasis); accommodation for far vision
Parasympathetic	Edinger-Westphal nucleus (oculomotor nerve—III)	Ciliary ganglion	Pupillary constriction (miosis); accommodation for near vision
Lacrimal gland			
Sympathetic	Cord segments T1 to T2	Superior cervical ganglion	Vasoconstriction
Parasympathetic	Lacrimal part of superior salivatory nucleus (facial nerve—VII)	Sphenopalatine ganglion	Tear secretion and vasodilation
Parotid, submandibular, and sublingual salivary glands			
Sympathetic	Upper thoracic cord segments	Superior cervical ganglion	Salivary secretion (mucus—low enzyme); vasoconstriction
Parasympathetic			
Parotid gland	Inferior salivatory nucleus (glossopharyngeal nerve—XI)	Otic ganglion	Salivary secretion (watery—high enzyme), vasodilation
Submandibular and sublingual glands	Superior salivatory nucleus (facial nerve—VII)	Submandibular ganglion	Same as above
THORACIC VISCERA			
Heart			
Sympathetic	Cord segments T1 to T4	Upper thoracic to superior cervical chain ganglia	Acceleration of heart rate and force of contraction; coronary dilation
Parasympathetic	Dorsal motor nucleus (vagus nerve—X)	Cardiac plexus	Deceleration of heart rate and force of contraction; coronary vasoconstriction
Esophagus			
Sympathetic	Thoracic cord segments	Thoracic and cervical chain ganglia	Vasoconstriction
Parasympathetic	Dorsal motor nucleus (vagus nerve—X)	Intramural plexuses	Peristalsis and secretion

Lungs			
Sympathetic	Cord segments T2 to T6	Thoracic chain ganglia	Bronchial dilation
Parasympathetic	Dorsal motor nucleus (vagus nerve—X)	Pulmonary plexus	Bronchial constriction
ABDOMINAL VISCERA			
Stomach and intestine			
Sympathetic	Cord segments T5 to T12 (thoracic splanchnic nerves)	Celiac and superior mesenteric ganglia	Inhibition of peristalsis and secretion; sphincter contraction
Parasympathetic	Dorsal motor nucleus (vagus nerve—X)	Intramural plexuses	Peristalsis and secretion
Adrenal medulla			
Sympathetic	Cord segments T8 to T11 (thoracic splanchnic nerves)	The adrenomedullary cells are derived from neural crests but have no dendrites nor axons. They are endocrine cells.	Secretion of epinephrine and norepinephrine directly into the blood
Parasympathetic (none)	—	—	—
Descending colon			
Sympathetic	Cord segments T12 to L2 (lumbar splanchnic nerves)	Inferior mesenteric ganglion	Inhibition of peristalsis and secretion; vasoconstriction
Parasympathetic	Cord segments S2 to S4 (pelvic splanchnic nerves)	Intramural plexuses	Peristalsis and secretion
PELVIC VISCERA			
Sigmoid colon, rectum and anus, bladder, gonads, and associated ducts and organs, and erectile tissue			
Sympathetic	Cord segments T12 to L2 (lumbar splanchnic nerves)	Inferior mesenteric ganglion (hypogastric nerves)	Inhibition of peristalsis and secretion; anal and bladder sphincter contraction; vasoconstriction; ejaculation
Parasympathetic	Cord segments S2 to S4 (pelvic splanchnic nerves)	Intramural or specific organ plexuses	Peristalsis and secretion; bladder detrusor muscle contraction; penile and clitoral erection

From J. Sundsten, The Autonomic Nervous System. In H. D. Patton, et al. *Introduction to Basic Neurology.* Philadelphia: Saunders, 1976. Reprinted with permission.

intermediolateral cell column of the spinal cord (preganglionic neurons) between T1 and L2. The axons from these neurons leave the ventral roots via myelinated fibers (white rami communicantes) to synapse in a series of paravertebral ganglia forming the sympathetic chain. The postglanglionic neurons rejoin the peripheral nerves via the gray rami communicantes and are distributed to the blood vessels, sweat glands, and hair cells (erector pili muscles) of the skin and muscles of the limbs and trunk. Other sympathetic fibers innervating subdiaphragmatic structures pass directly to a series of prevertebral ganglia (celiac, aorticorenal, superior, and inferior mesenteric) lying ventral to the abdominal aorta. Postganglionic fibers from these ganglia as well as from the superior cervical ganglion of the sympathetic chain innervating cranial structures travel along arteries to arrive at their sites of termination.

The **parasympathetic system** is concerned with the conservation of energy and restoration of homeostasis. Its cranial division arises from nuclei within the brainstem (Edinger-Westphal, superior and inferior salivatory, and dorsal vagal) and is carried by cranial nerves III, VII, IX, and X. Its sacral division arises from spinal segments S2–S4. Parasympathetic excitation causes salivation, pupillary constriction, slowing of the heart, defecation, evacuation of the urinary bladder, and erection of the penis.

There is also an **enteric component** to the ANS consisting of intrinsic neurons and ganglia located within the walls of the intestine that can function independently of central control. Parasympathetic preganglionic neurons contact the ganglia lying close to the organs innervated (e.g., ciliary, sphenopalatine, submandibular, and otic ganglia plus the cardiac and intramural intestinal plexuses).

There are also pharmacological differences between the two systems. **Acetylcholine** is elaborated by both parasympathetic and sympathetic preganglionic neurons and targets nicotinic receptors. Parasympathetic postganglionic neurons also elaborate acetylcholine, which targets muscarinic receptors. **Norepinephrine** is used by sympathetic postganglionic neurons to activate alpha or beta receptors, though the cholinergic sympathetic fibers that innervate sweat glands are an exception to this. The anatomy and pharmacology of the sympathetic system (in conjunction with adrenal medullary hormone secretion) are conducive to a much more diffuse and prolonged response to stimulation than is the parasympathetic system.

DIAGNOSIS OF AUTONOMIC DYSFUNCTION

The major symptoms of autonomic dysfunction are orthostatic hypotension, pupillary abnormalities, dry mouth due to decreased saliva production, sweating abnormalities (increased or decreased), disturbed temperature regulation, neurogenic bladder dysfunction, and impotence in men. There are both physiological and pharmacological methods for testing the intactness of the sympathetic and parasympathetic systems as well as for distinguishing central from peripheral dysfunction (Table 22-2). Clues to the underlying disorder can also be obtained from the patient's history. For example, in a patient seen because of syncope, the presence of nausea, pallor, and cold sweat prior to fainting suggests the intactness of the sympathetic system. Wrinkling of the skin over the fingers and toes after prolonged immersion in water suggests the intactness of the sympathetic efferents. Thermoregulatory sweating may also be absent or excessive in patients with autonomic disorders. Excessive sweating over the face may compensate for decreased sweating over the extremities. Bladder, bowel, and sexual function are other important areas to inquire about when taking the patient's history.

BLOOD PRESSURE AND ORTHOSTATIC HYPOTENSION

Blood Pressure Control

The long-term regulation of blood pressure depends on the renal, adrenal, and cardiac control of normal fluid and sodium balance. The ANS regulates moment-to-moment changes in blood pressure by influencing peripheral vascular resistance, cardiac output, and heart rate in re-

Table 22-2. Tests of Autonomic Function

Noninvasive tests	Invasive tests
Sympathetic system	Plasma norepinephrine level
Change in blood pressure and heart rate with standing from lying (blood pressure falls less than 30/15 mm Hg; heart rate increases approximately 10 beats/min)	on tilting from horizontal to vertical
Blood pressure change with mental arithmetic + harassment, cold pressor test, or isometric exercise	
Valsalva ratio (>1.4)	
Sweat test (increase body core temperature by 1°C; quinizarin hydrochloride powder turns from blue to purple in contact with sweat)	
Wrinkling of skin when hand soaked in water	
Presence of piloerection (gooseflesh)	
Parasympathetic system	Cystometry
Heart rate variation with breathing (heart rate increase ≥20% with atropine, 0.02 mg/kg IV)	
Valsalva ratio (>1.4)	
Pupillary light reaction	

sponse to changes in position, exercise, or stress. The afferent limb of the reflex arc arises from baroreceptors located in the chambers of the heart and in the walls of the aorta and other large arteries. These project to the nucleus tractus solitarii of the medulla. The efferent side of the arc includes sympathetic fibers that project to resistance arterioles, especially within the splanchnic arteriolar bed, capacitance venules, and the heart. The vagus nerves send parasympathetic fibers to postganglionic fibers in the heart that supply the sinoatrial and atrioventricular nodes. Central integration takes place at the cortical, limbic, and hypothalamic levels.

There is normally a rapid increase in the plasma norepinephrine level upon assuming the upright position. With standing, the normal response is a brief decline in blood pressure that is followed by a minor overshoot above resting levels and accompanied by a transient tachycardia (increase of 5–15 beats/min).

Orthostatic Hypotension

Orthostatic hypotension is arbitrarily defined as either a fall in the systolic blood pressure of more than 30 mm Hg or a fall in the diastolic blood pressure exceeding 15 mm Hg, both upon assuming the standing position after 3 minutes of lying horizontally. For the most accurate re-

sults, the patient should be kept supine for 15 to 30 minutes and then the standing blood pressure measured immediately and during each of the next 3 minutes. Orthostatic hypotension is often accompanied by symptoms ranging from blurred vision to lightheadedness or giddiness to syncope. It may be an intermittent phenomenon that is not readily reproducible when the patient is examined. Commonly symptoms are most marked upon arising in the morning, with exercise, or with conditions that promote vasodilation such as a hot environment or alcohol ingestion.

When orthostatic hypotension is due to primary autonomic dysfunction, and not to a decrease in the effective blood volume, the normally seen compensatory tachycardia accompanying the fall in blood pressure is lacking. If a tachycardia of 20 beats per minute or more occurs, the cause of the orthostatic hypotension is not primary autonomic failure. A decreased effective blood volume (e.g., arising because of blood loss, dehydration, Addison's disease, or varicose veins) and drugs (e.g., antihypertensives, phenothiazines, tricyclic antidepressants, and nitrates) are the most common causes of orthostatic hypotension. Peripheral neuropathies affecting small fibers or ganglion cells, such as occur in the context of diabetes mellitus, tabes dorsalis, amyloidosis, Guillain-Barré syndrome, and porphyria, or as a remote effect of carcinoma, may produce orthostatic hypotension as well as other autonomic disturbances. The autonomic reflexes in elderly or poorly conditioned individuals may be inadequate, leading to symptoms of orthostatic hypotension. Patients with autonomic instability accompanying a migraine attack or with prolapsed mitral valve, or both, may exhibit orthostatic hypotension. Finally, primary autonomic failure with orthostatic hypotension may occur in patients with Parkinson's disease, olivopontocerebellar degeneration, or striatonigral degeneration.

The Shy-Drager Syndrome

Primary autonomic failure in conjunction with extrapyramidal, pyramidal, and cerebellar motor systems degeneration has been termed *progressive autonomic failure with multiple-system atrophy,* or the Shy-Drager syndrome. This rare disorder is mainly encountered in men and begins in middle age. Orthostatic hypotension, often severe, is the usual presenting symptom. Other evidence of autonomic failure in these patients includes absence of sweating, pupillary abnormalities, and sexual dysfunction. The plasma resting norepinephrine levels are also low. Parkinsonism, corticospinal and corticobulbar signs, and cerebellar dysfunction appear after a few years. Lower motor neuron degeneration and vocal cord abductor paralysis with sleep apnea are occasional problems. The condition is usually fatal within 5 to 10 years of onset. The pathogenesis is uncertain, but both peripheral and central degeneration of nervous structures has been observed in many patients. The intermediolateral cell column in the spinal cord, locus ceruleus, substantia nigra, hypothalamus, and dorsal motor nucleus of the vagus have all shown involvement, and this consists of a central depletion in the norepinephrine and dopamine stores in these areas. A more minor involvement of cholinergic activity has also been noted.

Management of Orthostatic Hypotension

Symptomatic severe orthostatic hypotension is not only inconvenient but may precipitate myocardial infarction or stroke, and therefore pose a threat to life. Attention in such patients should first be directed toward improving venous return and preventing pooling in the standing position. Specially fitted elastic leotards or body garments or, in severe cases, special pressurized suits can be worn. These should ideally be donned before the patient arises in the morning. Keeping the head of the bed elevated at night by about 12 inches (30 cm) improves sympathetic reflexes, favors expansion of the intravascular volume, and may improve the autoregulation of cerebral blood flow. A high-sodium diet promotes volume expansion. Pharmacological management is often unsuccessful and leads to recumbent hypertension. 9-Alpha-fluorohydrocortisone has been widely employed for the purposes of volume expansion. Alpha sympathomimetics such as ephedrine have also been used with some success, but cause supine hypertension, tachycardia, and central nervous system stimulation. The new drug midodrine is a selective alpha agonist possessing fewer side effects, and may become the drug of choice for initial treatment.

OTHER AUTONOMIC DISORDERS

Familial Dysautonomia (Riley-Day Syndrome)

Familial dysautonomia is an autosomal recessive disorder that is encountered almost exclusively among Jews. It is seen at birth, and affected infants exhibit poor sucking and swallowing plus an absence of overflow tears. The most consistent additional features mainly reflect widespread impairment of autonomic function and include absence of fungiform papillae on the tongue with lack of taste, vasomotor disturbances that produce skin blotching and acrocyanosis, hyperhydrosis, incoordination, cyclic vomiting, emotional lability, growth impairment, labile blood pressure, kyphoscoliosis, absent deep tendon reflexes, and insensitivity to pain. Intradermal histamine injection does not elicit the flare response. These patients exhibit supersensitivity to both cholinergic and adrenergic agents. Both small unmyelinated C fibers and large myelinated fibers are missing in the peripheral nerves. Inconsistent changes have also been noted in the central nervous system and involve the intermediolateral cell columns and the reticular formation of the brainstem.

The pathogenesis of the disorder may possibly relate to a disturbance involving nerve growth factor. Many patients die in childhood, usually as the result of aspiration or other complications.

Acute or Subacute Pandysautonomia

A relatively pure and severe noradrenergic (and less commonly cholinergic) autonomic dysfunction has been described in the form of acute or subacute pandysautonomia. This disorder probably represents an immunologically mediated attack on small peripheral autonomic nerves. The CSF protein level is often elevated. Patients usually experience a relatively good recovery over a period of months.

Other Conditions with Prominent Autonomic Impairment

Various peripheral neuropathies, because of their predilection for small and unmyelinated fibers, characteristically lead to autonomic impairment in addition to sensory and motor involvement. Guillain-Barré syndrome, chronic inflammatory polyradiculoneuropathy, porphyria, amyloidosis, Tangier disease, diabetes mellitus, uremia, the remote effects of carcinomas, and acrylamide toxicity are the best examples of such disorders. Pain is also a major symptom of many of these neuropathies.

Patients with diabetic autonomic neuropathy classically suffer orthostatic hypotension, impotence, sweating disturbances, nocturnal diarrhea, and a neurogenic bladder. Its appearance in a patient with diabetes mellitus is generally considered a bad prognostic sign. Other disorders possessing prominent autonomic features include botulism, tabes dorsalis, syringomyelia, Wernicke's encephalopathy, and "diencephalic" epilepsy. It may prove difficult to distinguish "diencephalic" epilepsy, which is rare, from pheochromocytoma or panic attacks.

Dopamine-β-hydroxylase deficiency is a recently described condition that produces a selective failure of sympathetic noradrenergic function. These patients suffer from severe orthostatic hypotension and retrograde ejaculation, and may exhibit ptosis, nasal stuffiness, and hyperextensible joints. Epinephrine and norepinephrine are absent in plasma and CSF specimens.

NEUROGENIC BLADDER

Normal Bladder Function

The normally functioning urinary bladder stores from 350 to 500 ml of urine without a substantial rise in intravesicular pressure and then empties completely on demand. The detrusor muscle of the bladder contracts during urination and this opens up the bladder neck area as well as the smooth muscle of the proximal urethra to form a "facilitating funnel." The internal sphincter, consisting of the smooth muscle of the bladder neck which is contiguous with the urethral smooth muscle, comprises the primary continence mechanism. When intraurethral pressure exceeds intravesicular pressure, urination ceases and the proximal urethra closes. Although the intrinsic elastic properties of the bladder wall and urethra plus the intrinsic rhythmic contractions of the detrusor muscle play a role in these events, they are largely dependent on adequate coordination of nervous impulses, which are both under segmental and suprasegmental reflex control.

The **reflex voiding center** lies in the sacral spinal cord at the S2–S4 levels. Neurons in the intermediolateral cell column supply parasympathetic excitatory input to the detrusor muscle via the pelvic nerves and plexuses. These fibers synapse in ganglia near or within the bladder wall. Afferent inputs are also transmitted via the pelvic nerves mainly through the S2–S3 roots. Sensations of proprioception (distention), pain, and temperature are conveyed by these fibers. Connections to higher brain centers, which give rise to the sensation of the desire to void, are carried by the spinothalamic tracts as well as the posterior columns.

Sympathetic input to the bladder arises from the T11–L4 sympathetic centers of the spinal cord and travels via the hypogastric nerves. Sympathetic activation causes the detrusor muscle to relax, blocks parasympathetic transmission at the pelvic ganglia, and promotes an increase in urethral sphincter tone as the bladder fills. The sympathetic supply to the urethral sphincter also prevents retrograde ejaculation. The striated muscles of the urethra and pelvic floor (e.g., urogenital diaphragm and levator ani muscles), comprising the external urinary sphincter, receive somatic input from anterior horn cells in the S2–S4 segments via the pudendal nerves. These same nerves also contain afferent fibers that play a role in the "guarding reflex." Voiding normally can be voluntarily interrupted by the contraction of the external sphincter.

The act of voluntary voiding is initiated at higher levels through a complex interplay of influences from the inhibitory and excitatory micturition centers. Most important are the **pontine micturition center** in the reticular formation, which may be involved in a long-loop reflex during normal voiding, and the **paracentral lobule** and **anterior central gyrus** of the frontal lobe. Descending influences are carried mainly by the lateral reticulospinal tracts lying near the corticospinal tracts.

Assessment of Bladder Function

The primary symptoms of a neurogenic bladder are urinary incontinence, residual urine after voiding, inability to sense the need to void, and urinary tract infection. The last is a consequence of incomplete bladder emptying. In the later stages of a neurogenic bladder, repeated infection and fibrosis of the bladder wall cause a chronically contracted bladder with a markedly decreased capacity. In addition, ureteral and kidney function may ultimately be compromised because of high bladder pressures that interfere with normal ureteral filling as well as infection.

The anatomical level of the lesion causing a neurogenic bladder can be diagnosed fairly precisely on the basis of the concomitant neurological findings (e.g., the presence of the bulbo-cavernous reflex, resting anal sphincter tone and reflex contraction, sensation in the S2–S4 dermatomes), the EMG of the pelvic floor muscles or anal sphincter, and the results of cystometry. Cystometry is a method of measuring bladder pressure-volume relationships during filling and voiding after the gradual instillation of carbon dioxide or water into the bladder through a catheter. During this procedure, the volume at the first desire to void, the total bladder capacity, the presence of uninhibited contractions, the completeness of bladder emptying, the ability to voluntarily interrupt voiding, and the response to parasympathomimetic drugs such as bethanechol chloride (Urecholine) can all be determined. Cinefluoroscopic studies can yield additional information concerning the status of the bladder and urethra during voiding. Once the type of neurogenic bladder is known, treatment can be planned and an ultimate prognosis made.

Types of Neurogenic Bladder

An **uninhibited neurogenic bladder** occurs in patients whose cortical control over the sacral reflex voiding centers is impaired. Cystometry reveals uninhibited detrusor contractions, and these patients are unaware of bladder filling until detrusor contraction has already begun. They exhibit urgency incontinence, and the prevention of incontinence depends on the intactness of the guarding reflex employing the external sphincter. Because of the relative outlet obstruction, urinary infection is common. The vesicourethral control in these patients is essentially the same as that in young children or infants before bladder control is established. This form of neurogenic bladder is most common in patients suffering from the dementia of Alzheimer's disease. It may also be seen in patients with cerebral infarction, multiple sclerosis, Parkinson's disease, falx meningioma, or normal-pressure hydrocephalus. Anticholinergic agents such as propanthelene bromide may lessen the incontinence but can also worsen the mental status in demented patients. Condom catheters are often used in men.

The **reflex neurogenic bladder** occurs when both sensory and motor bladder pathways in the spinal cord are interrupted above the sacral segments. Bladder sensation is absent in the presence of lesions above the lower thoracic cord. The detrusor shows uninhibited contractions and the external sphincter may relax either in a physiological fashion, leading to incontinence, or it may relax incompletely. It may also contract inappropriately and produce bladder–external sphincter dyssynergia. This leads to increased residual urine, which then increases the risk of infection and eventually brings about upper urinary tract deterioration. Multiple sclerosis and spinal cord trauma are the most common disorders associated with this form of bladder dysfunction.

Management strategies in patients with a reflex neurogenic bladder are aimed at reducing the detrusor hyperactivity through the use of anticholinergic agents such as propantheline bromide or smooth muscle relaxants; in extreme cases, sacral rhizotomy may be called for. When necessary, the external sphincter hyperactivity can be treated either pharmacologically (less effective) or by sphincterotomy. In many cases, intermittent self-catheterization is necessary to overcome the outlet obstruction. In cases where this is impractical, a permanent indwelling catheter may need to be installed or a urinary diversionary procedure performed.

Lesions in the sacral spinal cord causing denervation of the detrusor muscle and failure of detrusor contraction are responsible for causing the **autonomous neurogenic bladder.** If some degree of sphincter function is retained, continence may be preserved. Overflow incontinence is commonly seen and bladder sensation is absent in these patients. This form of bladder may occur in the context of lower spinal cord trauma, tumor, meningomyelocele, or multiple sclerosis. To deal with the incontinence, voiding can be done according to a fixed schedule using the Credé maneuver (voluntary lower abdominal pressure), but intermittent self-catheterization, which also removes residual urine, is usually the best solution.

Patients with tabes dorsalis or diabetes mellitus may have problems with a "sensory paralytic bladder," consisting of a large capacity, delayed desire to void, and increased residual urine. A "motor paralytic bladder" can occur when there is selective involvement of efferents to the bladder or their motor neurons such as in poliomyelitis or Guillain-Barré syndrome. In these pathological states, the bladder is atonic with an enlarged capacity, and there is residual urine but bladder sensation is intact. In many cases of a neurogenic bladder, there are combined lesions that affect both the upper and lower motor neuron supply to the bladder or that involve combinations of peripheral sensorimotor supply as well as the sacral spinal cord.

BIBLIOGRAPHY

Appenzeller, O. *The Autonomic Nervous System,* 3rd ed. Amsterdam: Elsevier, 1982.

Appenzeller, O., and Atkinson, R. Autonomic Disorders: Assessment and Management. In A. K. Asbury and R. W. Gilliatt (editors). *Peripheral Nerve Disorders.* London: Butterworths, 1984.

Appenzeller, O., and Kornfeld, M. Acute pandysautonomia. Clinical and morphologic study. *Arch. Neurol.* 29:334–339, 1973.

Bannister, R. (editor). *Autonomic Failure: A Textbook of Clinical Disorders of the Autonomic Nervous System.* New York: Oxford University Press, 1983.

Bannister, R., and Oppenheimer, D. R. Degenerative diseases of the nervous system associated with autonomic failure. *Brain* 95:457–474, 1972.

Biaggioni, I., et al. Dopamine-β-hydroxylase deficiency in humans. *Neurology* 40:370–373, 1990.

Blaivas, J. G. Management of bladder dysfunction in multiple sclerosis. *Neurology* 30(2):12–18, 1980.

Bradley, W. E. (editor). Aspects of diabetic autonomic neuropathy. *Ann. Intern. Med.* 92(Part 2):289–342, 1980.

Bradshaw, M. J., and Edwards, R. T. M. Postural hypotension—pathophysiology and management. *Q. J. Med.* 60:643–657, 1986.

Brunt, P. W., and McKusick, V. A. Familial

dysautonomia: a report of genetic and clinical studies with a review of the literature (Riley-Day). *Medicine* 49:343–370, 1970.

Chobanian, A. V., et al. Mineralocorticoid-induced hypertension in patients with orthostatic hypotension. *N. Engl. J. Med.* 301:68–73, 1979.

Chokroverty, S. Autonomic Dysfunction in Olivopontocerebellar Atrophy. In R. C. Duvoisin and A. Plaitakis (editors). *The Olivopontocerebellar Atrophies.* New York: Raven, 1984.

Henrich, W. L. Autonomic insufficiency. *Arch. Intern. Med.* 142:339–344, 1982.

Johnson, R. H., et al. Autonomic failure with orthostatic hypotension due to intermediolateral column degeneration. *Q. J. Med.* 35:276–292, 1966.

Johnson, R. H., and Spalding, J. M. K. *Disorders of the Autonomic Nervous System.* Oxford: Blackwell, 1974.

Koff, S. A., Diokno, A. C., and Lapides, J. Neurogenic bladder dysfunction. *Am. Fam. Phys.* 19:100–109, 1979.

Low, P. A. Autonomic neuropathy. *Semin. Neurol.* 7:49–57, 1987.

Low, P. A., et al. Acute panautonomic neuropathy. *Ann. Neurol.* 13:412–417, 1983.

McLeod, J. G., and Tuck, R. R. Disorders of the autonomic nervous system: Part I. Pathophysiology and clinical features. *Ann. Neurol.* 21:419–430, 1987.

McLeod, J. G., and Tuck, R. R. Disorders of the autonomic nervous system: Part 2. Investigation and treatment. *Ann. Neurol.* 21:519–529, 1987.

Onrot, J., et al. Management of chronic orthostatic hypotension. *Am. J. Med.* 80:454–464, 1986.

Polinsky, R. J., et al. Pharmacological distinction of different orthostatic hypotension syndromes. *Neurology* 31:1–7, 1981.

Riley, C. M. *Living with a Child with Familial Dysautonomia.* New York: Dysautonomia Association, 1967.

Shy, G. M., and Drager, G. A. A neurological syndrome associated with orthostatic hypotension. *Arch. Neurol.* 2:511–527, 1960.

Siegler, M. G., Lake, R., and Kopin, I. J. Deficient sympathetic nervous response in familial dysautonomia. *N. Engl. J. Med.* 294:630–633, 1976.

Siroky, M. B., and Krane, R. J. Rehabilitation of the patient with neurogenic bladder dysfunction. *Semin. Neurol.* 3:122–134, 1983.

Spokes, E. G. S., Bannister, R., and Oppenheimer, D. R. Multiple system atrophy with autonomic failure. Clinical, histological and neurochemical observations on four cases. *J. Neurol. Sci.* 43:59–82, 1979.

Strittnatter, W. J. Autonomic Nervous System. In S. Appel (editor). *Current Neurology,* New York: Wiley, 1986, Pp. 73–90.

Thomas, J. E., et al. Orthostatic hypotension. *Mayo Clin. Proc.* 56:117–125, 1981.

Thomson, P. D., and Melmon, K. L. Clinical assessment of autonomic function. *Anesthesiology* 29:724–731, 1968.

Young, R. R., et al. Pure pandysautonomia with recovery. Description and discussion of diagnostic criteria. *Brain* 98:613–636, 1975.

Cerebrovascular Disorders

Stroke is the most common serious condition encountered by neurologists, and, in recent years, has received greater attention from neurosurgeons as well. Stroke can be defined simply as a focal neurological deficit, usually of acute or subacute onset, stemming from ischemic or hemorrhagic cerebrovascular disease. The subsequent discussion considers cerebral ischemia due to occlusive cerebrovascular disease separately from intracranial hemorrhage, because the pathogenesis and management of these two entities differ. Despite the declining incidence of stroke in recent decades, attributable to the better recognition and control of risk factors such as hypertension, it remains the third leading cause of death in Western countries. The importance of stroke is also founded on the fact that many of the patients who survive are left with chronic severe neurological deficits that require long-term rehabilitation or institutional care, and this has profound psychosocial and financial implications.

The incidence of stroke increases dramatically with age, which itself constitutes a major independent risk factor. The average annual incidence of atherothrombotic brain infarction increases from 2 per 1,000 in males and 1.3 per 1,000 in females aged 55 to 64 to five times these levels two decades later. In males aged 75 to 84, the average annual incidence of strokes of all types (including hemorrhages) is one in 50. The young are not spared, however, and an increasing number of specific causes and syndromes have been linked to stroke in children, adolescents, and young adults.

Recently, new techniques such as positron emission tomographic (PET) scanning, Doppler flow and imaging studies, and magnetic resonance imaging (MRI) scanning and spectroscopy have yielded information that has contributed to our understanding of the pathophysiology of stroke. Unfortunately, the approach to therapy in the stroke patient remains largely empirical and symptomatic, with the main focus on prevention through the management of known risk factors. Future advances in the management of the stroke patient depend on a further understanding of the underlying pathophysiology and subsequent application of this knowledge to individual patients.

ISCHEMIC CEREBROVASCULAR DISEASE

Pathophysiology

Blood flow is supplied to the anterior portions of the cerebral hemispheres and retina by the carotid (anterior) circulation and to the posterior cerebral hemispheres and hindbrain by the vertebrobasilar (posterior) circulation (Figs. 23-1 to 23-4). The cortical watershed between the two circulations takes place at the temporo-parietal–occipital junction and the deep watershed, at the level of the thalamus. Hippocampal and mesial temporal structures are supplied mainly by the posterior circulation (see Fig. 23-

3). The internal carotid artery gives rise to the anterior cerebral artery and middle cerebral artery and, in 15 percent of normal individuals, supplies flow to the posterior cerebral artery. The vertebrobasilar circulation has the unusual feature of possessing two smaller arteries (vertebrals) that join to form a larger artery (basilar); this feature explains why emboli tend to lodge at the top of the basilar artery. The two circulations are linked at the base of the brain through the posterior communicating arteries, which are either missing or underdeveloped in a small percentage of individuals. The most important collateral channel is the circle of Willis, which is formed by the distal portions of the internal carotid arteries and basilar artery plus posterior and anterior communicating arteries located at the base of the brain that link not only the anterior and posterior circulations but also the right- and left-sided circulations. The

Fig. 23-1. *Diagram of the lateral aspect of the cerebral hemisphere showing the middle cerebral artery and its cortical branches. (A = artery; Ant. = anterior; Post. = posterior; Sup. = superior; Inf. = inferior; PO = parietal operculum [conduction aphasia]; PPR = posterior parietal region [alexia with agraphia].) (Reprinted with permission from R. D. Adams and M. Victor, Cerebrovascular Diseases. In R. D. Adams and M. Victor [editors]. Principles of Neurology, 3rd ed. New York: McGraw-Hill, 1985, Pp. 569–640.)*

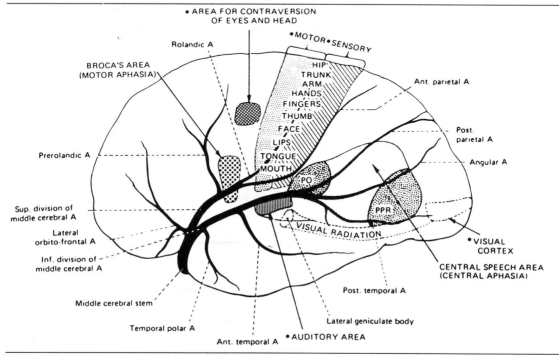

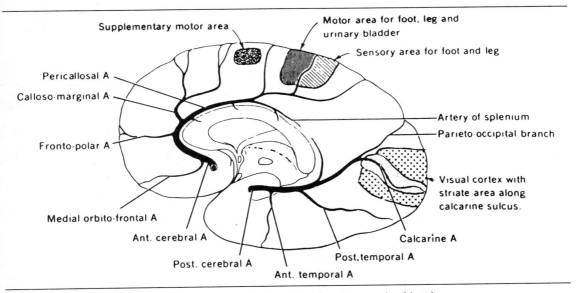

Fig. 23-2. *Diagram of medial aspect of cerebral hemisphere showing anterior* (Ant.) *cerebral and posterior* (Post.) *cerebral arteries* (A) *and their branches. (Reprinted with permission from R. D. Adams and M. Victor, Cerebrovascular Diseases. In R. D. Adams and M. Victor [editors].* Principles of Neurology, *3rd ed. New York: McGraw-Hill, 1985, Pp. 569–640.)*

anterior and middle plus middle and posterior cerebral arteries have the potential to form collateral connections over the surface of the brain.

Extracranial to intracranial anastomoses also assume importance in the presence of stenosis or occlusion of the internal carotid or vertebral artery. Reversal of flow through the ophthalmic artery, which forms anastomoses to superficial temporal branches, frequently allows blood to reach the carotid siphon and its distal branches when there is a proximal internal carotid artery occlusion or high-grade stenosis. Occipital artery–vertebral connections can also provide extracranial-intracranial collateral flow if needed. In addition, several smaller arteries within the neck, such as the maxillary and ascending thyrocervical arteries, may permit an extracranial vertebral artery occlusion to be bypassed.

Collateral Flow

The degree of collateral flow in the face of occlusive intracranial or extracranial cerebrovascular disease depends on the rate at which the occlusive process is developing. For example, when stenosis develops gradually in the extra-

cranial artery, often a rich collateral network forms that allows the maintenance of fully adequate cerebral blood flow. By contrast, the abrupt blockage of an extracranial vessel by a thrombus in a younger person whose vasculature exhibits little atherosclerosis may result in a major cerebral infarction. The establishment of collateral flow may be seriously hindered in some individuals because of congenital developmental variations. These temporal and anatomical factors explain, at least partly, why it is often difficult to predict the pattern of occlusive disease, revealed by angiography, solely on the basis of the neurological deficits manifested by the stroke patient.

Atherosclerosis and Transient Ischemic Attacks

Atherosclerosis is the underlying process giving rise to occlusive vascular disease in the vast majority of stroke patients, especially the elderly. Atherosclerosis tends to affect the larger vessels at the base of the brain and in the neck at bifurcations where the flow patterns can inflict intimal arterial damage. The internal carotid artery at its origin from the common carotid

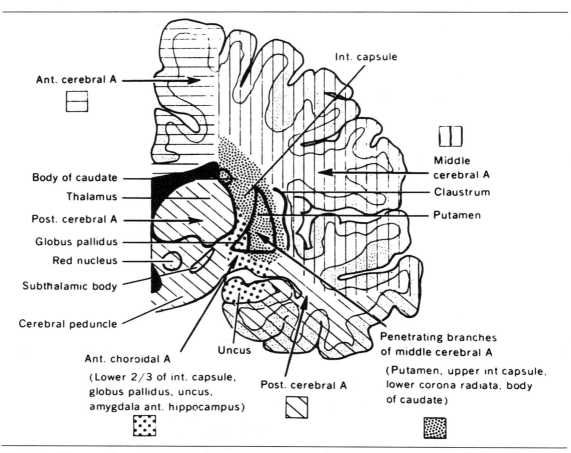

Fig. 23-3. *Diagram of coronal section of a cerebral hemisphere showing the territories of the major cerebral arteries. (A = artery; Ant. = anterior; Post. = posterior; Int. = internal.)*

artery, the carotid siphon, the proximal middle cerebral artery, the vertebral arteries at their origins, and the basilar artery are all prime sites for atherosclerotic narrowing. Atherosclerotic plaque, cholesterol debris, and eventually small intraplaque hemorrhages, platelet-fibrin clots, and thrombus collect at these and other sites. Hemorrhage into a plaque may convert a high-grade stenosis into a complete occlusion. Flow is not significantly affected distal to a stenotic lesion until the lumen is 75 percent blocked or is narrowed to a critical diameter of 2 mm.

Transient cerebral ischemic attacks (TIAs) or transient retinal ischemia producing amaurosis fugax is thought to be due to platetlet-fibrin or cholesterol emboli that are carried distally to lodge temporarily in cerebral and retinal arterioles. These may be visualized on ophthalmoscopy as "bright plaques" located at arteriolar bifurcations in the retina. Temporary slowing of flow through a stenosed artery, secondary to hypotension, and reversible thrombus formation are other possible mechanisms responsible for TIAs. Once the importance of extracranial, particularly carotid, occlusive disease in the pathogenesis of TIAs and stroke was recognized, this spawned the widespread use of endarterectomy in patients with high-grade carotid stenosis or ulcerated plaques in an attempt to restore flow or remove the source of emboli. Surgical bypass procedures have also been used, but with limited success.

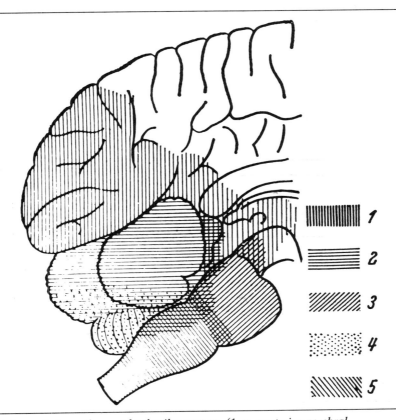

Fig. 23-4. *Arterial supply from the vertebrobasilar system. (1 = posterior cerebral artery; 2 = superior cerebellar artery; 3 = basilar artery and superior cerebellar artery; 4 = posterior inferior cerebellar artery; 5 = vertebral artery [posterior inferior cerebellar artery, anterior spinal artery, posterior spinal artery].)*

Autoregulation

Study of the regional metabolic alterations and cellular events that attend cerebral ischemia has yielded clues to the mechanisms of neuronal injury that operate in stroke, and has also pointed the way to potentially useful therapeutic interventions.

The normal cerebral oxygen consumption in healthy young men is 3.5 ml/100 gm of brain/min, which represents approximately 20 percent of the total body oxygen consumption. The brain depends on a continuous supply of glucose, which is normally metabolized at an average rate of 30 ml/100 gm of brain/min. Normal cerebral blood flow is 55 ml/100 gm of brain/min, with higher flows in gray matter than in white matter.

Through the process of autoregulation cerebral blood flow is kept relatively constant within a range of mean systemic arterial pressures of 60 to 130 mm Hg. This mechanism also links regional cerebral blood flow to metabolic demand. Autoregulation takes place at the level of the precapillary resistance vessels, which automatically alter their caliber in response to changes in the extracellular pH. This keeps flow relatively constant despite changes in cerebral perfusion pressure.

Ischemia can affect autoregulation, such that cerebral blood flow is influenced by relatively small fluctuations in systemic arterial pressure. In the stroke patient, long-standing hypertension may produce a shift in the pressure-flow relationship, so that, at normotensive pressures, cerebral blood flow is barely maintained.

[handwritten annotations: PₐO₂ <3 → ↓LOC; circ arrest → LOC 10-15 sec; blood flow 15-20/100 → ...]

Metabolic Events

Neurons require energy for the maintenance and restoration of ionic membrane potentials, the synthesis of neurotransmitters and cellular elements, and the maintenance of intracellular transport. Complete oxidation of 1 mole of glucose yields 38 moles of ATP, the cell's main energy store, compared with only 2 moles of ATP generated by glycolysis under anaerobic conditions. A systemic arterial PO_2 of less than 30 mm Hg precipitates loss of consciousness. Circulatory arrest in humans causes loss of consciousness within 10 to 15 seconds. Cerebral blood flow below 15 to 20 ml/100 gm/min usually leads to cerebral infarction within 30 minutes to 2 hours. The mitochondrial PO_2 may have to fall as low as 0.6 mm Hg before energy depletion occurs.

Using PET scanning techniques, the regional metabolic rates for oxygen and glucose can be measured during an acute cerebral ischemic event. Increased blood volume can be demonstrated within mildly ischemic areas where autoregulation is still intact. An increased oxygen extraction fraction is thought to reflect a second level of compensation for the falling blood flow, but, if reduced, this is believed to indicate irreversible cell damage. With complete ischemia, the phosphocreatine store is depleted within about 1 minute, but compensatory mechanisms, including the utilization of ketone bodies, can furnish some energy for up to 5 to 7 minutes.

The accumulation of lactic acid during anaerobic glucose metabolism precipitates cellular acidosis, which may be an important determinant of cell death. When blood glucose levels are higher preceding ischemia, this contributes to greater neuronal damage in adults than do lower levels of glucose, due to the greater lactic acid production in the former case. In addition, animals appear to recover better from total cerebral ischemia than from subtotal ischemia with blood flows of less than 10 percent of normal, a condition that would favor more lactic acidosis because glucose is still provided in this situation. The application of these findings to the clinical setting is still controversial.

One of the interesting features of cerebral infarction that has been verified by PET scanning is the concept of **diaschisis**, which is a metabolic dysfunction somewhat remote from the actual area of ischemic damage that is likely due to reduced afferent or efferent flow to or from the area secondarily affected. For example, homologous contralateral hemispheric sites, subcortical sites such as the thalamus, or the contralateral cerebellar hemisphere may exhibit reduced glucose and oxygen metabolism in the presence of large cerebral cortical infarcts.

Ultrastructural Damage

Ultrastructurally, the earliest evidence of failure of energy supply is disruption and swelling of the mitochondria, which imparts a microvacuolated appearance to the cytoplasm. There are also clumping of nuclear chromatin and fragmentation of microtubules. As ischemia progresses, the astrocytes swell, endothelial blebs form, and there is disruption of the capillaries. If damage is extensive enough, even restoration of an adequate perfusion pressure cannot restore flow—the "no-reflow" phenomenon. Brain cells show a variable susceptibility to hypoxia and ischemia. Neurons, oligodendroglia, and astrocytes are more susceptible than endothelial and supporting cells. There is also a gradation in the regional susceptibility to global ischemia and hypoxia, which is, descending from higher to lower, the deeper cortical layers, basal ganglia, thalamus, hippocampus, and Purkinje cells of the cerebellum.

Biochemical Mechanisms of Ischemic Cell Damage

A number of secondary consequences, in themselves destructive, result from cellular energy failure and acidosis. There is a rapid accumulation of extracellular potassium, which induces swelling in the astroglia, thus further compromising blood flow. There is also a massive influx of calcium and sodium into the cell. An increased intracellular calcium concentration leads to cell destruction through lipolysis, proteolysis, and protein phosphorylation, and this further impedes energy production. Free fatty acids accumulate within the cell due to the breakdown of membrane phospholipids, and this imposes further adverse effects on cell membranes. Increased amounts of arachidonic acid, in particular, are metabolized to form

[handwritten at bottom: ↑ glu → ↑ lactic acid → ↑ neuronal damage]

prostacyclin (PGI$_2$) and thromboxane A$_2$ (TXA$_2$). Active oxygen species, or free radicals, accumulate as a result of stimulation of this metabolic pathway and other effects of ischemia. These substances, which adversely affect cell membranes, may be important mediators of cell damage. Under normal conditions, PGI$_2$, which serves as a vasodilator and inhibitor of platelet aggregation, and TXA$_2$, formed mainly in platelets, have directly opposite physiological actions. During ischemia, however, the balance is distributed in favor of TXA$_2$ formation, thereby compounding the effects of reduced blood flow. Changes in neurotransmitter concentrations such as those of gamma-aminobutyric acid, an inhibitor of neuronal function, and serotonin, which possesses vasoactive properties, undoubtedly also play a role in the complex chain of events succeeding ischemia. More important, excitotoxic neuronal damage is likely triggered by excessive release of glutamate and excitation of NMDA and AMPA receptors.

Around the area of an infarct where irreversible neuronal damage has already been incurred lies an area of reversible ischemia (the ischemic "penumbra"), where neurons are functionally impaired and electrically inactive but their energy supplies are not yet depleted enough to cause cell death. Still farther away from the center of an ischemic area lies an area where cerebral blood flow is actually increased ("luxury perfusion"), created by the diffusion of lactate and other acidic end products into this area. Strategies directed toward minimizing the damage from an acute stroke focus on restoring flow and preserving the function of those neurons lying within the ischemic penumbra. Blood flow and PO$_2$ within this area must be maintained by whatever means possible.

Risk Factors

There has been increasing recognition in recent years of the importance of the heart in the production of TIAs and stroke through the operation of embolic mechanisms. Rheumatic valvular disease, atrial fibrillation of any cause, mitral valve prolapse, prosthetic heart valves, ischemic heart disease (e.g., acute myocardial infarction), cardiomyopathy, and atrial myxomas are among the cardiac conditions that predispose to the formation of cerebral emboli.

Besides age, various other risk factors contribute to an increased incidence of stroke. Hypertension is the most important risk factor for all forms of stroke, including large cerebral infarcts, lacunar infarction, and intracerebral hemorrhage. Besides accelerating the atherosclerotic process, hypertension produces lypohyalinosis in the walls of small penetrating end-arterioles; this predisposes to occlusion, which can then lead to lacunar infarction. Additional risk factors include TIAs, heart disease, as mentioned previously, diabetes mellitus, elevated hematocrit, tobacco smoking, oral contraceptive use, and possibly alcoholism.

Clinical Diagnosis of Stroke and TIA

The diagnosis of stroke and management decisions can be facilitated by answering a series of sequential questions in each patient.

Is a Stroke or TIA Present?

Certain conditions other than stroke must first be considered in any patient presenting with the acute or subacute onset of a neurological deficit localized to the brain or visual system. **Classic migraine** is one of the conditions most commonly construed as a stroke, especially in younger patients. Hemiplegia, hemianesthesia, aphasia, or hemianopia usually precedes the onset of the headache in these cases and lasts less than 30 minutes. Accompanying headache (not always present) and march of the deficit over the ensuing several minutes may help to distinguish migraine from TIA or stroke. Migraine can, however, rarely cause ischemic brain damage in younger patients. Some authors have entertained the concept of "migraine equivalents" as a common cause of unexplained TIA-like episodes in elderly patients.

Hypoglycemia and hyperosmolar nonketotic states may give rise to transient focal deficits such as aphasia or hemiparesis, which are usually reversible with correction of the underlying metabolic abnormality. A **postictal** transient neurological deficit (Todd's paralysis) in a patient with antecedent focal brain damage may be confused with a stroke, particularly if the seizure went unobserved. In some patients the deficits may take several days to resolve.

Multiple sclerosis can produce focal brain abnormalities appearing subacutely, especially in younger patients, although hemiplegias and aphasias are unusual. Intracranial space-occupying lesions such as **meningiomas** may manifest TIA-like symptoms, possibly mediated by effects on local cerebral autoregulation. A **subdural hematoma** is an important treatable cause of progressing neurological deficits that mimic stroke or TIA-like symptoms. Cerebral involvement by HIV and other forms of **encephalitis**, including herpes simplex encephalitis and Creutzfeldt-Jakob disease, may occasionally show confusing strokelike presentations.

Is the Stroke Resulting from Ischemia or an Intracranial Hemorrhage?

Typically an intracerebral hemorrhage presents as a catastrophic event, with the abrupt onset of severe headache, hemiplegia, and a diminished level of consciousness. Experienced gained from the use of neuroimaging techniques such as computed tomographic (CT) scanning has shown that differentiating between an infarct and a small encapsulated hemorrhage can be extremely difficult on a clinical basis. For this reason, early CT scanning is recommended in all stroke patients. Headache and an impaired level of consciousness may not occur in patients with small intracranial hemorrhages, but are usually present along with nuchal rigidity in those with subarachnoid hemorrhage. Hemorrhagic cerebrovascular disease is discussed later.

What Is the Temporal Profile of the Ischemic Stroke: TIA, Progressing Stroke, or Completed Stroke?

By definition, a TIA completely resolves within 24 hours, although most TIAs last only a matter of minutes. When a patient is seen initially, it is usually too early to predict whether the deficit will resolve within hours, although major deficits are less likely to do so. Those deficits that resolve completely or nearly so within days are called **reversible ischemic neurologic deficits** (RINDs). In fact, the pathogenesis of an RIND is not substantially different from that of a TIA. Stroke within the carotid distribution may progress in a stepwise fashion over about 24 hours and in the vertebrobasilar distribution for up to 3 days. A **completed stroke** is a stroke that is no longer progressing, and does not refer to the degree of the neurological deficit. Therapeutic intervention is more likely to be beneficial in patients with a TIA or progressing stroke, but can do relatively little in those with an already completed stroke.

Is the Ischemia Arising from the Anterior or Posterior Circulation and What Vascular Territory Is Involved?

In many but not all cases, the neurological signs and symptoms can fairly accurately delineate the ischemic territory affected. The following signs or syndromes imply ischemia in the anterior circulation: aphasia, especially when combined with right-sided weakness; hemiparesis with contralateral eye deviation; left hemiparesis with anosognosia (i.e., unconcern or unawareness of deficit); and amaurosis fugax or blindness in one eye that may be associated with aphasia or contralateral hemiparesis. Amaurosis fugax is often experienced as the sudden sensation of a curtain rising or falling, which obscures vision in one eye, later receding in the opposite direction. Vertebrobasilar system involvement is strongly indicated by the following signs or syndromes: total bilateral visual loss or "gray out"; hemianopia (may occur with anterior as well as vertebrobasilar involvement because the posterior cerebral artery is supplied by the carotid system in 15% of individuals and hemianopia is part of the anterior choroidal artery syndrome); diplopia; internuclear ophthalmoplegia; bilateral weakness or sensory loss (however, anterior cerebral artery territory ischemia may also produce bilateral leg weakness when both anterior cerebral arteries arise from a common stem); loss of consciousness at the onset of the stroke that cannot be attributed to an epileptic seizure; isolated amnesia of the Korsakoff type; thalamic syndromes; top-of-the-basilar syndrome; "crossed" syndromes (i.e., cranial nerve involvement on one side with contralateral hemiparesis); locked-in syndrome; various other defined brainstem syndromes (e.g., Wallenberg's); and cerebellar limb ataxia. Table 23-1 lists some of the better-defined ischemic stroke syndromes. The nature of the lesions in some of the more common brainstem stroke syndromes is illustrated in Figures 23-5 to 23-7.

The term *vertebrobasilar insufficiency* is often used to refer to a variety of symptoms suggesting the existence of posterior circulation ischemia, including recurrent spells of vaguely described "dizziness" or vertigo, fainting or faintness, drop attacks, and memory disturbances. This rubric often serves to mask our ignorance of the actual underlying pathogenesis of such symptoms, many of which are not vascular in origin. When there are more definite symptoms of posterior circulation ischemia, transient or otherwise, it may be appropriate to deem this condition vertebrobasilar insufficiency, with the understanding that a wide variety of underlying pathogenetic factors may be responsible. These include cardiac arrhythmias, cardiac emboli, stenotic atherosclerotic disease within the intracranial vertebral or basilar arteries, and the subclavian steal syndrome.

It is important to determine whether the stroke is large or small because this has both prognostic and therapeutic implications. Since neuroimaging studies are often normal in the acute phase, this judgment depends on the neurological findings. For example, contralateral hemiparesis, hemisensory loss, ipsilateral conjugate eye deviation, stupor, and global amnesia point to a large dominant hemisphere stroke. Anticoagulation is not usually recommended in the acute phases of large embolic strokes because of the danger of hemorrhage, but may be safely instituted in patients with small embolic strokes.

Where Is the Vascular Pathology That Accounts for the Ischemia?

Although localization of the ischemic deficit within the brain is often related to pathology within specific arterioles or arteries supplying that territory, the pathological process frequently exists more proximally within the large vessels of the neck or even the heart. For example, a lateral medullary syndrome is most frequently due to thrombosis within the intracranial vertebral artery from which the posterior inferior cerebellar artery arises. Middle cerebral artery territory ischemia is less often due to atherosclerotic disease within the middle cerebral artery than to stenosis or occlusion at the origin of the internal carotid artery or an embolus from the heart.

The **subclavian steal syndrome** refers to a hemodynamic alteration leading to the reversal of blood flow within the vertebral artery, which may or may not spawn symptoms of brainstem ischemia. The most common pattern stems from atherosclerotic stenosis of the left subclavian artery proximal to the origin of the left vertebral artery. When the left arm is exercised, the increased demand for blood may shunt blood away from the brainstem down the left vertebral artery to supply the left brachial artery. Diagnosis can be confirmed by Doppler studies. There is a low risk of brainstem stroke in these patients and limitation of activity involving the left arm may be the only therapy required.

Although clinical clues such as bruits in the neck can help answer this question, the direct evidence furnished by ultrasound studies and angiography is often necessary. It is important to determine the site of the vascular pathology because surgical therapy for the prevention of stroke is done only on extracranial vessels and principally on the internal carotid artery. The identification of potential embolic sources also has important therapeutic implications.

The **lacunar syndromes** arise from the occlusion of deep penetrating arterioles within the brain affected by lipohyalinosis in hypertensive patients. Occlusion within these end-arterioles produces infarcts that are 0.5 to 15 mm in diameter. These appear as discrete hypodense areas on CT scans (Fig. 23-8) or as hyperintense areas on T_2-weighted MRI scans. In cut sections of brain, they consist of small cavities or "lakes"— hence the term *lacunae*. These lesions are often multiple and tend to affect mainly subcortical white matter, the thalamus, pons, and cerebellum. The syndromes they most commonly produce are listed in Table 23-2. Although it was originally thought that these syndromes were quite specific to a lacunar pathology, it is now

Table 23-1. Some Ischemic Stroke Syndromes

Syndrome	Localization
CAROTID TERRITORY INFARCTION	
Contralateral hemiplegia (arm mainly), lower facial weakness, aphasia (dominant hemisphere), ipsilateral eye deviation, possibly hemianopia, anosognosia (non-dominant hemisphere), visuospatial disorder, dressing difficulty, prosopagnosia	Middle cerebral artery territory (large)
Contralateral leg weakness, transcortical motor aphasia, hypophonia, "supplementary motor area" seizures (contralateral head and eye deviation plus arm elevation)	Anterior cerebral artery territory (supplementary motor area)
Bilateral leg weakness, "frontal" syndrome (including disinhibition)	Bilateral frontal in anterior cerebral artery territory (origin from common stem)
Mutism, dysphagia, markedly impaired voluntary buccal, lingual/facial, and extraocular movements	Bilateral frontal/parietal opercular syndrome (Foix-Chavany-Marie)
Mutism at onset (aphemia), oral/buccal/lingual/facial apraxia, minimal aphasia, variable right-arm weakness	Broca's area (embolic)
Isolated Wernicke's aphasia	Wernicke's area (embolus to inferior division of middle cerebral artery)
Right hemiparesis, apraxia of left arm	Left frontal (middle cerebral artery territory) with anterior corpus callosum involvement
Contralateral hemiplegia, hemianesthesia (variable), homonymous hemianopia (variable), visuospatial neglect (nondominant), ipsilateral head and eye deviation, reduced fluency (dominant)	Posterior part of posterior limb of internal capsule (anterior choroidal artery)
Contralateral hemiplegia (arm predominant), facial weakness, nonfluent aphasia (dominant), neglect (variable)	Striatocapsular infarction (lenticulostriate arteries)
Isolated Gertsmann's syndrome (agraphia), acalculia, left-right disorientation, finger agnosia	Dominant parietal near supramarginal gyrus (branch embolus to inferior division of middle cerebral artery)
VERTEBROBASILAR TERRITORY INFARCTION	
Alexia without agraphia, right hemianopia (variable), visual agnosia (variable), color-naming difficulty	Left occipital lobe and splenium of corpus callosum (posterior cerebral artery)
Agitated delirium and visual loss (often cortical blindness)	Bilateral or unilateral medial temporooccipital (posterior cerebral artery)
Balint's syndrome: optic ataxia, disturbance of spatial attention (visual disorientation, simultanagnosia), psychic paralysis of gaze (ocular apraxia)	Bilateral occipitoparietal infarction (e.g., posterior border zone infarction)
"Top of the basilar" syndrome consisting of variable combination of impaired vertical and horizontal gaze; pupillary disturbances (e.g., midbrain corectopia); behavioral abnormalities (somnolence, peduncular hallucinosis, amnesia, agitated delirium); sensory and motor deficits (often bilateral); visual defects (hemianopia, cortical blindness, Balint's syndrome)	Basilar occlusion near bifurcation
Déjerine-Roussy syndrome: contralateral hemianesthesia and thalamic pain, choreoathetosis, mild transient hemiparesis, ataxia, homonymous hemianopia (due to simultaneous medial occipital infarction)	Thalamogeniculate artery
Midbrain syndromes (Weber, Benedikt, Claude): ipsilateral third nerve palsy and contralateral lower facial and limb paresis, gaze palsy, tremor, choreoathetosis or ataxia	Mesencephalic penetrating branches of basilar artery
Medial pontine infarct (Millard-Gubler): contralateral hemiparesis, loss of touch and position sense, ipsilateral facial palsy, ataxia, sixth nerve palsy	Paramedian branch of basilar artery
Lateral superior pontine infarct. Ipsilateral: limb and gait ataxia, Horner's syndrome, tremor. Contralateral: loss of pain and temperature sensation over body and face, loss of position sense in limbs, decreased hearing	Superior cerebellar artery territory

Table 23-1 (Continued).

Syndrome	Localization
Lateral inferior pontine infarct. Ipsilateral: limb ataxia, facial weakness, deafness, vertigo and nystagmus, gaze palsy, Horner's syndrome, loss of pain and temperature sensation over face. Contralateral: loss of pain and temperature sensation over body	Anterior inferior cerebellar artery territory
Locked-in syndrome: alert, quadriplegia, muteness, blinking and vertical eye movements preserved, ocular bobbing	Bilateral ventral pons (basilar penetrating branches)
Lateral medullary syndrome (Wallenberg's): vertigo, hoarseness, dysphagia, hiccups, ipsilateral facial pain. Ipsilateral: limb ataxia, loss of pain and temperature sensation on face, reduced corneal reflex, Horner's syndrome, palatal and vocal cord weakness, occasionally mild facial weakness. Contralateral: loss of pain and temperature sensation over body. Other: lateropulsion of eyes (especially with blink) to side of lesion, contralateral torsional nystagmus, contralateral gaze weakness	Lateral medulla posterior to olivary body and inferior cerebellar hemisphere (posterior inferior cerebellar artery territory due to blockage of intracranial vertebral artery), ipsilateral inferior cerebellum may be involved
Medial medullary syndrome: ipsilateral tongue weakness, atrophy, and fibrillations; contralateral hemiplegia and loss of vibratory and joint position sensation	Occlusion of anterior spinal or vertebral artery

Fig. 23-5. *Schematic section of midbrain at level of superior colliculus illustrating lesions (shaded) in the various midbrain syndromes: Parinaud's (paralysis of upward gaze, ptosis, pupillary dilatation); sylvian aqueduct (paralysis of vertical gaze, convergence-retraction nystagmus); Claude (ipsilateral third nerve, contralateral cerebellar signs), Benedikt (ipsilateral third nerve, contralateral tremor or choreoathetosis), Weber (ipsilateral third nerve, contralateral hemiplegia). (MLF = medial longitudinal fasciculus.)*

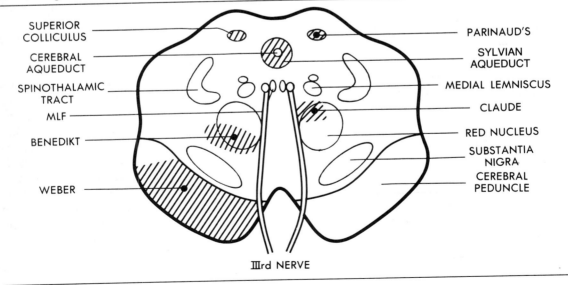

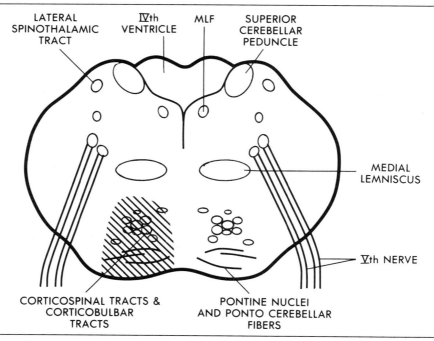

Fig. 23-6. *Schematic section of mid-pons illustrating lesion (shaded) in paramedian midpontine syndrome (ipsilateral ataxia, contralateral paralysis, variable contralateral sensory loss). (MLF = medial longitudinal fasciculus.)*

[handwritten: thrombotic: ⓛ prior TIAs]

known that identical syndromes can occur in the context of underlying atherothrombotic or embolic strokes. The lacunar syndromes carry a good prognosis for recovery and therapy consists of the careful management of hypertension.

What Is the Mechanism of the Stroke: Thrombotic, Embolic, Hypotensive, Lacunar, or Venoocclusive?

Although the clinical differentiation between embolic and thrombotic infarction is difficult, a presumptive diagnosis of embolus can often be made if there is an identifiable source of embolization, such as a stenotic lesion or ulcerated plaque at the origin of the internal carotid artery, mitral stenosis, atrial fibrillation, or subacute bacterial endocarditis. Embolic strokes tend to be abrupt with deficits maximal soon after onset. Preceding TIAs are more common with thrombotic strokes. When there is a history of dozens or hundreds of stereotyped TIAs preceding a stroke, a cardiac embolic source is less

likely; however, emboli from proximal sources tend to be carried repeatedly to the same vascular territory due to laminar flow and thus embolism cannot be ruled out entirely in these instances.

Because emboli are often, but not always, relatively small and travel to distal cortical arterial branches, there is a relatively high incidence of seizures at the onset of stroke due to the irritation of cortical gray matter. Several patterns of arterial involvement or neurological deficit are strongly correlated with an embolic cause. Examples are strokes involving the posterior cerebral artery territory, occlusions at the origin of the middle cerebral artery, and branch occlusions of the middle cerebral artery producing discrete syndromes such as isolated Wernicke's or Broca's aphasia.

Ischemia within multiple vascular territories also indicates the possibility of emboli originating from a proximal source. Embolic infarcts also tend to be hemorrhagic, which may be ap-

[handwritten notes at bottom left: embolic = ⓛ TIAs due - stenotic lesion / ulcerated plaque / mitral stenosis / afib / subac bact endocard]

[handwritten notes at bottom right: ① abrupt, max such after onset / ② high incdn of sz / ③ hemorrhagic - bc even more distal; blood flow to area if ischem when embol loosens → damage to bv]

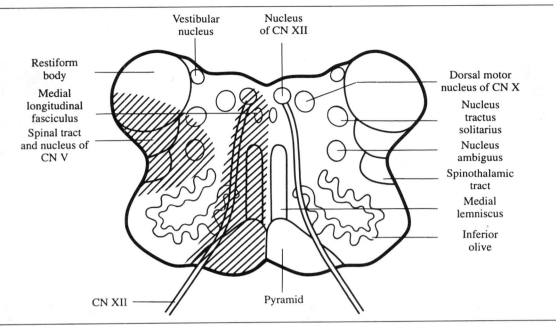

Fig. 23-7. *Schematic section of medulla at the level of the inferior olive illustrating lesions (shaded) in the lateral medullary syndrome of Wallenberg (ipsilateral loss of facial sensation, contralateral loss of pain and temperature sensation over body, ipsilateral Horner's syndrome, vertigo, hiccups, dysphagia, ipsilateral ataxia of limbs) and medial medullary syndrome (ipsilateral twelfth nerve, contralateral hemiplegia, contralateral loss of posterior column sensation). (CN = cranial nerve.)*

parent on CT or MRI scans. When an embolus breaks up and moves distally, the abrupt restoration of blood flow to areas where ischemia has damaged the blood-brain barrier may explain the relatively high incidence of hemorrhagic infarction in these cases. One of the best, although less common, indicators of cardiogenic cerebral emboli is the simultaneous occurrence of systemic embolization.

The presence of lacunar infarction is often inferred from a typical lacunar syndrome arising in a hypertensive patient, although this is a far from absolute conclusion. Prolonged systemic hypotension, such as follows cardiac arrest, produces a picture of **border zone infarction** with variable cortical deficits, including bilateral weakness predominating in the hip and shoulder girdle muscles, aphasia, and often seizures with periodic lateralized epileptiform discharges in the electroencephalogram. These infarcts may also be hemorrhagic.

Cortical venous and sinus thromboses tend to occur in a variety of clinical settings, but are especially linked to the use of oral contraceptive agents, pregnancy, and puerperium (Table 23-3). They may occur as early as the sixth week of gestation but most cases occur during the puerperium. The clinical picture is somewhat variable but headache is a universal feature. This is followed by the subacute evolution of focal signs, including aphasia, bilateral long-tract signs, stupor, seizures, raised intracranial pressure, and coma. A contrast-enhanced CT scan may show the empty delta sign with nonfilling of the cortical veins in the sagittal or other sinuses. MRI scanning is the best way to establish the diagnosis because the usual signal void of flowing blood within the veins and sinuses is replaced by a high-intensity signal arising from the existence of clotted blood (Fig. 23-9). The mortality in this disorder is approximately 30 percent. Findings from recent studies have suggested that heparin therapy may be effective, but

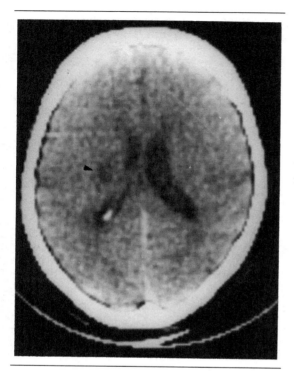

Fig. 23-8. *CT scan showing lacunar infarction in the left internal capsule* (arrowhead) *in a 62-year-old hypertensive woman presenting with a right-sided pure hemiparesis. She had a good recovery.*

this is controversial in view of the danger of hemorrhagic infarcts.

What Is the Etiology of the Stroke?

Localization of the stroke in the brain; delineation of the vessel involved through clinical means and with ultrasound and angiographic

studies; and determining whether the stroke is thrombotic, embolic, lacunar, or hypotensive in origin all provide important clues to the etiology. If the patient is older than 50, atherosclerosis or hypertension, or both, are implicated in the vast majority of cases. If the patient has other evidence of atherosclerotic vascular disease, such as ischemic heart disease, intermittent claudication, or bruits over the neck or other vessels, then atherosclerotic disease can often be deemed the cause.

It is the younger stroke patient, below age 50, who poses a challenge. A large number of potential causes must be rigorously sought through the process of history-taking, examination, and special testing so that specific therapy can be instituted to reduce the chances of recurrence of stroke or permanent deficits in the patient suffering from TIAs (see Table 23-3). In some cases, a **hypercoagulable state** is implied by the patient's history or a family history of thromboembolic disease (e.g., protein C or S deficiency, anti–thrombin III deficiency, paroxysmal nocturnal hemoglobinuria, antiphospholipid antibodies, or lupus anticoagulant).

Cerebral **vasculitis** may be part of an underlying collagen disease that displays classic serological and systemic features (e.g., lupus erythematosus or polyarteritis nodosa). It may also stem from drug abuse, occur as a remote effect of malignancy, or be due to a number of other systemic conditions (see Table 23-3).

Isolated **CNS granulomatous angiitis** is a rare disorder with a diverse and often obscure etiology. Patients usually present with headache,

Table 23-2. Lacunar Syndromes

Symptoms	Localization
Pure motor hemiplegia	Contralateral internal capsule or basis pontis
Pure hemisensory stroke	Contralateral thalamus
Dysarthria—clumsy hand syndrome	Contralateral basis pontis or contralateral internal capsule
Ataxic hemiparesis	Contralateral basis pontis or contralateral internal capsule
Transient coma, vertical gaze abnormalities, Korsakoff-like memory deficit, hypersomnia	Bilateral paramedian thalamic infarction (common thalamosubthalamic perforating branch of proximal posterior cerebral artery)

Table 23-3. Causes of Ischemic Stroke
in Young People

Hypertension

Emboli
  Cardiac
    Rheumatic valvular heart disease
    Atrial fibrillation
    Prosthetic heart valve
    Prolapsed mitral valve
    Cardiac transplantation
    Mural thrombus (postmyocardial infarction,
      cardiomyopathy)
    Angiography (cardiac or cerebral)
    Atrial myxoma
    Infective endocarditis
    Marantic endocarditis
    Congenital cyanotic heart disease
    Libman-Sacks endocarditis
  Aortic
  Paradoxical
    Deep leg or pelvic veins and patent foramen in
      heart
    Osler-Weber-Rendu syndrome with lung shunt
  Other
    Fat
    Air
    Tumor
    Bone marrow
    Amniotic fluid
    Thrombus within berry aneurysm

Vasculitis
  Polyarteritis nodosa group of systemic necrotizing
    vasculitis
  Hypersensitivity vasculitis and variants
  Giant-cell arteritis
    Temporal arteritis
    Takayasu's arteritis
  Isolated granulomatous angiitis of CNS
  Miscellaneous vasculitides
    Heroin and amphetamine abuse
    Ulcerative colitis
    Sarcoidosis
  Possibly infectious-related
    Tuberculosis and other meningitides
    Syphilis
    AIDS

Juvenile atherosclerosis/familial
      hyperlipoproteinemia

Oral contraceptives, pregnancy

Hematological abnormalities
  Polycythemia
  Thrombocytosis
  Thrombotic thrombocytopenic purpura,
      disseminated intravascular coagulation
  Sickle cell disease
  Leukemia

Hyperviscosity syndromes
  Multiple myeloma
  Waldenstrom's
Cryofibrinogenemia
Paroxysmal nocturnal hemoglobinuria
Protein S and C deficiencies
Anti–thrombin III deficiency
Antiphospholipid antibodies/lupus anticoagulant

Dissection and trauma
  Dissecting aortic aneurysm
  Dissection of other major neck vessels (plus
      trauma)
  Other—prolonged extreme neck flexion or
      extension (e.g., yoga)
    Excessive manipulation of neck (e.g.,
      chiropractic)
    Dental anesthesia
    "Lollipop" injuries

Metabolic diseases affecting vessels
  Fabry's disease
  Homocystinuria; heterozygote for homocystinuria
  Mitochondrial encephalomyopathy, lactic acidosis
      and strokelike episodes (MELAS syndrome)

Cerebral venous thrombosis from various causes
  Pregnancy and oral contraceptives
  Ulcerative colitis
  Leukemia
  Severe head trauma
  Severe dehydration
  Sinusitis/otitis media

Miscellaneous
  "Crack" cocaine
  Moyamoya
  Migraine
  Retropharyngeal abscess
  Remote effect of systemic cancer
  Microangiopathy of the brain, cochlea, and retina
  Eales disease
  Sneddon's syndrome

mild CSF pleocytosis and elevated protein levels, and often multiple cerebral infarctions. It affects adults, but rare cases have been encountered in children. The patients are usually acutely ill and other clinical findings include an elevated sedimentation rate, fever, and encephalopathy. Rare patients may suffer progressive dementia. The prognosis appears to be poor, although most confirmed cases have been ascertained only by postmortem examination. The diagnosis can be confirmed by angiography, which may show irregular beading or constriction of intracranial arteries, and meningeal biopsy specimen may be obtained to permit histological confirmation before cyclophosphamide treatment is begun.

A variety of **embolic sources** can be responsible for strokes and may be difficult to detect, particularly when they are cardiac in origin. These include mitral valve prolapse (present in up to one third of young stroke patients and four to five times more common in young patients with stroke than in young controls); a mural thrombus following recent myocardial infarction; cardiomyopathy; subacute bacterial endocarditis; marantic endocarditis, seen most commonly in patients with lung carcinoma or other serious pulmonary diseases; or atrial myxoma. Atrial myxoma is a rare, usually left-sided, intracardiac tumor with a strong tendency to embolize. It may produce chest pain, symptoms of congestive heart failure, and a mitral insufficiency murmur, as well as systemic symptoms of fever, fatigue, anorexia, weight loss, and an elevated sedimentation rate. It is now recognized that **atrial fibrillation,** even without underlying rheumatic heart disease poses as high as a fivefold increased risk for stroke, but the use of prophylactic long-term anticoagulation in these patients is controversial. **Artificial cardiac valves** are also a frequent source of emboli and impart a risk for embolization of approximately 1 percent per year.

In many cases in which embolization is presumed, a source is not readily apparent. In such instances, platelet-fibrin or cholesterol emboli may be originating from an atherosclerotic aortic arch. Another possibility is a small cardiac thrombus that can be easily missed on ultrasound and even more sensitive studies. Once emboliza-

Fig. 23-9. *A 19-year-old man with a history of sinusitis presenting with headache, papilledema, and a sixth nerve palsy who was thought to have pseudotumor cerebri. This T₁-weighted MRI scan showed a clot in the posterior part of the sagittal sinus (arrow). The patient responded well to anticoagulation.*

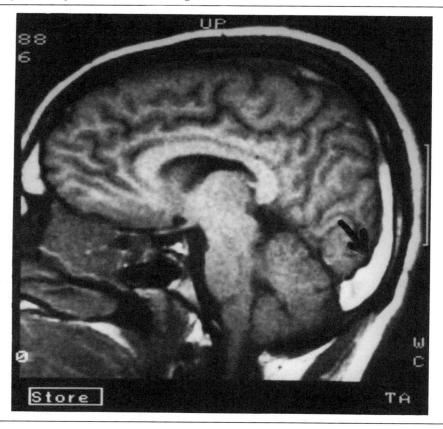

ion takes place, such thrombi may be no longer detectable in the heart. **Paradoxical embolization** from deep leg or pelvic veins, traversing a right-to-left intracardiac shunt, should be considered in such cases, especially if attacks are recurrent. A contrast study that includes the injection of small intravenous air bubbles and the performance of a Valsalva maneuver during echocardiography can reveal occult right-to-left cardiac shunts. Use of **"crack" cocaine** has not only been implicated as a cause of intracranial hemorrhage but has also been associated with acute intracranial arterial occlusive disease.

Moyamoya disease, with the name derived from the Japanese word for "puff of smoke," appears on angiograms as a network of small collateral vessels in the basal ganglia located at the base of the brain. This anomaly is related to bilateral intracranial narrowing of the internal carotid arteries and their major branches, the anterior cerebral and middle cerebral arteries. Although most commonly seen in the Japanese population, it is encountered worldwide. About half of the cases present in childhood, often with recurrent hemiplegias. Adults with the disease more commonly present with intracerebral or subarachnoid hemorrhage. The pathogenesis of this usually progressive condition is obscure, and diverse inflammatory causes probably play a role. External carotid–internal carotid bypass procedures have been carried out in some cases, but with limited success. **Takayasu's aortitis** ("pulseless disease") is another possibly inflammatory condition seen most commonly in young Japanese patients. The aorta and the origin of major cervical arteries are affected.

Dissection of the extracranial and intracranial arteries has been recognized with increasing frequency as a cause of stroke in young people, with the average age ranging from 40 to 45 years. Carotid dissection accounted for 2.5 percent of the strokes in one large prospective series. In some cases, trauma arising from a blunt blow to the neck, whiplash injury, chiropractic manipulation, carrying heavy weights on the shoulder, and prolonged neck flexion with yoga are implicated as causes. In spontaneous cases, minor trauma cannot be excluded. About 15 percent of patients have underlying arterial wall abnormalities that affect the media; these in-

clude fibromuscular hyperplasia, cystic medial necrosis, or Marfan's syndrome.

Dissection may have various consequences such as obliteration of the lumen due to hematoma formation in the wall of the vessel, intraluminal thrombosis, and possibly distal embolization. Subarachnoid hemorrhages stemming from penetration through the adventitia may occur in patients with dissections beginning or extending intracranially. The clinical picture almost invariably includes headache and less commonly neck pain near the site of dissection. Antecedent TIAs and an intermittent course are relatively common.

Oculosympathetic paralysis is a frequent component of carotid dissection in the neck. Neurological deficits are variable. Hemiparesis, aphasia, and other major hemispheric deficits are seen in the presence of carotid dissections, and lateral medullary and cerebellar deficits occur with vertebral dissection.

A double lumen or pseudoaneurysm on cerebral angiograms confirms the diagnosis (Fig. 23-10). Although an irregular or tapering occlusion is suggestive, the distinction from embolus, spasm, or vasculitis is not always clear-cut. Characteristic involvement 2 to 5 cm distal to the origin of the internal carotid artery or at the C1–C2 level in the vertebral artery indicates dissection. Although some authors have claimed a relatively benign prognosis in the disorder, others have documented that major cerebral infarcts with residua or even early death may result. In the event of extracranial dissections, a treatment regimen consisting of short-term heparinization and long-term anticoagulation with warfarin for 6 months is generally recommended to reduce the risk of distal embolization.

Once the specific etiologies of stroke have been sought, a significant number of patients will still have no identifiable apparent cause. Some of these patients will have known risk factors, such as migraine or oral contraceptive use (especially in combination with cigarette smoking), which may then be deemed of etiological importance. Certainly such patients should be encouraged to reduce the risk of subsequent strokes by eliminating any potential risk factors.

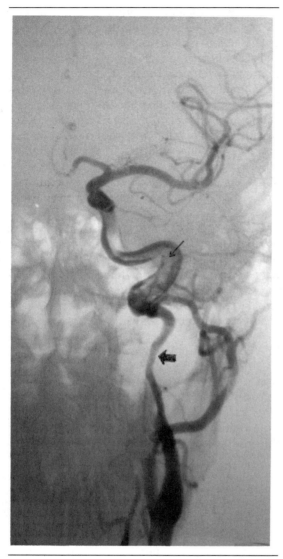

Fig. 23-10. *Left carotid subtraction angiogram in a 42-year-old hypertensive man presenting with a generalized headache that had lasted for 2 days and word-finding difficulties. There was no history of trauma. The study shows an area of narrowing in the extracranial internal carotid artery (large arrow)* due to dissection as well as a clot within the artery more superiorly. The next day he suffered the sudden onset of right hemiplegia, muteness, and blindness in the left eye due to distal embolization from the intraarterial thrombus. With heparin treatment he experienced a good recovery from all his deficits, except the left eye blindness.

Binswanger's disease (subcortical arteriosclerotic encephalopathy) is an ischemic syndrome encountered mainly in older hypertensive patients that has recently been more clearly defined. Patients suffer from multiple white matter lesions that are a reflection of patchy ischemia, and these can be visualized on CT or MRI scans, particularly in the periventricular areas (Fig. 23-11). These patients are often demented and may exhibit stepwise neurological deterioration in conjunction with multiple strokes. Some patients are normal neurologically even though CT or MRI scanning shows periventricular white matter involvement (leukoaraiosis). Typical autopsy findings consist of atherosclerotic involvement of the penetrating end-arterioles supplying the deep white matter along with destruction of the white matter, sparing of the subcortical U fibers, and often accompanying lacunar infarcts. The entity is now considered to be more common than was previously thought and probably accounts for a significant proportion of patients with vascular dementia.

Investigations in the Acute Stroke Patient

Computed Tomography and Magnetic Resonance Imaging

An unenhanced CT scan should be done early in all stroke patients to differentiate infarct from hemorrhage, to help diagnose hemorrhagic infarction, and to detect lesions such as intracranial tumors or subdural hematomas that can cause strokelike syndromes (Fig. 23-12). Edema and brain shifts are also well visualized on CT scans, but fresh infarcts are unlikely to be detected before 12 hours have passed following the ictus. Early-appearing, well-defined infarcts represent residua from previous strokes. Hemorrhagic areas within embolic infarcts may not appear for several days. Within days or weeks following infarction, gray matter enhancement may be seen, and this represents a sign of ischemia (Figure 23-13). In some cases, volume averaging and other effects may obscure the infarct, which seems to disappear on the CT scan for several days; this phenomenon has been termed "CT fogging."

Some major limitations of CT in delineating ischemic cerebrovascular disease are its inability to detect most lesions smaller than 5 mm and its reduced capacity to pick up small lesions in the brainstem or near the bony base of the skull. Some of these limitations are overcome by MRI, which may reveal infarcts as early as 2 hours after the onset of symptoms (Fig. 23-14). However, MRI is not available at all centers and it requires a degree of patient cooperation, which acute stroke patients are not often capable of, or heavy sedation, which is not usually desirable in the acute stroke patient.

CT and MRI are neuroimaging methods that aid in the localization and differential diagnosis of stroke. They are also useful in the investigation of TIA, because they may reveal the presence of unsuspected silent infarction, tumor, aneurysm, or subdural hema-toma. The pathogenesis of the stroke or TIA is best delineated by studies directed at the intracranial and extracranial vasculature.

Cerebral Angiography

Traditional cerebral angiography, or the more recently introduced digital subtraction angiography, is the "gold standard" for the visualization of the cerebral circulation (Fig. 23-15). Magnetic resonance angiography has recently shown some promise as a noninvasive method for demonstrating cerebral vessels. Cerebral angiography can often identify the site of arterial occlusion or stenosis and may give clues that can establish the diagnosis of cerebral embolus, vasculitis, venous thrombosis, or cerebral aneurysm.

Full four-vessel angiography is essential for preoperative planning but carries about a 1 percent risk of complications, including stroke

Fig. 23-11. *T₂-weighted MRI scans showing severe white matter changes* (arrows) *in a 76-year-old man with hypertension and dementia due to ischemic small vessel disease. This likely represents a case of Binswanger's disease.*

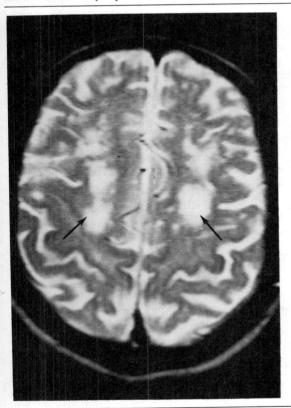 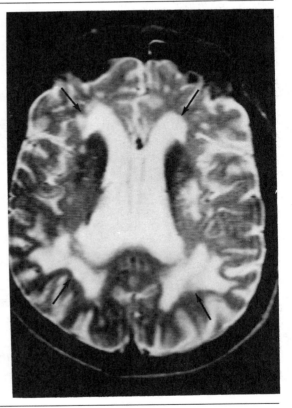

(usually embolic), allergic reactions (less common with nonionized contrast agents), cardiac arrhythmia or myocardial infarction, hematomas at the site of arterial puncture, and possibly emboli to arteries of the lower extremities. These complications are most commonly encountered in elderly patients with widespread atherosclerotic disease. Generally, angiography is indicated in the investigation of all younger patients with stroke or TIAs, including clear-cut vertebrobasilar TIAs. Most elderly patients with vertebrobasilar insufficiency symptoms do not require angiography because surgical therapy is not usually a consideration. However, when long-term anticoagulation is being considered in the treatment of vertebrobasilar TIAs, angiographic evidence of posterior occlusive disease should be sought. In older patients with acute cerebral infarction, angiography should be contemplated if the recovery from stroke and the overall cardiac prognosis are good enough to

Fig. 23-12. *Unenhanced CT scan showing an infarct* (arrowheads) *in the chronic stages, involving the whole distribution of the left posterior cerebral artery.*

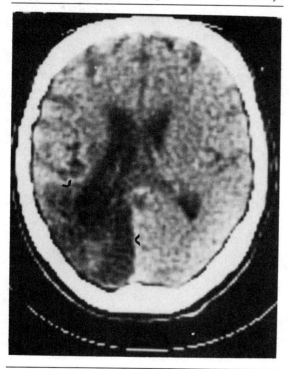

permit consideration of carotid endarterectomy for future prophylaxis.

Digital intravenous subtraction angiography may be substituted for intraarterial angiography in high-risk patients in certain cases. The large volumes of contrast media that are necessary and the need for patient cooperation are limitations to the technique, however. The timing of angiography in the acute stroke patient is somewhat controversial. It is usually prudent to delay angiography at least one week in the acute ischemic stroke patient because findings are unlikely to prompt immediate changes in management.

Doppler Ultrasound

Doppler ultrasound techniques including duplex, supraorbital, and transcranial Doppler, provide information that complements the angiographic findings. They give a much better depiction of the flow through a stenosed vessel. These techniques all have limitations, which must be clearly understood, and the choice of investigations must be tailored to each patient.

Additional Methods

Additional investigations are undertaken, particularly in younger patients, to search for specific causes, as mentioned earlier. When ultrasound studies or angiography has shown clear neck vessels in the patient with a presumed embolic stroke or repeated TIAs, attention must then be directed to the heart. Two-dimensional, but ideally transesophageal, echocardiography should be done in such cases, even when there are no symptoms or clinical indices such as arrhythmia, murmur, or midsystolic click to point to a cardiac source. In such cases, an occult cardiac problem such as prolapsed mitral valve, small intraventricular clot, or akinetic segment may be found. However, a negative study does not rule out a left atrial or atrial appendage thrombus. In such cases, transesophageal echocardiography should be performed. A contrast-enhanced study should be obtained when paradoxical embolus is a consideration. Holter monitoring is worth doing to look for unsuspected arrhythmias in TIA patients when the findings from other studies are

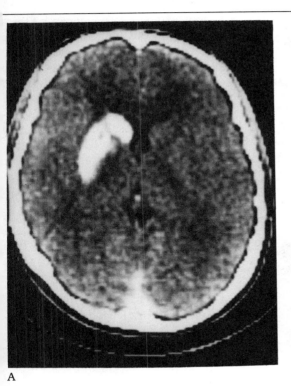

A

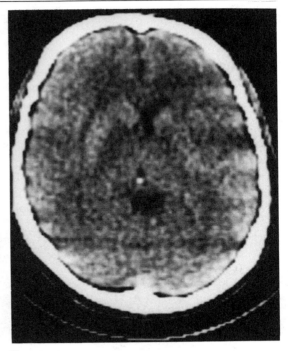

B

Fig. 23-13. *Serial CT scans showing the evolution of a striatocapsular infarct in a 16-year-old boy. (A) Enhanced scan 8 days after infarct revealing marked contrast uptake in ischemic gray matter. (B) Unenhanced scan 2 days later revealing only a faintly increased density in the area of the infarct due either to residual contrast or some hemorrhage. (C) Unenhanced scan 16 months after the infarct showing residual striatal damage and dilatation of the adjacent lateral ventricle.*

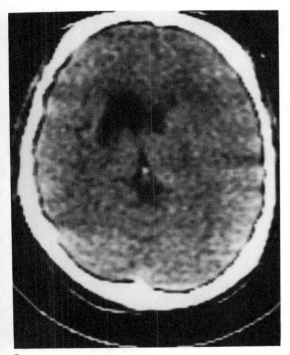

C

negative, even though the yield of this method is small.

Management of Ischemic Cerebrovascular Disease

TIAs or RINDs

Studies of the natural history of cases of untreated TIAs have shown that approximately one third of patients with TIAs continue to have

attacks without adverse consequence, one third experience spontaneous remission, and one third subsequently suffer brain infarction. Most patients that do develop an infarct do so within 3 to 6 months following the onset of TIAs and the number of TIAs preceding an infarct is quite variable. Management is therefore directed toward reducing the risk of subsequent stroke by carefully delineating the underlying pathogenesis and using medical or surgical means, or both, to treat the pathology. In some cases, all that

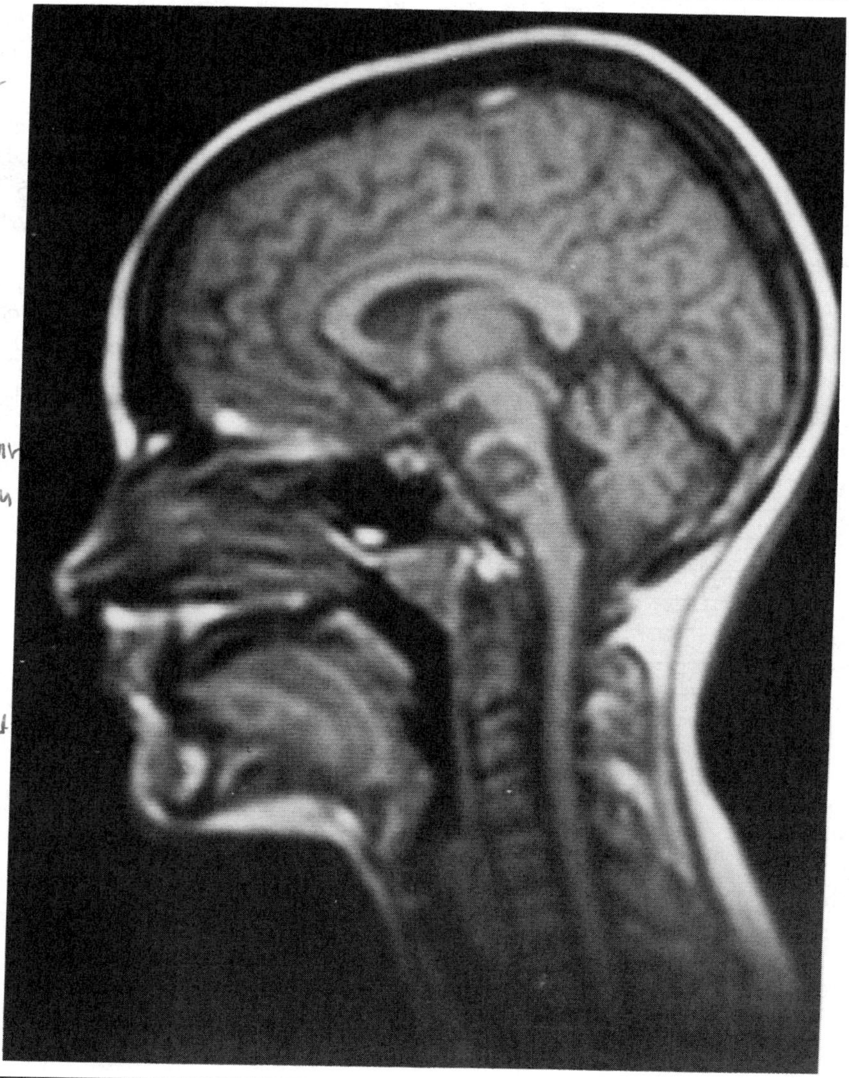

Fig. 23-14. *T₁-weighted MRI scan from a 16-year-old girl with basilar artery thrombosis and a locked-in syndrome. Note the large infarct within the ventral pons.*

is needed is the better management of systolic and diastolic hypertension. Cessation of smoking, stopping the use of oral contraceptive agents, and control of cardiac arrhythmias should all be undertaken.

Because the risk of stroke is highest within the first 6 months following the appearance of TIAs, investigations and the institution of definitive treatment must be carried out without delay to be of benefit. The nature of the TIA also has some bearing on the prognosis, and therefore the urgency for therapeutic intervention. Long-lasting (more than one-half hour) attacks resulting in major neurological deficits such as aphasia or hemiplegia are more likely to lead to serious strokes than are short and less severe attacks. Amaurosis fugax also has a

more benign prognosis, especially in patients under 40. In the vertebrobasilar system, TIAs which include long motor or sensory tract involvement should be managed with greater urgency than attacks with symptoms such as vertigo, perioral numbness, or ataxia. In most cases, TIAs are a sign of generalized atherosclerotic disease and point to an increased risk of myocardial infarction, which in fact is actually the most common cause of death in this group of patients. Thorough examination of the heart, including, perhaps, stress testing or even coronary angiography, is recommended.

In certain instances when TIAs are frequent and disabling (e.g., aphasia and loss of consciousness), reducing the number of attacks becomes a goal of treatment, but, in the vast

Fig. 23-15. *Angiogram showing critical stenosis* (arrowhead) *due to an atherosclerotic plaque at the origin of the right internal carotid artery.*

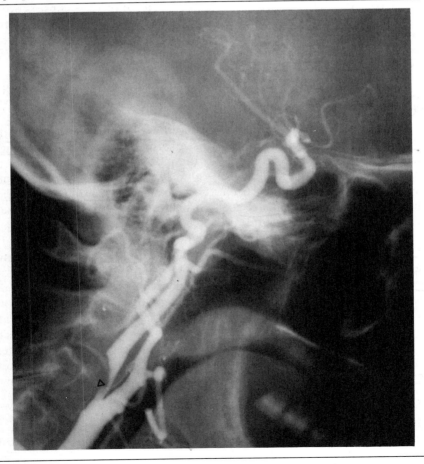

majority of cases, the prevention of subsequent stroke and myocardial infarction is the focus of management.

Aspirin. The most widely used medical therapy for TIAs is aspirin. At low doses, it is an irreversible inhibitor of cyclooxygenase, which leads to reduced thromboxane production and diminished platelet aggregability. At higher doses, it reduces prostacyclin generation within the vessel wall, a theoretically undesirable effect because prostacyclin is a vasodilator. Most studies have shown that aspirin taken in doses ranging from 80 to 1300 mg per day spawns a modest reduction in stroke or death following TIAs, which reached 48 percent for men in the Canadian Cooperative Study. The benefits for women are questionable. In addition, there is evidence that aspirin therapy may also lower the risk of myocardial infarction in these patients. Many clinicians routinely prescribe aspirin (enteric-coated) for patients suffering from TIAs or small strokes because the potential benefits outweigh the minimal risk of serious side effects such as gastrointestinal hemorrhage. There is still controversy concerning whether low or high doses should be prescribed.

Ticlopidine. Ticlopidine (250 mg b.i.d.) is a newer platelet-inhibiting agent, which, in preliminary trials, appears to be even more effective than aspirin in preventing stroke. In addition, it is the only agent that has been shown to reduce significantly the risk of recurrent stroke when therapy is instituted after an initial stroke. It seems to have a higher incidence of side effects, including diarrhea, jaundice, mild elevation of the serum cholesterol level, and rarely reversible neutropenia within the first 3 months of therapy. At the present time it is often recommended in patients who cannot tolerate aspirin or continue to have TIAs on aspirin.

Oral Anticoagulants. Oral anticoagulants have been used to prevent stroke in TIA patients for at least thirty years, but have never been investigated in an adequately designed trial. Despite their unproved benefit in preventing stroke, they do appear to reduce the

frequency of recurrent TIAs, as does aspirin. The long-term risks of serious hemorrhagic complications are significant, but many clinicians recommend warfarin therapy for 6 to 12 months, with the prothrombin time adjusted to 16 to 18 seconds, if TIAs continue to occur despite aspirin or ticlopidine therapy. In addition, anticoagulation appears to reduce the risk of stroke due to cardiac emboli in patients with TIAs who have atrial fibrillation, valvular disorders, or mural thrombi. In the context of crescendo TIAs, which are TIAs that are increasing in frequency or severity, or both, over a space of days, heparin therapy is commonly instituted. These patients usually have a high-grade internal carotid stenosis in imminent danger of becoming occluded and producing a major neurological deficit.

Carotid Endarterectomy. The surgical management of TIAs consists principally of carotid endarterectomy. Although this procedure has been used extensively, only recently has a systematic trial been carried out to determine its effectiveness compared with medical therapy. The multicenter randomized trial showed that symptomatic patients with over 70 percent stenosis demonstrated by angiography experienced a 17 percent reduction in their risk for stroke over the 2 years following endarterectomy. Relative contraindications to the procedure consist of TIAs that do not correspond to the angiographically demonstrated stenosis, significant atherosclerotic disease around the carotid siphon or in the proximal intracranial branches of the internal carotid artery, advanced cardiac disease, and age over 80. Risks include those that are usually associated with angiography, intraoperative or postoperative stroke, hemorrhage at the operative site, or myocardial ischemia. In the hands of experienced surgeons, however, serious morbidity or mortality is less than 1 percent. Results are still being analyzed to determine whether surgery is beneficial in patients with intermediate-grade stenosis.

Progressing Stroke
Heparin has been used empirically in many cases of a progressing stroke in either the ca-

rotid or vertebrobasilar distribution. Once the patient's condition is stabilized, heparin is temporarily stopped if angiographic studies are to be done to determine whether there are any surgically correctable lesions.

Completed Stroke

Management of the acute stroke patient involves several considerations. An immediate goal is to reduce the degree of damage in the ischemic area and particularly to preserve tissue in the "ischemic penumbra" zone. Although various pharmacological approaches (such as calcium channel blockers, vitamin E, and barbiturates) have been tried in an attempt to alter the sequence of events leading to cell damage following cerebral ischemia, no agent has been shown to be effective in this regard.

General measures to maintain circulation and oxygenation are important. Oxygen should be delivered by mask or nasal cannula, and pulmonary complications such as edema, atelectasis, or aspiration pneumonia must be treated. Blood pressure must be maintained within reasonable limits, and hypotension or extreme hypertension prevented. Many patients, often previously hypertensive, have very high blood pressures acutely, but pressures up to approximately 190/110 mm Hg should not ordinarily be treated because of the dangers of hypotension in patients with cerebral ischemia and autoregulatory disturbances. Mild sedation in the agitated patient or the administration of nitropaste to the patient experiencing angina may help to reduce the blood pressure.

Any cardiac arrhythmias should be managed appropriately. Hyperglycemia should be avoided and blood glucose levels kept within the normal range.

If the patient presents with generalized or partial convulsive seizures, vigorous attempts should be made to stop the epileptic activity with intravenous phenytoin (15–18 mg/kg delivered at less than 50 mg/min) or lorazepam, or both agents. Ongoing seizure activity may worsen the cerebral ischemia through the operation of several mechanisms. Raised intracranial pressure due to cerebral edema may occur in the presence of large infarcts, usually after 24 to 48 hours. Steroids are not useful in this context. Occasionally mannitol must be administered as a life-saving measure.

Many patients with large strokes are admitted to intensive care units. In this setting, adequate attention can be given to cardiopulmonary support, fluid and electrolyte balance, the prevention of pulmonary emboli, the close monitoring of neurological status, and the control of elevated intracranial pressure.

Mortality in the period after an acute cerebral infarction is approximately 15 percent in the first 30 days. The 5-year survival following a cerebral infarct is about 50 percent. Causes of death in the setting of acute stroke include cerebral edema with brain herniation (especially within the first week), cardiac ischemia and arrhythmias (peaking in the second week), and systemic complications such as pneumonia, pulmonary embolus, and sepsis (peaking around the second week).

Management in the chronic recovery phase consists of preventing further systemic complications, providing adequate nutrition, a vigorous physiotherapy and rehabilitation program instituted in the early phases (including passive range-of-motion exercises to prevent frozen shoulder and contractures), attention to bladder and skin care, and proper positioning to prevent bed sores from forming. Attention must also be given to controlling hypertension, reducing risk factors, and treating the epileptic seizures, which occur in up to 10 percent of cases. Ticlopidine is the only drug that has been shown to reduce the risk of recurrent stroke (by 33%) after a major thromboembolic stroke.

Cardiogenic Embolism

Up to one fifth of cerebral infarcts are caused by emboli originating from a cardiac source. Nonvalvular atrial fibrillation accounts for approximately 50 percent of such cases, acute myocardial infarction for 20 percent, rheumatic heart disease for 15 percent, prosthetic heart valves for 10 percent, and miscellaneous causes (e.g., cardiomyopathy, left atrial myxoma, mitral valve prolapse, infective endocarditis, paradoxical emboli, and marantic endocarditis) for 5 percent. In the Framingham study, nonvalvular atrial fibrillation was associated with a five- to sixfold increase of stroke (not necessarily embolic). The age-associated risk was increased about 18 times in the presence of rheumatic heart disease and concurrent atrial fibrillation.

The risk of stroke is especially high in the first month after the onset of atrial fibrillation, reaches 13 percent in the first year, and remains at 5 percent per year thereafter. Many of the strokes associated with emboli due to atrial fibrillation are major. The recurrence rate following an initial embolic stroke is approximately 20 percent in the first year.

Five factors have been linked to an increased risk of emboli in the context of atrial fibrillation: a previous embolic event, left atrial enlargement, coexisting congestive heart failure or low-output syndrome, new-onset sustained atrial fibrillation, and conversion to sinus rhythm.

In view of these statistics, long-term anticoagulation with warfarin has been recommended for most patients with cardiogenic brain embolism, provided there are no major contraindications such as gastric ulcer, uncontrolled hypertension, poor compliance, extreme old age, or tendency to fall. This decision must be balanced against the likelihood of a hemorrhagic complication while on long-term warfarin, which is approximately 4 percent per year. In patients with cardiac conditions predisposing to emboli but no history of TIA or stroke, aspirin is often used rather than long-term anticoagulation.

The management of an acute infarct caused by a cardiogenic embolus is controversial because early heparinization entails an approximate 4 percent risk of a bland infarct being converted to a hemorrhagic infarct or frank hematoma with deterioration. Current recommendations include a 2- to 3-day delay in heparinization in patients with large cardiogenic embolic infarcts and immediate anticoagulation in those with small infarcts, in both instances after a CT scan is obtained to rule out hemorrhage.

Asymptomatic Carotid Bruits

Bruits in the neck may arise from various sources: venous structures, external carotid arteries, or internal carotid arteries. Noninvasive tests such as Doppler flow and imaging studies can now readily establish whether a bruit is the result of stenosis of the internal carotid artery. However, the management problem facing clinicians is what to do about an asymptomatic internal carotid artery stenosis. Population-based followup studies have shown that asymptomatic bruits increase in incidence with age and hypertension and carry a risk for causing subsequent stroke of 1 to 2 percent per year. The stroke incidence is also greater in patients with over 75 percent stenosis or with known concurrent heart disease. Most significantly, the strokes that do occur are frequently not atherothrombotic and occur contralateral to the bruit. These patients are also at significant risk for suffering myocardial infarction.

Asymptomatic carotid bruits and stenosis should therefore be viewed as signs of generalized atherosclerotic disease, and thus endarterectomy for asymptomatic carotid stenosis is unlikely to bring about a long-term risk reduction in terms of either stroke or overall mortality. The best strategy in these patients is therefore to instruct them to report TIAs should they occur and to attempt to eliminate risk factors such as smoking, uncontrolled hypertension, and elevated serum cholesterol levels. Sequential noninvasive studies may also furnish additional important information, as they can identify progressing stenosis, which appears to carry a higher risk of leading to stroke.

If TIAs do appear, more extensive investigations (e.g., cerebral angiography) are called for, with a view toward possible endarterectomy. It has not yet been established whether certain subgroups of patients with asymptomatic carotid bruit or stenosis might benefit from early endarterectomy, and, until the results of large multicenter studies become available, the best approach may be to put such patients on long-term aspirin treatment.

HEMORRHAGIC CEREBROVASCULAR DISEASE

Intracranial hemorrhage, including intracerebral or subarachnoid hemorrhage, or both, constitutes 10 to 20 percent of all cases of stroke. Experience with CT scanning has made it apparent that intracerebral hemorrhage cannot be reliably distinguished from ischemic infarcts on the basis of clinical criteria alone. Small encapsulated hemorrhages may mimic ischemic deficits in all aspects, including absence of headache and no red blood cells in the CSF. Precise diagnosis is, however, vital because of the specific etiological considerations in intracranial hemorrhage and the different management strategies involved.

Intracerebral Hemorrhage

Pathophysiology and Etiology

Hypertension, as with ischemic infarcts, is the primary risk factor for intracerebral hemorrhage (Table 23-4). Pathogenesis is likely re-

Table 23-4. Causes of Intracerebral/Subarachnoid Hemorrhage

Chronic hypertension
Hypertensive crisis
    Hypertensive encephalopathy
    Eclampsia
    Pheochromocytoma
Ruptured saccular aneurysm or mycotic aneurysm
Ruptured AVM (including spinal cord AVM)
Osler-Weber-Rendu disease
Blood dyscrasias
    Hemophilia
    Thrombocytopenia
    Disseminated intravascular coagulation
    Administration of anticoagulants
Tumors
    Primary (e.g., glioblastoma, oligodendroglioma,
        pituitary adenoma, choroid plexus papilloma)
    Secondary (e.g., melanoma, renal cell carcinoma,
        choriocarcinoma)
Trauma
Drugs (sudden hypertension)
    MAO inhibitors plus foods containing tyramine
    Cocaine
    PCP ("angel dust")
    Amphetamines, methylphenidate
    Phenylpropanolamine
Intracranial dissections
Moyamoya disease
Vasculitis
Cerebral amyloid angiopathy

AVM = arteriovenous malformation; MAO = monoamine oxidase; PCP = phencyclidine.

lated to the formation of Charcot-Bouchard microaneurysms on small penetrating arterioles that have undergone hyaline degeneration (Figs. 23-16 to 23-18).

Ruptured angiomas or arteriovenous malformations are often implicated in otherwise unexplained hemorrhages that occur in younger age groups. They are only one tenth as common as aneurysms. Microangiomas may be obliterated at the time of the hemorrhage, accounting for negative radiographic findings and even the lack of findings at autopsy in some cases. Arteriovenous malformations are congenital lesions that are often furnished with a complex blood supply consisting of many "feeders." They are frequently located in the temporo-parieto-occipital areas. Pathologically, arteriovenous malformations can be divided into capillary telangiectasias, cavernous hemangiomas, venous angiomas, and true arteriovenous malformations. Before rupture they may be manifested by long-standing epileptic seizures, headaches (which may mimic classic migraine except that they are always on the same side), progressive neurological deficits (possibly due to an intracerebral steal syndrome), an intracranial bruit, or increased extracranial vascular flow on the side of the malformation. Arteriovenous malformations may enlarge with time. They most commonly bleed in affected patients between the ages of 20 and 40 years. Unlike aneurysmal hemorrhages, when rupture occurs, blood escapes at a lower pressure, and therefore the deficits are less devastating and the patient more likely to survive.

Cerebral tumors may first present as an intracerebral hemorrhage. Those types of metastatic tumors that are most likely to bleed include melanomas, choriocarcinomas, and hypernephromas. Of the primary tumors, glioblastoma, oligodendroglioma, pituitary adenoma, and choroid plexus papilloma have a tendency to bleed.

Hemorrhagic diathesis, either congenital or acquired, is a relatively common cause of intracerebral hemorrhage. Large intracerebral hemorrhages can occur in patients with hemophilia after trivial head trauma. Thrombocytopenia, with platelet counts below 10,000 to 20,000, significantly augments the risk of intracerebral

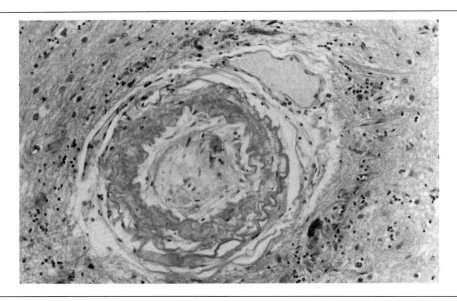

Fig. 23-16. *Microscopic cross section of a brain arteriole undergoing hyaline degeneration in a hypertensive patient. Note thickening of the media and disruption of the elastic membrane. (Original magnification, ×140.)*

Fig. 23-17. *Coronal section of brain showing a typical large basal ganglion hypertensive hemorrhage that has ruptured into the lateral ventricle.*

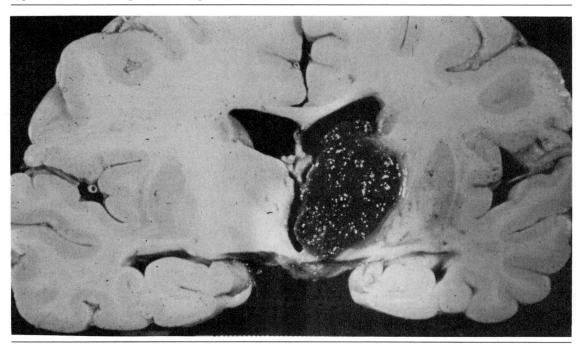

hemorrhage. Anticoagulant therapy can also predispose to intracranial hemorrhage, including massive subdural hematomas. The prothrombin time in these patients is often excessively prolonged, and many are also hypertensive.

Other causes of intracerebral hemorrhage include amphetamine or "crack" cocaine abuse, eclampsia, vasculitis, mycotic aneurysms, moyamoya disease, and head trauma. Cerebral amyloid "congophilic" angiopathy is an increasingly recognized cause of intracerebral hemorrhage, at times multiple, in patients over age 65. A progressive dementia may precede the hemorrhage. Lobar hemorrhages, often occurring in unusual locations and particularly at the junction of gray and white matter, are seen most commonly.

Clinical Picture and Diagnosis

The classic picture of intracerebral hematoma is well known and consists of the sudden onset of severe headache followed by "collapse," with loss of consciousness, hemiplegia, and, in some cases, a seizure. There are many variations to this picture, depending on the size and location of the hemorrhage and whether intraventricular rupture or subarachnoid leakage has taken place. Bleeding into or adjacent to the ventricular system may lead to acute hydrocephalus and rapid demise stemming from raised intracranial pressure and herniation. However, intraventricular rupture does not invariably indicate a poor prognosis. Small, deep encapsulated hemorrhages can manifest surprisingly few signs and leave the patient fully alert.

The most common locations where hematomas form are the putamen, thalamus, subcortical white matter (lobar hemorrhage), pons, and cerebellum (see Figs. 23-17 and 23-18). In patients with deep thalamic hemorrhages, their eyes may peer down toward the nose because of pressure on the midbrain tectal plate. Patients with pontine hemorrhage present a catastrophic picture consisting of coma or the locked-in syndrome, pinpoint pupils, horizontal

Fig. 23-18. *Large pontine hemorrhage seen at autopsy.*

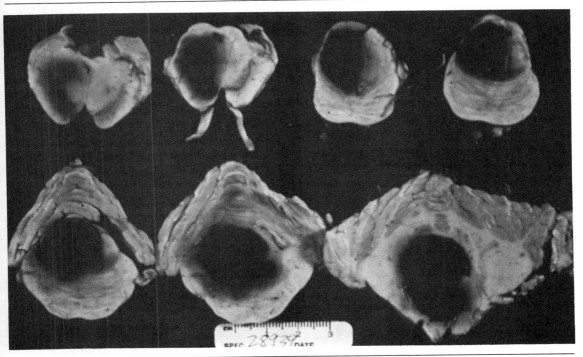

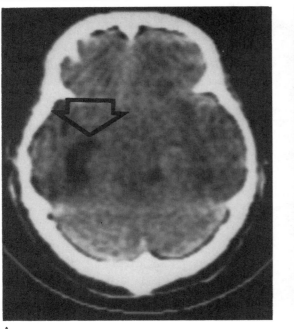
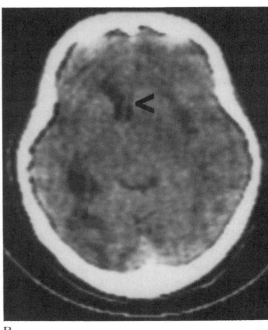

A   B

Fig. 23-19. *This 82-year-old woman had a past history of hypertension and spells of dysequilibrium thought to represent vertebrobasilar transient ischemic attacks. She suffered the sudden onset of severe headache and incoherent speech, and, a few hours later, coma with left hemiplegia and eyes conjugately deviated to the right. (A, B) Note the marked right-to-left shift of the lateral ventricles* (arrowhead) *and dilatation of the left temporal horn due to obstructive hydrocephalus* (open arrow).

gaze paralysis, decerebrate posturing, and, at times, fever. Patients with cerebellar hemorrhage may also manifest a catastrophic picture that includes the rapid onset of coma and severe brainstem compromise, or it can evolve more subacutely beginning with headache, hemiataxia or total inability to stand, severe vertigo and vomiting, and a contralateral conjugate eye deviation.

CT or MRI scanning offers a ready means of diagnosing and localizing the hemorrhage, as well as of determining whether acute hydrocephalus or intraventricular rupture has occurred (Fig. 23-19). The specific etiology such as an arteriovenous malformation or tumor may also be identified by neuroimaging procedures.

Arteriovenous malformations are usually apparent on CT scans (see Fig. 9-1). MRI scans can also distinguish recent from remote hemorrhage by the presence of methemoglobin and

hemosiderin in the latter. Cavernous hemangiomas, which can arise in unusual locations such as the brainstem, display a characteristic appearance on MRI scanning, consisting of a high-intensity core surrounded by an area of lower-intensity signal, which imparts a "target" appearance to T_2-weighted images. They may be multiple, have a familial basis, and generally do not bleed (Fig. 23-20).

Small hemorrhages around the base of the skull are best visualized by MRI because artifacts from bony structures are eliminated. Prior to the advent of these neuroimaging techniques, cerebral angiography was frequently performed in the acute stage in these patients to obtain evidence of a possible "mass effect" resulting from the various displacements and distortions of arterial and venous structures. Angiography may now be performed to detect arteriovenous malformations, aneurysms, or vasculitis. Lumbar

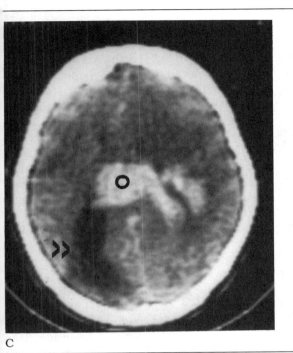 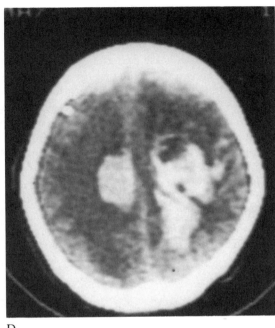

C   D

Fig. 23-19. *(C, D) These unenhanced CT scans show a large right lobar white matter hemorrhage that has ruptured into the ventricles* (circle). *(C) The double arrowhead points to a preexisting infarct in the left posterior cerebral artery territory.*

puncture was also formerly done to detect red blood cells in the CSF, but should now be avoided because it can provoke brain herniation.

Management and Prognosis

Initial management in most patients with intracranial hemorrhage is approached medically, except in certain patients showing acute deterioration who have accessible hematomas or acute hydrocephalus. These patients may undergo emergency surgery as a life-saving measure. Initially, respiratory and cardiac function must be stabilized and excessively high blood pressures should be lowered. However, the levels to which blood pressure should be lowered are controversial since many patients require high pressures so that cerebral perfusion can be maintained in the face of elevated intracranial pressure. Excessively high pressures should be gently lowered to approximately 200/110 mm Hg, especially in patients without preexisting hypertension. Coagulation deficits should be corrected when possible. Edema begins to form

around the hematoma at 6 to 8 hours and progresses over the ensuing 24 to 48 hours. Attention should be directed mainly toward the rapid control of intracranial pressure in comatose or deteriorating patients with large hematomas in the cerebrum or cerebellum (see Chapter 20). Intubation and hyperventilation together with the administration of mannitol are primary measures. Fluid administration should consist of less than 50 ml of normal saline per hour. Intraventricular drainage can be instituted in patients with acute hydrocephalus. Phenytoin (18 mg/kg) may be given intravenously (at a rate of less than 50 mg/min) to prevent seizures, which can substantially worsen elevated intracranial pressure.

The indications for and timing of surgical intervention to remove intraparenchymal hematomas is controversial. Some advocate the early removal of relatively superficial hemispheric hematomas in patients whose condition has stabilized and who have not incurred severe brain damage. This measure may avoid prolonged comatose or stuporous states and the accompanying morbidity. Cerebellar hematomas in stable patients who are not comatose can be managed expectantly with repeated CT scans. However, in comatose patients or those showing acute deterioration, the emergency removal of a cerebellar hematoma can be a life-saving measure. Brainstem hematomas are generally not treated surgically, although there are a few isolated reports of good results following the heroic removal of a pontine hematoma in younger patients.

The treatment of vascular malformations ideally entails complete excision, but, when they are in inaccessible locations, or cases are otherwise inoperable, specialized interventional radiological techniques have been employed to

Fig. 23-20. *T₂-weighted MRI scan showing numerous discrete areas of low signal intensity representing multiple cavernous hemangiomas. Hemosiderin deposition accounts for these low-intensity signals.*

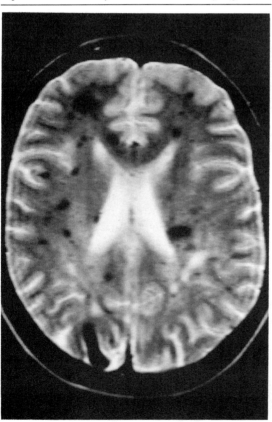

obliterate feeding vessels with a variable degree of success. These techniques include proton-beam therapy, conventional x-ray therapy, embolization of the feeding vessels, and the insertion of various detachable balloons or specialized glues through precisely placed catheters. These highly specialized techniques are performed only at a few centers and carry a relatively high risk of complications, such as focal ischemic brain damage or hemorrhage.

The management of unruptured arteriovenous malformations that have been detected, for example, by CT or MRI in patients undergoing investigation for headache or epilepsy, is controversial. The annual rate of rupture of arteriovenous malformations is about 2 to 3 percent, and the first hemorrhage is fatal in about 10 percent of these patients. However, the surgical mortality is approximately 5 to 10 percent. The age of the patient, size and location of the malformation, and local morbidity and mortality of the procedure must all be considered in these cases. In general, a nonsurgical approach is indicated.

The prognosis of intracerebral hemorrhage is very variable and depends on such factors as its size and location, the degree of elevated intracranial pressure, the extent of midline shift on the CT scan, and the patient's age. Rebleeding after an initial intracerebral hemorrhage is rare in cases that do not involve an aneurysm or arteriovenous malformation. The overall mortality is approximately 50 percent in the first month. Some patients, particularly in younger age groups, do surprisingly well once their condition stabilizes. Some patients ultimately do better than would be expected with comparable infarcts, since hematomas may cause less destruction of neurons and neuronal pathways. In survivors, control of chronic hypertension and definitive treatment of aneurysms or arteriovenous malformations should be carried out to lessen the risk of recurrent hemorrhage.

Subarachnoid Hemorrhage

Subarachnoid hemorrhage accounts for 6 to 8 percent of the cases of strokes. Primary subarachnoid hemorrhage is due to the release of blood directly into the subarachnoid space; secondary subarachnoid hemorrhage is defined as the leakage of blood into the subarachnoid space from a primary intracerebral hematoma. The most common cause of blood in the subarachnoid space is a cerebral contusion due to head trauma. However, usually when the term *subarachnoid hemorrhage* is used, it refers to the hemorrhage resulting from the spontaneous rupture of an intracranial saccular aneurysm or arteriovenous malformation, an event that produces a fairly stereotyped clinical picture.

The etiological factors mentioned in the discussion of intracerebral hematoma also pertain to primary subarachnoid hemorrhage. Dissection, particularly of the vertebral artery in the neck, may produce a subarachnoid hemorrhage. Arteriovenous malformations of the spinal canal and spinal cord tumors can also cause subarachnoid hemorrhage, and a pituitary adenoma or other tumor may bleed into the subarachnoid space. Discussion in the rest of this section focuses on aneurysmal subarachnoid hemorrhage, which has a yearly incidence of 15 to 20 cases per 100,000 population, accounts for 70 to 82 percent of all cases of subarachnoid hemorrhage, and represents a medical emergency that poses management problems which are both challenging and controversial.

Pathogenesis

Intracranial saccular aneurysms, which tend to occur at the bifurcation of large arteries at the base of the brain around the circle of Willis, are found during 3 to 5 percent of routine autopsies. Although not usually present at birth, and therefore not congenital in the strict sense, they are thought to be due to congenital defects in the arterial wall involving the media and elastic membrane. This allows a thin-walled sac composed of a layer of muscle fibers and fibrous tissue to form a balloonlike pouch on the vessel. The aneurysm may enlarge with time and eventually rupture, sending a high-pressure jet of blood into the subarachnoid space and the brain parenchyma, or occasionally into the subdural space, producing a subdural hematoma. Often there is evidence of small hemorrhagic leaks surrounding the aneurysm with hemosiderin staining, which can be picked up on MRI scans. A thrombus may form within the aneurysmal

sac and calcification of the walls can take place. The most common locations for berry aneurysms are the internal carotid–posterior communicating junction, the anterior communicating artery, the middle cerebral artery, the posterior communicating artery, the posterior inferior cerebellar artery, and the tip of the basilar artery. Other types of aneurysm, such as mycotic (due to infectious emboli) or atherosclerotic ones, may also occasionally rupture and cause subarachnoid hemorrhage. Aneurysms are multiple in 20 percent of cases; may occur in conjunction with other vascular anomalies such as arteriovenous malformations, cervicocephalic fibromuscular hyperplasia, and moyamoya disease; and are found with increased incidence in patients with Ehlers-Danlos syndrome, coarctation of the aorta, Marfan's syndrome, and polycystic kidney disease. Occasional familial cases are encountered. Giant aneurysms over 2.5 cm in diameter often present as mass lesions and require special management (Fig. 23-21).

Clinical Picture and Diagnosis

The peak age for aneurysmal rupture is 40 to 50 years and aneurysmal subarachnoid hemorrhage is rare before age 20. About 50 percent of patients with aneurysms experience a "sentinel" headache prior to a major rupture. This headache is typically sudden and severe, and may be accompanied by some neck stiffness, nausea, and vomiting. In such patients, especially those who have not been subject to previous recurrent headaches, this history should prompt the performance of a lumbar puncture to search for blood or xanthochromia as well as a cranial CT scan.

The classic picture of a full-blown aneurysmal subarachnoid hemorrhage is well known and consists of the explosive onset of severe headache (often during activity, straining, or coitus), nausea, vomiting, and photophobia; the initial loss of consciousness in approximately 20 percent of cases; and the development of nuchal rigidity within a few hours. Epileptic seizures occur at the onset in 4 percent of patients and overall throughout the course in 25 percent of cases. Obtundation and confusion are common. Occasionally patients may exhibit an agitated delirium. Back pain at the onset strongly suggests an intraspinal cause.

On examination, nuchal rigidity is a frequent but not invariable finding. Fever may be present and blood pressure is usually elevated. The level of alertness may vary initially from fully alert to deeply comatose, and is a very important predictor of prognosis. Subhyaloid retinal hemorrhages are frequently seen and can be an important clue to diagnosis, especially in patients found deeply comatose without an available history.

Focal neurological findings include a third or sixth cranial nerve palsy due to the direct pressure effects of the aneurysm (or a sixth nerve palsy as a sign of elevated intracranial

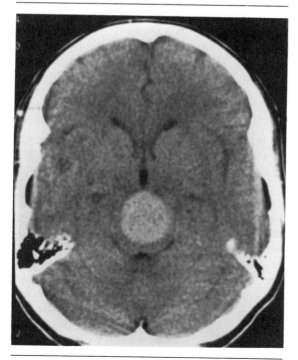

Fig. 23-21. *This 28-year-old woman had been observed since her midteens, because of spells consisting of vivid visual hallucinations which were originally treated as complex partial seizures but were more likely to represent peduncular hallucinosis. She then developed extreme emotional lability over a period of weeks with uncontrolled outbursts of laughter, and also exhibited bilateral corticobulbar and corticospinal tract signs. (A) Unenhanced CT scan revealed a giant basilar tip aneurysm in the interpeduncular region of the midbrain.*

pressure) and signs such as conjugate eye deviation or hemiplegia due to the accumulation of an intracerebral hematoma, a subdural hematoma, or the early development of arterial spasm. Occasionally early hydrocephalus due to impaired CSF flow and absorption from subarachnoid blood may produce stupor and impaired up-gaze.

Other conditions that can bring about sudden, explosive headache, and thus enter into the differential diagnosis, include migraine, viral meningitis, acute hydrocephalus (e.g., due to a colloid cyst of the third ventricle causing intermittent ventricular obstruction), and pheochromocytoma. Occasionally an aneurysmal rupture producing a small intracerebral clot may mimic the picture of a brain abscess, since severe headache, fever, and elevated peripheral white blood cell count are common to both conditions. Herpes simplex encephalitis may also produce a picture resembling that of aneurysmal subarachnoid hemorrhage.

The electrocardiogram in the setting of subarachnoid hemorrhage frequently shows abnormalities, including elevated S-T segments, U waves, flattened or inverted T waves, and arrhythmias such as ventricular tachycardia, the tachy-brady syndrome, atrioventricular conduction defects, or torsades de pointes. These changes are believed to be autonomically mediated by the effects of blood on the hypothalamus.

CT scanning reveals positive findings in up to 95 percent of cases, if done within the first 24 hours (Fig. 23-22). The aneurysm itself may appear as an enhancing round structure located at the base of the brain or in the sylvian fissure, if it is large enough or calcification is present. Blood is frequently noted in the basal cisterns, sylvian fissures, intrahemispheric fissure, over the cerebral convexities, or in the parenchyma in the case of an intracerebral hematoma. The location of the subarachnoid blood offers a fairly reliable clue to the location of the aneurysm and, in the case of multiple aneurysms, correlates with the site of rupture. In addition, the extent of the blood may predict the future development of vasospasm.

An MRI scan is even more sensitive for demonstrating aneurysms, particularly if they have bled previously, and can identify small intracerebral hematomas missed on CT because of their proximity to bone at the base of the skull.

Apart from the sentinel headache, a small proportion of patients with aneurysms may suffer neurological or other symptoms prior to rupture (see Fig. 23-21). Chronic headaches are rarely due to aneurysms. An isolated third nerve (usually with pupillary involvement) or sixth nerve palsy must always be cause for suspecting a cerebral aneurysm. Large aneurysms around the sella turcica may precipitate endocrine abnormalities such as galactorrhea and amenorrhea. Rarely an aneurysm can cause distal embolization from an intraluminal clot, thus leading to TIAs. Also rarely, an aneurysm can produce epilepsy due to the irritation of surrounding brain tissue, perhaps resulting from the leakage of blood.

Examination of the CSF frequently shows the existence of gross blood (or xanthochromia if more than 8 hours have elapsed since the ictus), an elevated protein level, elevated pressure, and elevated white count due to a secondary inflammatory response. The CSF glucose level may occasionally be low.

Cerebral angiography is the definitive test for identifying cerebral aneurysms and delineating their shape prior to surgery. All studies should include examination of the four major vessels. Using digital subtraction techniques, magnification, and oblique views, angiography can reveal an aneurysm in 80 to 90 percent of cases of subarachnoid hemorrhage. Studies may be negative if there is arterial spasm or an intraluminal clot that interferes with visualization of the aneurysm. If the angiogram is initially negative, re-

Fig. 23-21. *(B) Vertebral angiogram demonstrating the giant aneurysm. Following an attempt to clip the aneurysm, she remained in a chronic vegetative state with bilateral thalamic infarction.*

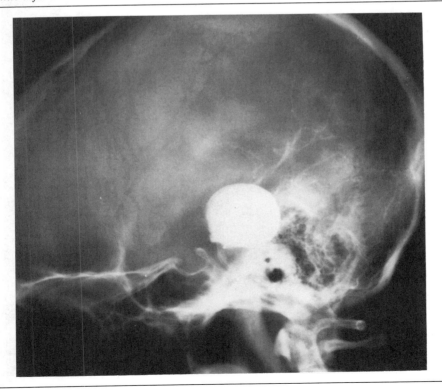

peat studies should be done at 2 weeks and 6 months and may show the aneurysm in an additional 5 to 10 percent of cases. If the angiogram continues to be negative, then the chances of rebleeding are considerably less than in those cases in which an aneurysm has been demonstrated.

Spinal cord MRI or myelography can be used to detect spinal tumors or arteriovenous malformations that are causing subarachnoid hemorrhage, and transcranial Doppler studies have been useful for detecting arterial spasm following a subarachnoid hemorrhage.

Prognosis and Management

Despite advances in diagnostic and surgical techniques, a ruptured aneurysm remains a devastating condition. The results of large studies, in which patients have been followed for 6 months after rupture of an aneurysmal subarachnoid hemorrhage, have shown that only approximately half of all patients and two thirds of patients who undergo surgery recover well. Mortality is 25 percent in the first 24 hours.

A ruptured aneurysm constitutes a neurological emergency, and several possible conse-

Fig. 23-22. *This 42-year-old man was brought to the emergency room after being found comatose at home. When examined, he showed marked nuchal rigidity, withdrew all four extremities equally to pain, had bilateral Babinski's signs and full roving eye movements, and pupils were 2 mm and unreactive bilaterally. (A) Unenhanced CT scan revealing blood in the cisterns around the midbrain extending into the sylvian fissures, dilatation of the temporal horns* (horizontal arrow) *indicating hydrocephalus, a basilar tip aneurysm* (circle), *and a right middle cerebral artery aneurysm* (oblique arrowhead).

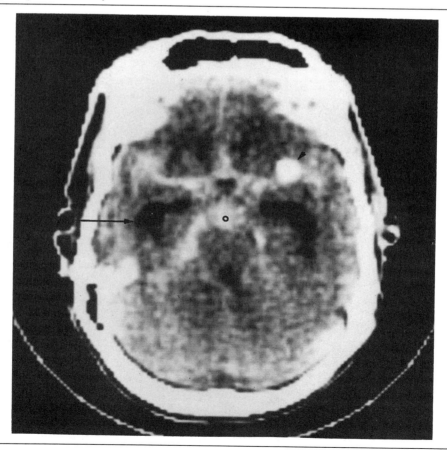

quences must be anticipated and prevented if possible. If aneurysms are untreated, **rebleeding** occurs in 20 percent of patients within 2 weeks, 40 percent by 6 months, and 3 percent per year thereafter. A rebleed in the early weeks is fatal in 50 percent of cases. The first 24 hours represents the time when the risk for rebleeding is greatest, and a second peak occurs between days 5 and 9. Medical measures to reduce the threat of rebleeding include lowering of blood pressure below levels of approximately 180/100 mm Hg, adequate analgesia to control headaches, sedation, and the administration of phenytoin (18 mg/kg intravenously) to prevent seizures. The patient's head is elevated to lower intracranial pressure and mannitol may be given if patients exhibit signs of herniation. The use of epsilon-aminocaproic acid or tranexamic acid, which inhibit fibrinolysis, lowers the incidence of rebleeding, but routine use has been abandoned because these agents do not improve outcome because they cause peripheral venous thrombosis and predispose to cerebral ischemia.

The other feared and common complication of subarachnoid hemorrhage is cerebral **arterial spasm.** Spasm develops in approximately one fourth of patients and is caused by the presence of blood breakdown products such as vasoactive amines and prostaglandins in the subarachnoid space. Cerebral angiography shows narrowing of the major cerebral arteries and their branches in these cases, and spasm is confined to the intracranial portions of these major arteries. Spasm is maximal between days 3 and 10 and is often manifested clinically as a diminished level of consciousness, with or without focal neurological signs. It may be transient or prolonged, often but not always involves the vessels near the site of the aneurysmal rupture, and may lead to cerebral ischemia and focal infarction. For example, infarction may be seen

Fig. 23-22. (B) Carotid angiogram showing the left middle cerebral artery aneurysm (arrow).

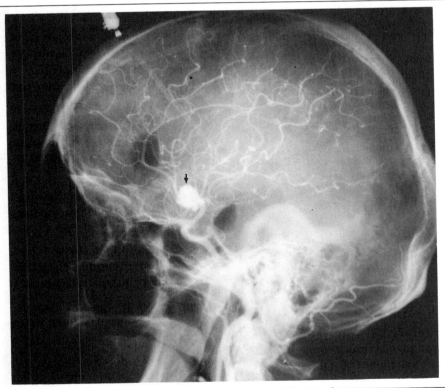

in the medial frontal regions due to spasm in the pericallosal branches of the anterior cerebral artery following an anterior communicating artery aneurysm rupture.

Craniotomy is generally not performed in patients during spasm. Transcranial Doppler testing is a convenient way to detect and monitor spasm and can be performed repeatedly. No treatment for spasm has been definitively proven effective, but nimodipine, a calcium-channel blocker that crosses the blood-brain barrier, appears to work. It is administered orally, 60 mg every 4 hours. Standard treatment also includes avoidance of dehydration and hypotension. Intravenous volume expansion and administration of pressor agents such as dopa-mine, which are more safely carried out once the aneurysm has been clipped surgically, are measures used to treat vasospasm.

These considerations have sparked a great deal of controversy concerning the appropriate timing of neurosurgical intervention. As microsurgical techniques, instrumentation, and anesthesia have been refined, ever earlier operations have been the trend in order to forestall rebleeding, especially in patients who are alert or only mildly stuporous. However, surgical clipping of an aneurysm that has freshly bled is a technically demanding procedure in the best of hands, and many neurosurgeons prefer to wait 24 to 48 hours even in less severely compromised patients to permit the aneurysm and sur-

Fig. 23-22 *(Continued). (C) Vertebral angiogram revealing the second aneurysm* (arrow) *at the tip of the basilar artery. The patient eventually died due to rebleeding, severe vasospasm, and bilateral cerebral infarction.*

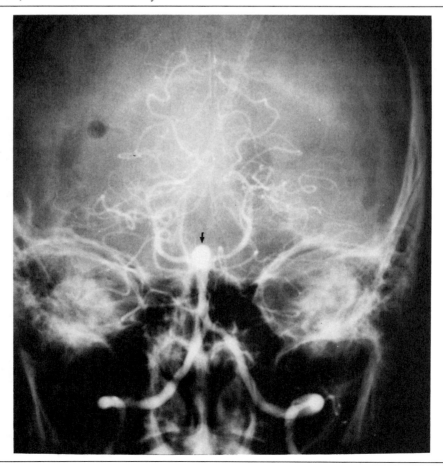

rounding brain tissue a chance to "settle down" and to ensure optimal operating conditions (e.g., a rested team of experienced surgeons, nurses, and anesthesiologists). In more severe cases, operation toward the end of the first week, before spasm is likely to develop, has been recommended. In cases in which there is a substantial intracerebral hematoma or early hydrocephalus, surgical removal of the hematoma or placement of a ventricular shunt (or ventriculostomy) is carried out.

The criteria for surgical clipping of unruptured aneurysms discovered incidentally during angiography, CT scanning, or MRI scanning for reasons other than subarachnoid hemorrhage are still controversial. Some of the considerations that enter into the decision of whether to clip the aneurysm include its size, location, shape, whether it is producing compressive symptoms such as third nerve palsy, and the age and overall medical condition of the patient. Some studies have suggested that aneurysms greater than 1 cm in diameter are at greater risk of rupture and therefore should be tackled surgically. Accessible aneurysms in younger healthy patients should generally be clipped.

BIBLIOGRAPHY

General

Adams, R. D., and Victor, M. Cerebrovascular Diseases. In R. D. Adams and M. Victor (editors). *Principles of Neurology*, 3rd ed. New York: McGraw-Hill, 1985, Pp. 569–640.

Barnett, H. J. M. (editor). Cerebrovascular disease. *Neurol. Clin.* 1:1–358, 1983.

Barnett, H. J. M., and Hachinski, V. C. (editors). Cerebral ischemia: treatment and prevention. *Neurol. Clin.* 10:1–299, 1992.

Biller, J. (editor). Cerebrovascular disorders in the 1990's. *Clin. Geriatr. Med.* 7:401–643, 1991.

Caplan, L. R. Stroke. *CIBA-GEIGY Clin. Symp.* 40:2–32, 1990.

Caplan, L. R. Diagnosis and treatment of ischemic stroke. *JAMA* 266:2413–2418, 1991.

Caplan, L. R., and Stein, R. W. (editors). *Stroke, a Clinical Approach.* Boston: Butterworths, 1986.

Hachinski, V., and Norris, J. W. (editors). *The Acute Stroke.* Philadelphia: Davis, 1985.

Harrison, M. J. G., and Dyken, M. L. (editors). *Cerebral Vascular Diseases.* London: Butterworths, 1983.

Norris, J. W., and Hachinski, V. C. (editors). *Prevention of Stroke.* New York: Springer-Verlag, 1991.

Yatsu, F. M., Grotta, J. C., and Pettigrew, L. C. (editors). Stroke. *Semin. Neurol.* 6:243–331, 1986.

Pathophysiology of Ischemic Cerebrovascular Disease

Hakim, A. M. Hemodynamic and metabolic studies in stroke. *Semin. Neurol.* 9:286–292, 1989.

Hakim, A. M. The cerebral ischemic penumbra. *Can. J. Neurol. Sci.* 14:557–559, 1987.

Kricheff, I. I. Arteriosclerotic ischemic cerebrovascular disease. *Radiology* 162:101–109, 1987.

Raichle, M. The pathophysiology of brain ischemia. *Ann. Neurol.* 13:2–10, 1983.

Scheinberg, P. The biologic basis for the treatment of acute stroke. *Neurology* 41:1867–1873, 1991.

Diagnosis of Ischemic Cerebrovascular Disease

Ackerman, R. H. Noninvasive diagnosis of carotid disease in the era of digital subtraction angiography. *Neurol. Clin.* 2:263–278, 1983.

Come, P. C., Riley, M. F., and Bivas, N. K. Roles of echocardiography and arrhythmia monitoring in the evaluation of patients with suspected systemic embolism. *Ann. Neurol.* 13:527–531, 1983.

Damasio, H. A computed tomographic guide to the identification of cerebral vascular territories. *Arch. Neurol.* 40:138–142, 1983.

Faught, E., Trader, S. D., and Hanna, G. R. Cerebral complications of angiography for transient ischemia and stroke: prediction of risk. *Neurology* 29:4–15, 1979.

Kinkel, P. R., Kinkel, W. R., and Jacobs, L. Nuclear magnetic resonance imaging in patients with stroke. *Semin. Neurol.* 6:43–52, 1986.

Kistler, J. P., et al. Diagnostic approaches to cerebrovascular disease. *Semin. Neurol.* 6:254–261, 1983.

Little, J. R., et al. Digital subtraction angiography in cerebrovascular disease. *Stroke* 13:557–566, 1982.

Petty, G. W., Wiebers, D. O., and Meissner, I. Transcranial Doppler ultrasonography: clinical applications in cerebrovascular disease. *Mayo Clin. Proc.* 65:1350–1364, 1990.

Management of TIAs

Amaurosis Fugax Study Group. Current management of amaurosis fugax. *Stroke* 21:201–208, 1990.

Barnett, H. J. M. Evaluating methods for prevention in stroke. *Ann. R. Coll. Phys. Surg. Can.* 24:33–42, 1991.

Biller, J., and Love, B. B. Recent therapeutic options for stroke prevention. *Hosp. Phys.* 27:13–24, 1991.

Bogousslavsky, J., et al. Cardiac and arterial lesions in carotid transient ischemic attacks. *Arch. Neurol.* 43:223–228, 1986.

Bogousslavsky, J., et al. Clinical predictors of cardiac and arterial lesions in carotid transient ischemic attacks. *Arch. Neurol.* 43:229–233, 1986.

Canadian Cooperative Study Group. A randomized trial of aspirin and sulfinpyrazone in threatened stroke. *N. Engl. J. Med.* 299:53–59, 1978.

The Dutch TIA Trial Study Group. A comparison of two doses of aspirin (30 mg vs 283 mg a day) in patients after a transient ischemic attack or minor ischemic stroke. *N. Engl. J. Med.* 325:1261–1266, 1991.

Hass, W. K., et al. A randomized trial comparing ticlopidine hydrochloride with aspirin for the prevention of stroke in high-risk patients. *N. Engl. J. Med.* 231:501–507, 1989.

Hurwitz, B. J., et al. Comparison of amaurosis fugax and transient cerebral ischemia: a prospective clinical and arteriographic study. *Ann. Neurol.* 698–704, 1985.

Norris, J. Outcome of transient ischemic attacks and stroke. *Drugs* 42(Suppl. 5):10–15, 1991.

Management and Prevention of Ischemic Stroke

Biller, J., and Love, B. B. Medical management of acute cerebral ischemia in the elderly. *Clin. Geriatr. Med.* 7:455–473, 1991.

Bornstein, N. M., and Korczyn, A. D. Prevention of Recurrent Stroke. In J. W. Norris and V. C. Hachinski (editors). *Prevention of Stroke.* New York: Springer-Verlag, 1991, Pp. 261–268.

Davis, P. H., et al. Risk factors for ischemic stroke: a prospective study in Rochester, Minnesota. *Ann. Neurol.* 22:319–327, 1987.

Easton, J. D. Antiplatelet therapy in the prevention of stroke. *Drugs* 42(suppl. 5):39–50, 1991.

Grotta, J. C. Current medical and surgical therapy for cerebrovascular disease. *N. Engl. J. Med.* 317:1505–1516, 1987.

Hershey, L. A. Stroke prevention in women: role of aspirin versus ticlopidine. *Am. J. Med.* 91:288–292, 1991.

Kistler, J. P., Ropper, A. H., and Heros, R. C. Therapy of ischemic cerebral vascular disease due to atherothrombosis. *N. Engl. J. Med.* 311:27–34;100–105, 1984.

Shuaib, A., and Hachinski, V. C. Mechanisms

and management of stroke in the elderly. *Can. Med. Assoc. J.* 145:433–443, 1991.

Syndromes and Localization

Ajax, E. T., Schenkenberg, T., and Kosteljanetz, M. Alexia without agraphia and the inferior splenium. *Neurology* 27:685–688, 1977.

Alexander, M. P., and Schmitt, M. A. The aphasia syndrome of stroke in the left anterior cerebral artery territory. *Arch. Neurol.* 37:97–100, 1985.

Amarenco, P. The spectrum of cerebellar infarctions. *Neurology* 41:973–979, 1991.

Ameri, A., and Bousser, M. G. Cerebral venous thrombosis. *Neurol. Clin.* 10:87–111, 1992.

Ausman, J. I., et al. Vertebrobasilar insufficiency. A review. *Arch. Neurol.* 42:803–808, 1985.

Baloh, R. W., Furman, J. M., and Yee, R. D. Dorsal midbrain syndrome: clinical and oculographic findings. *Neurology* 35:54–60, 1985.

Bladin, P. F., and Berkovic, S. Striatocapsular infarction: large infarcts in the lenticulostriate arterial territory. *Neurology* 34:1423–1430, 1984.

Bogousslavsky, J., and Regli, F. Anterior cerebral artery territory infarction in the Lausanne stroke registry. *Arch. Neurol.* 47:144–150, 1990.

Bogousslavsky, J., and Regli, F. Capsular genu syndrome. *Neurology* 40:1499–1502, 1990.

Bogousslavsky, J., Regli, F., and Uske, A. Thalamic infarcts. Clinical syndromes, etiology and prognosis. *Neurology* 38:837–848, 1988.

Caplan, L. R. "Top of the basilar" syndrome. *Neurology* 30:72–79, 1980.

Caplan, L. R. Intracranial branch atheromatous disease: a neglected, understudied, and underused concept. *Neurology* 39:1246–1250, 1989.

Caplan, L. R., et al. Lateral thalamic infarcts. *Arch. Neurol.* 45:959–964, 1988.

Fisher, C. M. Lacunar strokes and infarcts: a review. *Neurology* 32:871–876, 1982.

Fisher, M., and McQuillen, J. B. Bilateral cortical border-zone infarction. A pseudobrainstem stroke. *Arch. Neurol.* 38:62–63, 1981.

Guberman, A., and Stuss, D. The syndrome of bilateral paramedian thalamic infarction. *Neurology* 33:540–546, 1983.

Hankey, G. J., and Warlow, C. P. Lacunar transient ischemic attacks: a clinically useful concept? *Lancet* 337:335–338, 1991.

Helgason, C., et al. Anterior choroidal artery-territory infarction. Report of cases and review. *Arch. Neurol.* 43:681–686, 1986.

Hennerici, M., Klemm, C., and Routenberg, W. The subclavian steal phenomenon: a common vascular disorder with rare neurologic deficits. *Neurology* 38:669–673, 1988.

Kase, C. S., et al. Cerebellar infarction in the superior cerebellar artery distribution. *Neurology* 35:705–711, 1985.

Kinkel, W. R., et al. Subcortical arteriosclerotic encephalopathy (Binswanger's disease). Computed tomographic, nuclear magnetic resonance, and clinical correlations. *Arch. Neurol.* 42:951–959, 1985.

Lhermitte, F., Gauthier, J. C., and Derouesné, C. Nature of occlusions of the middle cerebral artery. *Neurology* 20:82–88, 1970.

Mao, C. C., Coull, B. M., and Golper, L. A. C. Anterior operculum syndrome. *Neurology* 39:1169–1172, 1989.

Medina, J. L., Chokroverty, S., and Rubino, F. A. Syndrome of agitated delirium and visual impairment: a manifestation of medial temporo-occipital infarction. *J. Neurol. Neurosurg. Psychiatry* 40:861–864, 1977.

Miller, V. T. Lacunar stroke: a reassessment. *Arch. Neurol.* 40:129–134, 1983.

Mohr, J. P., et al. Broca aphasia: pathologic and clinical. *Neurology* 28:311–324, 1978.

Roeltgen, D. P., Sevush, S., and Heilmann, K. M. Pure Gertsmann's syndrome from a focal lesion. *Arch. Neurol.* 40:46–47, 1983.

Sypert, G., and Alvord, E. C., Jr. Cerebellar infarction. A clinicopathological study. *Arch. Neurol.* 32:357–363, 1975.

Tuszynski, M. H., Petito, C. K., and Levy, D. E. Risk factors and clinical manifestations of pathologically verified lacunar infarctions. *Stroke* 20:990–999, 1989.

Ward, T. N., Bernat, J. L., and Goldstein, A. S. Occlusion of the anterior choroidal artery. *J. Neurol. Neurosurg. Psychiatry* 47:1048–1049, 1984.

Etiology of Stroke and Stroke in Young People

Amarenco, P., et al. The prevalence of ulcerated plaques in the aortic arch in patients with stroke. *N. Engl. J. Med.* 326:221–225, 1992.

Asherson, R. A., et al. The "primary" antiphospholipid syndrome: major clinical and serological features. *Medicine* 68:366–373, 1989.

Boers, G. H. J., et al. Heterozygosity for homocystinuria in premature peripheral and cerebral occlusive arterial disease. *N. Engl. J. Med.* 313:709–715, 1985.

Bogousslavsky, J., and Regli, F. Ischemic stroke in adults younger than 30 years of age: cause and prognosis. *Arch. Neurol.* 44:479–482, 1987.

Bogousslavsky, J., and Pierre, P. Ischemic stroke in patients under age 45. *Neurol. Clin.* 10:113–124, 1992.

Bogousslavsky, J., et al. Migraine stroke. *Neurology* 38:223–227, 1988.

Calabrese, L. H., and Mallek, J. A. Primary angiitis of the central nervous system: report of 8 new cases, review of the literature, and proposal for diagnostic criteria. *Medicine* 67:20–39, 1987.

Caselli, R. J., Hunder, G. G., and Whisnant, J. P. Neurologic disease in biopsy-proven giant cell (temporal) arteritis. *Neurology* 38:352–359, 1988.

Covill, B. M., and Goodnight, S. H. Antiphospholipid antibodies, prethrombotic states and stroke. *Stroke* 21:1370–1374, 1990.

Easton, J. D., and Hart, R. G. Underestimated causes of stroke. *Ann. R. Coll. Phys. Surg. Can.* 16:37–43, 1983.

Hankey, G. J. Isolated angiitis/angiopathy of the central nervous system. *Cerebrovasc. Dis.* 1:2–15, 1991.

Hart, R. G., and Miller, V. T. Cerebral infarction in young adults. A practical approach. *Stroke* 14:110–114, 1983.

Hilton-Jones, D., and Warlow, C. P. Non-penetrating arterial trauma and cerebral infarction in the young. *Lancet* 1:1435–1438, 1985.

Lechat, P., et al. Prevalence of patent foramen ovale in patients with stroke. *N. Engl. J. Med.* 318:1148–1152, 1988.

Levine, S. R., et al. "Crack" cocaine–associated stroke. *Neurology* 37:1849–1853, 1987.

Lhermitte, F., et al. Ischemic accidents in the middle cerebral artery territory: a study of the causes in 122 cases. *Arch. Neurol.* 19:248–256, 1968.

Luscher, T. F., et al. Arterial fibromuscular dysplasia. *Mayo Clin. Proc.* 62:931–952, 1987.

Marshall, J. The cause and prognosis of strokes in people under 50 years. *J. Neurol. Sci.* 53:473–488, 1982.

Natowicz, M., and Kelley, R. I. Mendelian etiologies of stroke. *Ann. Neurol.* 22:175–192, 1987.

Schafer, A. I. The hypercoagulable states. *Ann. Intern. Med.* 102:814–828, 1985.

Sloan, M. A., et al. Occurrence of stroke associated with use/abuse of drugs. *Neurology* 41:1358–1364, 1991.

Suzuki, J., and Kodama, N. Moyamoya disease—a review. *Stroke* 14:104–109, 1983.

Younger, D. S., et al. Granulomatous angiitis of the brain: an inflammatory reaction of diverse etiology. *Arch. Neurol.* 45:514–518, 1988.

Cerebral Embolism

Albers, G. W., et al. Stroke prevention in non-valvular atrial fibrillation: a review of prospective randomized trials. *Ann. Neurol.* 30:511–518, 1991.

Behar, S., et al. Cerebrovascular accident complicating acute myocardial infarction: incidence, clinical significance and short- and long-term mortality rates. *Am. J. Med.* 91:45–50, 1991.

Biller, J., et al. Paradoxical cerebral embolism: eight cases. *Neurology* 36:1356–1360, 1986.

The Boston Area Anticoagulation Trial for Atrial Fibrillation Investigators. The effect of low-dose warfarin on the risk of stroke in patients with nonrheumatic atrial fibrillation. *N. Engl. J. Med.* 323:1505–1511, 1990.

Cerebral Embolism Task Force. Cardiogenic brain embolism. *Arch. Neurol.* 43:71–84, 1986.

Cerebral Embolism Task Force. Cardiogenic brain embolism. The second report of the Cerebral Embolism Task Force. *Arch. Neurol.* 46:727–743, 1989.

Edmunds, L. H., Jr. Thromboembolic complications of current cardiac valvular prostheses. *Ann. Thorac. Surg.* 34:96–106, 1982.

Hart, R. G., et al. Stroke in infective endocarditis. *Stroke* 21:695–700, 1990.

Laureno, R., Shields, R. W., Jr., and Narayan, T. The diagnosis and management of cerebral embolism and hemorrhagic infarction with sequential computerized cranial tomography. *Brain* 110:93–105, 1987.

Nadeau, S. Stroke due to cardiogenic embolism. *Semin. Neurol.* 6:277–284, 1986.

Petersen, P. Thrombo-embolic complications in atrial fibrillation. *Stroke* 21:4–13, 1990.

Scheibel, M., et al. Cardiac disease in patients with reversible cerebral ischemic events. *Acta Med. Scand.* 217:417–421, 1985.

Stroke Prevention in Atrial Fibrillation Study Group. Preliminary report of the stroke prevention in atrial fibrillation study. *N. Engl. J. Med.* 322:863–868, 1990.

Wolf, P. A., Abbott, R. D., and Kannell, W. B. Atrial fibrillation: a major contributor to stroke in the elderly. *Arch. Intern. Med.* 147:1561–1564, 1987.

Yatsu, F. M. et al. Anticoagulation of embolic strokes of cardiac origin: an update. *Neurology* 38:314–316, 1988.

Arterial Dissection

Bogousslavsky, J., Despland, P. A., and Regli, F. Spontaneous carotid dissection with stroke. *Arch. Neurol.* 44:137–140, 1987.

Hart, R. G. Vertebral artery dissection. *Neurology* 38:987–989, 1988.

Mokri, B., et al. Spontaneous dissection of the cervical internal carotid artery. *Ann. Neurol.* 19:126–138, 1986.

Yamaura, A., Watanabe, Y., and Saeki, N. Dissecting aneurysms of the intracranial vertebral artery. *J. Neurosurg.* 72:183–188, 1990.

Asymptomatic Bruit

Bogousslavsky, J., Desplant, P. A., and Regli, F. Asymptomatic tight stenosis of the internal carotid artery: long-term prognosis. *Neurology* 36:861–863, 1986.

Bornstein, N. M., and Norris, J. W. Management of patients with asymptomatic neck bruits and carotid stenosis. *Neurol. Clin.* 10:269–280, 1992.

Chambers, B. R., and Norris, J. W. Outcome in patients with asymptomatic neck bruits. *N. Engl. J. Med.* 315:860–865, 1986.

Ford, C. S., et al. Asymptomatic carotid bruit and stenosis. A prospective follow-up study. *Arch. Neurol.* 43:219–222, 1986.

Mohr, J. P. Asymptomatic carotid artery disease (editorial). *Stroke* 13:431–433, 1982.

Yatsu, F. M. Asymptomatic carotid bruit and stenosis. *Semin. Neurol.* 6:262–266, 1986.

Surgical Management of Occlusive Cerebrovascular Disease

Barnett, H. J. M. Stroke prevention by surgery of symptomatic disease in carotid territory. *Neurol. Clin.* 10:281–292, 1992.

North American Symptomatic Carotid Endarterectomy Trial Collaborators. Beneficial effect of carotid endarterectomy in symptomatic patients with high-grade carotid stenosis. *N. Engl. J. Med.* 325:445–453, 1991.

Intracerebral and Cerebellar Hemorrhage and Arteriovenous Malformations

Adams, H. P., Jr., and Marsh, E. E. Intraparenchymal hemorrhage. *Curr. Opin. Neurol. Neurosurg.* 2:52–60, 1989.

Aminoff, M. Treatment of unruptured cerebral arteriovenous malformations. *Neurology* 37:815–819, 1987.

Batjer, H. H., et al. Failure of surgery to improve outcome in hypertensive putamenal hemorrhage. A prospective randomized trial. *Arch. Neurol.* 47:1103–1106, 1990.

Drake, C. G., Friedman, A. H., and Peerless, S. J. Posterior fossa arteriovenous malformations. *J. Neurosurg.* 64:1–10, 1986.

Farmer, J. P., et al. Intracerebral cavernous angiomas. *Neurology* 38:1699–1704, 1988.

Heros, R. C., and Tu, Y. K. Is surgical therapy needed for unruptured arteriovenous malformations? *Neurology* 37:279–286, 1987.

Marshall, L. F., and El-Hefnawai, M. Spontaneous intracranial hemorrhage. *Semin. Neurol.* 4:422–429, 1984.

Ondra, S. L., et al. The natural history of symptomatic arteriovenous malformations of the brain: a 24-year follow-up assessment. *J. Neurosurg.* 73:387–391, 1990.

Rigamonti, D., et al. Cerebral cavernous malformations. Incidence and familial occurrence. *N. Engl. J. Med.* 319:343–347, 1988.

Ropper, A. H., and Davis, K. R. Lobar cerebral hemorrhages: acute clinical syndromes in 26 cases. *Ann. Neurol* 8:141–147, 1980.

Stein, B. M., and Wolpert, S. M. Arteriovenous malformations of the brain. (Current Concepts and Treatment). *Arch. Neurol.* 37:1–5, 1980.

Steinberg, G. K., et al. Stereotactic heavy-charged-particle Bragg-peak radiation for intracranial arteriovenous malformations. *N. Engl. J. Med.* 323:96–101, 1990.

Vinters, H. V., Lundie, M. J., and Kauffmann, J. C. E. Long-term pathological follow-up of cerebral arteriovenous malformations treated by embolization with bucrylate. *N. Engl. J. Med.* 314:477–483, 1986.

Aneurysmal Subarachnoid Hemorrhage

Adams, H. P., Jr., et al. Intracranial operation within seven days of aneurysmal subarachnoid hemorrhage. Results in 150 patients. *Arch. Neurol.* 45:1065–1069, 1988.

Adams, H. P., Jr., et al. CT and clinical correlations in recent aneurysmal subarachnoid hemorrhage. A preliminary report of the Cooperative Aneurysm Study. *Neurology* 33:981–988, 1983.

Drake, C. G. Management of cerebral aneurysm. *Stroke* 12:273–283, 1981.

Heros, R. C. Preoperative management of the patient with a ruptured intracranial aneurysm. *Semin. Neurol.* 4:430–438, 1984.

Heros, R. C., Zervas, N. T., and Varsos, V. Cerebral vasospasm after subarachnoid hemorrhage: an update. *Ann. Neurol.* 14:599–608, 1983.

Kassell, N. F., and Thorner, J. C. The international co-operative study on the timing of aneurysm surgery—an update. *Stroke* 15:566–570, 1984.

Mullan, S., Hanlon, K., and Brown, F. Management of 136 consecutive supratentorial berry aneurysms. *J. Neurosurg.* 49:794–804, 1978.

Nishioka, H., et al. Cooperative study of intracranial aneurysms and subarachnoid hemorrhage: a long-term prognostic study. II. Ruptured intracranial aneurysm managed conservatively. *Arch. Neurol.* 41:1142–1146, 1984.

Nishioka, H., et al. Cooperative study of intracranial aneurysms and subarachnoid hemorrhage: III. Subarachnoid hemorrhage of undetermined etiology. *Arch. Neurol.* 41:1147–1151, 1984.

Sahs, A. L., et al. Cooperative study of intracranial aneurysms and subarachnoid hemorrhage: a long-term prognostic study. I. Introduction. *Arch. Neurol.* 41:1140–1141, 1984.

Sahs, A. L., and Adams, H. P., Jr. (editors). Aneurysmal subarachnoid hemorrhage. *Semin. Neurol.* 4:271–389, 1984.

Solomon, R. A., and Fink, M. E. Current strategies for the management of aneurysmal subarachnoid hemorrhage. *Arch. Neurol.* 44:769–774, 1987.

Weir, B. *Aneurysms Affecting the Nervous System.* Baltimore: Williams & Wilkins, 1987.

Wiebers, D. O., Whisnant, J. P., and O'Fallon, W. M. The natural history of unruptured intracranial aneurysms. *N. Engl. J. Med.* 304:696–698, 1981.

Infectious Disorders

BACTERIAL MENINGITIS

Bacterial meningitis has remained a prominent cause of morbidity and mortality, especially in children and in the populations of developing countries. The importance of early diagnosis and the institution of appropriate therapy make this condition a true neurological emergency.

Pathophysiology and Etiology

Underlying conditions that predispose to the development of bacterial meningitis are listed in Table 24-1. Bacterial organisms gain access to the meninges primarily by the blood-borne route. Meningeal infection may also be due to spread from contiguous sites of infection (e.g., paranasal sinusitis, mastoiditis, otitis, or osteomyelitis of the skull or vertebrae) or direct implantation (e.g., neurosurgery, penetrating cranial wounds, or lumbar puncture), or infection may be introduced to the meninges via preexisting connections between the CSF and

the surface (e.g., dural defects, congenital sinuses, or occult encephaloceles). An underlying pneumonia is found in about half the cases of pneumococcal meningitis. *Haemophilus influenzae* and meningococcal meningitis are occasionally acquired through household contacts. Meningococcal meningitis may also be acquired from asymptomatic carriers and can occur in epidemics.

The bacteria causing meningitis secrete IgA proteases, which facilitate their attachment to mucous epithelium. The organisms then enter the bloodstream where their capsular polysaccharides protect them from inactivation by complement. Once bacteria gain access to the arachnoid membranes by somehow crossing the blood-brain barrier, rapid proliferation can ensue because opsonization and phagocytosis are relatively poor in the CSF.

Much of the damage done by the invading bacteria is secondary to a brisk inflammatory response prompted by the production of cell-wall lipopolysaccharide or gram-negative endotoxin. The blood-brain barrier is further com-

419

Table 24-1. Conditions Predisposing to Bacterial Meningitis

Condition	Common organisms
Underlying infection (e.g., upper respiratory, pneumonia, otitis, sinusitis, purulent conjunctivitis, bacterial endocarditis, septicemia, osteomyelitis)	Dependent on primary focus (e.g., *H. influenzae* with otitis)
Malignancy (especially of head and neck)	Gram-neg., staphylococci
Splenectomy, sickle-cell anemia	*Strep. pneumoniae*
Immunological deficits: AIDS, immunosuppressant agents, diabetes, alcoholism, uremia	*Listeria*, gram-neg., *Strep. pneumoniae*, unusual organisms
Neurosurgery, penetrating head trauma, ventricular shunts	Gram-neg., *S. aureus*, *Staph. epidermidis*
Neonatal	Hemolytic streptococci, *E. coli*, *Listeria*
Congenital sinuses connecting to subarachnoid space; acquired dural defects (e.g., basilar skull fracture) with rhinorrhea	*Strep. pneumoniae*, staphylococci

promised, and cytokines such as interleukin-1 and tumor necrosis factor, which mediate inflammation, are released from cells in the CNS. The blood-brain barrier is further impaired, neutrophils cross into the CSF, and cerebral edema occurs. The cascade of inflammation and edema continues with the degranulation and subsequent release of toxic substances from neutrophils. Bacterial lysis therefore triggers further inflammation. Pus forms within the meningeal spaces, envelops cranial nerves at the base of the brain, and spreads over the cortical surface.

Although the pia and the brain itself are relatively resistant to bacterial invasion, cerebritis arises in the superficial cortical layers through the infiltration of the organisms into the Virchow-Robin spaces around vessels. Ventriculitis or ependymitis may also occur, particularly in infants. Bacterial toxins may also interfere with cortical function. In severe cases, necrosis and demyelination of the subcortical white matter can take place. An arteritis is seen, especially in cases of *H. influenzae, Streptococcus pneumoniae*, and *Mycobacterium tuberculosis* meningitis. Cerebral infarction may result from vasculitis, or from cortical venous or sinus thrombosis, or both. Hydrocephalus, either communicating or obstructive, is another potential consequence of pus formation, and, in addition to the brain edema, accounts for the raised intracranial pressure. Focal collections

of pus, either in the subdural space (subdural empyema) or as an intraparenchymal abscess, occasionally act as mass lesions and produce focal deficits and brain shifts. However, brain abscess is relatively uncommon as a complication of bacterial meningitis.

In most series, *S. pneumoniae, Neisseria meningitidis*, and *H. influenzae* account for at least 80 percent of the cases. The incidence of individual organisms is strongly related to age (Table 24-2). Unusual organisms can be responsible for infection in special clinical situations, often involving immunological deficits (see Table 24-1). Certain clinical features are rela-

Table 24-2. Most Common Bacteria Causing Meningitis Related to Age of Patient

Age	Bacteria
Neonates	Beta-hemolytic streptococci *Escherichia coli* *Listeria monocytogenes*
Childhood (3 mo to 5 yr)	*Haemophilus influenzae*, type B *Neisseria meningitidis* *Streptococcus pneumoniae*
Older childhood to adulthood	*Streptococcus pneumoniae* *Neisseria meningitidis* *Haemophilus influenzae*

tively specific to infection with particular organisms, and offer clues to both the diagnosis and potential complications (Table 24-3).

Clinical Picture

The classic clinical features of fever, headache, nuchal rigidity, and other signs of meningeal irritation (e.g., Kernig's and Brudzinski's signs; see Chapter 2) and an altered mental state are well known. There are, however, relatively common atypical presentations, particularly in the very young and elderly or those with severe systemic illness who may not show fever and signs of meningeal irritation. The neonate may present with a bulging fontanelle, high-pitched weak cry, lethargy, poor feeding, vomiting, hypothermia, hypoglycemia, and subtle seizures (e.g., apneic spells). Meningeal irritation in children can be so severe as to cause opisthotonos. An agitated delirium is common and may precede stupor or coma.

Focal neurological signs, apart from cranial nerve palsies, are unusual in the early phases. Occasional patients present with gait ataxia and seizures occur in up to 50 percent of the cases. Even though intracranial pressure is commonly raised, papilledema is not usually observed in the early phase. Petechiae, purpura, or, less commonly, a morbilliform rash strongly suggest *N. meningitidis* infection. These findings, however, can also be encountered in less life-threat-

ening bacterial or viral infections such as ECHO 9. Petechiae may be seen earliest over the conjunctiva, especially with down-gaze. The syndrome of inappropriate antidiuretic hormone secretion (SIADH) is common and contributes to the formation of cerebral edema. Hyponatremia, when severe, may precipitate seizures. Disseminated intravascular coagulation is most commonly associated with *N. meningitidis* infection. Other causes of death include cerebral edema with herniation, shock, or fulminant meningococcemia.

Diagnosis

The following guidelines can be used for determining the need for lumbar puncture in the patient with fever, particularly the pediatric patient:

1. Disproportionate headache or alteration in mental status
2. Nuchal rigidity or other signs of meningeal irritation
3. Focal neurological signs or seizures, provided the seizures are not the "typical" febrile seizures seen in pediatric patients

Lumbar puncture should be carried out when there is the least suspicion of meningitis in the immunocompromised patient, while remaining

Table 24-3. Clinical Features Suggesting Specific Bacterial Cause of Meningitis

Bacteria	Clinical features
Streptococcus pneumoniae	Focal neurological signs
	Recurrent meningitis
	Subdural empyema
Haemophilus influenzae	Subdural effusions
Neisseria meningitidis	Skin rash
	Shock, overwhelming systemic illness, disseminated intravascular coagulation
	Epidemic occurrence
	Deafness
	Pericardial and joint effusions
Listeria monocytogenes	Negative Gram's-stained CSF preparations and culture
	Focal brainstem signs
Gram-negative organisms	Absence of classic signs
	No organisms seen on Gram's-stained CSF preparations

cognizant of the risks associated with lumbar puncture in patients with coagulation deficits.

Lumbar puncture is the definitive diagnostic technique and should not be delayed if bacterial meningitis is suspected. However, when concurrent brain abscess is suspected because of focal neurological signs or marked brain swelling indicated by papilledema and other signs of elevated intracranial pressure, a CT scan should be done before lumbar puncture, as long as lumbar puncture is not delayed by more than one hour. As a general rule, blood cultures should be drawn in all cases of suspected meningitis. *S. pneumoniae* and *Listeria monocytogenes* are particularly likely to be grown from blood cultures. Antibiotic treatment should be instituted immediately, based on the most probable infecting organism, even if lumbar puncture is delayed. If raised intracranial pressure is suspected and a CT scan cannot be obtained within a reasonable time, lumbar puncture should be done (always using the smallest possible needle and an atraumatic technique), mannitol therapy begun, and the CT scan obtained as soon as possible.

In the presence of established bacterial meningitis, the CSF often appears cloudy and the opening pressure is moderately elevated. White cell counts are usually greater than 1,000 cells/mm³; in fulminant cases, counts exceed 10,000. Neutrophils constitute over 80 percent of the cells, except occasionally early in the course when lymphocytes predominate. A second lumbar puncture, 8 to 12 hours later, can confirm the predominance of polymorphs in these cases.

The protein level in the CSF is moderately elevated and the glucose concentration depressed to levels less than half of the blood levels, and often much lower. Gram's staining of CSF sediment is a rapid way of establishing a probable diagnosis, although the results are often nonspecific and may even be negative with certain organisms. *Listeria,* an intracellular gram-positive organism, is often missed on Gram's staining or mistaken for a gram-negative organism. Rarely in patients with pneumococcal infection who were previously normal, numerous organisms are found in the CSF but the cell count is minimal. A similar picture is common in immunosuppressed individuals and underlines the importance of performing Gram's staining in suspected cases even when the cell count is normal.

Within 24 to 48 hours, CSF culture will yield a specific etiological answer in about 80 percent of cases. The importance of immediate plating of the CSF and special cultures for anaerobes, which are being increasingly recognized as the cause in meningitis, cannot be overemphasized. It has been repeatedly shown that prior treatment with antibiotics in doses lower than those used for meningitis does not interfere with the accuracy of CSF examination in the vast majority of cases. There are now several techniques that yield a rapid specific diagnosis before the results of CSF culture are available. Counter current immunoelectrophoresis and latex agglutination tests performed on serum and CSF can detect and quantify specific bacterial antigens for a limited number of commonly encountered organisms. Results of the limulus lysate test, which detects bacterial endotoxins, are positive in gram-negative meningitis but also occasionally in meningococcal and *Haemophilus* meningitis.

The CT scan may reveal enhancement of inflamed meninges over the cortical surface, around the base of the brain, and of the ependymal lining of the ventricles when ventriculitis is present. Hydrocephalus, intraparenchymal abscess formation, diffuse brain swelling, and areas of infarct due to vascular involvement are other changes that CT can detect. An unusual MRI picture of thickened meninges is shown in a case of idiopathic chronic granulomatous meningitis in Figure 24-1.

Conditions to consider in the differential diagnosis of bacterial meningitis are meningitis due to other organisms (see later discussion), systemic viral infection with meningismus, parameningeal infection (e.g., sinusitis or retropharyngeal abscess) with meningismus, migraine with secondary neck muscle contraction, herpes simplex encephalitis, and subarachnoid hemorrhage.

Management and Prognosis

Early antibiotic treatment is the most important principle of management and should be insti-

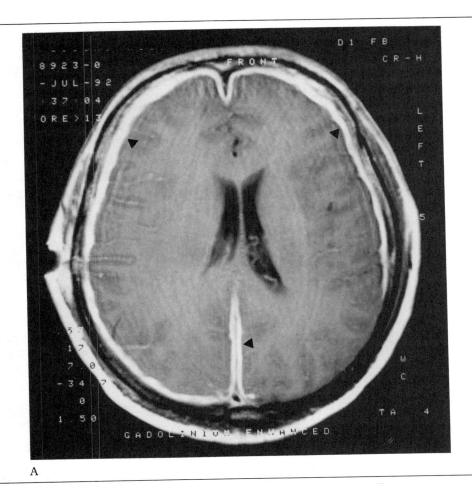

A

Fig. 24-1. *(A, B) Gadolinium-enhanced T_1-weighted MRI scans showing markedly thickened meninges (arrowheads) due to a chronic idiopathic meningitis of unknown cause. Meningeal biopsy showed a granulomatous pattern but no evidence of tuberculosis. The patient presented with headache and papilledema. Note the sparse gyral pattern and cerebellar tonsillar herniation.*

tuted as soon as the most likely organism is determined on the basis of the patient's age, the clinical setting, and the CSF findings. Antibiotics such as chloramphenicol, which cross the blood-brain barrier best, are theoretically preferable but the ability to penetrate through the inflamed meninges is generally adequate for most antibiotics. Bactericidal agents have a theoretical advantage over bacteriostatic drugs.

In general, drugs are administered intravenously in high doses. Certain agents such as the aminoglycosides, used for treating gram-negative meningitis, are most effective when administered intrathecally via an Ommaya res-

ervoir. The initial choices of antibiotics are given in Table 24-4. Once the results of culture and sensitivity tests are known, the treatment regimen may be altered accordingly.

The wide spectrum of action and good ability to penetrate the CSF possessed by the third-generation cephalosporins are making them increasingly popular for the management of meningitis. In general, in the initial phases when the etiology is unknown, it is better to err on the side of overtreatment that covers all the potential pathogens, rather than to use an inadequate number of drugs. Treatment is continued for a minimum of 14 days and may have to be prolonged for 5

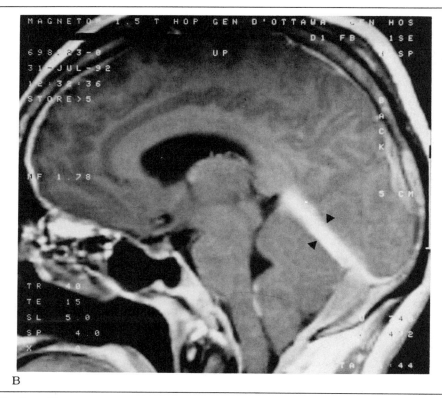

B

Fig. 24-1 (Continued).

Table 24-4. Initial Choice of Antibiotic Treatment for Meningitis Based on Clinical Setting

Patient group	Primary	Alternative
Adult or child over 5 yr	Penicillin G + chloramphenicol	3rd-generation cephalosporins* + ampicillin
Neonate or child under 5 yr	Ampicillin + chloramphenicol	Ampicillin + 3rd-generation cephalosporins
Immunosuppressed patient (not AIDS)	Ampicillin + 3rd-generation cephalosporins	Chloramphenicol + vancomycin
Suspected *Staphylococcus*	Nafcillin, cloxacillin, or methicillin	Vancomycin (for resistant strains and penicillin allergy)
Suspected gram-neg. (including *Pseudomonas*)	3rd-generation cephalosporins	Gentamicin C + tobramycin
Suspected anaerobes	Penicillin + metronidazole	3rd-generation cephalosporins + metronidazole

*Cefotaxime or ceftriaxone.

days after the fever subsides. Low glucose levels may persist for several weeks despite an absence of bacteria in the CSF.

In addition to appropriate antibiotic therapy, management must be aimed at maintaining fluid and electrolyte balances (i.e., anticipation of SIADH), reducing intracranial pressure, and controlling seizures. Placement of ventricular shunts for managing the hydrocephalus, repeated taps of subdural effusions, and the surgical removal of a subdural empyema may be required if these complications supervene. Intracranial pressure monitoring may be a useful adjunct in the control of intracranial pressure. Recent studies have shown that the use of dexamethasone in the initial 4 days of treatment in cases of childhood meningitis led to a more rapid resolution of fever and the incidence of permanent hearing loss dropped from approximately 15 to 3 percent. Steroids are now also recommended by some in adults to try to reduce the severe inflammatory response consequent to bacterial lysis, although this is still a controversial point.

Despite the various approaches to management that are now at our disposal, the mortality associated with acute bacterial meningitis still approaches 20 to 30 percent. The factors listed in Table 24-5 are linked to an adverse prognosis. Approximately 20 to 30 percent of patients are left with sequelae, including deafness (in 10–15%), other cranial nerve palsies, epilepsy, hemiplegia, hydrocephalus, mental retardation, and more subtle learning or behavioral deficits.

TUBERCULOSIS OF THE CENTRAL NERVOUS SYSTEM

Tuberculous meningitis, although uncommon in developed countries, is an important source of morbidity in immunosuppressed individuals and in the populations of developing countries. In most cases, there is no apparent primary focus of the tuberculosis outside the nervous system, but miliary or late generalized tuberculosis is very common with tuberculous meningitis. Meningitis likely occurs secondarily to an ependymal focus or in some cases a focus involving the skull or vertebrae.

Table 24-5. Factors Associated with an Adverse Prognosis in Bacterial Meningitis

Delay in treatment
Organism
   Streptococcus pneumoniae
   Mixed infection
   Unusual organisms (e.g., gram-neg. *Listeria*)
Underlying illness
   Life-threatening systemic illness
   Diabetes
Immunosuppression, e.g.,
   AIDS
   Lymphoreticular malignancy
   Alcoholism
   Renal transplantation
Age
   Neonates
   Elderly
Clinical state
   Coma on presentation
   Seizures
Laboratory findings
   Low white blood cell count in CSF
   High bacterial antigen content in CSF
   Low peripheral white blood cell count
   Bacteremia

The clinical picture is usually subacute and differs little from that described for bacterial meningitis. However, chronic cases exhibiting nonspecific prodromal features of headache and malaise do occur. The CSF typically shows a moderate cell count, lymphocytic predominance, and a low glucose and very high protein level. However, in rare cases, no cells are found in the CSF and polymorphonuclear leukocytes may dominate in the early stages. A careful search for acid-fast staining bacilli, ideally done on several CSF specimens, may establish a diagnosis but most frequently yields negative findings.

Because of the marked inflammatory and allergic components of the tissue response to the tuberculous bacillus, spinal block or hydrocephalus and vasculitis arising from arachnoiditis and leading to infarction are relatively more frequent in tuberculous than in other forms of bacterial meningitis. Patients with tuberculous meningitis may also have tuberculomas and parenchymal abscesses or these may occur independently. These lesions are most commonly found in the cerebellum.

A strongly positive skin test for tuberculosis or chest x-ray findings suggestive of tuberculosis may facilitate diagnosis but neither of these findings is reliably positive.

Therapy must be started in suspected cases while awaiting culture results, which may take up to 6 weeks. Mortality is high in untreated cases. Because of the increasing incidence of resistant strains, a triple-pronged antimicrobial therapy that includes isoniazid, rifampin, and either ethambutol or pyrazinamide is recommended. Pyridoxine must be given with the isoniazid to prevent neuropathy. Isoniazid, rifampin, and pyrazinamide are all hepatotoxic, and this effect may be additive. Hepatotoxicity is a particular problem in the elderly. Ethambutol causes optic neuritis when given in higher doses. Double-pronged antimicrobial therapy must be continued for at least 9 months once sensitivities have been determined. The addition of corticosteroids to the treatment regimen to reduce the inflammation is controversial.

VIRAL AND ASEPTIC MENINGITIS

In aseptic meningitis, no bacterial organism can be readily demonstrated or grown, usually because the source of the infection is viral. The syndrome is most common in children and young adults. The clinical picture consists of headache, neck stiffness, low-grade fever, and symptoms of a systemic or upper respiratory viral illness, which may occur as a prodrome. The CSF obtained by lumbar puncture is usually clear with a white cell count typically ranging between 50 and several hundred cells per cubic millimeter, predominantly composed of mononuclear cells. Occasionally neutrophils predominate in the initial specimens, but a lymphocytic pleocytosis is found in specimens obtained 24 to 48 hours later. The glucose level is normal, but may be mildly depressed in rare cases of mumps or herpesvirus infection. The protein generally ranges between 50 and 100 mg/dl (0.5–1.0 gm/L).

The specific viruses implicated most commonly include the enteroviruses (ECHO, Coxsackie, and polio), herpes simplex virus type 2, Epstein-Barr virus, lymphocytic choriomeningitis virus, and the arbor viruses, but no specific virus is identified in most cases. HIV infection can present as aseptic meningitis, especially at the time of seroconversion. Occasionally, enteroviruses, mumps, lymphocytic choriomeningitis virus, or herpes simplex virus type 2 can be cultured from the CSF. However, the clue to a specific viral etiology is based on (1) a rise in the specific serum antibody titer between the acute and convalescent stages, the latter specimen obtained 4 weeks later, which is by then helpful only in retrospect; (2) the results of specific tests such as the monospot test; or (3) the occurrence of meningitis in conjunction with a recognizable viral illness such as mumps or infectious mononucleosis.

Parameningeal foci of infection such as sinusitis or brain abscess can manifest a similar clinical picture. A CT scan should be performed whenever a picture of aseptic meningitis includes focal neurological signs, stupor, or papilledema (Fig. 24-2). Other nonviral disorders causing a similar syndrome include *Mycoplasma* infections, sarcoidosis, chemical meningitis (e.g., resulting from a ruptured cholesteatoma or from the intrathecal injection of contrast material for radiological or radionuclide procedures), systemic lupus erythematosus, and carcinomatous or lymphomatous meningitis. Use of the drug ibuprofen and some other nonsteroidal antiinflammatory agents has also rarely been the cause of aseptic meningitis.

All patients with viral meningitis recover spontaneously within a week or two. Only those with concurrent encephalitis are at risk for suffering neurological sequelae. The problem faced by the physician in these cases is to be certain that a bacterial, tuberculous, or fungal etiology is not missed. Typical mild cases of viral meningitis can be managed outside the hospital, but those patients who are in extreme discomfort, or with excessive vomiting, may have to be hospitalized for symptomatic treatment. If the diagnosis is doubtful or there are signs of concurrent encephalitis, patients should be hospitalized so that they can be closely observed or can receive initial coverage with antibiotics for the treatment of possible bacterial meningitis while culture results are awaited.

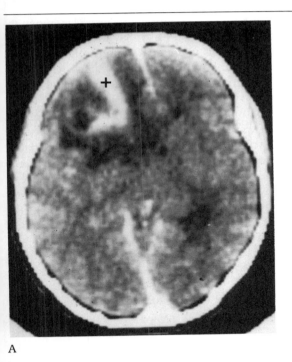

A

Fig. 24-2. *This healthy 17-year-old woman was admitted following a 1-week history of headache, nausea, and vomiting but no fever. She exhibited mild drowsiness and nuchal rigidity on admission. The initial diagnosis was aseptic meningitis and a lumbar puncture was done that showed a normal opening pressure, 6 red blood cells/mm³, 22 mononuclear white blood cells/mm³, and a mildly elevated protein (82 mg/dl). She was about to be discharged 2 days later when a CT was done because of persistent drowsiness. Later that same day, deepening stupor, mild papilledema, a dilated right pupil, and a right hemiparesis, worse in the lower extremity, developed. She then suffered a generalized tonic-clonic seizure and exhibited a full left third-nerve palsy, bilateral decorticate posturing, Cheyne-Stokes respirations, and bradycardia. At surgery, a left frontal abscess was drained and the capsule removed. Culture grew* Staph. epidermidis, Peptostreptococcus, Bacteroides, *and* Actinomyces. *(A) Enhanced CT scan showing an irregular ring enhancement around the abscess (cross), marked edema surrounding the abscess, obscuration of the ventricles, and midline shift with bowing of the falx to the right. (B) EEG showing high-voltage rhythmic delta activity seen mainly over the left frontal area but also over the right frontal region.*

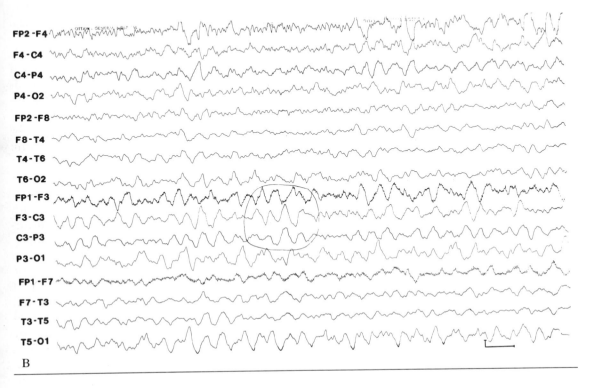

B

The patient who has recurrent bouts of aseptic meningitis over the course of months or years poses a special diagnostic challenge (Table 24-6). Some of these cases fit into specific syndromes such as Behçet's, recurrent chemical meningitis from a parameningeal focus, or recurrent herpesvirus infection. Those idiopathic cases that recur over the course of months or many years as self-limited bouts in otherwise healthy individuals are deemed Mollaret's meningitis. CSF examination in the first 24 hours in these patients may reveal the existence of large fragile epithelioid cells containing a foamy cytoplasm (Mollaret's cells).

FUNGAL INFECTIONS

Fungi are ubiquitous in the environment and most infections are acquired through inhalation. Certain fungi, such as *Coccidioides immitis,* which is found mainly in the southwestern United States, have a specific geographical distribution.

The diagnosis of fungal infection of the CNS is often difficult because the clinical symptoms may be minimal and the infection can be indolent. The presence of disseminated fungal involvement of the skin, lungs, vital organs, and other areas is enough to suggest a presumptive diagnosis in a patient with signs of meningoencephalitis or brain abscess. Most, but not all, cases occur in immunocompromised patients with lymphoreticular malignancies, AIDS, diabetes, or sarcoidosis, or following renal or cardiac transplantation or steroid treatment. Often the fungal infection is the terminal event in these settings. The syndromes include occult asymptomatic CNS infection, mild headache alone, chronic meningitis, acute or subacute meningitis, meningoencephalitis, brain abscess, multiple microabscesses, CNS granulomata, or myelitis (rarely). The clinical expression of the disorder varies according to the immunological status of the host and the specific fungus.

Aspergillosis (Fig. 24-3) and mucormycosis tend to invade the cerebral arteries and cause ischemic infarcts. Mucormycosis typically occurs in the context of diabetic ketoacidosis. It invades and causes necrosis of the paranasal sinuses (giving rise to a dark, bloody nasal discharge) and the orbit. An attack is often rapidly fatal. Histoplasmosis only rarely attacks the nervous system. CNS blastomycosis tends to cause the formation of abscesses and occurs in the context of disseminated infection. *Candida* represents one of the most common fungal pathogens to involve the CNS, usually in individuals with disseminated candidiasis. *Candida albicans* is a normal constituent of the flora of the mucosa but disseminated infections occur when host resistance is altered, such as stemming from intravenous drug abuse, prolonged antibiotic or corticosteroid use, or intravenous hyperalimentation. The yeast may be seen on smears of CSF.

Cryptococcal CNS infection is the most notable cause of fungal meningitis in adults. About half of the cases occur in hosts with conditions predisposing to impaired cell-mediated immunity, such as lymphoreticular malignancies, AIDS, or diabetes mellitus. The clinical picture may resemble that of classic acute bacterial meningitis or may consist of little more than a chronic headache and mental deterioration. The base of the brain and cerebellum are often the areas most affected by the exudate, and this typically leads to hydrocephalus, ataxia, and cranial nerve palsies. India ink staining of a drop of CSF to demon-

Table 24-6. Etiologies of Recurrent Meningitis

Bacterial causes
    Acquired anatomic defects: basal skull fracture with or without rhinorrhea, post craniotomy
    Congenital anatomic defects: sinus, myelomeningocele, neurenteric cyst
    Parameningeal focus: chronic otitis, sinusitis, epidural abscess, subdural empyema, osteomyelitis of skull or vertebrae
    Immune deficits: agammaglobulinemia, complement deficiency, splenectomy
Aseptic causes
    Tumors: epidermoid/dermoid, third ventricular hemangioma, ependymoma, craniopharyngioma
    Behçet's syndrome
    Systemic lupus erythematosus
    Enteroviruses
    Mollaret's meningitis (? herpes simplex)

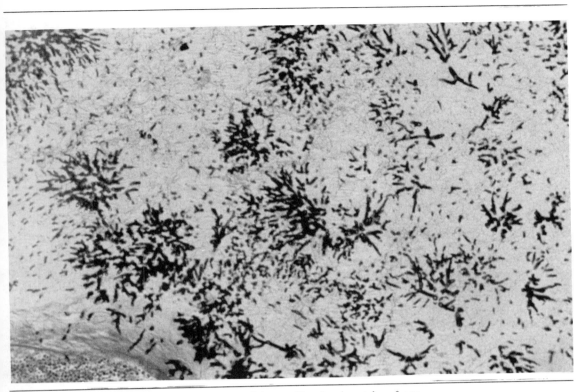

Fig. 24-3. *Typical microscoping appearance of* Aspergillus *hyphae taken from material obtained from a brain abscess. (Giemsa, ×200.)*

strate the encapsulated yeast may establish diagnosis. The organism grows well on standard media for fungi, but large volumes of CSF increase the yield of culture. Urine cultures may also be positive. The latex agglutination test, which detects cryptococcal antigen in the CSF, is very helpful in the diagnosis and false-positive results are rare.

The mainstay of specific therapy for fungal infections has been amphotericin B, which is given intravenously and at times also intrathecally (through an Ommaya reservoir). Approximately 0.5 to 1 mg/kg is given daily for several weeks, to a total dose of approximately 1.5 to 2 gm. Nephrotoxicity, chills, fever, nausea, vomiting, hypokalemia, anemia, and localized phlebitis are potential side effects. Intrathecal administration commonly gives rise to pain in the back and legs as well as aseptic meningitis. Careful monitoring of renal function is mandatory throughout a course of amphotericin. 5-

Flucytosine is often combined with amphotericin in the treatment of cryptococcosis, candidiasis, or mucormycosis. Its ability to penetrate the CSF is excellent but it cannot be used alone because this may foster the development of resistant organisms. Miconazole, ketoconazole, and fluconazole are other antifungal agents, but the indications for their use are still not well defined.

BRAIN ABSCESS

Pathophysiology and Etiology

Brain abscesses are most prevalent in patients under the age of 40 and are encountered twice as often in males as in females. An abscess originally forms from a focus of cerebritis, often within an area of brain ischemia. Within about 14 days, there is a localized collection of central pus and necrotic tissue surrounded by a fibro-vascular capsule and a surrounding area of edema. Most abscesses are formed through the contiguous spread of infection from paramen-ingeal foci such as sinusitis, otitis media, dental abscess, or osteomyelitis. Abscesses may also result from the direct implantation of organisms following penetrating head trauma or during neurosurgical procedures, including ventricular shunt installation. Metastatic spread from re-mote sources of infection (e.g., bronchiectasis, pulmonary abscess, and bacterial endocarditis) often spawns multiple abscesses with a predilec-tion for forming at the gray matter–white matter junction. Congenital cyanotic heart disease (es-pecially tetralogy of Fallot) predisposes chil-dren to brain abscesses, usually in those over the age of 3. Meningitis is rarely the source of localized abscess formation.

The exact location of the abscess as well as the organism involved depends mainly on the primary source of the infection. In approx-imately 20 percent of the cases, however, no primary source is identified. The ever-increasing population of immunosuppressed patients accounts for a rising incidence of brain abscess and a wider range of unusual organisms responsible, such as fungi and *Tox-oplasma*. The most common organisms en-countered are various types of streptococci (including anaerobes), other anaerobes, *Staphylococcus aureus*, gram-negative organ-isms, *Actinomyces*, *Nocardia*, and fungi such as *Cryptococcus*, *Aspergillus*, and *Candida*. Because of the increasing recognition of the prevalence of anaerobes and the use of meticu-lous techniques for the collection and culture of specimens, specific organisms have been identified in 80 percent of the patients who underwent operations. In about half of the cases, multiple organisms are found.

Clinical Picture and Diagnosis

The most common clinical presentation of a brain abscess consists of headache and signs of raised intracranial pressure that develop sub-acutely. Focal neurological signs are common and reflect the location of the abscess. Seizures

occur in about one third of the patients. Fever is a component in a minority of cases and a peripheral leukocytosis and elevated sedimen-tation rate are common. The primary infection may give a clue not only to the presence of an abscess but also its location. Otitis media and mastoiditis are associated with temporal lobe or cerebellar abscesses and frontal sinusitis with frontal lobe abscess.

CT scanning has facilitated the diagnosis of brain abscess. Cerebritis appears on CT scans as an area of localized hypodensity with indistinct margins. A typical abscess appears as a strongly enhancing ring-shaped regular capsule sur-rounding a hypodense core (Figs. 24-2 and 24-4). There is usually a moderate amount of edema around the abscess. The capsule may be thicker and better formed toward the cortical surface. Ring enhancement on a CT scan is not a finding specific to abscesses, but may also appear with primary and secondary tumors, granulomas, hematomas, infarcts, and large de-myelinating plaques.

The electroencephalogram (EEG) character-istically reveals high-voltage delta activity in the region of an abscess (see Fig. 24-2). Radionu-clide brain scanning is useful for demonstrating abscesses if CT is unavailable.

Lumbar puncture should be avoided when an abscess is suspected, not just because the yield of useful information is usually low but also because of the great danger of its causing herniation due to brain shifts. CSF pressure is elevated, protein levels are moderately in-creased, and there are usually between 100 to 300 white blood cells per cubic millimeter, mostly lymphocytes. The results of Gram's staining and culture are negative except in the rare instance of concurrent meningitis. The dif-ferential diagnosis of brain abscess includes meningitis, herpes simplex encephalitis, brain tumor, and cortical venous thrombosis.

Subdural empyema produces a clinical pic-ture resembling brain abscess except that pa-tients are almost always febrile and more ill appearing. Most cases result from sinusitis or meningitis. Venous sinus thrombosis is a fre-quent complication and is associated with high morbidity. Treatment includes a combination of antibiotics and surgical evacuation.

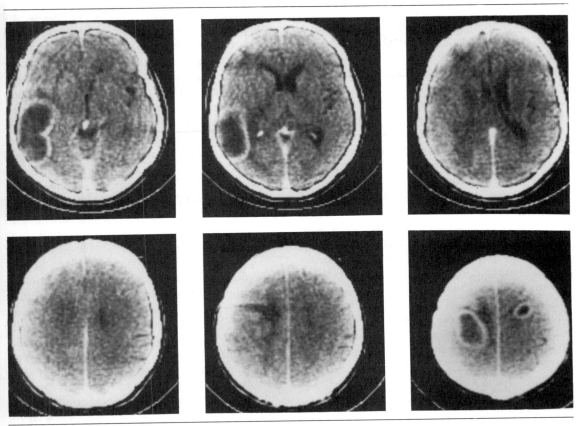

Fig. 24-4. *Enhanced CT scans showing multiple ring-enhancing brain abscesses in a 63-year-old man with bronchiectasis. The patient had undergone surgical removal of a left frontal abscess 4 years before. He now presented with aphasia, right hemiparesis, and right focal seizures.*

Management and Prognosis

Although the management of brain abscess has been simplified by the ability to monitor the lesion with CT scanning and the mortality reported in recent studies has dropped to less than 10 percent, the exact role of surgery is still controversial. Cerebritis may be treated by antibiotics alone. Aspiration and drainage through a burrhole is commonly performed when the abscess is well defined and encapsulated. This permits a specimen to be obtained for precise bacteriological analysis. Repeated aspirations are done in some cases. When a single abscess is located near the cortical surface

in a noncritical area, it may be excised to reduce the risk of recurrence.

In all cases, appropriate antibiotics are initiated in high doses and continued for a period of 4 to 8 weeks, depending on the CT evidence for resolution of the abscess. The improvement documented by CT may lag behind the clinical improvement by several weeks. One of the main problems in relying solely on drug treatment is that antibiotics generally penetrate poorly into an abscess, partly because of the capsule and the edema. The initial choice of antibiotics is governed by the clinical setting and the underlying primary infection. The traditional combination of penicillin G and chloramphenicol is a time-honored treatment that is effective in most cases. The combination of metronidazole and a third-generation cephalosporin such as cefotaxime provides good coverage for anaerobe infection and gram-negative organisms and is less toxic than chloramphenicol. Nafcillin or cloxacillin is an appropriate choice when *Staph. aureus* infection is suspected. Management in patients with elevated intracranial pressure consists of monitoring and the administration of dexamethasone or mannitol. Steroids should only be used sparingly because they can reduce the patient's resistance to infection. Seizures should be treated appropriately.

About 40 percent of survivors are left with some neurological sequelae, including possible epilepsy. One of the hazards in treating brain abscess is mistaking a temporary clinical improvement, due to walling off of the abscess, for resolution. Before the advent of CT scanning, such cases were difficult to diagnose. Rupture of an abscess, which leads to a meningoencephalitis or ventricular empyema, is a feared but rare complication.

VIRAL ENCEPHALITIS

Pathophysiology and Clinical Features

The clinical syndromes attributable to viral CNS invasion vary widely and depend on the virulence of the virus, the immune competence of the host, and any predilection the virus may have for particular brain areas. The viral invasion of the CNS more often gives rise to a meningoencephalitis than to a pure encephalitis. Most commonly, encephalitis is a transient syndrome accompanying a systemic viral illness, and symptoms comprise headache and altered mental status. A more fulminant illness occurs with viruses such as herpes simplex or eastern equine encephalitis and the clinical picture consists of headache, behavioral change, seizures, stupor or coma, and multifocal neurological signs. Brainstem encephalitis produces stupor or coma and multiple signs of brainstem dysfunction, which are often reversible. The clinical presentation of viral cerebellitis in chil-

dren consists of acute ataxia and at times mental changes. Direct viral cerebellar invasion has not been proved in these cases. Infectious mononucleosis or varicella virus infection seems to have a relatively high association with this syndrome. A small percentage of these children are left with permanent learning disabilities.

The classic pathological features of viral encephalitis include infiltration of the meninges and perivascular areas with round cells, foci of neuronophagia, and microglial nodules. Inclusion bodies are seen in these areas in the context of infection with viruses such as herpes, measles, and rabies.

Diagnosis

Diagnosis of viral encephalitis is based on the clinical picture, which often occurs in conjunction with signs of a specific systemic viral illness or in an epidemic setting. However, no specific viral etiology is determined in most cases. The enteroviruses, ECHO, Coxsackie, and polio, may cause a gastroenteritis accompanied by fever and headache prior to CNS invasion, and often organisms are detected in stool cultures. Poliomyelitis, which is rare now because of widespread immunization, produces an asymmetrical paralysis and loss of reflexes, especially affecting the lower extremities. In severe cases, bulbar palsy and respiratory paralysis develop. Other enterovirus infections may exhibit a similar paralytic picture.

The CSF from patients with viral encephalitis characteristically exhibits a lymphocytic pleocytosis with moderately elevated protein and normal glucose levels, findings very similar to those seen in aseptic meningitis and a number of other nonviral inflammatory conditions. The electroencephalogram often reveals widespread slowing, which is disproportionately severe considering the clinical state of the patient. Serological diagnosis depends on the demonstration of a fourfold rise in specific antibody titer, but often is not evident in the acute phase.

Types of Viral Encephalitis

Mumps and measles are the most common childhood exanthematous diseases to cause enephalitis, at times in epidemics. **Mumps encephalitis,** which is usually mild, is seen most commonly in late winter. **Measles encephalitis,** with a mortality as high as 15 percent, has declined in incidence because of the widespread use of measles vaccines.

Epidemic viral encephalitis is often seasonal and confined to certain geographic locations, where the virus is endemic in a particular animal reservoir, and is transferred to humans via specific insect vectors. In temperate climates, children and older adults are the most common victims. **Arbor virus encephalitis,** which is due to mosquito transmission, is most prevalent in late summer and fall. Tick-borne viruses may be implicated in cases of viral encephalitis from spring until the first frost. Eastern equine encephalitis and Japanese B encephalitis are among the most fulminant forms in this group (Table 24-7). Japanese B encephalitis, found throughout the Orient, is the most common form of epidemic viral encephalitis in the world.

In the immunosuppressed population, **cytomegalovirus** is one of the most common causes of encephalitis. It produces a variable syndrome, often presenting as a subacute encephalopathy with or without focal signs. Discrete areas of enhancement may be seen on CT scans. The diagnosis is confirmed by the isolation of the pathogen from multiple peripheral sites, including the blood, urine, or tissue obtained by biopsy. Serology may also be helpful.

The varicella-zoster virus, which frequently causes herpes zoster in the immunosuppressed patient, rarely becomes a disseminated skin infection followed by diffuse CNS invasion. The resultant encephalitis is often indolent and accompanied by signs of cranial nerve, peripheral nerve, spinal cord, or cerebellar involvement. Ganciclovir is used to treat disseminated cytomegalovirus infection and acyclovir for herpes zoster, but resistant strains have now emerged.

Rabies virus exists in a variety of wild animal reservoirs, including bats, foxes, skunks, and squirrels. Humans acquire the virus most commonly from the bites of dogs or cats that have contracted the virus by coming in contact with saliva from wild animals. The rabies virus, an RNA-containing enveloped virus of the rhabdovirus group, is neurotropic and invades the CNS after ascending the peripheral nerves via axoplasmic flow. There is a variable incubation period before neurological symptoms appear, ranging from 10 days to over a year (mean, 1–2 months). A prodromal phase with nonspecific symptoms of headache, fever, gastrointestinal upset, myalgias, and sore throat lasts for 1 to 4 days. An acute encephalitic phase then ensues with manifestations of delirium, later followed by stupor and coma, muscle spasms, meningeal signs, seizures, and focal neurological signs. Other features include high fever, autonomic abnormalities, and hypersensitivity to sensory stimuli. The brainstem is particularly affected, producing vocal cord paralysis, dysphagia, facial paralysis, ocular movement problems, and optic neuritis. Many cases show "hydrophobia," in which violent muscle spasms of the diaphragm, pharynx, and larynx are precipitated by swallowing liquids or even the sight of water. In occasional cases, there is a flaccid paralysis, leading to a misdiagnosis of Guillain-Barré syndrome. The disease is universally fatal if untreated.

Pathological changes in the brain consist of neuronophagia, microglial cell proliferation, and round-cell infiltration, findings typical of any viral encephalitis. In addition, eosinophilic inclusions containing viral particles, known as Negri bodies, are particularly conspicuous in the cerebral cortex, hippocampus, and brainstem.

Diagnosis is based on the known history of an animal bite which is then followed by the appearance of local symptoms of paresthesias and spasms at the wound site and later by the just described neurological picture. A fourfold rise in the serum titer of neutralizing antibodies is diagnostic if the patient has not undergone immunization after exposure. The presence of high titers of neutralizing antibodies in serum or of such antibodies in CSF, even in patients who have been immunized, suggests the diagnosis. If necessary, the diagnosis can be confirmed by the demonstration of Negri bodies and rabies virus antigen in a brain biopsy specimen.

An important step in deciding whether to carry out postexposure prophylaxis is to capture the animal responsible for the bite. Any such wild animals or domestic animals that exhibit abnormal behavior should be killed and their

Table 24-7. Arthropod-borne Viruses Causing Epidemic Encephalitis

Encephalitis	Insect vector	Season	Geographic location	Severity	Specific features
Eastern equine	Mosquito	Late summer, early fall	Eastern and Gulf coasts of U.S., Caribbean	Severe	High WBC in CSF, 50% mortality
Western equine	Mosquito	Late summer, early fall	West and southwestern U.S.	May be severe	25% less than 1 year old: highest attack rate over 55 years old
Venezuelan	Mosquito	Late summer, early fall	South and Central America; Florida and southwestern U.S.	Mild	—
St. Louis	Mosquito	Late summer, early fall	Widespread in U.S.	May be severe	Dysuria, often affects older adults, specific IgM in serum or CSF for early diagnosis
California	Mosquito	Late summer, early fall	Widespread in U.S., mainly North Central states	Mild and severe forms	Early diagnosis with LaCrosse virus IgM antibody in serum and CSF, seizures common, temporal lobe predominance
Japanese	Mosquito	Late summer, early fall	Japan, China, Siberia, Southeast Asia, India	Severe	Mortality 7–33%
Powassan	Tick	Late spring, summer	Canada and northern U.S.	Mild	—
Colorado tick fever	Tick	Late spring, early summer	Rocky Mountain area	Mild	—

brains appropriately examined. Healthy cats and dogs should be isolated and observed for 10 days for any signs of illness or abnormal behavior. Rabies prophylaxis is administered when the involved animal has a confirmed diagnosis of rabies or when a person is bitten by an uncaptured animal suspected to be rabid in an area where rabies is prevalent. Postexposure prophylaxis consists of thorough wound cleansing, passive immunization with antirabies serum (preferably human rabies immune globulin), and active immunization with vaccine prepared from inactivated rabies virus grown in human diploid cell cultures. This regimen is virtually universally successful in the prevention of clinical rabies. Vaccination occasionally causes mild systemic reactions or more severe hypersensitivity reactions.

Differential Diagnosis

A picture of encephalitis or meningoencephalitis, which is virtually identical to that seen with viruses, can be exhibited by a variety of other conditions, some specifically treatable. These include tuberculous meningitis, multiple cerebral microabscesses, bacterial endocarditis, brucellosis, leptospirosis, *Mycoplasma* pneumonia, rickettsial infections (e.g., Rocky Mountain spotted fever), Lyme disease (*Borrelia burgdorferi*), toxoplasmosis, Behçet's disease, Whipple's disease, and sarcoidosis. Several noninfectious conditions may also produce a similar picture, including acute disseminated encephalomyelitis, acute hemorrhagic necrotizing leukoencephalitis, multiple sclerosis, CNS vasculitis, multiple cerebral emboli from an atrial myxoma, or meningeal carcinomatosis or lymphomatous involvement of the CNS.

HERPES SIMPLEX ENCEPHALITIS

Pathophysiology and Etiology

Herpes simplex encephalitis represents the most common form of sporadic viral encephalitis and is fatal in up to 70 percent of untreated cases. The human herpesvirus is a DNA-containing virus possessing a nucleocapsid and envelope. It consists of type 1 and 2 antigenic groups. Type 2 is responsible for causing genital ulcers and can be the source of aseptic meningitis or neonatal encephalitis. Type 1 is associated with recurrent oral ulcerations and causes the vast majority of cases of herpes encephalitis after the neonatal period.

Neurotropism, which is a tendency for the virus to invade the CNS along peripheral nerves, is a common characteristic of this group of viruses. It has been postulated that the herpesvirus gains access to the brain through the nose and then ascends via the olfactory bulb and tracts to the basal forebrain. An alternative explanation for the orbitofrontal and temporal distribution typical of herpes simplex encephalitis is the reactivation of latent virus within the trigeminal ganglion, after which it ascends along the trigeminal afferents supplying the meninges of the anterior and middle fossae. Latent herpesvirus is often reactivated by some type of stress, such as a concurrent viral infection, surgery, or immunosuppressant drugs; the stress accomplishes this by weakening the immunological defenses.

The pathological effects of herpes simplex encephalitis consist of hemorrhagic necrosis of the mesial temporal, orbitofrontal, and other limbic structures, which may be quite marked (Fig 24-5). Neuronophagia, microglial nodules, and perivascular mononuclear cuffing are typically found in less involved areas. Intranuclear eosinophilic viral inclusions (Cowdry type A) are seen within neurons, astrocytes, and oligodendroglia. Edema is often marked and herniation of the uncus is one of the common causes of death in this disorder.

Clinical Picture and Diagnosis

There is likely a wide spectrum of clinical involvement in herpes simplex encephalitis, with milder cases frequently unproved. Typically a patient with a more severe case initially exhibits nonspecific behavioral disturbances and then becomes delirious with visual hallucinations (Table 24-8). Amnesia may be an early feature but is often overshadowed by confusion. Fever, and in some cases headache and meningeal signs, supervene and the level of conscious-

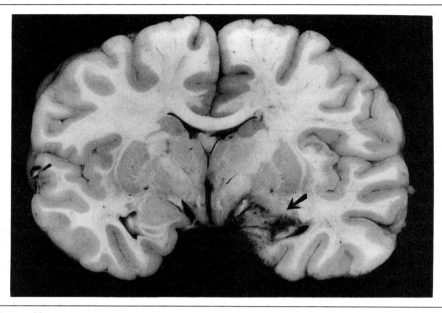

Fig. 24-5. *Coronal brain section at autopsy in a patient who died from herpes simplex encephalitis, showing hemorrhagic necrosis in the medial temporal area* (arrow).

Table 24-8. Diagnosis of Herpes Simplex Encephalitis

Clinical findings
  Acute/subacute change in behavior, delirium,
    hallucinations
  Headache
  Fever
  Early memory impairment
  Focal neurological deficits, seizures, raised
    intracranial pressure
Laboratory findings
  CSF: moderate lymphocytic pleocytosis, elevated
    RBCs, moderately elevated protein level
  EEG: generalized and temporal slowing,
    unilateral or bilateral temporal periodic
    lateralized epileptiform discharges
  CT: may be normal or show temporal lesions with
    edema
  MRI: temporal and orbitofrontal increased signal
    on T_2-weighted images
Special tests
  Herpesvirus DNA in CSF identified by
    polymerase chain reaction
  Detection of herpes antigen in brain biopsy
    specimens

ness declines. Focal signs such as hemiparesis and aphasia often occur and temporal lobe or generalized seizures are common. Elevated in-

tracranial pressure is a major problem in severe cases.

The diagnosis is made on the basis of the clinical picture and confirmatory studies. CSF shows a moderate lymphocytic pleocytosis, often in conjunction with a significant number of red cells and a moderately elevated protein level. The virus is almost never recovered from the CSF. Recently the polymerase chain reaction has been used to isolate herpesvirus DNA from the CSF. This method should allow early, specific diagnosis, although false negatives may be a rare problem. A CT scan may show evidence of brain destruction in the temporal areas but findings can also be normal. MRI scanning is more sensitive for detecting earlier signs of orbitofrontal and temporal inflammation and has become an important initial test in suspected cases (Fig. 24-6). An EEG showing periodic discharges in one or both temporal lobes also supports the diagnosis. The differential diagnosis includes brain abscess, tuberculous meningitis, and acute hemorrhagic necrotizing leukoencephalitis.

Temporal lobe biopsy and the use of immunohistofluorescent and electron microscopic techniques to examine the tissue, as well as the

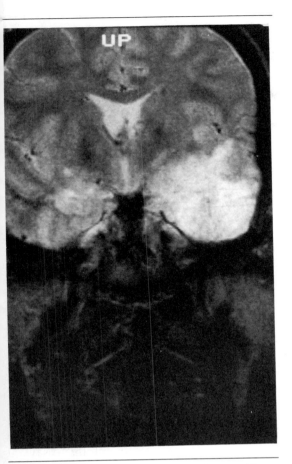

Fig. 24-6. *T$_2$-weighted MRI scan in a 32-year-old man with herpes simplex encephalitis. Note the abnormal signal intensity in both temporal regions, particularly the left. CT scan was normal.*

inoculation of tissue into a cell-culture medium for growth of the virus, constitute the only sure way to confirm the diagnosis of herpes simplex encephalitis. There are two reasons to perform brain biopsy: it can disprove the existence of the encephalitis, thereby avoiding the potential adverse effects of unnecessary treatment, and it may also reveal an unsuspected treatable condition other than herpes simplex encephalitis. Now that acyclovir, a specific antiviral agent for herpes with very low toxicity, is available for treatment, biopsy primarily serves the second purpose. A certain diagnosis is always the ideal objective before treatment of an infectious illness is instituted, as the excessive use of antimicrobial agents can invite the development of

microbial resistance. However, the availability of noninvasive diagnostic techniques such as MRI and the definite morbidity associated with brain biopsy in usually ill patients make the decision to perform a biopsy a difficult one in individual cases. The significant incidence of falsely negative biopsy findings is another consideration.

In practice there are few treatable conditions mimicking herpes simplex encephalitis closely enough to cause confusion, and acyclovir treatment is often begun without a tissue diagnosis. Biopsy is instead reserved for those instances in which the diagnosis is reasonably uncertain or the patient is not responding to the acyclovir. The outcome in patients with herpes simplex encephalitis depends on the early institution of specific antiviral therapy.

Management and Prognosis

Acyclovir (10 mg/kg given intravenously every 8 hours) has become the drug of choice. It is phosphorylated by herpes simplex virus–encoded thymidine kinase and this inhibits the subsequent synthesis of viral DNA. However, resistant mutant strains of the virus have now been identified in immunocompromised patients (e.g., those with AIDS). In these cases, vidarabine, an older drug with a proven efficacy, can be used instead. Other therapeutic measures consist of monitoring the intracranial pressure and using appropriate measures to reduce elevations as well as the administration of antiepileptic drugs such as phenytoin. With the advent of modern management approaches the mortality from the disease has dropped to about 20 percent. About 30 percent of the survivors of severe cases are left with residua such as severe amnesia, aphasia, or epilepsy.

ACUTE DISSEMINATED ENCEPHALOMYELITIS AND ACUTE HEMORRHAGIC NECROTIZING LEUKOENCEPHALITIS

Acute disseminated encephalomyelitis (ADEM) is a parainfectious neurological syndrome caused by a delayed hypersensitivity reaction that is presumably triggered by a viral antigen and is most commonly seen in children over 2 years of age. The pathological changes consist of a perivenular mononuclear inflammatory infiltration and demyelination. The syndrome characteristically arises 4 to 14 days after a bout of a specific childhood exanthematous infection such as measles, varicella, or rubella, but is also commonly associated with nonspecific upper respiratory infections, *Mycoplasma* pneumonia infections, and vaccinations. In former years, smallpox vaccinations and antirabies serum prepared from animal spinal cord tissue were implicated relatively frequently. Rarely ADEM precedes the systemic manifestations of a viral infection. Measles is the most important specific viral offender worldwide, although its incidence has declined dramatically in North America as a result of the measles vaccination program. It occurs in about one out of every 1,000 children who get measles over the age of 2, carries a mortality rate of 10 to 20 percent, and tends to leave survivors with neurological sequelae.

The clinical picture exhibited by ADEM can be indistinguishable from that of viral encephalitis. An interval of several days following the onset of a systemic viral infection, accompanying signs of transverse myelitis, peripheral, or cranial neuropathies, and the paucity of CSF findings are helpful distinguishing features. A CT scan may show cortical enhancing lesions, low-density areas in the deep white matter and basal ganglia, and edema of the brainstem. Treatment with corticosteroids has never been definitively shown to alter the outcome, but nevertheless is frequently employed.

Acute hemorrhagic necrotizing leukoencephalitis is a rare hyperacute form of ADEM that is distinguished in pathological terms by the findings of widespread fibrinoid necrosis of capillaries and small cerebral vessels and multiple small cerebral hemorrhages. Red cells are not usually found in the CSF. It may present as a cerebral mass lesion and elevated intracranial pressure is a major feature. Although corticosteroids and measures to reduce elevated intracranial pressure may improve the patient's outcome, most cases are rapidly fatal.

NEUROSYPHILIS

The protean manifestations of neurosyphilis and its high prevalence in the last century and early part of this century have given this disorder an important niche in the history of clinical neurology. In recent years, however, the incidence of the disease appears to be rising, and new, more aggressive forms of the illness are emerging in patients with AIDS.

The spirochete *Treponema pallidum*, which is transmitted through sexual contact, invades the nervous system and produces symptoms in about 7 percent of patients with untreated primary syphilis. The pathogen most frequently invades the meninges but may also attack the brain parenchyma. This may even give rise to granulomatous formations known as *gummata*, which can create localized mass effects. Asymptomatic neurosyphilis, revealed by a pleocytosis and positive serological findings in the CSF, occurs within the first 2 years of infection in about 25 percent of cases. A small fraction of patients exhibit an acute meningitis picture, often with cranial nerve involvement, hydrocephalus, elevated intracranial pressure, and accompanying arteritis. The **meningovascular syphilis** that appears within months to several years following initial infections reflects a predilection of the spirochete for vessel walls. Strokes may result, particularly in younger victims and most commonly in the middle cerebral artery distribution. Spinal vascular involvement is also seen. Late complications include **tabes dorsalis** and **general paresis.** However, there are intimations that the neurological involvement in present-day cases is shifting away from the classic syndromes to more subtle, ill-defined manifestations.

Tabes dorsalis classically includes lightning pains (severe, lancinating, shocklike pains, usually in the extremities) and loss of posterior column sensation (including joint position sense, vibration, and deep pain, especially in the lower extremities) that leads to sensory ataxia, areflexia, and Argyll Robertson pupils (usually small pupils that react better to accommodation than to light). It succeeds the primary infection after a mean interval of 10 to 15 years.

A neurogenic bladder, optic atrophy, and Charcot joints (principally affecting the lower extremities) are other manifestations.

General paresis represents a dementia that stems from diffuse parenchymal involvement and consists of prominent deterioration of personality. Outwardly it tends to mimic the characteristics of various psychiatric syndromes. Other features also seen are tremor and Argyll Robertson pupils. It occurs 5 to 30 years after the primary phase.

The diagnosis of neurosyphilis is based on serological findings and signs of active inflammation in the CSF. Laboratory diagnosis must be heavily relied on in atypical clinical forms, which appear to be relatively common. The VDRL test, which is directed against a cardiolipin-lecithin antigen, is a common screening test. Although the results are relatively nonspecific, they do give an idea of the activity of the disease when measured in serum and CSF. The fluorescent treponemal antibody absorption (FTA-ABS) test or the microhemagglutination assay–*Treponema pallidum* test is much more specific and sensitive, but the test results remain positive for the lifetime of the patient once syphilis is acquired, even with treatment. Therefore, an unreactive serum FTA-ABS effectively excludes the diagnosis of neurosyphilis. The significance of the FTA-ABS in CSF is controversial. The most important indicator of active neurosyphilis is an elevated lymphocyte count (and usually elevated protein level) in the CSF. Although a negative VDRL in the CSF does not rule out neurosyphilis, a normal cell count virtually does. Therefore, the decision to treat is based on the occurrence of a typical neurological picture in conjunction with either cells in the CSF or appropriate serological evidence. Because neurosyphilis may be latent, there is good reason to perform a lumbar puncture to look for pleocytosis in anyone either known to have had syphilis (treated or untreated) or exhibiting positive serological findings in the absence of known previous infection.

The best treatment for active neurosyphilis consists of the intravenous administration of aqueous penicillin G every 4 hours for 2 weeks. Repeat CSF examination should be done at 6 months and one year. Although symptoms of parenchymal involvement are generally not reversed by treatment, it can prevent further progression of the disease. A falling VDRL titer may be evidence of successful therapy.

LYME DISEASE

Lyme disease is a spirochetal multisystem disease acquired in the endemic forested areas of North America and Europe. It is caused by the organism *Borrelia burgdorferi*, which is transmitted by the bite of the deer tick *Ixodes dammini*. The annual incidence of the disease in the United States has increased from 226 cases in 1980 to over 7,000 cases in 1989 to 1990, but this largely reflects greater recognition of the illness. About 25 to 50 percent of the cases have afflicted children less than 16 years of age. The disease typically occurs in the summer months from May to August, when the tick is in its nymph phase and feeding on blood. The initial phase of the resulting illness often resembles a flu-like illness with the patient characteristically exhibiting skin lesions termed *erythema chronicum migrans*. The skin lesions begin as a red macule and papule that gradually enlarges to a typical size of 15 cm or more in diameter. Atrioventricular block is the most frequent consequence of cardiac involvement.

Neurological manifestations develop after an interval of 1 to 6 months in about 10 to 15 percent of cases and consist of meningoencephalitis with prominent headache, cranial nerve palsies (especially the seventh), radiculopathies, plexopathies, a neuropathy resembling Guillain-Barré syndrome, or myelopathy. Arthritis can be an early or late manifestation, appearing as much as years after the initial infection. The findings are usually subjective in the initial phases with migratory arthralgias and pain when moving the joints. Typically the knee and temporomandibular joints are affected.

There are a variety of "late" neurological manifestations, including a multiple sclerosis–like syndrome. Diagnosis is based on the clinical picture and the results of serological studies for IgG antibodies to *Borrelia*. Serological testing almost invariably yields positive results once the initial stages have passed.

A variety of antibiotics, including doxycycline (100 mg b.i.d. for 10–30 days) or amoxicillin (500 mg q.i.d. for 10–30 days), have been used to treat the initial manifestations in adults. Intravenous penicillin in full meningeal doses or ceftriaxone (2 mg intravenously daily for 14–21 days) is used to treat the neurological aspects of the disease (except the seventh nerve palsy, which responds to oral therapy) or to manage severe disease in general.

MISCELLANEOUS CONDITIONS

Sarcoidosis

Sarcoidosis is a systemic idiopathic granulomatous disease whose infectious nature has not been proved. It afflicts blacks ten times more often than whites and women twice more frequently than men. Typically patients have lung lesions that consist of hilar "eggshell" calcifications. A more diffuse reticular pattern is often seen on x-ray studies. Ophthalmic involvement (uveitis and lacrimal gland involvement), parotitis, and skin involvement (erythema nodosum) are other classic features. Hypercalcemia and cutaneous anergy are common.

Neurological involvement occurs in about 5 to 10 percent of the cases and is the presenting symptom in about half of these. A chronic basilar meningitis due to the granulomatous and vasculitic changes at the base of the brain is commonly encountered. Cranial nerve involvement, especially bilateral seventh nerve palsies and cerebellar deficits, is frequent. A more acute picture of aseptic, at times recurrent, meningitis is manifested in about 20 percent of those patients with neurosarcoidosis. The hypothalamic-pituitary area is particularly prone to attack, and involvement precipitates diabetes insipidus or other neuroendocrine disturbances. Hydrocephalus may result from the basilar involvement. Other manifestations consist of a myelopathy, radiculopathy, multiple mononeuropathy, and, in rare cases, a granulomatous polymyositis–like syndrome. Cases with minimal systemic manifestations may be misdi-

agnosed as multiple sclerosis because of the multifocal nervous system involvement, which may be relapsing and remitting, and the elevated immunoglobulin levels in the CSF. The coexistence of neurotuberculosis or progressive multifocal leukoencephalopathy may rarely confuse the picture.

Diagnosis is largely based on the clinical picture in conjunction with the identification of noncaseating granulomata on a tissue biopsy specimen. Muscle biopsy has a high yield even in the absence of symptomatic myositis. The CSF shows nonspecific findings of pleocytosis, together with an elevated protein and occasionally reduced glucose level. Sometimes meningeal or brain biopsy is necessary to confirm the diagnosis. A biopsy specimen from an enlarged lymph node, conjunctiva, salivary gland, mucocutaneous lesion, or the liver may also reveal the existence of characteristic granulomata. Elevated serum levels of angiotensin-converting enzyme also constitute a helpful finding. The overall prognosis varies widely depending on the severity of the CNS and systemic involvement. Corticosteroid treatment for several months seems to be effective in many cases and immunosuppressant agents have been used as an alternative. In patients with a positive skin test or history of tuberculosis, antituberculosis therapy should be added.

Tetanus

Clostridium tetani is an anaerobic gram-positive rod-shaped organism whose spores may remain dormant in soil and fecal matter for long periods. Tetanus results from a localized infection caused by the vegetative form of the organism, which elaborates a soluble exotoxin that interferes with the presynaptic release of acetylcholine. The toxin acts at the level of the neuromuscular junction, spinal interneurons, the brain, and the sympathetic nervous system.

Classically, the disease is acquired through the contamination of either deep puncture wounds or wounds involving extensive tissue destruction. It can also result from bowel surgery or abortions. In many cases, the wound is relatively trivial and some patients may not recall an antecedent wound. Some cases arise in intravenous drug abusers due to contaminated needles or supplies. Neonatal cases are particularly prevalent in developing countries where poor hygienic conditions persist.

Incubation usually takes 3 to 21 days, although this may stretch to several months. There may be localized muscle spasms at the site of infection. **Cephalic tetanus** may result from injuries to the head or otitis media. It manifests in the form of cranial nerve palsies, particularly the seventh, as well as trismus (spasm of the jaw muscles), which often progresses to become generalized muscle spasms. Most cases of generalized tetanus begin with trismus, dysphagia, and pain and stiffness in the neck and back muscles. Generalized muscle spasms are painful and often result in opisthotonos. Patients suffer from hyperthermia and urinary retention and exhibit autonomic signs of sympathetic overactivity. Consciousness is preserved but true epileptic seizures may be seen. The differential diagnosis includes hysteria, malignant hyperthermia, tonic status epilepticus, decerebrate spasms, and dystonic reactions to medication. Diagnosis is based primarily on the clinical picture with laboratory findings adding little useful information.

With proper intensive care management, the mortality in patients with tetanus is currently less than 10 percent. Glottal or laryngeal spasm leading to asphyxia, cardiac arrhythmias due to autonomic instability, and electrolyte and fluid imbalances are all important contributors to the disease's morbidity and mortality.

The early placement of a tracheostomy, paralysis with neuromuscular blocking agents, and ventilation are important measures in generalized cases. Intravenous diazepam in large doses reduces the muscle spasms, provides sedation, and decreases the likelihood of epileptic seizures. It is important to avoid overstimulation, and patients should be kept as quiet as possible; caregivers should refrain from undue suctioning or manipulation of the patient. The local wound site should be properly cleansed and debrided of dead tissue.

Penicillin in large doses, administered parenterally, and human hyperimmune globulin (3,000 to 6,000 units intramuscularly) are routine measures. Antitoxin may also be instilled locally around the wound site if it cannot be debrided. Active immunization is also carried out later with tetanus toxoid because the disease does not confer humeral immunity. The average duration of paralysis in severe cases is 21 days, with some cases persisting for 6 weeks.

The key to treatment is prevention. A primary series of vaccinations should be given to all infants and at 2, 4, 6, and 18 months, followed at 5 years, and thereafter every 10 years for life. In the event of an injury, the protocol for tetanus prevention should be rigorously applied.

Behçet's Disease

Behçet's disease is an inflammatory disorder, with an uncertain etiology that is found mainly in the Middle Eastern population. It causes recurrent oral-genital ulceration, uveitis, and neurological manifestations in 10 to 25 percent of the cases. A wide variety of CNS syndromes are exhibited, but the most common is a recurrent aseptic meningitis. Other features may include erythema nodosum, thrombophlebitis, arthralgias, pericarditis, and epididymitis. Mortality is relatively high when there is CNS involvement. Recently azathioprine has been shown to slow progression of the disease.

Cerebral Whipple's Disease

Whipple's disease is a chronic bacterial infection that affects multiple organs whose causal agent has not been identified. Men over 35 years old are the most frequent victims. Macrophages that stain positively with periodic–acid Schiff (PAS) and intracellular and extracellular rod-shaped organisms are seen in the tissues of affected patients, particularly the jejunum. Early manifestations include pneumonia, nondeforming arthritis, fever, malaise, and leukocytosis, with malabsorption appearing later.

The neurological complications that have been described include dementia, supranuclear gaze palsies, myoclonus and other movement disorders, ataxia, and hypothalamic dysfunction, which may be relapsing. Examination of jejunal biopsy specimens occasionally yields negative findings in patients with neurological involvement, particularly if there has been prior antibiotic treatment. PAS-positive macrophages may occasionally be found in the CSF or the diagnosis can be confirmed by a brain biopsy, although false negatives may occur. MRI scanning may show involvement of the hypothalamus and adjacent medial temporal areas. Neurological symptoms may be slow to respond to antibiotics such as chloramphenicol.

Cysticercosis

Cysticercosis is the systemic expression of infection by the larval stage of *Taenia solium,* the pork tapeworm. It is the most common parasitic infection of the nervous system and is especially prevalent in the populations of Mexico and Central and South America, where it constitutes one of the major causes of epilepsy. The infection is acquired from the consumption of undercooked pork that contains the larval cysts or from the ingestion of contaminated fecal material. Autoinfection is also a possibility.

The ova hatch in the small intestine of the host and the larvae then enter the bloodstream and lodge in muscle, eye, subcutaneous areas, meninges, or the brain, where they enlarge over a period of years to form cysts. The resulting neurological manifestations include meningitis, focal deficits, seizures, and hydrocephalus. Multiple cysts are common and are arranged in grapelike clusters that sometimes form at the base of the brain, thereby obstructing CSF pathways. Cysts may reach a size of several centimeters and frequently become calcified.

The inflammatory reaction produced when the larvae die contributes to the symptomatology. Diagnosis is made on the basis of a CT scan that shows the cystic lesions, which are often multiple and exhibit a characteristic appearance, in a patient who is living in or has migrated from an endemic area. Subcutaneous cysts, muscle calcifications, eosinophilia in the blood and CSF, and serological abnormalities may help confirm the diagnosis.

Therapy consists of antiepileptic drugs, shunting to control the hydrocephalus, and the surgical removal of any large and accessible solitary cysts. Praziquantel is a new drug that can eradicate the cysts. Steroids should also be administered during praziquantel treatment to reduce the inflammatory response as the larvae are killed by the drug.

AIDS

The acquired immune deficiency syndrome was first recognized in 1981. Since then, its incidence has reached epidemic proportions worldwide, but particularly in the United States and Central West Africa.

Pathophysiology and Etiology

The disease is due to infection by a specific RNA-containing retrovirus—the human immunodeficiency virus (HIV), of which two types have been identified: HIV-1 and HIV-2 (in West Africa). The virus is transmitted through intimate contact with body fluids, especially blood and semen. Currently the disease is mainly confined to certain high-risk groups, including homosexual and bisexual males, intravenous drug abusers, hemophiliacs and other blood transfusion recipients, and the sexual partners of those who are at high risk or from a region of high endemicity. Increasingly, however, the disease is being spread by heterosexual contact.

Through its reverse transcriptase enzyme, the virus manufactures DNA, which is then integrated into the host chromosome following infection. It has a specific lymphotropism that allows it to infect and selectively destroy CD4 (helper) lymphocytes. The depletion of T4 lymphocytes impairs cellular immunity; this indirectly interferes with B-lymphocyte antibody production and causes macrophage dysfunction. Patients exhibit a lymphopenia, decrease in CD4 lymphocytes, increase in CD8 (suppressor) lymphocytes, and hypergammaglobulinemia. The full-blown AIDS picture develops in at least 50 percent of HIV-positive patients within 10 years of infection.

Clinical Picture and Diagnosis

The illness includes the appearance of an opportunistic infection such as *Pneumocystis carinii* pneumonia or a neoplasm highly associated with AIDS such as Kaposi's sarcoma in a previously well patient who exhibits serological evidence of HIV infection. Serious opportunistic infection does not tend to occur until the CD4 lymphocyte counts fall below 250/mm³. Common early symptoms of HIV infection include chronic lymphadenopathy, weight loss, fatigue, night sweats, and behavioral changes. Such symptoms in a patient in one of the high-risk groups should always suggest the possibility of HIV infection.

Neurological symptoms, arising from both the central and peripheral nervous system, are being increasingly recognized in AIDS patients and probably occur in at least 75 percent of the cases. The HIV virus itself demonstrates neurotropism and may gain entry to the CNS via infected lymphocytes and macrophages. Neurons and glia are damaged by unknown mechanisms. Subacute HIV encephalopathy can be thought of as a "slow" virus syndrome stemming from the presence of HIV within the brain and is the most important neurological syndrome caused by the HIV virus. Microglial nodules are prominent, along with patchy demyelination, subcortical gliosis, and spongiform changes but little inflammation. The neurological presentation of AIDS exhibits a variety of focal findings as well as a chronic or subacute encephalopathy. This consists of a personality change, apathy, hallucinations, delirium, and eventually dementia. The symptoms may occasionally remit and relapse. The CT scan shows atrophy and possibly focal enhancing areas. AIDS dementia is discussed further in Chapter 4.

The pathogenesis of the acute and chronic inflammatory polyneuropathies seen in AIDS may also be directly related to HIV involvement of peripheral nerves. One form of subacute lumbosacral neuropathy has been found to stem from cytomegalovirus infection and responds to ganciclovir treatment. A vacuolar myelopathy affecting the posterior and lateral columns and presenting as an ataxic-spastic paraparesis has also been attributed to HIV virus and is seen in about 20 percent of AIDS patients. An atypical aseptic meningitis, which is discussed earlier in this chapter, is another neurological manifesta-

tion of HIV involvement and may occur at the time of seroconversion. The HIV virus itself may also cause an inflammatory myopathy resembling polymyositis and zidovudine, which is the primary agent in the treatment of AIDS, has been shown to cause a mitochondrial myopathy.

A variety of other viruses can infect the CNS in AIDS patients, including cytomegalovirus (causing encephalitis as well as a variety of other syndromes), herpes simplex encephalitis, and Epstein-Barr virus (possibly responsible for lymphoma). AIDS has become the most common setting for progressive multifocal leukoencephalopathy due to a papovavirus (J-C virus) (Fig. 24-7). The clinical picture is one of a subacute dementing illness with visual loss, focal motor signs, and ataxia. CT scanning discloses the presence of low-density nonenhancing areas in the white matter, which are often located periventricularly in the centrum semio-

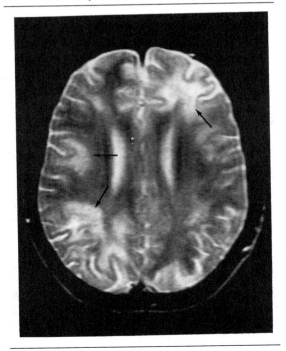

Fig. 24-7. *T₂-weighted MRI scan in a 31-year-old man with AIDS who presented with subacutely developing changes in his personality and unusual behavior. The arrows indicate patchy areas of demyelination typical of progressive multifocal leukoencephalopathy. CT scan showed only mild abnormalities.*

vale (especially parietooccipitally) as well as within the cerebellum.

Fungal infections, particularly with *Cryptococcus, Candida,* and *Aspergillus,* may cause meningitis or abscesses, as they do in other immunosuppressed patients. Unusual bacteria, particularly *Mycobacterium avium–intracellulare,* reactivated tuberculosis, and a particularly aggressive form of syphilis, may also attack the nervous system in AIDS patients.

Of the opportunistic organisms invading the brain, *Toxoplasma gondii* is particularly common and its detection is important because of its treatability. This protozoal organism often produces multifocal abscesses affecting structures in both the cortex and the basal ganglia. A wide variety of symptoms may appear, including headache, multifocal signs, seizures, cerebellar signs, dementia, or stupor. CT scanning is particularly useful for the diagnosis of this disorder and often reveals the presence of multiple discrete ring-enhancing lesions (Fig. 24-8). Occasionally nonenhancing or uniformly enhancing lesions are seen. Serological studies of specific IgG and IgM titers are less useful diagnostically in AIDS patients than in other groups of immunosuppressed patients who also occasionally suffer from *Toxoplasma* infections.

Other intracranial lesions in AIDS patients that may show up as discrete enhancing lesions on CT scans include lymphomas (Fig. 24-9) and more rarely Kaposi's sarcoma of the brain. In addition, there is a significant occurrence of cerebral hemorrhages (due to platelet defects) and cerebral infarcts (due to marantic endocarditis or vasculitis) in AIDS patients.

Management

At present, patients with full-blown AIDS or CD4 counts less than 500/mm³ are treated with zidovudine (AZT; 60–1,200 mg/day), which is a reverse transcriptase inhibitor. Therapy is maintained indefinitely, unless side effects supervene such as anemia, granulocytopenia, nausea, vomiting, or headache. Dideoxyinosine is an alternative agent that can cause peripheral neuropathy or pancreatitis as side effects. These agents have lengthened the life span and reduced the number of opportunistic infections in AIDS patients.

When an enhancing lesion is discovered on a CT scan from an AIDS patient with neurological deficits, the approach to management often includes trial treatment for toxoplasmosis with pyrimethamine and sulfadiazine or clindamycin. If the lesion does not resolve within 1 to 2 weeks and there are no definite clues to its etiology, a trial of antifungal therapy with amphotericin may be undertaken. If the lesion persists, biopsy should probably be done, provided the lesion is accessible. If a lymphoma is discovered, then radiotherapy may bring about regression of the lesion and prolong overall survival. In some advanced cases, the poor prognosis and social considerations may dictate a more conservative approach. Therapy for the toxoplasmosis must be life-long to effectively prevent recurrence of the disease.

SLOW VIRUSES

Sigurdsson first elaborated the concept of slow virus infections in the 1950s based on his study of the neurological diseases scrapie, visna, and maedi, which affect Icelandic sheep. These infections are characterized by a long latency (months to years), an irregular protracted course resembling a degenerative condition after the first appearance of signs, and usual limitation to a single host species and single organ system. The findings from transmission and other studies have now made it clear that the criteria pertaining to host and organ limitation are not usually applicable.

The mechanisms by which the so-called slow viruses remain latent or persistent and can escape eradication by normal cellular and humoral immune mechanisms is still unclear. HIV viral infection, the most recently recognized slow virus infection of the brain (discussed in the previous section), exhibits the unique feature of causing specific immunological impairment through the selective destruction of T4 lymphocytes. In the absence of immunosuppression, a virus may persist by existing in a degenerated, incomplete form that is not recognized by host immune mechanisms. The con-

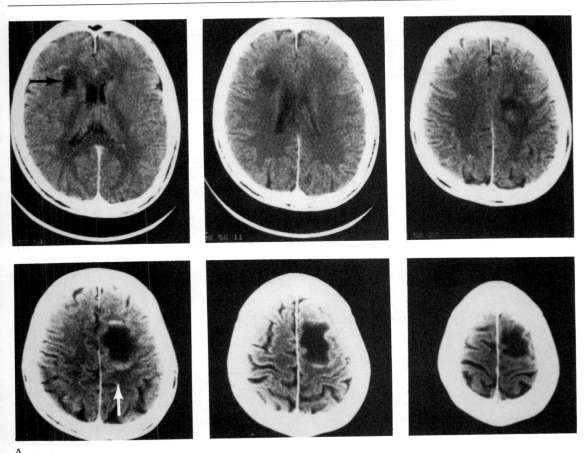

A

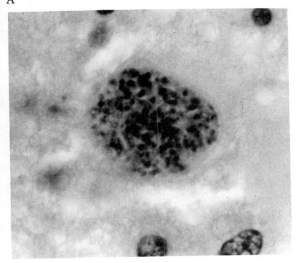

B

Fig. 24-8. *(A) Enhanced CT scans in a 33-year-old homosexual man who was known to have been HIV-positive for 4 years but was asymptomatic until he developed word-finding difficulties, headache, and incoordination of the right hand. Two abscesses (arrows),* one in the left parietal area, which is mildly enhancing, and a second smaller ill-defined one in the right frontal area, are seen. Biopsy revealed *Toxoplasma and he has responded well to treatment with sulfadiazine and pyrimethamine. (B) Typical microscopic appearance of* Toxoplasma *pseudocysts. (Hematoxylin-eosin,* ×250.)

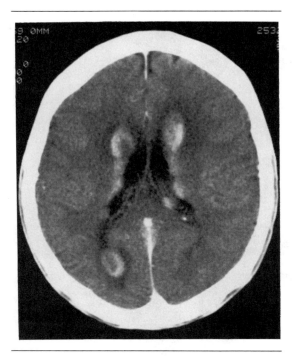

Fig. 24-9. *Enhanced CT scan in a patient with AIDS, showing subependymal enhancing lymphoma.*

cept of the brain as an immunologically privileged site because of the poor lymphocytic penetration of the blood-brain barrier and an absent lymphatic circulation may also account for viral persistence within the CNS.

The slow viruses fall into two main categories. The "conventional" slow virus infections cause neuropathological changes that suggest viral infection, such as perivascular lymphocytic cuffing and inclusion bodies, often some evidence of an immunological response in the serum, and the existence of viral antigen, which can be detected by conventional methods. This group of disorders includes subacute sclerosing panencephalitis (SSPE), progressive rubella panencephalitis, and progressive multifocal leukoencephalopathy (PML). The "unconventional" slow virus infections in humans include kuru and the Creutzfeldt-Jakob disease and the Gerstman-Straussler syndrome. These spongiform encephalopathies have been discussed (see Chapter 4). Although these disorders are transmissible to a variety of animal species, histological and serological studies have furnished no further clues to their infectious nature. The concept of prions (proteinaceous infectious particles) has been advanced by Prusiner on the basis of findings yielded by extensive chemical and virological investigations of the transmissible scrapie agent. Chemical and physical agents such as formalin, the nucleases, alkylating agents, and ultraviolet light do not inactivate these infectious particles, and their mode of replication remains unknown. These agents, which resemble a form of cerebral amyloid, are possibly the etiological agent responsible for Creutzfeldt-Jakob disease and kuru.

Subacute Sclerosing Panencephalitis

SSPE was formerly known as *Dawson's inclusion body encephalitis,* and is known to be a late protracted form of measles encephalitis. The patient invariably has a history of childhood measles (usually in the first 2 years of life), but rarely cases occur after a live measles vaccination. The disease is seldom seen and is diminishing in incidence because of the widespread measles vaccination program. Males afflicted by SSPE outnumber females by 3 to 1. The mean latency of onset following measles infection is 7 years (range, 2–32 years).

The disease is a panencephalitis that affects both gray and white matter and causes gross atrophy. There is a loss of neurons in the gray matter as well as subcortical demyelination and gliosis. Perivascular mononuclear cell cuffing, microglial nodules, neuronophagia, and intranuclear inclusions (Cowdry type A), plus intracytoplasmic inclusions within neurons, astrocytes, and oligodendrocytes, constitute the constellation of findings exhibited by a conventional slow virus infection. Electron microscopic examination discloses the existence of typical myxovirus structures within the intranuclear inclusions and immunofluorescent studies reveal measles antigen. Using special cocultivation techniques, investigators have been able to culture the measles virus from the brains of patients with SSPE.

The disease presents in its early stages as an insidious dementia which is manifested as a decline in school performance, behavioral disturbances, alterations in the sleep cycle, and hallucinations. Later, myoclonus, seizures, involuntary movements, cortical blindness, dysphagia, and progressive spasticity appear. Retinitis and optic atrophy can be helpful clues to the diagnosis, if present. At this stage, the EEG shows characteristic periodic sharp and slow complexes that occur every 3 to 7 seconds (Fig. 24-10). These tend to be very stereotyped in a given patient and may or may not coincide with the myoclonus. These complexes may disappear later in the disease as the EEG background is progressively decimated. In the late stages the patient is severely demented with quadriplegia in flexion. In the terminal stage, there are autonomic and hypothalamic disturbances. Diagnosis is usually evident from the clinical picture, but can be confirmed by very high serum levels of measles antibody, elevated CSF titers of measles antibody, elevated CSF gamma globulin levels, and the presence of oligoclonal bands. A serum-to-CSF antibody ratio of less than 50 indicates that measles antibody is being produced in the CSF.

The disease is almost invariably fatal within several months to a year of onset, but in rare instances patients experience remission and survive several years. There is no known specific treatment, though valproic acid or clonazepam may prove useful for controlling the myoclonus and seizures.

Progressive Rubella Panencephalitis

Patients infected with rubella in utero may be born with cataracts, retinal pigmentation, deafness, cardiac anomalies, and microcephaly, and are also mentally retarded from birth. Rarely there may be later neurological deterioration in the second decade due to a rubella panencephalitis that is causing worsening of the dementia, ataxia, and spasticity resembling that seen in SSPE.

Fig. 24-10. *Periodic EEG complexes typical of subacute sclerosing panencephalitis seen in a previously well 15-year-old boy with a 3-year history of deteriorating school performance, dementia, myoclonus, and seizures.*

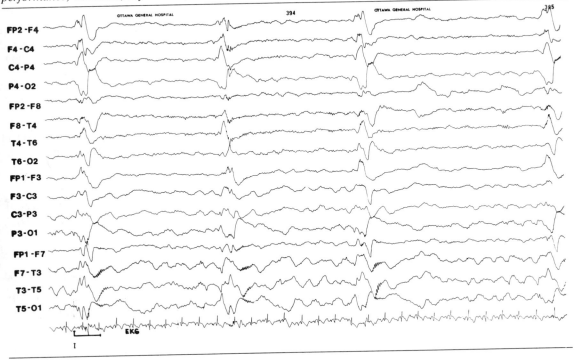

Progressive Multifocal Leukoencephalopathy

PML is a relatively rare slow virus infection of the brain that is seen in individuals with impaired cellular immunity. Formerly PML was encountered most commonly in the lymphoproliferative disorders such as Hodgkin's disease, with smaller numbers of cases seen in patients with systemic lupus erythematosus or sarcoidosis or in patients following renal transplantation. The disease is now most frequently observed in AIDS patients.

A papovavirus of the J-C variety is the usual causative agent. There is multifocal involvement of the brain in the disorder, particularly affecting the white matter. Inclusions are seen within oligodendroglial nuclei and the oligodendroglia are eventually destroyed. Multifocal demyelinated areas form that are surrounded by enlarged bizarre-appearing astrocytes which resemble neoplastic cells. There is little inflammatory response because of the immunosuppression of the host.

The clinical presentation is widely variable, often including a subacute dementia, cortical blindness, spastic hemiparesis, and infrequently seizures. The CSF is usually normal. CT or MRI scanning can reveal the presence of multiple areas of demyelination, often in both parietal or both frontal regions and in the cerebellum (see Fig. 24-7). Occasionally discrete low-density areas are seen deep in the brain. In AIDS patients, cerebral involvement with HIV virus or other infectious agents is a not uncommon additional finding. There is no specific treatment for this disorder except to do everything possible to enhance the patient's immune status. Survival for more than 18 months is unusual.

BIBLIOGRAPHY

Bacterial Meningitis

Anderson, M. Bacterial Meningitis. In W. B. Matthews and G. H. Glaser (editors). *Recent Advances in Clinical Neurology*. Edinburgh; Churchill Livingstone, 1984, Vol. 4, Pp. 87–121.

Bolan, G. and Barza, M. Acute bacterial meningitis in children and adults. A perspective. *Med. Clin. North Am.* 69:231–241, 1985.

Feigin, R. D., and Dodge, P. R. Bacterial meningitis: newer concepts of pathophysiology and neurologic sequelae. *Paediatr. Clin. North Am.* 23:541–565, 1976.

Granoff, D. M. and Squires, J. E. *Hemophilus* meningitis: new developments in epidemiology, treatment and prophylaxis. *Semin. Neurol.* 2:151–165, 1982.

Greenlee, J. E. Bacterial meningitis. In R. T. Johnson (editor). *Current Therapy in Neurologic Disease 1985–1986*. St. Louis: Mosby–Year Book, 1985, Pp. 123–128.

Lavetter, A., et al. Meningitis due to *Listeria monocytogenes*. A review of 25 cases. *N. Engl. J. Med.* 285:598–603, 1971.

Lebel, M. H., et al. Dexamethasone therapy for bacterial meningitis. Results of two double-blind, placebo-controlled trials. *N. Engl. J. Med.* 319:964–971, 1988.

LeFrock, J. L., Smith, B. R., and Molavi, A. Gram-negative bacillary meningitis. *Med. Clin. North Am.* 69:243–256, 1985.

Quagliariello, V., and Scheld, W. M. Bacterial meningitis: pathogenesis, pathophysiology and progress. *N. Engl. J. Med.* 327:864–872, 1992.

Roos, K. L. Management of bacterial meningitis in children and adults. *Semin. Neurol.* 12:155–164, 1992.

Swartz, M. N., and Dodge, P. R. Bacterial meningitis—review of selected aspects. *N. Engl. J. Med.* 272:725–731; 779–787; 842–848; 898–902, 1965.

Tuomanen, E. Partner drugs: a new outlook for bacterial meningitis. *Ann. Intern. Med.* 109:690–692, 1988.

Tuberculosis of the Nervous System

Harder, E., Al-Kawi, M. Z., and Carney, P. Intracranial tuberculoma: conservative management. *Am. J. Med.* 74:570–576, 1983.

Matthai, K. V., and Chandy, J. Tuberculous

infections of the central nervous system. *Clin. Neurosurg.* 14:145–177, 1967.

Molavi, A., and LeFrock, J. L. Tuberculous meningitis. *Med. Clin. North Am.* 69:315–331, 1985.

Sheller, J. R., and Des Prez, R. M. CNS tuberculosis. *Neurol. Clin.* 4:143–158, 1986.

Aseptic and Recurrent Meningitis

Goldstein, R., et al. Mollaret's meningitis: a case with circulating natural killer cells. *Ann. Neurol.* 20:359–361, 1986.

Hermans, P. E., Goldstein, N. P., and Wellman, W. E. Mollaret's meningitis and the differential diagnosis of recurrent meningitis. *Am. J. Med.* 52:128–140, 1972.

Ratzan, K. R. Viral meningitis. *Med. Clin. North Am.* 69:399–413, 1985.

Silverstein, A., Steinberg, G., and Nathanson, M. Nervous system involvement in infectious mononucleosis. *Arch. Neurol.* 26:353–365, 1972.

Wilhelm, C., and Ellner, J. J. Chronic meningitis. *Neurol. Clin.* 4:115–141, 1986.

Fungal Infections of the Nervous System

Bell, W. E. Treatment of fungal infections of the central nervous system. *Ann. Neurol.* 9:417–422, 1981.

Bennett, J. E., et al. A comparison of amphotericin B alone and combined with flucytosine in the treatment of cryptococcal meningitis. *N. Engl. J. Med.* 301:126–131, 1979.

Bouza, E., et al. Coccidioidal meningitis: an analysis of thirty-one cases and review of the literature. *Medicine* 60:139–172, 1981.

Lewis, J. L., and Rabinovich, S. The wide spectrum of cryptococcal infections. *Am. J. Med.* 53:315–322, 1972.

Lyons, R. W., and Andriole, V. T. Fungal infections of the CNS. *Neurol. Clin.* 4:159–170, 1986.

Medoff, G., and Kobayashi, G. S. Strategies in the treatment of systemic fungal infections. *N. Engl. J. Med.* 302:145–154, 1980.

Sabetta, J. R., and Andriole, V. T. Cryptococcal infection of the central nervous system. *Med. Clin. North Am.* 69:333–344, 1985.

Salaki, J. S., Louria, D. B., and Chmel, H. Fungal and yeast infections of the central nervous system. *Medicine* 63:108–132, 1984.

Walsh, T. J., Hier, D. B., and Caplan, L. R. Aspergillosis of the central nervous system: clinicopathological analysis of 17 patients. *Ann. Neurol.* 18:574–582, 1985.

Wilhelm, C. S., and Marra, C. M. Chronic meningitis. *Semin. Neurol.* 12:234–247, 1992.

Brain Abscess

Berg, B., et al. Non-surgical cure of brain abscess: early diagnosis and follow-up with CT. *Ann. Neurol.* 3:474–478, 1978.

Black, P., Silverberg, A. L., and LeFrock, J. L. Management of brain abscess. In R. T. Johnson (editor). *Current Therapy in Neurological Disease, 1985–1986.* St. Louis: Mosby–Year Book, 1985, Pp. 129–133.

Chun, C. H., et al. Brain abscess. A study of 45 consecutive cases. *Medicine* 65:415–431, 1986.

Kaplan, K. Brain abscess. *Med. Clin. North Am.* 69:345–360, 1985.

Kaufman, D. M., Miller, M. H., and Steigbigel, N. H. Subdural empyema: analysis of 17 recent cases and review of the literature. *Medicine* 54:485–498, 1975.

Morgan, H., and Wood, M. W. Cerebellar abscess: a review of seventeen cases. *Surg. Neurol.* 3:93–96, 1975.

Sarwar, M., Falkoff, G., and Naseem, M. Radiologic techniques in the diagnosis of CNS infections. *Neurol. Clin.* 4:41–68, 1986.

Wispelwey, B., and Scheld, W. M. Brain abscesses. *Semin. Neurol.* 12:273–278, 1992.

Neurosyphilis and Lyme Disease

Bayne, L. L., Schmidley, J. W., and Goodin, D. S. Acute syphilitic meningitis. Its occurrence after clinical and serologic cure of secondary syphilis with penicillin G. *Arch. Neurol.* 43:137–138, 1986.

Coyle, P. K. Neurologic Lyme disease. *Semin. Neurol.* 12:200–208, 1992.

Finkel, M. F. Lyme disease and its neurologic complications. *Arch. Neurol.* 45:99–104, 1988.

Halperin, J. J., et al. Lyme borreliosis–associated encephalopathy. *Neurology* 40:1340–1343, 1990.

Halperin, J. J., et al. Lyme disease: cause of a treatable peripheral neuropathy. *Neurology* 37:1700–1706, 1987.

Hook, E. W., III and Marra, CM. Acquired syphilis in adults. *N. Engl. J. Med.* 326:1060–1068, 1992.

Logigian, E. L., Kaplan, R. F., and Steere, A. C. Chronic neurologic manifestations of Lyme disease. *N. Engl. J. Med.* 323:1438–1444, 1990.

Simon, R. Neurosyphilis. *Arch. Neurol.* 42:606–613, 1985.

Sparling, P. F. Diagnosis and treatment of syphilis. *N. Engl. J. Med.* 284:642–652, 1971.

Steere, A. C. Lyme disease. *N. Engl. J. Med.* 321:586–596, 1989.

Viral Encephalitis

Baringer, J. R. Human herpes simplex virus infections. In R. A. Thompson and J. R. Green (editors). *Advances in Neurology.* New York: Raven, 1974, Pp. 41–51.

Ho, D. D., and Hirsch, M. S. Acute viral encephalitis. *Med. Clin. North Am.* 69:415–429, 1985.

Jemsek, J., et al. Herpes zoster–associated encephalitis: clinicopathologic report of 12 cases and review of the literature. *Medicine* 62:81–97, 1983.

Johnson, R. T. *Viral Infections of the Nervous System.* New York: Raven, 1982.

Johnson, R. T., et al. Measles encephalomyelitis—clinical and immunologic studies. *N. Engl. J. Med.* 310:137–141, 1984.

Laskin, O. L. Acyclovir. Pharmacology and clinical experience. *Arch. Neurol.* 144:1241–1246, 1984.

Longson, M. Herpes simplex encephalitis. In W. B. Matthews and G. H. Glaser (editors). *Recent Advances in Clinical Neurology.* Edinburgh: Churchill Livingstone, 1984, Vol. 4, Pp. 123–139.

Monath, T. P. Japanese encephalitis—a plague of the Orient. *N. Engl. J. Med.* 319:641–643, 1988.

Rubeiz, H., and Roos, R. P. Viral meningitis and encephalitis. *Semin. Neurol.* 12:165–177, 1992.

Schroth, G., et al. Early diagnosis of herpes simplex encephalitis by MRI. *Neurology* 37:179–183, 1987.

Skoldenberg, B., et al. Acyclovir versus vidarabine in herpes simplex encephalitis. Randomised multicentre study in consecutive Swedish patients. *Lancet* 2:707–711, 1984.

Varvghese, P. V. Rabies in Canada in 1985. *Can. Med. Assoc. J.* 136:1277–1280, 1987.

Whitley, R. J. Viral encephalitis. *N. Engl. J. Med.* 323:242–248, 1990.

Whitley, R. J., et al. Vidarabine versus acyclovir therapy in herpes simplex encephalitis. *N. Engl. J. Med.* 314:144–149, 1986.

Whitley, R. J., et al. Herpes simplex encephalitis. Clinical assessment. *JAMA* 247:317–320, 1982.

Miscellaneous Infections of the Nervous System; Parainfectious Conditions; Sarcoidosis

Adams, M., et al. Whipple's disease confined to the central nervous system. *Ann. Neurol.* 21:104–108, 1987.

Dalakas, M. C., et al. A long-term follow-up study of patients with post-poliomyelitis neuromuscular symptoms. *N. Engl. J. Med.* 314:959–963, 1986.

De Ghetaldi, L. D., Norman, R. M., and Douville, A. W., Jr. Cerebral cysticercosis treated biphasically with dexamethasone and praziquantel. *Ann. Intern. Med.* 99:179–181, 1983.

Edmonson, R. S., and Flowers, M. W. Intensive care in tetanus: management, complications and mortality in 100 cases. *Br. Med. J.* 1:1401–1404, 1979.

Feurle, G. E., Volk, B., and Waldherr, R. Cerebral Whipple's disease with negative jejunal histology. *N. Engl. J. Med.* 300:907–908, 1979.

Hart, M. N., and Earle, K. M. Haemorrhagic and perivenous encephalitis: a clinico-pathological review of 38 cases. *J. Neurol. Neurosurg. Psychiatry* 38:585–591, 1975.

Herskovitz, S., Lipton, R. B., and Lantos, G. Neuro-Behçet's disease: CT and clinical correlates. *Neurology* 38:1714–1720, 1988.

Luke, R. A., et al. Neurosarcoidosis: the long-term clinical course. *Neurology* 37:461–463, 1987.

McCormick, G. F., Zee, C. S., and Heiden, J. Cysticercosis cerebri. Review of 127 cases. *Arch. Neurol.* 39:534–539, 1982.

Miller, H. G., Stanton, J. B., and Gibbons, J. L. Para-infectious encephalomyelitis and related syndromes: a critical review of the neurological complications of certain specific fevers. *Quart. J. Med.* 25:427–505, 1956.

Nash, T. E., and Neva, F. A. Recent advances in the diagnosis and treatment of cerebral cysticercosis. *N. Engl. J. Med.* 311:1492–1496, 1984.

O'Duffy, J. D., and Goldstein, N. P. Neurological involvement in seven patients with Behçet's disease. *Am. J. Med.* 61:170–178, 1976.

Shakir, R. A., et al. Clinical categories of neurobrucellosis. A report of 19 cases. *Brain* 110:213–223, 1987.

Sharma, O. P., and Sharma, A. M. Sarcoidosis of the nervous system: a clinical approach. *Arch. Intern. Med.* 151:1317–1321, 1991.

Stern, B., et al. Sarcoidosis and its neurological manifestations. *Arch. Neurol.* 42:909–917, 1985.

Thomas, J. E., and Howard, F. M., Jr. Segmental zoster paresis—a disease profile. *Neurology* 22:459–466, 1972.

Wadia, N., Desai, S., and Blatt, M. Disseminated cysticercosis. New observations including CT scan findings and experience with treatment by praziquantel. *Brain* 111:597–614, 1988.

Weinstein, L. Tetanus. *N. Engl. J. Med.* 289:1293–1298, 1973.

Wittner, M., and Tanowitz, H. B. Neurologic complications of parasitic disease. *Med Clin. North Am.* 8:770–782, 1984.

Infections in the Immunocompromised Host and Neurological Complications of AIDS

Berenger, J., et al. Tuberculous meningitis in patients with the human immunodeficiency virus. *N. Engl. J. Med.* 326:668–672, 1992.

Berger, J. R., et al. Progressive multifocal leukoencephalopathy associated with human immunodeficiency virus infection. A review of the literature with a report of sixteen cases. *Ann. Intern. Med.* 107:78–87, 1987.

Chernik, N. L., Armstrong, D., and Posner, J. B. Central nervous system infections in patients with cancer. *Cancer* 40:268–274, 1977.

Fenelon, G., Bolgert, F., and Dehen, H. Les manifestations neurologiques du syndrome d'immuno-dépression acquise (SIDA). *Rev. Neurol.* 142:97–106, 1986.

Ho, D. D., Pomerantz, R. J., and Kaplan, J. C. Pathogenesis of infection with human immunodeficiency virus. *N. Engl. J. Med.* 317:278–286, 1987.

Ho, D. D., et al. Isolation of HTLV-III from cerebrospinal fluid and neural tissues of patients with neurologic syndromes related to the acquired immunodeficiency syndrome. *N. Engl. J. Med.* 313:1493–1497, 1985.

Johns, D. R., Tierney, M., and Felsenstein, D.

Alteration in the natural history of neurosyphilis by concurrent infection with the human immunodeficiency virus. *N. Engl. J. Med.* 316:1569–1572, 1987.

Koralnik, I. J., et al. A controlled study of early neurologic abnormalities in men with asymptomatic human immunodeficiency virus infection. *N. Engl. J. Med.* 323:863–870, 1990.

Leehey, M., and Gilden, D. Neurologic disorders associated with the HIV and HTLV-1 viruses. In S. H. Appel (editor). *Current Neurology*. Chicago: Mosby–Year Book, 1990.

Miller, R. G., Storey, J. R., and Greco, C. M. Ganciclovir in the treatment of progressive AIDS-related polyradiculopathy. *Neurology* 40:569–574, 1990.

Levy, R. M., Bredesen, D. E., and Rosenblum, M. L. Neurological manifestations of the acquired immuno-deficiency syndrome (AIDS): experience of UCSF and review of the literature. *J. Neurosurg.* 62:475–495, 1985.

Lukes, S. A., et al. Bacterial infections of the CNS in neutropenic patients. *Neurology* 34:269–275, 1984.

Navia, B. A., et al. The AIDS dementia complex: II. Neuropathology. *Ann. Neurol.* 20:289–295, 1986.

Navia, B. A., et al. Cerebral toxoplasmosis complicating the acquired immune deficiency syndrome: clinical and neuropathological findings in 27 patients. *Ann. Neurol.* 19:224–238, 1986.

Powderly, W. G., et al. A controlled trial of fluconazole or amphotericin B to prevent relapse of cryptococcal meningitis in patients with the acquired immune deficiency syndrome. *N. Engl. J. Med.* 326:793–798, 1992.

Price, R. W., and Brew, B. Infection of the central nervous system by human immunodeficiency virus. Role of the immune system in pathogenesis. *Ann. NY Acad. Sci.* 540:162–175, 1988.

Rubin, R. H., and Hooper, D. C. Central nervous system infection in the compromised host. *Med. Clin. North Am.* 69:281–296, 1985.

Snider, W. D., et al. Neurological complications of acquired immune deficiency syndrome: analysis of 50 patients. *Ann. Neurol.* 14:403–418, 1983.

Slow Virus and Related Infections

Becker, L. E. Slow infections of the central nervous system. *Can. J. Neurol. Sci.* 4:81–88, 1977.

Brooks, B. R., and Walker, D. L. Progressive multifocal leukoencephalopathy. *Neurol. Clin.* 2:299–313, 1984.

Brown, P., et al. Creutzfeldt-Jakob disease: clinical analysis of a consecutive series of 230 neuropathologically verified cases. *Ann. Neurol.* 20:597–602, 1986.

Dyken, P. R. Subacute sclerosing panencephalitis. Current status. *Neurol. Clin.* 3:179–196, 1985.

Haywood, A. M. Patterns of persistent viral infections. *N. Engl. J. Med.* 315:939–948, 1986.

Houff, S. A., and Sever, J. L. Slow virus diseases of the central nervous system. *Disease-a-Month* 1985, Pp. 1–70.

Prusiner, S. B. Prions and neurodegenerative disease. *N. Engl. J. Med.* 317:1571–1581, 1987.

Ravilochan, K., and Tyler, K. L. Human transmissible neurodegenerative diseases (Prion diseases). *Semin Neurol.* 12:178–192, 1992.

Robertson, W. C., Jr., Clark, D. B., and Markesbery, W. R. Review of 38 cases of subacute sclerosing panencephalitis: effect of amantadine on the natural course of the disease. *Ann. Neurol.* 8:422–425, 1980.

Townsend, J. J., et al. Progressive rubella panencephalitis. Late onset after congenital rubella. *N. Engl. J. Med.* 292:990–998, 1975.

Multiple Sclerosis

Multiple sclerosis (MS) is a disease in which apparently normal myelin in the central nervous system (CNS) becomes damaged at multiple sites. Initially patients suffer relapses and remissions, although the disease may begin as a chronically progressive disorder or it may become progressive after an initial remitting phase. It can also be clinically silent. Many clues suggest an autoimmune pathogenesis, but the actual cause of MS remains unknown and the immune abnormalities observed in patients with MS may represent only epiphenomena.

EPIDEMIOLOGY

MS is a major cause of disability in young adults. Its prevalence is 60 to 100 per 100,000 in the populations of temperate regions, but has been increasing in recent years due, in part, to longer survival, but more importantly to enhanced recognition. Its incidence may be increasing in some geographic areas but appears to be decreasing in others.

Both acquired and genetic factors likely play a role in the etiology of MS. The low incidence in tropical areas where relatively poor socioeconomic and hygienic conditions prevail suggests an infectious etiology, in that exposure to the putative infectious agent early in life in these areas might confer life-long immunity, as happens with polio. The findings from migration studies conducted in Afro-Asians who went to Israel and British who moved to South Africa support an acquired, possibly infectious etiology, in that migration after the age of 15 from a high to low prevalence region was associated with a high risk of developing MS, which was not seen in people who migrated before age 15. An environmental agent, such as a virus that remains latent in the nervous system, has been hypothesized to explain these data. However, the recent reexamination of these findings has cast some doubt on the validity of this conclusion. The geographic distribution may instead mirror genetic and ethnic differences, and not environmental ones. These studies did not entirely account for possible genetic heterogeneity within the migrant population and among the members of the indigenous population, however. An "epidemic" of multiple sclerosis in the Faroe Islands, located between Norway and Iceland, supports the environmental hypothesis, and suggests that an infectious agent which was introduced to these islands by British troops stationed there in the 1940s may be responsible.

Genetic factors clearly seem to play a role in the acquisition of MS. Approximately 15 percent of patients have a positive family history. The relative risk in first-degree relatives is increased by a factor of 20- to 40-fold compared to the risk for the general population. The concordance rate for the disease is nearly 30 percent among monozygotic twins, as compared to approximately 2 percent in dizygotic twins. Certain histocompatibility antigens are more common in patients with MS. Racial differences in the occurrence of MS are also seen, with low rates in blacks, Orientals, and American Indians living in high-prevalence areas. The disease is relatively frequent in those of Northern European origin. The female-to-male ratio is 1.8 : 1, and the age of onset is 10 to 50 years in the vast majority of patients, with a peak in the third decade.

PATHOPHYSIOLOGY AND ETIOLOGY

Myelin is composed of 70 percent lipid and 30 percent protein. Cholesterol, phospholipid, and glycolipid (including the specific marker galactocerebroside) constitute the lipids. The major structural proteins are myelin basic protein and proteolipid protein. Myelin-associated glycoprotein (part of the immunoglobulin gene superfamily) is also a constituent.

The myelin sheath surrounding larger CNS axons is fashioned from oligodendrocyte membranes that wrap around axons to create as many as ninety concentric layers. In the CNS, one oligodendrocyte forms many segments of myelin on different axons, whereas, in the peripheral nervous system, one Schwann cell relates to one internodal segment on a single axon. The inner and outer plasmalemma membranes of the oligodendrocyte fuse to form the

major dense line, as seen in cross section on electron micrographs. The minor dense line is formed by the opposition of two adjacent outer cellular membrane surfaces. The cytoplasm is squeezed out to the periphery to create a thin rim, which forms paranodal loops that make contact with the axonal membrane. Short bare segments of axonal membrane that are flanked by the paranodal loops from adjacent myelin segments are known as *nodes of Ranvier*. The axonal membrane at these sites contains a particularly high concentration of excitatory sodium channels that enable saltatory conduction to take place. These highly specialized myelin and axonal structural adaptations allow the rapid and efficient node-to-node conduction of nervous impulses along central pathways.

The typical plaque of MS is formed by the breakdown of myelin in discrete regions of the white matter with the relative preservation of axons (Fig. 25-1). In advanced cases, there are acute and chronic plaques of varying size and activity throughout the white matter and to a certain extent in the gray matter as well. The spinal cord, optic nerve, and periventricular white matter including the corpus callosum are particularly prevalent sites. Acute plaques are often periventricular and contain a mixture of T lymphocytes, inflammatory cells, and macrophages. Macrophages in the plaque contain neutral lipid. More chronic plaques are almost acellular and consist mainly of astrocytic gliosis, and some axonal breakdown occurs in the larger ones.

Disruption of the myelin sheath has a variable effect on axonal conduction, depending on the degree of myelin breakdown, the length of the damaged segment, or segments, and the extent of secondary axonal damage. In the earliest phases, conduction is slow in some axons of a particular pathway and the temporal dispersion of impulses within that pathway is increased. When axons still conduct but in a slow or out-of-phase manner, the patient experiences symptoms such as dysesthesias or sensory distortions, incoordination, and weakness. The safety factors that operate to preserve neural conduction may ordinarily compensate for any losses, and only when these factors are diminished under certain circumstances, such as hyperthermia,

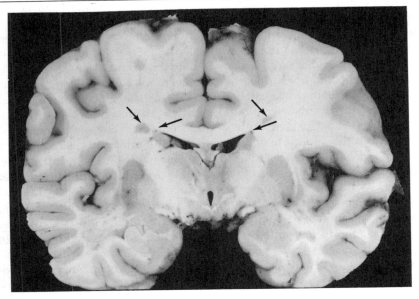

A

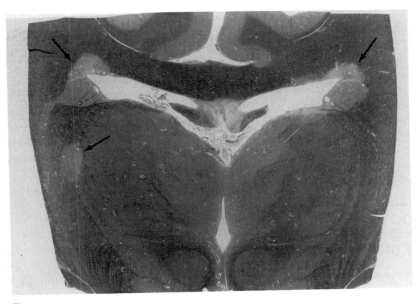

B

Fig. 25-1. *(A) Coronal section of brain showing periventricular plaques involving the corpus callosum* (arrows) *as well as a plaque lying at the junction of the internal capsule and putamen. (B) Hematoxylin-eosin–stained whole brain mount in the same patient showing the pale appearance of multiple sclerosis plaques* (arrows).

do symptoms emerge. These pathogenetic factors have been used to explain some of the transient fluctuations seen in the context of MS, such as Uhthoff's phenomenon, which is a transient worsening of the visual deficit following exercise or an elevation in body temperature in patients who have recovered from optic neuritis.

After severe disruption of the myelin sheath, conduction block occurs. If enough fibers in a particular pathway are affected, then the function of that pathway is completely disrupted. Ephaptic conduction (cross-talk) may also occur in adjacent demyelinated fibers, thereby causing short-circuiting. This may account for some of the "positive" or irritative symptoms seen in patients with MS, such as Lhermitte's sign (see the section on the clinical features), trigeminal neuralgia, or painful tonic spasms.

Whether it takes one or more plaques within a particular pathway to produce a neurological deficit depends on the number of axons affected and the functional organization of the pathway. Even a single small plaque in the optic nerve could give rise to symptoms due to the density of information conveyed by its axons ("eloquence").

Once demyelination has occurred, recovery may take place through the operation of poorly understood mechanisms, including resolution of the acute inflammation and edema in the short term and partial remyelination or reorganization of the axonal membrane in the long term. The process of remyelination, which is likely accomplished through the formation of oligodendrocytes from undifferentiated cells, produces thin myelin with short internodal segments. In addition, intact pathways may assume the functions of affected pathways or the nervous system may adapt to deficits through other compensatory mechanisms.

IMMUNOLOGY

Structure of the Immune System

To appreciate the putative role of the immune system in MS, it is important to have a basic understanding of the structure of the immune system and its regulation in general and in the brain in particular. The immune system is composed of cellular elements, primarily lymphocytes, that detect foreign antigens (i.e., recognizable amino acid sequences). Each activated lymphocyte multiplies or expands clonally and either attacks the antigen directly or helps other cells to do so, or to produce antibodies that attack the antigen.

The immune system can be understood in terms of its afferent recognition functions, its efferent effector functions, and the control elements that restrict antigen recognition and regulate the strength of the immune response. The recognition elements are T lymphocytes, which bear CD4 and CD8 proteins. These cells "see" antigens by means of a specific receptor (T-cell receptor) residing on antigen-presenting cells, which are primarily macrophages. Nervous system elements can act as antigen-presenting cells in MS and other neurological diseases. T-lymphocytes can only "see" antigens when they are "presented by" (attached to) major histocompatibility (MHC) proteins, of classes I and II, on the surface of antigen-presenting cells.

MHC proteins, which were initially recognized in experiments that made use of alloantisera obtained from multiparous women who had been repeatedly immunized to fetal (nonself) antigens, play an important role in immune system recognition. These proteins enhance antibody production and delayed-type hypersensitivity in such processes as graft rejection. They are encoded on chromosome 6 in humans and are also known as *HLA antigens*. T-helper cells (T cells bearing the CD4 marker) recognize antigen when attached to MHC class II proteins on antigen-presenting cells, and T-cytotoxic cells (T cells bearing the CD8 marker), which are important effectors of immune-mediated damage, recognize the antigen of their target when attached to MHC class I proteins on the surface of the target.

In addition to antigen-specific restriction, the strength of the immune response may be determined by several mechanisms, among which are the relative balance of T-helper and T-suppressor cell activity, and lymphokines, which are chemicals produced by lymphocytes that either up-regulate or down-regulate the strength of the immune response.

The Brain and the Immune System

The brain has traditionally been thought of as an immune-privileged organ, given the paucity of lymphocytes in the CNS, the tight junctions in cerebral endothelial cells which bar lymphocytes from the CNS, and the lack of class I and

II proteins, which are recognition elements for the immune systems, on the surface of neuroglial cells. The only MHC antigens normally expressed in the CNS are class I antigens located on the surface of cerebral endothelial cells.

It is now known that T cells activated by brain antigens can traverse the blood-brain barrier to reach their targets. In disease processes such as MS, brain cells can express class I and II proteins on endothelial cells and astrocytes, both locally at the site of inflammation and beyond these sites into histologically normal brain tissue. Recently, oligodendrocytes have been induced to express class I antigens as well.

Multiple Sclerosis and the Immune System

When considering the putative role of the immune system in disease, it is important to distinguish between truly important abnormalities and secondary epiphenomena. This is an especially important consideration in MS, given the plethora of reported immune abnormalities involved. As in any immune process, immune function in MS should be considered in terms of:

1. Susceptibility: why does MS occur more frequently in some ethnic groups and families than in others?
2. The trigger: is there a foreign antigen that may deceive the immune system into believing it is a myelin antigen, or could an endogenous antigen have been altered by a remote infection?
3. Maintenance of disease: why is the inflammatory process restricted in anatomical extent and frequency of occurrence in some patients but is fulminant and occasionally fatal in others?

As previously noted, antigen-specific recognition and effector functions are restricted by class II and I MHC molecules, respectively. These molecules are highly polymorphic, in that their structure varies from individual to individual. Each variation in a coding region of DNA in an individual results in a different allele. The frequency of different allelic polymorphisms varies according to ethnic group. If some of these genetically determined alleles promote greater susceptibility to MS than do others, then this serves as a plausible explanation for the familial and ethnic clustering typical of MS. Several class I and II MHC alleles, most notably the class II alleles DR2 and Dqw1, are relatively more common in MS patients than in control subjects. Furthermore, preliminary evidence suggests some association between certain germline polymorphisms of the T-cell receptor and the occurrence of MS in particular families. The results of other studies suggest that there are differences in the usage of different building-block components of the T-cell receptor (the T-cell receptor repertoire) in the lymphocytes in plaques of MS patients, and in myelin basic protein–reactive lymphocyte clones, compared to other lymphocytes of the same patients. It is still highly speculative whether these differences mediate or are important to MS susceptibility. If this were true, then it might be possible to devise immune-mediated specific therapy consisting of monoclonal antibodies directed against the offending clones, identified by their specific T-cell receptor.

Generally, identification of a putative antigen is a prerequisite to understanding the triggering process responsible for immune-mediated disease. The number of immune cells that respond to a given antigen represents only a very small proportion of the total population of immunocompetent cells, however, and studying the immune reactivity to irrelevant antigens or mitogens bears questionable relevance to the definition of the disease process. Myelin basic protein has been suspected to be an important antigen, as it is able to induce an MS-like disease in animals, experimental allergic encephalomyelitis. However, most studies, with the possible exception of one, have not documented a myelin basic protein reactivity in appropriate control lymphocytes that significantly differs from that seen in the lymphocytes of MS patients. Hepatitis virus can induce myelin basic protein reactivity in the lymphocytes and experimental allergic encephalomyelitis–like lesions in the brains of mice. There is some antigenic cross-reactivity between the virus and myelin basic protein that share a common 6–amino acid residue. It may be that a foreign antigen can fool the immune system into reacting to CNS antigen, a process called *molecular mimicry*. However, to date, despite numerous reported isolations of virus and numerous positive serological studies, no virus has stood the test of time as a causal or triggering agent for MS. It is not even known whether the immune response is triggered primarily in the peripheral immune system; if this were so, the disease might respond to therapy such as total lymphoid irradiation, which has no direct effect on the brain. Total lymphoid irradiation has recently sparked interest as a therapy in patients with progressive MS.

Once the immune system is activated, the disease must be maintained. There are immunological mechanisms that may amplify and sustain the disease and others that may inhibit the immunological response, and in fact promote remyelination and recovery. CD8-positive T lymphocytes and functional suppressor-cell activity have been reported to diminish at the onset of an acute attack, and a persistent decrease in the number of CD4- and 2H4-positive suppressor/inducer subtype T-helper cells has been observed in patients with progressive MS.

Interferon-gamma, a lymphokine released by activated lymphocytes, stimulates the production of inflammatory mediators by mast cells; this event increases vascular permeability. It also induces class II antigens to appear on macrophages and on glial cells in the brain. This may promote antigen presentation in the brain and secondarily amplify the immune response. Other lymphokines such as tumor necrosis factor (TNF), which is produced by macrophages, are myelinotoxic. The levels of TNF have been reported to correlate with the prognosis in MS patients. Other lymphokines, such as interferon alpha and beta as well as transforming growth factor–beta (TGF-beta), down-regulate the immune response.

Lymphocytes congregate in a periventricular distribution in the brain. In active plaques, macrophages predominate in the center of plaques, along with immunoglobulin. CD8-positive cells are located on the periphery of plaques and CD4-positive cells are distributed beyond the margins of plaques and infiltrate into normal white matter. Class II antigen is expressed on the endothelium, and class I and II antigens are expressed on astrocytes. Recently, class I expression was recognized on the surface of oligodendrocytes. Interferon gamma is demonstrable in brain as well as the putative immunosuppressive lymphokines, interferon alpha and beta, which may dampen the immune response locally. In the peripheral blood, there are "activated" T cells bearing surface markers, which indicates that they have been activated by antigen and have expanded by clonal means. These markers include the receptor for IL2, which is a clonal proliferation-stimulating lymphokine. These lymphocytes migrate quickly and preferentially into the brain. The functional suppressor-cell activity is depressed and B cells produce excessive amounts of immunoglobulin in vitro in response to mitogen.

Immunological tests that are relevant to the diagnosis of MS include measurement of the IgG index and the intrathecal IgG production, both of which correct for leakiness of the blood-brain barrier, and CSF electrophoresis to detect the existence of oligoclonal bands; this test is discussed later in this chapter. Other tests are of no current clinical utility.

In the future, specific immunotherapy may be targeted at many different levels. There have been two trials that assessed the effectiveness of pan T-cell–specific monoclonal antibodies in the treatment of MS. Monoclonal antibodies directed against T-helper cell markers and class II antigens have aborted cases of experimental allergic encephalomyelitis induced in animals. Similar antibodies have not yet been tested in MS patients. T-cell receptor–specific monoclonal antibodies to myelin basic protein–reactive cells have blocked the development of experimental allergic encephalomyelitis in rodents. It remains to be seen if the immune response in humans is sufficiently restricted to a limited number of clones, such that a culprit clonotype can be identified based on a specific T-cell receptor. If so, the technology exists to tailor-make a specific antibody that can block the function of the offending clone.

CLINICAL PICTURE

The symptoms and signs of MS are largely in keeping with the particular involvement of the CNS white matter (Table 25-1). Subcortical (especially periventricular) white matter, corticospinal tracts, and posterior columns within the spinal cord, the optic nerve, and cerebellar pathways are favored sites. The early symptoms of MS, consisting of fleeting paresthesias, emotional lability, minor visual disturbances, and fatigability, are often nonspecific and are frequently mistaken for functional (psychiatric) disorders. The most common presenting symptom is weakness or sensory loss in the extremities. The symptoms and signs are those typical of a spinal cord or brain syndrome (hemiparesthesias, paraparesis) and not a root or nerve lesion. Quite often, one limb is disproportionately affected. In such cases, subtle findings in a second limb can confirm the presence of a CNS lesion.

Diplopia or subacute visual loss in one eye due to optic neuritis is also common.

Less common presenting symptoms are vertigo, deafness, a conus medullaris syndrome, and trigeminal neuralgia. In advanced stages of the disease, patients commonly manifest several of the following symptoms or signs: bilateral spastic paraplegia, neurogenic bladder, visual impairment, moderate dysarthria, intention tremor, ataxia, nystagmus, and a pseudobulbar syndrome with marked emotional lability. Neuropsychological deficits, including impaired short-term memory and concentration, are common. Depression is also a very common component and its presence often confounds interpretation of neuropsychological findings. Less commonly, patients exhibit indifference and euphoria, which herald dementia. Incapacitating dementia probably afflicts less than 5 percent of patients.

Epileptic seizures occur in 5 percent of cases and are probably due to superficial cortical plaques impinging on gray matter. Signs of pe-

Table 25-1. Common Clinical Features of Multiple Sclerosis and Their Anatomical Correlations

Signs	Symptoms	Plaque location
Central visual loss (occasional papillitis of optic disc), often temporal disc pallor	Subacute monocular visual loss, often with pain	Optic nerve
Weakness of adduction in one eye and nystagmus of the opposite abducting eye with gaze to one side (i.e., internuclear ophthalmoplegia)	Horizontal diplopia	Medial longitudinal fasciculus on side of adduction deficit
Diminished vibration and proprioception in one arm	Tingling paresthesias and clumsiness of the hand, "useless hand"	Ipsilateral fasciculus cuneatus of upper cervical spine
Loss of pain, temperature, vibration, and touch sensation below the waist; spastic paraparesis	Numbness and tingling below the waist, hyperalgesic band at level of lesion, urinary retention, weakness in the legs	Extensive demyelination in lower thoracic spinal cord (transverse cord lesion)
Sensory loss in trigeminal nerve distribution	Lancinating brief pains in face (trigeminal neuralgia)	Root entry zone of trigeminal nerve in pons
Spasticity, hyperreflexia, Babinski's sign in lower extremity	Weakness, heaviness in leg	Ipsilateral corticospinal tract in cord
Intention tremor, nystagmus, dysarthria	Dysarthria, ataxia	Cerebellar white matter and dentatorubral pathway
Lhermitte's sign	Shocklike paresthesias down the spine with neck flexion	Posterior columns of cervical spinal cord

ripheral nervous system involvement such as atrophy and loss of deep tendon reflexes are due to spinal cord plaques overlapping root entry zones or anterior horn cells.

Certain signs and symptoms, when encountered in a young person, are highly suggestive of MS. These include trigeminal neuralgia, bilateral internuclear ophthalmoplegia, worsening of neurological deficits with elevated body temperature, the "useless hand" syndrome (loss of proprioception in the hand leading to incoordination), Lhermitte's sign (shocklike sensations that shoot down the back and extremities provoked by neck flexion), and McArdle's sign (worsening weakness in the extremities with neck flexion). The latter two signs are not specific to MS and may be seen in the context of other cervical spine lesions such as cervical spondylosis or tumors.

Brief paroxysmal painful attacks of dystonic flexion that affect half the body or the lower extremities can be precipitated by hyperventilation and occur several times per day. These attacks are called painful tonic spasms. Rarely, they may occur at the onset of MS. Patients have mistakenly been labeled as having pseudoseizures when these spells have been induced by hyperventilation during EEG recordings, but with no EEG correlate. They often respond well to low doses of carbamazepine or phenytoin.

Neuromyelitis optica (Devic's disease) is thought to be a variant of MS. Affected patients present with both transverse myelitis and optic neuritis (unilateral or bilateral) that both arise within days or weeks of each other.

The neurological signs in a patient with MS are often more extensive than would be expected on the basis of symptoms because these may be residual from previous subclinical attacks for which the patient may not have corresponding symptoms. Evidence of a previous optic neuritis may be apparent from temporal optic disc pallor or an afferent pupillary defect (Marcus Gunn pupil). Subtle signs of an internuclear ophthalmoplegia (an incompleteness of eye adduction on the affected side and abducting nystagmus of the other eye on rapid saccadic refixation) may be elicited. An attempt should be made to elicit Lhermitte's sign through neck flexion. Facial myokymia consists

of a fine rippling movement of the facial muscles that the patient may perceive as a tightness and pulling of the face to the affected side. It can also be seen in patients with pontine glioma or undergoing regeneration following facial nerve damage. Hyperactive deep tendon jerks (including the jaw jerk), Babinski's signs, spastic quadriparesis, cerebellar signs, and sensory deficits are common in advanced cases.

The course of MS is highly variable and unpredictable in the early phases. Most early attacks resolve almost completely within 6 weeks, with or without treatment. A minority of patients pursue a chronic downhill course, with gradually worsening deficits or very closely spaced attacks starting from the time of onset. For unknown reasons, some patients may suffer numerous attacks over several years, yet recover completely from each without any or with very few residual deficits. However, most patients with recurrent attacks eventually tend to recover less and less completely, and are left with disabilities that accumulate gradually or in a stepwise fashion.

Although the course in any given patient is unpredictable in the early stages, there are certain clinical features indicative of a benign course, including early age at onset, female sex, and onset with sensory symptoms. In general, if the disability is only minimal or moderate after 5 years, the subsequent course is likely to be benign. Unfortunately, it is not uncommon to encounter patients whose clinical course violates this general rule.

In those patients who do become bedridden, the average time to reach this extreme disability is 20 to 25 years. Overall survival is about 50 percent by 30 years from the onset of MS. The mortality has decreased for severely affected patients in recent years because of better management of neurogenic bladder and the treatment of infections in general. However, studies from the Mayo Clinic have shown that the overall survival, though admittedly favorable, has not changed appreciably over the last century.

The prognosis in patients with an isolated acute optic neuritis but no apparent cause has been widely studied, with very different results. Approximately 60 to 70 percent of such patients eventually exhibit other signs of MS, some as long as 25 years after their visual loss. The findings from earlier studies suggested the contrary. However, MRI scans obtained at the time of presentation show cerebral lesions in up to 60 percent of these patients. It could be argued that some of these cases represent monophasic bouts of demyelination with a pathogenesis similar to that of MS, but possess modifying genes that limit the disease process. MRI has shown the existence of disseminated cerebral lesions consistent with MS in a majority of patients whose only neurological feature is an unexplained chronic myelopathy.

DIAGNOSIS

Multiple lesions of the white matter of the CNS occurring in discrete attacks separated by an interval of several weeks or months is the hallmark of MS (Table 25-2). MS is always a leading consideration when a neurological deficit appears subacutely in a young adult. Diagnosis poses a greater challenge in patients who are unusually young or old or who exhibit less common syndromes, particularly when that syndrome has a broad differential diagnosis, such as slowly pro-

Fig. 25-2. *(A) Visual evoked responses to a reversing checkerboard pattern in a normal subject and a patient with multiple sclerosis (MS). Each response is the summation of 200 responses that are time-locked to the visual stimulus. Two sets of responses are obtained for each eye. The latency of the main positive wave (P100) is normal (upper limit, 114 msec). Visual evoked responses in an MS patient (right) with only mild reduction in visual acuity in the left eye. Note the prolonged latency and reduced amplitudes of P100 in each eye, indicating demyelination in the visual pathways. (O_z = midline occipital electrode; F_z = midline frontal electrode; VA = visual acuity.)*

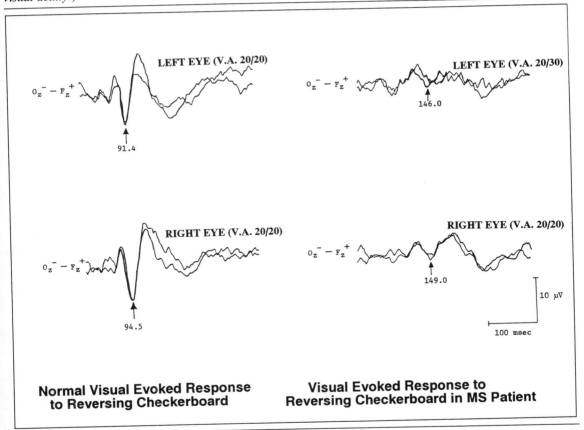

Normal Visual Evoked Response to Reversing Checkerboard

Visual Evoked Response to Reversing Checkerboard in MS Patient

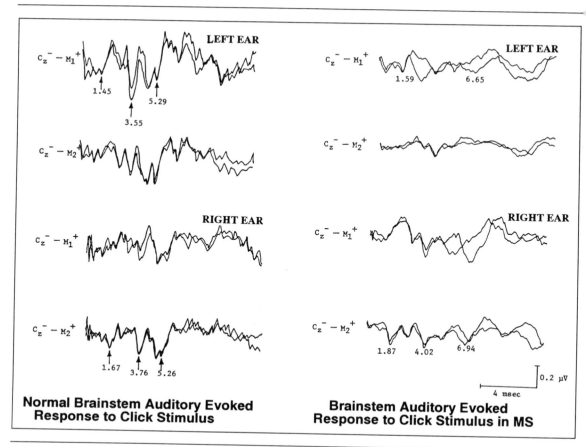

Fig. 25-2 *(Continued). (B) Brainstem auditory evoked responses to 2,000 repetitive click stimuli in each ear in a normal subject and MS patient. Note the short latencies of the main brainstem positive responses (I, III, V) compared to the visual evoked potentials. There are both increased latency and decreased amplitude in the MS patient, suggesting a demyelinating lesion in the brainstem auditory pathways. (C_z = vertex electrode; M_1 = left mastoid electrode; M_2 = right mastoid electrode.)*

gressive spastic paraparesis. In a young person, one might suspect adrenomyeloneuropathy and, in an older person, vitamin B_{12} deficiency or cervical spondylosis. MS remains primarily a clinical diagnosis with laboratory findings used as supportive evidence. There are no tests to provide absolute proof of the diagnosis, but when the clinical picture, CSF, and MRI findings are compatible, the diagnosis becomes highly probable. Diagnosis is also predicated on a negative search for alternative causes.

In the differential diagnosis, special consideration has to be given to other conditions, some treatable, that can produce remitting and relapsing CNS lesions in younger patients. The

differential diagnosis can be grouped into a number of categories according to their mode of presentation. Relapsing and remitting multifocal CNS disease can occur in the presence of vasculitides, Sjögren's syndrome, systemic lupus erythematosus, sarcoidosis, and Lyme disease. A progressive systems degeneration can be seen in olivopontocerebellar and other hereditary and sporadic cerebellar degenerations, hereditary spastic paraplegia, hereditary optic atrophies (e.g., Leber's), and subacute combined degeneration. Progressive or relapsing unifocal brainstem or spinal cord processes that can mimic MS include brainstem cavernous angioma, cervical spondylosis, and

Table 25-2. Diagnosis of Multiple Sclerosis

Clinical findings
　Two or more attacks of a neurological deficit
　　conforming to the existence of white matter
　　lesions (e.g., optic nerve or corticospinal tracts)
　　at different locations and presumably occurring
　　at different times
or
　Chronically progressive neurological white matter
　　deficits persisting for at least 6 months
and
　Without identifiable etiology
Additional clinical support
　Exacerbations and remissions of neurological
　　deficits
　Lhermitte's sign, painful tonic spasms, bilateral
　　internuclear ophthalmoplegia
　Young adult patient
　Northern European Caucasian descent
　Positive family history
Laboratory support
　Discrete white matter lesions seen on MRI or CT
　　neuroimaging of the brain or spinal cord
　Oligoclonal IgG bands in the CSF
　Elevated IgG turnover in the CSF
　Visual, somatosensory, or brainstem auditory
　　evoked potential abnormalities revealing the
　　presence of silent lesions

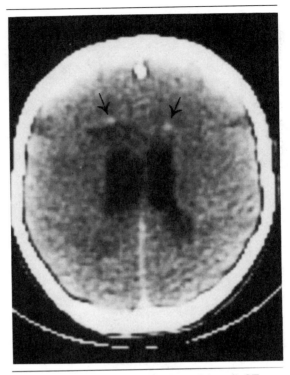

Fig. 25-3. *Enhanced (double-dose, delayed) CT scan in a patient with long-established multiple sclerosis. Note the enhancing plaques anterior to the frontal horns (arrows) as well as low-density lesions adjacent to the posterior portion of the ventricles.*

an Arnold-Chiari malformation. Hysteria and malingering are occasional considerations when suspicions are raised about the organic nature of symptoms and signs.

The cell count in the CSF of patients with MS is usually normal, but the CSF may contain up to 50 white cells/mm³, all mononuclear. A normal or mildly elevated CSF protein and an elevated gamma globulin (IgG) level occur in two thirds of the cases. Oligoclonal bands of IgG on agarose electrophoresis, which indicate clonal expansion of individual antibody-producing clones in the CSF, can be demonstrated in 90 percent of definite cases. However, oligoclonal bands are a sensitive but not entirely specific indicator of MS, as they may also be seen in other inflammatory CNS conditions such as sarcoidosis, lupus, Lyme disease, neurosyphilis, and AIDS.

Visual, brainstem auditory, and somatosensory evoked potentials may be useful for demonstrating subclinical involvement of sensory pathways in patients with suspected MS who present with a single central lesion (Fig. 25-2).

MS lesions occasionally appear on CT scans as small discrete enhancing or low-density lesions in the subcortical or periventricular white matter (Fig. 25-3). Occasionally larger plaques exhibit ring enhancement and can be mistaken for tumors (Fig. 25-4). In advanced disease, generalized cerebral atrophy is common. The MRI scan is a much more sensitive tool for detecting MS lesions, which appear as white matter low-intensity areas on T_2-weighted images (Fig. 25-5). Involvement of the corpus callosum is often seen on MRI scans and this is a typical location for plaques. Enhancement with gadolinium and other agents, which is seen in the presence of acutely forming or active plaques, increases the ability to demonstrate acute blood-brain barrier disruption, especially in the spinal cord. MRI often demonstrates asymptomatic plaques in the

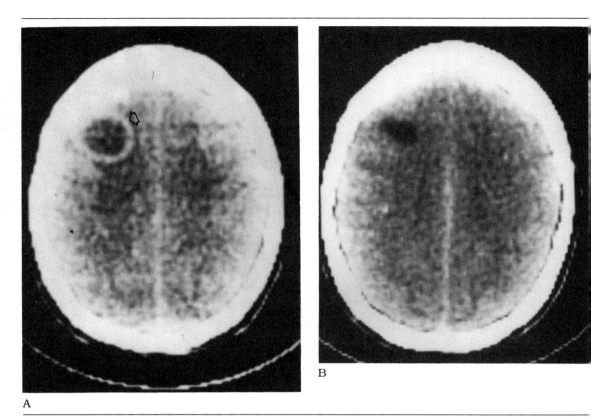

A

B

Fig. 25-4. *(A) Enhanced CT scan showing a ring-enhancing plaque in the left frontal area* (arrow) *in a 25-year-old woman with newly diagnosed multiple sclerosis. She presented with a transverse myelitis and the plaque shown was asymptomatic. (B) Follow-up unenhanced CT scan showing regression in the plaque's size 3 months later. Contrast was not used because she had experienced an allergic reaction to the dye with the initial scan.*

brains of MS patients presenting with evidence of spinal cord lesions and is the preferred test when laboratory documentation is desirable because of an uncertain diagnosis. Disseminated lesions on MRI scans, similar to those seen in MS, may be encountered in patients with vasculitides such as lupus or Sjögren's syndrome.

MANAGEMENT

A frequent problem for the neurologist is what to tell the patient in the early phases of the disorder, when diagnosis is only possible or probable and the patient has few disabilities. Just the mention of MS may have adverse psychological consequences. Therefore, one must be honest, but must show due regard for the potential psychological impact of the diagnosis. Occasionally it is preferable to describe the illness in more euphemistic terms, such as referring to it as an "inflammation of the insulation around the nerves possibly due to a virus." If patients pointedly ask about the possibility of MS, they should be told that the diagnosis is a possibility (or probability) and the variability of the course from one patient to another fully explained.

No specific treatment has been proved to alter the course of MS. Most therapeutic trials have concentrated on attempting to alter the presumed immune derangement underlying the disease. Both immune suppression, by such means as corticosteroids, ACTH, azathioprine, cyclophosphamide, cyclosporine, and total

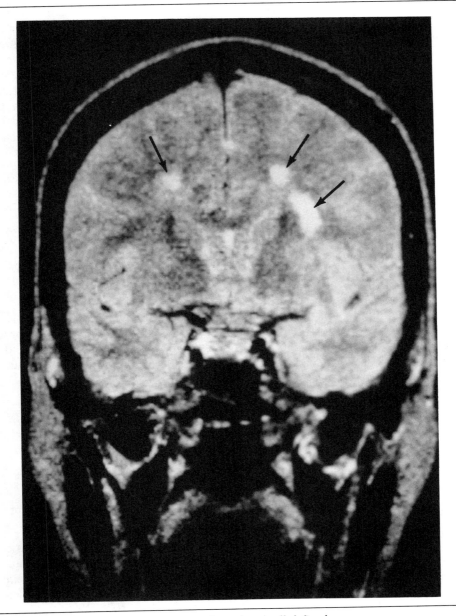

Fig. 25-5. *A T_2-weighted MRI image showing at least three well-defined periventricular plaques in a patient with multiple sclerosis.*

lymphoid irradiation, and immune enhancement, through the administration of transfer factor, have been attempted, but the results of these modalities have been either negative or equivocal. ACTH or high doses of methylprednisolone are often given intravenously for several days at the time of an acute exacerbation. However, these agents may abbreviate the attack but not necessarily influence the degree of recovery. This is currently the only widely accepted remittent treatment for MS.

Interferon-beta, administered intrathecally, has recently been shown to reduce the attack rate in relapsing cases of MS, but further experience is necessary before it can be recommended. Treatment with azathioprine has been widely studied, particularly because this agent is easily administered over long periods. Only modest benefits have accrued in patients participating in short-term studies conducted for 2 to 3 years, but some long-term studies seem to indicate benefit. The long-term risk of malignancy is a major concern. Cyclophosphamide has been employed with some success in patients with chronically progressive cases who show moderate disability and are still ambulatory. However, it is often associated with severe toxicity, including hemorrhagic cystitis. Its effectiveness is controversial and benefits are short-lived at best. Plasmapheresis has been studied as a possible treatment but is not yet accepted as effective.

Patients should pay careful attention to their life-style, especially regarding good nutrition, regular exercise, and control of stress levels. The advisability of women with MS bearing children is controversial. First, the mother's overall level of functioning and capacity to care for the baby must be considered. The effect of pregnancy on the course of the MS is probably minimal, although there is a tendency for exacerbations to occur in the postpartum period. Young mothers should try to minimize postpartum fatigue as much as possible.

The mainstay of management in MS is symptomatic and supportive. Spasticity and flexor spasms, one of the most troublesome symptoms in patients with more advanced MS, can be managed with agents such as baclofen, dantrolene sodium, and tizanidine, or, in extreme cases, with surgical or chemical radiculotomy. Recently intrathecal baclofen has shown promise in patients with severe spasticity. However, treatment of the spasticity often exacerbates the weakness and therefore should only be undertaken for the purposes of comfort, and to facilitate transfer of the patient and easier nursing care. Physiotherapy and occupational therapy play a major role in keeping the patient mobile and independent, as well as in preventing contractures in advanced cases. Bladder management is extremely important and has been discussed in a previous chapter. Many patients suffer temporary worsening of their symptoms when there is a bladder infection, which abates once the infection is treated. Psychological support and counseling in vocational matters and sexual functioning are extremely important. Despite an overwhelming disability, some patients are able to maintain a certain measure of independence and employment through the added help of technologically advanced aids such as battery-powered wheelchairs and voice-activated microcomputer-controlled devices.

BIBLIOGRAPHY

Antel, J. P. (editor). Multiple sclerosis. *Neurol Clin.* 1:571–785, 1983.

British and Dutch Multiple Sclerosis Azathioprine Trial Group. Double-masked trial of azathioprine in multiple sclerosis. *Lancet* 2:179–183, 1988.

Carter, J. L., et al. Immunosuppression with high dose IV cyclophosphamide and ACTH in progressive multiple sclerosis: cumulative 6 year experience in 164 patients. *Neurology* 38(suppl. 2):9–24, 1988.

Carter, J. L., and Rodriguez, M. Immunosuppressive treatment of multiple sclerosis. *Mayo Clin. Proc.* 64:664–669, 1989.

Compston, A. Methylprednisolone and multiple sclerosis. *Arch. Neurol.* 45:669–670, 1988.

Ebers, G. Optic neuritis and multiple sclerosis. *Arch. Neurol.* 42:702–704, 1985.

Ellinson, G. W., et al. A placebo-controlled randomized, double-masked, variable dosage clinical trial of azathioprine with and without methylprednisolone in multiple sclerosis. *Neurology* 39:1018–1026, 1989.

Farrell, M. A., et al. Oligoclonal bands in multiple sclerosis: clinical pathologic correlation. *Neurology* 35:212–218, 1985.

Franklin, G. M., et al. Cognitive loss in multiple sclerosis. Case reports and review of the literature. *Arch. Neurol.* 46:162–167, 1989.

Goodin, D. S. The use of immunosuppressive agents in the treatment of multiple sclerosis: critical review. *Neurology* 4:980–985, 1991.

Hart, R. G., and Sherman, D. G. The diagnosis of multiple sclerosis. *JAMA* 247:498–503, 1982.

Hashimoto, S. A., and Paty, D. W. Multiple sclerosis. *Disease-a-Month* 32:518–589, 1986.

Hauser, S. L., et al. Intensive immunosuppresion in progressive multiple sclerosis. A randomized three-arm study of high-dose intravenous cyclophosphamide, plasma exchange and ACTH. *N. Engl. J. Med.* 308:173–180, 1983.

Isaac, C., et al. Multiple sclerosis: a serial study using MRI in relapsing patients. *Neurology* 38:1511–1515, 1988.

Koopmans, R. A., et al. The lesion of multiple sclerosis: imaging of acute and chronic stages. *Neurology* 39:959–963, 1989.

Kurtzke, J. F. Optic neuritis or multiple sclerosis. *Arch. Neurol.* 42:704–710, 1985.

Matthews, W. B., et al. (editors). *McAlpine's Multiple Sclerosis.* Edinburgh: Churchill Livingstone, 1985.

McDonald, W. I. Multiple sclerosis: the present situation. *Acta Neurol. Scand.* 68:65–76, 1983.

McFarland, H. F. Immunology of multiple sclerosis. *Ann. NY Acad. Sci.* 540:99–105, 1988.

McFarlin, D. E., and McFarland, H. F. Multiple sclerosis. *N. Engl. J. Med.* 307:1183–1188;1246–1251, 1982.

Paty, D. W. Multiple Sclerosis with an Emphasis on MR Imaging. In S. H. Appel (editor). *Current Neurology.* St. Louis: Mosby–Year Book, 1991, Pp. Vol. 11, Pp. 169–198.

Paty, D. W., et al. MRI in the diagnosis of MS: a prospective study with comparison of clinical evaluation, evoked potentials, oligoclonal banding and CT. *Neurology* 38:180–185, 1988.

Petersen, R. C., and Kokmen, E. Cognitive and psychiatric abnormalities in multiple sclerosis. *Mayo Clin. Proc.* 64:657–663, 1989.

Rao, S. M., et al. Cognitive dysfunction in multiple sclerosis. I. Frequency, patterns and prediction. *Neurology* 41:685–691, 1991.

Rao, S. M., et al. Cognitive dysfunction in multiple sclerosis. II. Impact on employment and social functioning. *Neurology* 41:692–696, 1991.

Rodriguez, M. Multiple sclerosis: basic concepts and hypothesis. *Mayo Clin. Proc.* 64:570–576, 1989.

Rudick, R. A., and Herndon, R. M. (editors). Disorders of myelin. *Semin. Neurol.* 5:85–193, 1985.

Sadovnick, A. D., Baird, P. A., and Ward, R. H. Multiple sclerosis: updated risks for relatives. *Am. J. Med. Genet.* 29:533–541, 1988.

Sadovnick, A. D., Paty, D. W., and Ebers, G. C. Life expectancy and cause of death in multiple sclerosis. *Neurology* 39(suppl. 1):285, 1989.

Swanson, J. W. Multiple sclerosis: update in diagnosis and review of prognostic factors. *Mayo Clin. Proc.* 64:577–586, 1989.

Thompson, A. J., et al. Relative efficacy of intravenous methylprednisolone and ACTH in the treatment of acute relapse in MS. *Neurology* 39:969–971, 1989.

Tourtelotte, W. W., and Pick, P. W. Current concepts about multiple sclerosis (editorial). *Mayo Clin. Proc.* 64:592–596, 1989.

Troiano, R., Cook, S. D., and Dowling, P. C. Steroid therapy in multiple sclerosis. *Arch. Neurol.* 44:803–807, 1987.

Waksman, B. Autoimmunity in demyelinating disease. *Ann. NY Acad. Sci.* 540:13–24, 1988.

Warren, S. The role of stress in multiple sclerosis. In S. M. Rao (editor). *Neurobehavioral Aspects of Multiple Sclerosis.* New York: Oxford University Press, 1990, Pp. 196–209.

Waxman, S. G. Membranes, myelin and the pathophysiology of multiple sclerosis. *N. Engl. J. Med.* 306:1529–1532, 1982.

Weiner, H. L., and Hafler, D. A. Immunotherapy of multiple sclerosis. *Ann. Neurol.* 23:211–222, 1988.

Weinshenker, B. G., and Bass, B. Multiple

sclerosis: the approach to diagnosis. *Diagnosis* August 1987, Pp. 101–117.

Weinshenker, B. G., and Ebers, G. C. The natural history of multiple sclerosis. *Can. J. Neurol. Sci.* 14:255–261, 1987.

Weinshenker, B. G., et al. The natural history of multiple sclerosis: a geographically based study. I. Clinical course and disability. *Brain* 112:133–146, 1989.

Weinshenker, B. G., et al. The natural history of multiple sclerosis: a geographically based study. II. Predictive value of the early clinical course. *Brain* 112:1419–1428, 1989.

Weinshenker, B. G., et al. The natural history of multiple sclerosis: a geographically based study. III. Multivariate analysis of predictive factors and models of outcome. *Brain* (in press).

Molecular Genetic Aspects of Neurological Disease

The past two decades have witnessed dramatic progress in our ability to manipulate the genetic material, DNA. For the first time, specific DNA fragments can be purified in large numbers. Once purified, the precise chemical structure of such fragments can be elucidated; moreover, they can then be placed in one of a variety of host organisms and rendered biologically active. The impact of this molecular genetic revolution on all aspects of clinical medicine has been significant and will be profound. This chapter outlines the central concepts underlying molecular genetics, provides an update on the current status of molecular neurogenetics, and delineates some areas where progress is expected in the near future.

MOLECULAR GENETICS—A BRIEF BACKGROUND

The Physical Structure of DNA

DNA is a linear molecule made up of structural and informational components. The structural backbone of DNA is composed of organic phosphate groups that alternate with deoxyribose carbohydrate residues. The informational component of DNA consists of a nucleic acid residue, either guanine, cytosine, adenine, or thymidine, that is bonded to each of the deoxyribose residues. The specific sequence of nucleic acid residues in DNA determines the amino acid sequence of a given protein. Each nucleotide triplet codes one of the twenty amino acids found in human proteins.

The linear molecule formed by a single strand of the deoxyribose phosphate backbone together with the associated nucleic acids is called *single-stranded DNA* (ssDNA). In humans, and in most other organisms, the native form of DNA is a double-stranded helix with two ssDNA molecules oriented in opposite directions and linked together by hydrogen bonds between nucleic acids on opposing strands. There exists a specific complementarity between nucleotides in double-stranded DNA (dsDNA), in that a guanine residue bonds only to a cytosine residue in the opposing strand and an adenine residue bonds only to a thymidine residue in the opposing strand. dsDNA molecules in solution can be separated (or denatured) into single strands by altering the pH, temperature, or ionic strength of the solution, or a combination of these factors. Return of the buffer solution to its original conditions (renaturing conditions) leads to the reannealing of the complementary ssDNA fragments. The annealing of one ssDNA molecule to another to form dsDNA takes place with complete specificity and only between complementary ssDNA molecules. The specificity of ssDNA reannealing (or hybridization) to form dsDNA is analogous to the antigen–antibody interaction and forms the basis of many important modern molecular genetic techniques.

Human Genome Organization

The term *genome* refers to the entire genetic complement for a given species. The human genome is comprised of 3×10^9 nucleotide base pairs and is divided up into functional units known as *genes,* each of which encodes a different protein. The genome is contained in 23 pairs of long linear DNA molecules known as *chromosomes*. The estimated 100,000 genes in the human genome actually reside on only 5 percent of the total DNA. The function of the remaining 95 percent is the subject of ongoing debate. A gene is transcribed into messenger RNA (mRNA), which contains exons that specify the sequence of amino acids in the protein, and other intervening stretches, called *introns,* which are excised from the final mRNA product. In most instances, the role of these introns, which are usually larger than the exons, is unknown.

Molecular Genetic Methodologies

DNA Isolation

Rapid and efficient methods for extracting DNA from peripheral leukocytes, as well as virtually every other tissue, have been developed in the past decade. The term *genomic DNA* refers to the high-molecular-weight DNA that is isolated in this manner.

Restriction Endonucleases

Restriction endonucleases are bacterial enzymes that recognize and cleave specific DNA sequences. These molecular "scissors" are instrumental in almost all the molecular genetic methodologies. Fragments of DNA, generated by the restriction endonuclease digestion of genomic DNA, can be isolated on electrophoretic gels. These can then be inserted into (ligated) DNA from virus-like organisms (vectors) for further amplification and purification.

DNA Vectors and Cloning

Vectors are DNA molecules that are usually derived from bacterial viruses or plasmids. All share the same cardinal property: the direction of their own replication after their introduction into a bacterial host. Molecules of foreign DNA (e.g., human DNA) can be ligated to vector DNA and the altered vector can then be placed in a bacterial host. This generates an abundance of both the vector and the foreign piece of DNA that has been inserted into it.

Fragments of DNA which have been amplified in this manner can be readily extracted from the bacteria and purified for further analysis. This process of linking DNA to vector DNA and replicating it in bacterial hosts is one example of cloning.

A more sophisticated form of cloning involves the placement of DNA into more complex organisms and rendering it biologically active. An example of this is the placement of human disease–causing genes into mice to create animal disease models. This approach has also been used in the first attempts at gene therapy for human genetic diseases. A crude form of genetic therapy has already been tried in Duchenne's muscular dystrophy, wherein myoblasts containing the normal dystrophin gene are injected into the skeletal muscle of affected boys. In this instance, the myoblast genome serves as the vector carrying the dystrophin gene.

DNA Sequencing

Chemical and enzymatic techniques to determine the nucleotide sequence of DNA molecules were developed in the 1970s. These methods, now refined and optimized, are much in use today. Laboratories can elucidate up to 1,000 nucleotides of a DNA sequence in a day sing automated DNA sequencers. Nonetheless, given that there are 6×10^9 nucleotides in the human genome, it is evident that an increase in sequencing speed of at least one hundred-fold is necessary before a realistic attempt to sequence the human genome can be contemplated.

Polymerase Chain Reaction

Polymerase chain reaction, a method of in vitro DNA amplification, has revolutionized much of the practice of molecular genetics. It affords a means of rapidly generating millions of copies of a DNA fragment from as little material as one molecule, without having to resort to cloning. The methodology employs a thermostable DNA-synthesizing polymerase enzyme.

Southern Blotting

Southern blotting is the technique that was devised by Edwin Southern, whereby DNA sequence variations occurring in specifically defined regions of the human genome can be readily identified and tracked in families from generation to generation. A central problem faced by the molecular geneticist interested in a specific region of the human genome (often a region containing a disease-causing gene) is distinguishing the relatively tiny fraction of DNA coming from this region from the vast excess making up the rest of the genome. It is not feasible to purify DNA from one region of the genome for each individual being studied. Dr. Southern's elegant solution to this problem , based on the aforementioned property of ssDNA to reanneal exclusively and specifically to complementary ssDNA.

This method is of value in the detection of gross structural changes in regions of interest in the human genome. The banding pattern detected in Southern blotting can also be used in genetic linkage studies, a topic discussed in the next section.

RECENT PROGRESS IN MOLECULAR NEUROGENETICS

Gene Mapping and Cloning

All neurogenetic illnesses are caused by a defective gene or genes. Much of the recent progress in molecular neurogenetics has involved the chromosomal localization (or mapping) of these disease-causing genes. In some cases, the actual gene responsible for a disease has been identified. The mapping and identification of disease-causing genes has been achieved through the use of three separate approaches: genetic linkage analysis, the detection of chromosomal abnormalities, and direct-candidate gene analysis.

Linkage Analysis

In linkage analysis, modern methodologies are applied in the context of the classic genetic theory of linkage. The concept underlying linkage analysis can be illustrated with a simple example. In a study of 100 families, it is noted that every time an individual has blue eyes he or she has blond hair; conversely, every time he or she does not have blue eyes, he or she does not have blond hair. If this pattern is seen consistently in the majority of kindreds studied, then the genes encoding these two traits are said to be genetically linked. The demonstration of genetic linkage between two genes (or loci) maps them to the same chromosome. Moreover, the stronger the pattern of linkage observed, the physically closer are the two given loci (*locus* refers to a site in an organism's genome). Consequently, in the example given, if the "blue eyes" gene is known to be on chromosome 7 then it can be assumed a priori that the "blond hair" gene also maps to chromosome 7. In this example, the "blue eyes" gene and "blond hair" gene are referred to as *genetic markers*. In modern genetics, markers known as *restriction fragment length polymorphisms* (RFLPs) are used.

There exists in all DNAs, single nucleotide variations in sequence. These variations are known as *DNA polymorphisms* and occur in approximately every 300 nucleotides. DNA polymorphisms are stable variations, inherited from generation to generation, and are, in the vast majority of cases, clinically inconsequential. For any given polymorphism, a certain percentage (e.g., 50%) of the population has one DNA sequence and the remainder has the alternative sequence. DNA polymorphisms are a rich source of genetic markers, which have been used in the past decade in the localization of disease-causing genes.

For some DNA polymorphisms, a given restriction enzyme will cut one allele but not the other, or others. (The variant sequences at a polymorphic site are referred to as *alleles*.) This differential cutting permits the identification and tracking of such polymorphisms from generation to generation. Individuals can be heterozygous for these polymorphisms, in that one chromosome containing the allele is cut by the endonuclease and the other chromosome containing the allele is not (remembering that we all have two copies of each chromosome, one from our mother and one from our father). In these cases, digestion with the restriction enzyme generates distinct sizes of DNA fragment in the vicinity of the polymorphic site.

Unfortunately, the digestion of genomic DNA and the subsequent electrophoresis of the digestion products on an agarose gel results, predictably, in a smear consisting of the thousands of DNA fragments so generated. However, Southern blotting of the digested DNA followed by probing of the blot with a ssDNA probe complementary to the region containing the polymorphic restriction enzyme site provides a means of selectively visualizing the DNA fragments of that region. Chromosomes with the DNA sequence that encodes the restriction enzyme sites will therefore have shorter DNA fragments (i.e., lower bands on the developed Southern blot), whereas those containing the allele not cut by the restriction enzyme will have larger fragments (i.e., higher bands). These variably sized restriction enzyme fragments are examples of RFLPs.

In genetic linkage studies, an effort is made to map a disease-causing gene to a specific region of the genome. Such mapping is usually a prerequisite to the ultimate identification of the disease-causing gene itself. To start with, Southern blots are performed on individuals from a large number of kindreds affected by the illness in question. These blots are then hybridized with a variety of DNA probes from regions throughout the human genome that contain polymorphic restriction enzyme sites. If probes that cover all regions of the human genome are used systematically, a consistent co-segregation of a banding pattern with the disease phenotype and an absence of co-segregation of this banding pattern with the healthy phenotype will eventually be noted. If this pattern is seen in the majority of affected kindreds with, for example, a probe from the short arm of chromosome 3, the disease-causing gene in question is then effectively mapped to this region of the genome.

A statistical parameter that determines the odds of there being genetic linkage between two loci has been devised by the British geneticist Morton. The lod score, as it is known, is the log of the odds that two given loci are genetically linked. Consequently, if locus A is said to be linked to locus B with a lod score of 4, there are 10^4 or 10,000 : 1 odds that the two loci are linked, and therefore relatively near each other on the same chromosome. A lod score of 3 or more is considered relatively conclusive proof of linkage. The concept of utilizing RFLPs in linkage analysis to map disease-causing genes, first proposed in 1981, was successfully proved in 1983 with the observation of genetic linkage between the gene causing Huntington's disease and markers on the short arm of chromosome 4. The Huntington's gene has since been identified.

DETECTION OF CHROMOSOMAL ABNORMALITIES

It has been estimated that to search the entire genome for a polymorphic DNA marker showing linkage to a given disease would require the use of 300 probes. Clearly, employing linkage analysis to search blindly for a disease-causing gene represents a formidable challenge. However, the use of linkage to find a disease-causing gene can be obviated when a chromosomal abnormality (usually a translocation or a chromosomal deletion) is observed to either co-segregate with a disease phenotype, or arise anew in an individual who clearly has a new mutation presentation of a given disease. It is now possible, using molecular genetic techniques, to isolate and amplify the DNA from the region of such an observed chromosomal abnormality. The underlying assumption in such a situation is that the chromosomal abnormality has occurred in the region of the disease-causing gene, with the inactivation of the gene resulting in the disease. This approach has been instrumental in cloning the dystrophin and the NF-1 genes. Defects in these genes cause Duchenne's (or Becker's) muscular dystrophy and neurofibromatosis type 1, respectively.

DIRECT-CANDIDATE GENE ANALYSIS

The candidate gene approach constitutes another means of circumventing linkage analysis. Frequently biochemical data on a disease's pathophysiology exist that indicate the involvement of a protein in the causation of that condition. In such instances, when the gene encoding that protein has been cloned, linkage is searched for between polymorphisms close to or within the candidate gene and the disease in affected kindreds. The presence of such linkage is taken as strong evidence for such a causative role. Alternatively, the candidate gene present in an affected individual may be sequenced and compared with that from an unaffected individual. For example, research on periodic hyperkalemic paralysis implicated the sodium pump of adult muscle as the possible site of the causative defect. The gene for the alpha subunit of this enzyme complex was recently cloned. Sequencing of this gene from an individual with this condition resulted in the identification of the causative mutation.

The genes associated with the majority of significant neurogenetic disorders have been mapped in the past 5 years (Table 26-1). Furthermore, the genes that, when defective, cause Duchenne's (and Becker's) muscular dystrophy, neurofibromatosis, and malignant hyperthermia have been identified. The cloning of disease-causing genes is expected to increase dramatically in the coming decade.

The localization and identification of disease-causing genes have been the most conspicuous recent advances in molecular neurogenetics. The advantages resulting from the latter achievement are readily apparent. In one step, the precise underlying molecular defect causing

a condition is elucidated, thereby identifying the pathogenetic basis of the disease.

What advantages accrue from localizing a disease-causing gene? Although the localization of such a gene does not increase the understanding of the underlying pathology of an inherited illness, in many cases it does permit the unequivocal identification of disease-causing gene carriers, irrespective of their clinical profile. This permits the genotype and phenotype to be correlated for neurogenetic disorders. Such an approach is helpful in the delineation of conditions such as myotonic dystrophy, which displays a marked variability in both the severity of the disease as well as the organ systems involved. In such cases, the unequivocal diagnosis of the illness can be problematic. However, the molecular genetic–based diagnosis of myotonic dystrophy yields a clearer profile of the individual carrying this disease-causing gene.

DUCHENNE'S MUSCULAR DYSTROPHY

The cloning of the Duchenne's muscular dystrophy (DMD)–causing dystrophin gene stands out as a landmark achievement in the field of molecular neurogenetics. A brief history of the mapping and cloning of this gene illustrates the potential power of molecular genetic methodologies.

The X-linked pattern of inheritance of the condition resulted in the de facto mapping of the DMD-causing gene to the X chromosome long before the advent of modern molecular genetics. In the late 1970s and early 1980s, cytogenetic analyses of females affected with DMD revealed the existence of balanced chromosome translocations involving a variety of autosomal chromosomes, but always at the Xp21 region of the X chromosome, strongly suggesting that the DMD gene mapped to Xp21. Additional evidence for this mapping came with the demonstration of genetic linkage between an Xp21 RFLP and the disease phenotype in several DMD kindreds. Similar linkage was observed for Becker's muscular dystrophy (BMD), suggesting that the two conditions were allelic, in

Table 26-1. The Chromosomal Localization and Identity of Neurogenetic Disease-causing Genes

Disease	Gene	Chromosome location
Adrenoleukodystrophy		Xq28
Aicardi's syndrome		Xp22
Ataxia telangiectasia		11q22–23
Becker's muscular dystrophy	Dystrophin	Xp21.1–21.3
Benign familial convulsions		20q
Central core disease	Ryanodine receptor*	19q13.1
Centronuclear myopathy		Xq28
Charcot-Marie-Tooth disease		
Type Ia		17p11.2–q23
Type Ib		1q21.2–q23
X-linked		Xq13
Duchenne's muscular dystrophy	Dystrophin	Xp21.1–21.3
Emery-Dreifuss muscular dystrophy		Xq28
Familial Alzheimer's disease		19q13.1*, 21q21–q22.1*
Familial amyloid neuropathy		18
Fascioscapulohumeral muscular dystrophy		4q35–qter
Friedreich's ataxia		9cen–q21
Huntington's disease		4pter
Hyperkalemic periodic paralysis	Na⁺ channel, α subunit	17q
Krabbe's disease		14
Lesch-Nyhan syndrome		Xq27
Limb-girdle muscular dystrophy		15
Malignant hyperthermia	Ryanodine receptor	19q13.1
Menkes' syndrome		Xq13.2–q13.3
Myasthenia gravis (hereditary form)	Acetylcholine receptors	
	α subunit	2q24–q32
	β submit	17p11–p12
	δ subunit	2q33–qter
Myotonic dystrophy		19q13.3
Myotubular myopathy		Xq27–q28
Neurofibromatosis		
Type 1	GAP	17q11.2
Type 2		22q12–q13.1
Pelizaeus-Merzbacher disease		Xq21.3–q22
Spinal muscular atrophy		
Types I, II, III		5q13.1
X-linked	Androgen receptor	X-q21.3–q22
Spinocerebellar ataxia		p21.3–6p24
Torsion dystonia		9q32–34
Tuberous sclerosis		9q34, 11q14–q22, 12q22–24
Von Hippel–Lindau disease		3p25–26
Wilson's disease		13q14.1–q21.1
Fragile X syndrome	550 bp CpG island	Xq27.3

*Tentative identification or mapping.

that they resulted from different mutations in the same gene.

The cloning of the dystrophin gene was achieved nearly simultaneously by two groups of investigators in 1987. One laboratory isolated and sequenced the autosomal/X-chromosome breakpoint from a female patient with DMD; the second group used a novel DNA reassociation technique on DNA isolated from an affected boy with a deletion of Xp21. The latter workers were the first to publish the entire dystrophin sequence. The gene is one of the largest known, spanning two million nucleotides; the coding region itself consists of 14,000 base pairs, resulting in a very large protein of approximately 400 kDa.

The identification of the dystrophin gene has spawned a period of highly productive research on the genetics and biochemistry of DMD. The most relevant clinical results can be summarized as follows: (1) immunological testing for the dystrophin protein has improved the identification of female DMD gene carriers and of fetal diagnosis of the condition; (2) the diagnostic accuracy of detecting affected individuals has also increased significantly, such that a proportion of disorders previously deemed limb-girdle and spinal muscular atrophy have been shown to be BMD; (3) BMD and DMD have been shown to be allelic disorders; (4) a good correlation between the dystrophin concentration and the severity of BMD has been shown; and (5) a myoblast transfer approach has been introduced as a possible treatment for DMD.

BIBLIOGRAPHY

Davies, K. E. *Human Genetic Diseases; A Practical Approach.* Oxford, U.K.: IRL Press, 1986.

Hyser, C. L. Recombinant DNA Approach to Clinical Neurology. In R. J. Joynt (editor). *Clinical Neurology.* Philadelphia: Lippincott, 1989, Vol. 4, P. 17.

Kunkel, L. M., and Hoffman, E. P. Duchenne/Becker muscular dystrophy: a short overview of the gene, the protein, and current diagnostics. *Br. Med. Bull.* 45:630–643, 1989.

Payne, C. S., and Roses, A. D. The molecular genetic revolution; its impact on clinical neurology. *Arch. Neurol.* 45:1366–1376, 1988.

Watson, J. D., et al. *Molecular Biology of the Gene,* 3rd ed. Menlo Park, CA: Benjamin/Cummings, 1987.

Wessel, H. B. Dystrophin: a clinical perspective. *Pediatr. Neurol.* 6:3–12, 1990.

Inherited Metabolic and Developmental Disorders

This chapter deals with two ostensibly disparate groups of disorders: those in which an inherited metabolic disorder leads to the progressive loss of neurological function, and those in which the nervous system is formed abnormally with consequent stable neurological handicaps. In many of the degenerative metabolic disorders, the nature of the genetic biochemical defect has been deciphered and a specific enzyme is known to be missing or malfunctioning. The precise cause of most developmental nervous system disorders, on the other hand, remains a mystery. In a few instances, disordered brain development and degenerative neurological disease appear to coexist. In Zellweger syndrome, for example, an apparent failure to form intracellular peroxisomes with their attendant array of oxidative enzymes leads to abnormal gyral formation and neuronal heterotopias on the one hand, and progressive, global loss of neurological function on the other. Infantile sulfatide lipidosis (metachromatic leukodystrophy) is accompanied by both *dys*myelination (abnormal myelin formation) and *de*myelination (break-

down of myelin) in the central and peripheral nervous systems. These, and other, examples suggest that the distinction between degenerative metabolic and developmental disorders of the nervous system may be more apparent than real, at least at the biochemical level.

This chapter attempts to develop a conceptual framework that can aid in the understanding of the clinical aspects of these disorders.

INHERITED METABOLIC DEGENERATIVE DISORDERS

Basic Mechanisms

Inherited metabolic errors affecting the nervous system ultimately derive their effects from a mutant gene belonging to the chromosomal or mitochondrial genome. The abnormal gene either fails to mediate the production of adequate amounts of a specific protein (e.g., enzyme, membrane transport protein, receptor, or cytoskeletal protein), or causes the manufacture of a protein that is structurally defective and therefore does not function properly.

The absent or dysfunctional protein may, in turn, adversely affect the nervous system through the operation of one or more of the following mechanisms:

1. The absent compound is required for normal brain growth; for example, the failure to produce adequate amounts of thyroxine seen in patients with congenital hypothyroidism leads to impairment of normal developmental processes such as dendritic growth, synapse formation, and myelination.

2. A synthetic or degradative reaction blocked by a defective enzyme leads to the accumulation of neurotoxic precursors; for example, in phenylketonuria, because phenylalanine cannot be hydroxylated to tyrosine, neurotoxic compounds such as phenylpyruvic acid form by an alternate metabolic route, with ultimate adverse effects on brain maturation.

3. Disturbed cellular energy metabolism leads to difficulty coping with metabolic stresses and early neuronal death; for example, electron transport chain defects such as cytochrome C oxidase deficiency impair the production of high-energy phosphates; medium-chain acyl-CoA dehydrogenase deficiency, in turn, interferes with fatty acid oxidation.

4. Disturbed membrane transport mechanisms lead to failure of absorption or lack of renal conservation of a compound for brain maturation; for example, in Hartnup disease, impaired tryptophan absorption and conservation leads to nicotinamide adenine dinucleotide synthesis.

5. An accumulated compound is toxic to another organ, with resultant dysfunction that then affects the nervous system; for example, in homocystinuria, abnormally high levels of this sulfated amino acid damage the vascular endothelium; this precipitates intravascular thromboses, emboli, and cerebral strokes.

The clinical presentation of a given metabolic error depends on the type of biochemical reaction, or reactions, involved and their impact on normal neurological function, the extent to which enzymatic activity is compromised, the presence or absence of toxic precursor compounds, the chance occurrence of metabolic stresses (e.g., infections), and the presence or absence of alternative metabolic pathways (e.g., via maternal metabolism). When the biochemical deficit is severe, especially if multiple metabolic pathways are blocked simultaneously, a global neurological dysfunction is likely to arise, usually at an early stage in brain development. If maternal transplacental metabolism cannot compensate for these blocked functions, the disorder becomes manifest in utero, with some degree of cerebral dysgenesis likely, as in Zellweger syndrome. When maternal metabolism can compensate for a severe metabolic deficit (as in branched-chain ketoaciduria), the baby will appear normal at birth but exhibit catastrophic neurological symptoms almost immediately. When the biochemical deficit is less severe, with the partial preservation of enzymatic function, clinical onset usually occurs at a later age, with selective metabolically vulnerable neuronal or glial populations being involved and the remainder of the nervous system essentially intact (as in certain allelic forms of hexosaminidase A deficiency presenting as spinocerebellar syndromes or motor neuron disease).

Principal Clinical Patterns

Although there is an almost infinite variability in the clinical features of the known genetic metabolic errors that affect the nervous system, a number of discrete clinical patterns can be recognized, with inevitable overlaps. Each genetic defect has its favorite pattern of presentation; these are relatively specific collections of symptoms and signs that tend to emerge at about the same age in affected individuals. From the clinician's point of view, the recognition of specific clinical patterns is the most reliable way of approaching the differential diagnosis of neurological metabolic degenerative disease.

On the surface it would seem more logical to try to categorize hereditary metabolic disorders according to the specific enzyme defects or specific metabolic pathways involved. However, this approach is actually less than satisfactory because specific enzyme deficiencies may have quite variable clinical presentations, depending on the nature of the allele. Marked impairment in hexosaminidase A activity for its physiological substrate (GM$_2$ ganglioside) may lead to a classic picture of Tay-Sachs disease in one family, while a less severe disturbance in enzyme activity may produce a combination of spinocerebellar degeneration and dementia in another family.

Only the most common and distinctive patterns are considered in any detail here (Fig. 27-1), along with descriptions of exemplary disorders. These include (1) rapid deterioration in infancy; (2) progressive insidious regression; (3) intermittent, stepwise regression; and (4) system degenerations. For reasons already mentioned, specific enzyme deficiencies may appear in more than one clinical category.

Rapid Deterioration in Infancy

Infants with disorders that involve rapid deterioration are typically normal at birth. The consumption of milk, with its inadequately metabolized substrates (amino acids, monosaccharides, and the like) is followed by the relatively rapid onset of neurological symptoms.

Affected infants become lethargic and feed poorly; vomiting, irritability, and seizures typically ensue. Depending on the specific disorder, infants may show a marked delay in developmental milestones, become jaundiced, or rapidly lapse into a coma and die in respiratory failure. Table 27-1 outlines the clinical and laboratory data pertaining to some of the most important metabolic errors belonging to this group of disorders.

Given that the developing nervous system is initially intact, and that toxic substrates are derived from the diet, early diagnosis is essential if brain function is to be preserved. Biochemically specific diagnoses are facilitated by laboratory investigations that are reviewed later in this chapter. Many of these disorders are treatable using approaches summarized in a later section.

Phenylketonuria. Patients with phenylketonuria are unable to convert phenylalanine (PA) to tyrosine, an important initial step in the synthesis of several crucial monoamines (dopa-dihydroxyphenylalanine and norepinephrine) and of melanin. Several clinical forms of the

Fig. 27-1. *Graph illustrating the principal patterns of clinical progression of inborn metabolic errors affecting the nervous system. The hatched line represents the normal steady acquisition of new skills during the first few years of postnatal life. Curves A, B, C, and D demonstrate the four major patterns of clinical deterioration (i.e., loss of skills) described in the text.*

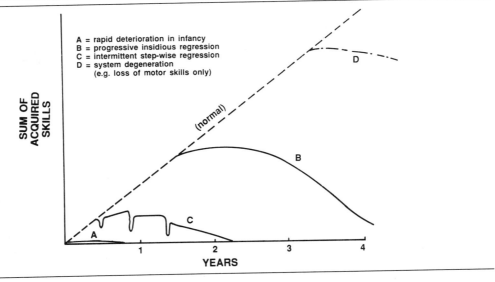

Table 27-1. Disorders Presenting with Rapid Deterioration in Infancy

Disorder (defective enzyme)	Inheritance pattern	Clinical features	Urine	Blood	Therapy
Phenylketonuria (PA hydroxylase)	AR	Irritability, vomiting, seizures, mental retardation, eczema, blond hair	+FeCl₃, ↑ PA	↑ Phenylalanine and metabolites	Low PA diet
Phenylketonuria (dihydropteridine reductase or deficient biopterin synthesis)	AR	Same	Same + ↓ HVA, ↓ 5-HIAA, ↓ VMA	Same	6-Methyltetra-hydrobiopterin
Branched-chain ketoaciduria (BCKA decarboxylase)	AR	Poor feeding, lethargy, seizures, coma, spasticity, ophthalmoplegia, bulbar palsy, urine odor of maple syrup	+FeCl₃, +DNPH, ↑ BCAA, ↑ BCKA	Acidosis, leukopenia, hypoglycemia	Low BCAA diet (oral or parenteral), exchange transfusion, peritoneal dialysis, thiamine
Isovaleric acidemia (isovaleryl-CoA dehydrogenase)	AR	Poor feeding, lethargy, seizures, coma, mental retardation, urine odor of sweaty feet	↑ Isovaleryl glycine, +DNPH	Acidosis, leukopenia, pancytopenia	↓ leucine intake, exchange transfusion, peritoneal dialysis, oral glycine
Propionic acidemia (propionyl-CoA carboxylase)	AR	Poor feeding, lethargy, seizures, coma, dysautonomia	↑ Propionic acid, +DNPH	Acidosis, leukopenia, hypoglycemia, hyperammonemia, hyperglycinemia	Protein restriction, exchange transfusion, peritoneal dialysis, oral biotin
Methylmalonic aciduria (methylmalonyl-CoA mutase)	AR	Same as propionic acidemia	+DNPH, ↑ methylmalonic acid	Same as propionic acidemia	Protein restriction, exchange transfusion, peritoneal dialysis, vitamin B₁₂
Nonketotic hyperglycinemia (glycine cleavage enzyme)	AR	Poor feeding, lethargy, seizures, coma, myoclonus, opisthotonos	↑ Glycine	Hyperglycinemia (↑ CSF glycine)	Strychnine sulfate, sodium benzoate, clonazepam, diazepam

Carbamoyl phosphate synthetase deficiency	AR	Poor feeding, lethargy, seizures, coma, hypotonia		Hyperammonemia, acidosis, hyperglycinemia	Protein restriction, sodium benzoate, peritoneal dialysis, exchange transfusion
Ornithine transcarbamoylase deficiency	XD	In males, same as for CPSD	↑ Orotic acid	Hyperammonemia	Same as for CPSD
Argininosuccinic aciduria (argininosuccinate lyase)	AR	Same as for CPSD; milder cases have ataxia, trichorrhexis, hepatomegaly	↑ Argininosuccinic acid	Hyperammonemia	Same as for CPSD
Galactosemia (galactose-1-phosphate uridyl transferase)	AR	Jaundice, hepatomegaly, edema, anorexia, vomiting, lethargy, hypotonia, cataracts, cirrhosis	+Benedict's test, −glucose oxidase, amino aciduria	Hyperbilirubinemia, hypoglycemia	Galactose-deficient diet (soy formula milk)
Hereditary fructose intolerance (fructose-1-phosphate aldolase)	AR	Jaundice, hepatomegaly, anorexia, vomiting, hypotonia, mental retardation	Same as for galactosemia	Same as for galactosemia	Fructose-deficient diet

PA = phenylalanine; AR = autosomal recessive; XD = X-linked dominant; DNPH = 2,4-dinitrophenylhydrazine; BCAA = branched-chain amino acids; BCKA = branched-chain ketoacids; HVA = homovanillic acid; 5-HIAA = 5-hydroxyindoleacetic acid; VMA = vanillylmandelic acid; CPSD = carbamoyl phosphate synthetase deficiency; ↑ = raised; ↓ = lowered; + = positive; − = negative.

disorder have been identified, in part related to distinct interlocked enzyme defects; examples include PA hydroxylase (classic phenylketonuria) and dihydropteridine reductase. Neurological compromise stems in part from the failure to synthesize tyrosine and in part from the accumulation of PA metabolites such as phenylpyruvic acid. The neuropathological consequences are principally those consonant with impaired brain maturation, consisting of reduced dendritic branching, synaptic spine formation, and myelination. Affected children are normal at birth, then irritability, vomiting, seizures (particularly infantile spasms), delayed motor and cognitive milestones, and a severe mental subnormality develop. Because of the lack of normal melanin formation, affected children are typically blond and blue-eyed with eczema.

An autosomal recessive condition without a distinct ethnic predilection, the disorder may be diagnosed in the neonatal period through the routine screening of newborns for the presence of elevated blood levels of PA. In the classic PA hydroxylase form of the disease, the clinical manifestations of the defect may be entirely prevented by the early institution of a PA-restricted diet; the dietary treatment of dihydropteridine reductase deficiency is less satisfactory. It is now fairly clear that the low-PA diet must be adhered to throughout life, with particular care during pregnancy, as high maternal blood PA levels have disastrous effects on fetal brain maturation. Stopping the diet in later childhood or adult life has been shown to lead to significant decrements in performance on neuropsychological testing.

Insidious Regression

Children with disorders that are associated with insidious regression negotiate the neonatal period well and initially appear to be developing normally. Then, at an age which is usually typical for the specific metabolic defect concerned, cognitive and motor development appear to be arrested, followed by the relentless and gradual loss of previously acquired abilities. Depending on the specific disorder, there may be rapid or gradual appearance of spasticity, blindness, and dementia. Although there is a considerable amount of overlap between the symptom patterns in this group of disorders, three subgroups can be distinguished, which are determined by the presence or absence of seizures and by the presence of dysostotic dwarfism.

Insidious Regression with Frequent Seizures.

In those patients afflicted with a disorder showing insidious regression accompanied by seizures, the seizures appear relatively early in the course and remain a major clinical symptom. The seizure patterns may include generalized tonic-clonic, generalized tonic, focal or multifocal clonic, and generalized or focal myoclonic; in addition, the same patient may exhibit multiple seizure patterns. As might be expected, the predominant pathology in these children resides in the cortical gray matter, and often involves the intraneuronal storage of an unmetabolized substrate, or substrates. Electroencephalograms typically show multifocal spike activity.

Table 27-2 and Figure 27-2 summarize the clinical and laboratory features of some of the more prominent disorders belonging to this group. As can be seen, the diagnosis can often be suspected on the basis of the age of symptom onset and a few characteristic clinical features. The clinical impression may be confirmed in some instances by documenting the presence of defective enzyme activity in cultured leukocytes (e.g., hexosaminidase A deficiency in Tay-Sachs disease), or by demonstrating the presence of intracytoplasmic stored material in biopsied tissues (e.g., the conjunctiva or sweat glands in ceroid lipofuscinosis).

GM₂ Gangliosidosis (Tay-Sachs Disease).

Tay-Sachs disease represents a classic example of a lysosomal enzyme defect leading to intraneuronal storage. Sphingolipid metabolism, which is abnormal in this as well as a number of other inherited disorders mentioned later, is depicted in Figure 27-3. An autosomal recessive trait common in Ashkenazi Jews and French Canadians, the metabolic error consists of an absent or defective function of the lysosomal enzyme hexosaminidase A (a variety of specific alleles have already been identified). There is a consequent inability to cleave an N-acetyl-galactosamine moiety from the carbohydrate side-chain

Table 27-2. Insidious Regression with Frequent Seizures

Disorder	Defective enzyme	Inheritance pattern	Symptom onset	Clinical features	Laboratory features
Tay-Sachs disease	Hexosaminidase A	AR	3–10 mo	Hyperacusis, hypotonia, blind, seizures (generalized, myoclonic, gelastic), macular cherry-red spot; later on, megalencephaly, spasticity	EEG: hypsarrhythmia, multifocal spike; stored material: GM_2 ganglioside
Sandhoff disease	Hexosaminidase A and B	AR	3–10 mo	Same as TSD plus hepatosplenomegaly	Same as TSD
Santavuori-Haltia disease	Unknown (NCL)	AR	9–19 mo	Rapid regression, ataxia, myoclonic seizures, blindness, brownish pigmentation in macula	↑ Urinary dolichols; EEG: decreased amplitude; ERG/VER absent; lymphocytes: granular osmophilic profiles
Bielschowsky disease	Unknown (NCL)	AR	2–4 yr	Seizures (generalized, myoclonic), ataxia, regression, blindness, optic atrophy	↑ Urinary dolichols; EEG: enhanced photic response; ERG/VER absent; lymphocytes: curvilinear profiles
Batten disease	Unknown (NCL)	AR	4–9 yr	Blindness, dementia, seizures usually later (myoclonic), pigmentary retinal degeneration	↑ Urinary dolichols; EEG: slow spike/wave; ERG/VER absent; lymphocytes: fingerprint profiles
Kufs' disease	Unknown (NCL)	AR, AD	Adult	Seizures (myoclonic), dementia, ataxia	Lymphocytes: granular osmophilic profiles; EEG, ERG, VER variable
Lafora's disease	Unknown	AR	7–14 yr	Generalized and myoclonic seizures, ataxia, progressive dementia, spasticity, myoclonic status	EEG: multifocal and synchronous spikes; muscle and sweat gland: polyglucosan storage; liver: Lafora's bodies

Table 27-2 (Continued).

Disorder	Defective enzyme	Inheritance pattern	Symptom onset	Clinical features	Laboratory features
Alpers' syndrome	Unknown, ?mitochondrial or slow virus	?AR, sporadic	Infancy	Developmental delay, failure to thrive, intractable multifocal seizures, liver failure	EEG: very high-amplitude polyspike–slow wave; VER absent; CT: diffuse atrophy, especially occipital lobe; liver: cirrhosis
Zellweger syndrome	Absent peroxisomes	AR	Neonate	High forehead, large fontanelles, hypoplastic supraorbital ridges, epicanthic folds, hypotonia, poor feeding, weakness, cataracts, glaucoma, pigmentary retinopathy, optic nerve dysplasia, frequent seizures from birth	Abnormal liver function; calcific stippling of long bones; abdominal ultrasound: renal cortical cysts; ↑ VLCFA, ↑ pipecolic acid; ↑ bile acid precursors

AR = autosomal recessive; VLCFA = very-long-chain fatty acids; AD = autosomal dominant; TSD = Tay-Sachs disease; NCL = neuronal ceroid lipofuscinosis; ERG = electroretinogram; VER = visual evoked responses; ↑ = raised.

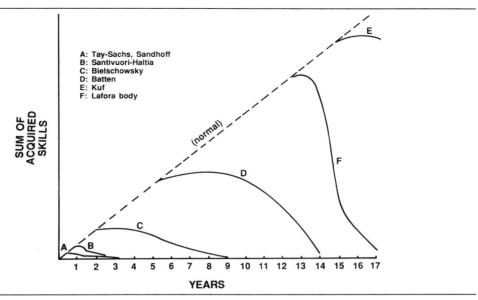

A: Tay-Sachs, Sandhoff
B: Santivuori-Haltia
C: Bielschowsky
D: Batten
E: Kuf
F: Lafora body

Fig. 27-2. *Graph illustrating the typical pattern of clinical progression of several metabolic disorders presenting with insidious regression and frequent seizures.*

of GM_2 ganglioside in neurons and glia. Pathologically, there is distortion and swelling of cortical dendrites, dysmyelination in the white matter, and the progressive ballooning of neurons with stored GM_2 ganglioside. Eventually there is marked loss of cortical and other telencephalic neurons, accompanied by cortical atrophy and diffuse cerebral gliosis. Affected children are ostensibly normal until the age of 5 to 6 months, although hyperacusis may already exist. Subsequently the infant is unable to achieve independent sitting, loses head control and the ability to roll over, loses visual function, exhibits a pronounced startle response to sound, develops tonic-clonic or myoclonic seizures, or both. When the disease is well established (at the age of 1 year), there are typically macrocrania, spasticity, blindness, and macular cherry-red spots. The child usually dies of cachexia and aspiration pneumonia by the age 2 to 5 years. The diagnosis may be confirmed by the assay of appropriate lysosomal enzymes in cultured leukocytes. Fortunately, the incidence of the disease is declining because of carrier detection and prenatal diagnosis in susceptible population groups.

Insidious Regression without Frequent Seizures. The group of disorders in which the course is insidiously regressive but frequent seizures are not a component, includes the majority of the lysosomal storage diseases. These disorders comprise a variety of defects in the orderly degradation of gangliosides and cerebrosides. These complex glycolipids play an important structural role in the formation of neuronal and glial cellular membranes, in that their intralysosomal accumulation leads inexorably to the degeneration of both gray and white matter structures.

In the case of ganglioside catabolism, it is principally the neurons, and hence the gray matter, that are involved in the degenerative process. Many of the ganglioside storage disorders, besides causing the insidious loss of cognitive function and generalized spasticity, are also associated with ganglioside deposition in the ganglion cell layer of the retina. This is manifested clinically as the macular cherry-red spot, which was already mentioned for Tay-Sachs disease. In addition, there may be storage of ganglioside in hepatocytes, presenting as hepatomegaly, or in the spleen and bone marrow.

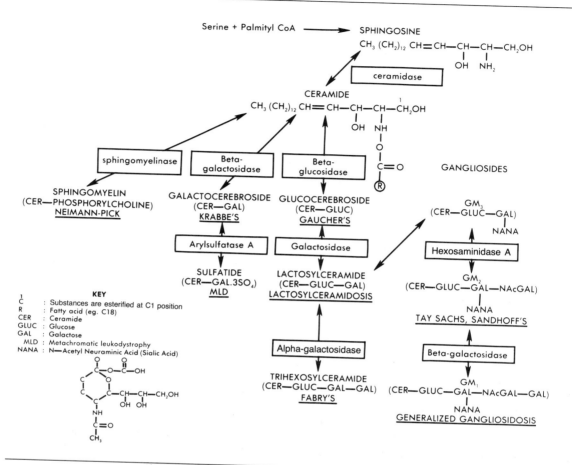

Fig. 27-3. *Scheme of sphingolipid metabolism.*

When cerebroside metabolism is defective, principally the central white matter and peripheral nerves are involved, hence the term *leukodystrophy*. Peripheral nerve degeneration can also produce hypotonic muscle weakness, wasting, and areflexia. At times, these peripheral features may appear prior to any loss of mental function or vision, and the disorder then mistaken for a subacute polyneuropathy. The eye findings in cerebroside storage disorders tend to consist of progressive optic atrophy rather than foveal changes, reflecting the primary involvement of myelinated axons.

The clinical and laboratory features of some of these disorders are summarized in Table 27-3 and Figure 27-4. As can be seen, seizures may be a factor in the clinical course of many disorders in this group, but are usually rare and seldom represent a significant therapeutic problem, unlike the situation in the disorders described in the previous section.

The rate of progression of these disorders is variable. Boys with adrenoleukodystrophy usually do not become symptomatic until around age 10 years, but the disease progresses rapidly with death in 1 to 2 years. Boys with Pelizaeus-Merzbacher disease are clinically impaired by the age of 3 months, but their condition deteriorates extremely slowly and they may survive with a remarkably intact intelligence for decades.

Sulfatide Lipidosis (Metachromatic Leukodystrophy). An autosomal recessive condition,

Table 27-3. Insidious Regression with Frequent Seizures

Disorder	Defective enzyme	Inheritance pattern	Symptom onset	Clinical features	Laboratory features
Krabbe's disease	Galactosylceramide β-galactosidase	AR	2–6 mo	Rapid regression, irritability, fever, blindness, opisthotonos, spasticity, optic atrophy, eventual hypotonia	↑ CSF protein; slowed motor/sensory nerve conduction; EEG: slow, high voltage
Metachromatic leukodystrophy	Arylsulfatase A	AR	1–2 yr	Hypotonia, weakness, ataxia → regression, blindness, spasticity, optic atrophy, muscle wasting	↑ CSF protein (late infantile); slowed motor and sensory nerve conduction; EEG: high-voltage slowing; nerve biopsy → demyelination with metachromatic granules
Metachromatic leukodystrophy (late infantile, juvenile, adult forms)			4–10 yr	School failure, dementia, spasticity, blindness	
			20–50 yr	Psychiatric disorders, insidious dementia	
Niemann-Pick disease (type A)	Sphingomyelinase	AR	1–4 mo	Failure-to-thrive, hepatosplenomegaly, macular cherry-red spot, rapid regression, spasticity, blindness, brown skin discoloration	Pulmonary infiltrates, vacuolated lymphocytes, bone marrow → sea-blue histiocytes
Gaucher's disease (infantile)	β-glucocerebrosidase	AR	1–2 mo	Rapid regression, marked hepatosplenomegaly, spasticity → flaccidity; hypersplenism	Bone marrow: Gaucher's (foam) cells; thrombocytopenia
Adrenoleukodystrophy	?lignoceroylCoA synthase	XR	5–20 yr	Behavioral disturbances, school failure, dysphasia, dyspraxia, blindness, spasticity, dysphagia, dementia, hyperpigmented skin	CT: hypodense parietooccipital white matter with contrast enhancement; MRI: ↑ T₂-weighted signal in white matter; ↑ VLCFA in blood

Table 27-3 (Continued).

Disorder	Defective enzyme	Inheritance pattern	Symptom onset	Clinical features	Laboratory features
Pelizaeus-Merzbacher disease	Unknown	XR	1–3 mo	Nystagmus, head titubation, trunk and limb ataxia, dysarthria, optic atrophy, spasticity; very slow progression with long plateau periods	MRI: patchy increased signal, T2-CT: progressive white matter atrophy; BAERs absent after wave I.
Canavan's disease	Aspartoacylase	AR	2–4 mo	Developmental arrest, spasticity, megalencephaly, optic atrophy, choreoathetosis, occasional seizures	Urine: ↑ N-acetylaspartate; CT: diffuse hypodensity of white matter
Alexander's disease	Unknown	AR	1–2 mo	Developmental arrest, spasticity, megalencephaly, occasional seizures	CT: attenuation of white matter with positive contrast enhancement; brain biopsy: Rosenthal's fibers
Cockayne's syndrome	Unknown	AR	1–2 yr	Progressive weakness, hypotonia, muscular atrophy, mental regression, optic atrophy	Nerve conduction studies: slowed; nerve biopsy: multiple axonal swellings with neurofilament aggregates
Rett's syndrome	Unknown	?XD (girls only)	1–2 yr	Loss of expressive language and purposeful hand use, microcephaly, hand-washing posture, autism, scoliosis, gait apraxia, ±seizures	CT: normal; EEG: active spikewave during sleep; CSF: ↓ monoamine metabolites

AR = autosomal recessive; XR = X-linked recessive; ?XD = X-linked dominant, lethal to males in utero?; VLCFA = very-long-chain fatty acids; ↑ = raised; ↓ = lowered; BAER = brainstem auditory evoked responses.

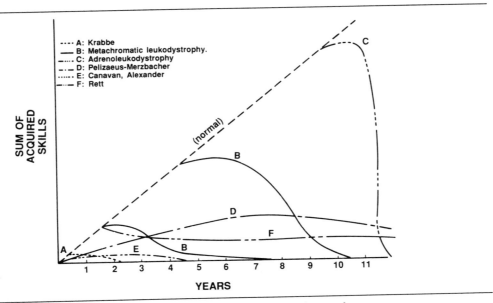

Fig. 27-4. *Graph illustrating the typical pattern of clinical progression of several metabolic disorders presenting with insidious regression* without *frequent seizures.*

sulfatide lipidosis stems from a deficiency in, or dysfunction of, the enzyme arylsulfatase A, leading to the impaired degradation of sulfated galactocerebrosides. Accumulation of the sulfated lipid causes oligodendroglial plus peripheral Schwann-cell dysfunction, with initial dysmyelination then generalized demyelination. As the myelin-forming cells die, sulfated galactocerebroside is stored in the macrophages, which exhibits a metachromatic appearance (brown) when stained with cresyl violet.

Sulfatides accumulate in the central white matter, peripheral nerve, kidneys, gallbladder, and liver. Characteristic cytoplasmic organelles containing stacked membranes may be seen on electron micrographs, a phenomenon observed for most lysosomal storage diseases.

There are several well-characterized alleles that are responsible for fairly distinctive clinical courses (see Fig. 27-4). A late-infantile form of the disease typically commences at approximately 18 months of age, with the relatively rapid onset of extremity weakness, ataxia, and areflexia. After a couple of months, affected children lose interest in the environment, stop speaking, develop spasticity, and become blind, with evidence of optic atrophy.

Peripheral nerve dysfunction is less obvious in the juvenile form, which usually debuts at the age of 4 to 6 years. These children typically exhibit progressive school failure, dementia, spasticity, and so on. There is also an adult form of the disease, usually beginning insidiously in late adolescence. Survival varies from 3 to 5 years in the infantile form to decades in the adult-onset form. The diagnosis may be seriously entertained if the motor nerve conduction velocities are slowed, and confirmed by arylsulfatase A assay performed in cultured leukocytes. Once the index case has occurred in a given family, prenatal diagnosis can prevent other cases.

Insidious Regression with Dysostotic Dwarfism. The clinical course in this subgroup, from a neurological standpoint, is similar to that of many of those disorders described in the preceding section, but with the typical additional features of progressive coarsening of facial features, growth failure, and skeletal malformations. The skeletal problems may predate the appearance of neurological symptomatology.

The mucopolysaccharidoses and mucolipidoses are the principal members of this subgroup of disorders. Facial and bony abnormalities stem from the storage of the accumulated compound or compounds, in soft tissues and bone. In some disorders, there may also be storage in other tissues, leading to clouding of the corneas, hypertrophy of the gums, and hepatosplenomegaly. The mucopolysaccharide (proteoglycan) or other compounds may also be found in the urine, a significant aid in reaching a specific diagnosis.

Table 27-4 outlines the clinical and laboratory characteristics of the main disorders in this subgroup. The neurological deterioration in these patients is a consequence of the intraneuronal accumulation of ganglioside, such that the enzyme defect simultaneously blocks the catabolism of both the proteoglycans (with soft tissue and bony consequences) and the gangliosides (with neurological sequelae). In some mucopolysaccharidoses, the nervous system is not involved (e.g., Morquio and Scheie syndromes; not shown in Table 27-4). The reason for this neurological sparing is not always biochemically apparent. In both the Hurler and Scheie syndromes, for example, there is a deficiency in the activity of alpha-iduronidase. Patients with either syndrome exhibit coarsening of their facial features, cloudy corneas, and dwarfism, but the former disorder also has relentless neurological regression while the latter does not. As with those disorders described in the previous section, seizures may occur in many of these conditions, but are rare and seldom pose a therapeutic problem.

Hunter's Syndrome. In Hunter's syndrome, a defect in the lysosomal enzyme sulfoiduronate sulfatase leads to impaired degradation of the mucopolysaccharides dermatan and heparan sulfate, as well as of the gangliosides. Unlike the examples given thus far, this disorder is a sex-linked recessive trait. Affected boys appear normal until the age of 2 to 3 years, then begin to show a decline in linear growth and coarsening of facial features, but not clouding of the corneas (Fig. 27-5). The long bones are short and broad with widened metaphyses and the ribs are thickened. Behavioral problems and hyperactivity are often the earliest symptoms of neurological compromise, followed gradu-

ally by loss of developmental milestones, spasticity, blindness, and dementia. Patients can suffer seizures, but this is a rare symptom. Most patients die in their late teens of cachexia and pneumonia. The diagnosis is suspected on the basis of the patient's sex, the clinical features, and the presence of dermatan and heparan sulfate in the urine. Confirmation of the diagnosis is made possible by leukocyte enzyme assay, which also makes prenatal diagnosis feasible.

Intermittent Stepwise Regression

We now turn to a group of disorders of varied etiology in which metabolic stresses provoke the dramatic appearance of neurological symptoms in a child who is otherwise normal. Depending on the nature of the defect, symptom onset may vary from early infancy to adult life. In a typical scenario, an intercurrent viral infection, accident, or surgical procedure is followed by the rapid development of irritability, vomiting, lethargy, seizures, ataxia, hemiplegia, quadriparesis, nystagmus, strabismus, psychosis, and coma, in varying combinations. Such symptoms and signs may peak in a matter of hours to days. A partial or complete clinical recovery may ensue, followed by an extended period of stability, during which the patient may continue to grow and acquire new skills. Eventually (weeks, months, or even years later), another neurological crisis occurs, again triggered by some sort of stress. With each crisis, neurological deficits may accumulate to the point where the patient becomes severely disabled and markedly regressed. In some instances, particularly in later-onset disorders, there is a minimal stepwise regression and patients continue to function fairly well between the acute crises.

Table 27-5 outlines the pertinent features of some of the best-defined members of this clinical group. As can be seen, alleles of many of those disorders exhibiting rapid deterioration in infancy belong to this category, that is, amino acid and urea cycle disorders. Also included are some disorders of membranal amino acid transport, as well as a group of defects in cellular energy metabolism that may affect entry to the tricarboxylic acid cycle or the electron transport chain. As a consequence, patients with diseases in this

Table 27-4. Insidious Regression with Dysostotic Dwarfism

Disorder	Defective enzyme	Inheritance pattern	Symptom onset	Clinical features	Laboratory features
GM$_1$ gangliosidosis	β-Galactosidase	AR	Birth	Coarse facies, edema, hepatosplenomegaly, dwarfism, skeletal dysplasia, macular cherry-red spot, seizures, developmental arrest, blindness	Blood: foam cells, vacuolated lymphocytes; urine: keratan sulfate; skeletal survey: similar to Hurler's disease
Hurler's disease	α-Iduronidase	AR	6–12 mo	Nasal congestion, corneal clouding, growth failure, coarse facies, hepatosplenomegaly, mental retardation, claw hands, gibbus, kyphosis, deafness, valvular heart disease	Blood: granulated lymphocytes; urine: dermatan and heparan sulfate; skeletal survey: beaked vertebrae, widened ribs and metacarpals, J-shaped sella, occasional hydrocephalus
Hunter's syndrome	Iduronosulfate sulfatase	XR	6–12 mo	Growth failure, coarse facies, hepatosplenomegaly, retinitis pigmentosa, papilledema, gibbus, occasional seizures	Blood: granulated lymphocytes; urine: dermatan and heparan sulfate; skeletal survey: similar to Hurler's disease
Sanfilippo's syndromes A, B, C, D	A. Heparan N-sulfatase B. N-acetyl-α-glucosaminidase C. Acetyl-CoA: α-glycosaminide-N-acetyltransferase D. N-acetyl-α-D-glycosaminide-β-sulfatase	AR	1–4 yr	Mental retardation, mild skeletal dysplasia, mild coarsening of facial features, mild hepatosplenomegaly, no significant ocular involvement	Blood: granulated lymphocytes; urine: heparan sulfate; skeletal survey: mild dysostosis

Table 27-4 (Continued).

Disorder	Defective enzyme	Inheritance pattern	Symptom onset	Clinical features	Laboratory features
Sly syndrome	β-Glucuronidase	AR	Infantile to adult	Coarse facies, dwarfism, gibbus, hepatosplenomegaly, corneal clouding, chronic pneumonia, mental retardation	Blood: granulated lymphocytes; urine: heparan and dermatan sulfate; x-ray: widened tubular bones
I-Cell disease (mucolipidosis II)	UDP-GlcNAc: glycoprotein, GlcNAc.yl phosphotransferase	AR	0–3 mo	Hurler phenotype and symptomatology plus gum hyperplasia	*No elevation of urine mucopolysaccharides*, inclusions in cultivated fibroblasts
Mannosidosis Type I	α-Mannosidase	AR	6–18 mo	Severe mental retardation, coarse features, cloudy corneas, cataracts, large tongue, kyphosis, hepatosplenomegaly, deafness	Blood: vacuolated lymphocytes, granulated neutrophils; skeletal survey: widened tubular bones
Type II			5–10 yr	Deafness, mild mental retardation, mild dysostosis	
Fucosidosis	α-Fucosidase	AR	3–12 mo	Coarse facies, severe regression, hypotonia → spasticity, hepatosplenomegaly, anhydrosis, cardiomegaly, mild dysostosis	Blood: vacuolated lymphocytes, ↑ sweat electrolytes; liver biopsy: foam cells

Sialidosis type II	Sialidase	AR	Birth–20 yr	Hurler phenotype, macular cherry-red spot	Blood: vacuolated lymphocytes; urine: ↑ sialyloligosaccharides
Multiple sulfatase deficiency	Arylsulfatases A, B, C, + other sulfatases	AR	1–4 yr	Mild Hurler phenotype, features of metachromatic leukodystrophy (Table 27-3), ichthyosis	Blood: granulated neutrophils; urine: dermatan and heparan sulfate; skeletal survey: mild dysostosis, slowed nerve conduction

AR = autosomal recessive; XR = X-linked recessive; UDP-GlcNAc = uridine diphosphate-*N*-acetylglucosamine; ↑ = raised.

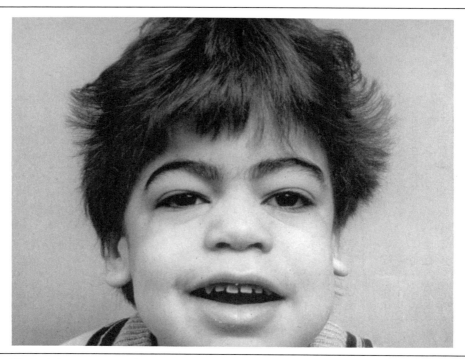

Fig. 27-5. *(A) Facial appearance of 6-year-old boy with Hunter's syndrome. Note the coarse, puffy facial features, the prominent eyebrows, and the lack of corneal clouding.*

group may exhibit varying combinations of hypoglycemia, lactic acidosis, hyperammonemia, and aminoaciduria during their neurological crises, with no apparent metabolic disturbance when they are well. Many of the potential treatments (e.g., dietary restriction) outlined for the group of disorders exhibiting a rapid deterioration in infancy also apply here.

Leigh's Disease (Subacute Necrotizing Encephalomyelopathy). Really a group of diseases possessing a similar neuropathology, Leigh's disease has a varied age of onset and a broad spectrum of symptomatology but with a number of common threads. The principal neuropathological changes consist of capillary proliferation, spongy changes in the neuropil, scattered neuronal loss, and gliosis affecting an array of structures in the central gray matter, including the putamen, caudate, globus pallidus, thalamus, subthalamic nucleus, substantia nigra, periaqueductal gray matter, oculomotor nuclei, and pontine/medullary tegmentum. Any or all of these structures may be involved in individual cases, and in varying combinations. In addition, the optic nerves, optic tracts, cerebral cortex, cerebellar nuclei, and even peripheral nerves may be affected. Symptoms characteristically begin during the first 2 years of life, often around the age of 4 to 6 months. The most common features include irregular respirations or even respiratory failure, gaze paralysis, choreoathetoid movements, dystonic quadriparesis, hypotonia, and dysphagia. Some patients become blind (with evidence of optic atrophy), suffer intractable multifocal seizures, or rapidly become comatose. Symptoms often appear very abruptly in association with febrile illnesses, followed by partial recovery and long plateau phases without further regression. Occasional patients appear hypotonic from birth, then their condition abruptly deteriorates at around 4 months of age; other patients suffer a rapid, relentless decline.

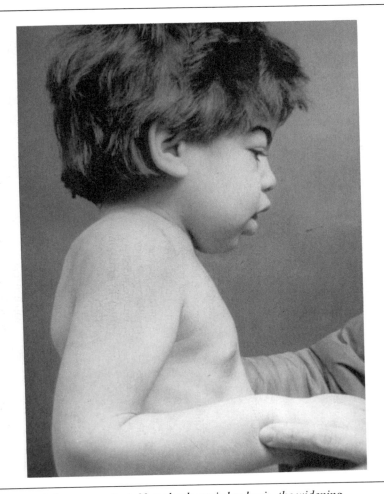

Fig. 27-5. *(B) Side view of the same patient. Note the thoracic kyphosis, the widening of the metaphysis at the wrist, and the broadened ribs.*

The diagnosis is often difficult to make on clinical grounds, and may only be revealed post mortem. In some patients, CT scanning (Fig. 27-6) or magnetic resonance imaging reveals the presence of focal abnormalities in the putamen, pallidum, thalamus, or brainstem. Metabolic acidosis with elevated lactate levels may occur during periods of acute symptomatic deterioration, but such changes are not consistent or necessary for the diagnosis. Various metabolic defects have been identified in specific cases, including a variety of deficiencies or malfunctions in the pyruvate dehydrogenase complex and in cytochrome C oxidase activity. Thus far,

all cases appear to represent autosomal recessive defects in the nuclear genome. Even though biochemically specific forms of Leigh's disease are being recognized with greater frequency, attempts to correct the defect (e.g., by the administration of cofactors) have proved ineffective.

System Degenerations

Whereas the previously discussed clinical patterns are the result of fairly widespread pathology in the nervous system, the system degenerations are characterized by degenerative changes that affect selective neuronal or

Table 27-5. Intermittent Stepwise Regression

Disorder	Defective enzyme	Inheritance pattern	Symptom onset	Clinical features	Laboratory features
Branched-chain ketoaciduria	BCKA decarboxylase	AR	Childhood	Irritability, stupor, ataxia, seizures, coma, urine odor of maple syrup during attacks, may be mentally retarded	See Table 27-1 (during acute attacks)
Propionic acidemia	Propionyl-CoA carboxylase	AR	Childhood	Anorexia, vomiting, seizures, hypotonia, spasticity, rigidity, mental retardation	See Table 27-1
Carbamoyl phosphate synthetase deficiency	Carbamoyl phosphate synthetase	AR	Childhood	Vomiting, lethargy, irritability (episodic, nonprogressive)	See Table 27-1
Ornithine transcarbamoylase deficiency	Ornithine transcarbamoylase	XD	Childhood	Vomiting, headache, lethargy, stupor, ophthalmoplegia (usually girls), may progress to mental retardation	See Table 27-1
Citrullinemia	Argininosuccinic acid synthetase	AR	Infancy to childhood	Recurrent vomiting, lethargy, ataxia, seizures; may have headaches, papilledema	Urine: ↑ orotic acid; blood: hyperammonemia during attacks
Hartnup disease	Unknown	AR	Childhood	Acute ataxia, pellagra-like rash, tremor, anxiety, psychotic symptoms, headaches; may be mentally retarded but improve with age	Urine: ↑ neutral amino acids, ↑ indoxyl sulfate, ↑ indole-3-acetate, ↑ indole-3-acrylglycine, ↑ indole-3-acetyl-L-glutamine; feces: ↑ neutral amino acids

Disease	Enzyme defect	Inheritance	Onset	Clinical features	Other findings
(Leigh's disease)	Pyruvate dehydrogenase complex; Cytochrome c oxidase, probably others	AR	Same	dysphagia, respiratory difficulties, nystagmus, ophthalmoplegia, vomiting, choreoathetosis, dystonia, ataxia, weakness, seizures, blindness plus optic atrophy, cognitive regression; some cases relentlessly progressive with intractable seizures, even though onset abrupt	generalized amino-aciduria; blood: intermittent lactic acidosis; muscle biopsy: ragged red fibers; CT scan/MRI: hypodensity or abnormal signal in caudate, putamen, globus pallidus, or midbrain
MELAS syndrome	Cytochrome c oxidase	AR	Childhood	Dwarfism, muscle weakness and wasting, retinitis pigmentosa, deafness, cardiomyopathy, recurrent strokelike episodes, seizures (intermittent)	Blood: marked lactic acidosis; muscle biopsy: ragged red fibers, myopathy; CT/MRI: multiple infarctions, vascular territories

BCKA = branched-chain ketoacids; AR = autosomal recessive; XD = X-linked dominant; MELAS = mitochondrial encephalopathy with lactic acidosis and stroke; ↑ = raised.

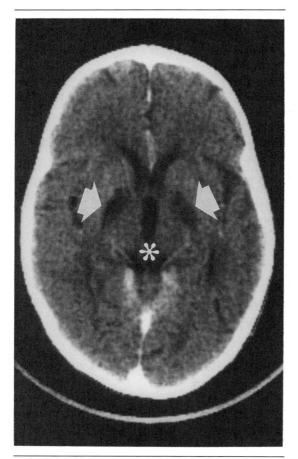

Fig. 27-6. *Contrast-enhanced axial CT scan of a 2-year-old boy with Leigh's disease. Note the bilateral hypodense lesions corresponding to the area of the globus pallidus (arrows). The caudate and putamen appear to be relatively preserved. There is enlargement of the third ventricle (star).*

glial populations, with most of the brain and spinal cord remaining more-or-less intact. The neuronal populations most often impacted are the anterior horn cells, dorsal root ganglia and posterior columns, Clarke's column and the spinocerebellar tracts, cortical Betz's cells and the corticospinal tracts, and the basal ganglia, all in varying combinations.

The system degenerations represent a very large and complex group of diseases, the most characteristic of which are considered in separate chapters. This section considers only those disorders possessing relatively well-defined metabolic or genetic defects. Because a system

degeneration (e.g., a spinocerebellar degenera tion pattern resembling Friedreich's ataxia may actually constitute a final common pathwa for a variety of inborn metabolic errors, an e: tensive search for a specific enzymatic def ciency is mandatory in each case.

Table 27-6 summarizes the key features c some of the principal disorders in this grouț Alleles of many specific enzyme defects in thos disorders typified by insidious regression reap pear in the system degenerations group. Th example given, however, is a distinctive meta bolic system degeneration that has no know parallel in the other clinical categories.

Wilson's Disease. More common than prϵ viously realized, Wilson's disease represents a autosomal recessive error in copper metabolisɪ that is associated with hepatic cirrhosis and de generative changes in the basal ganglia. A though the precise enzyme defect responsibl for the disorder remains to be identified, th best evidence suggests that there is a primar defect in the biliary excretion of copper leadin to the gradual accumulation of copper in th liver and secondary hepatocellular damage This, in turn, brings about diminished produc tion of copper transport protein (ceruloplas min), high levels of unbound cupric ion in th blood, and the deposition of large quantities c copper in the kidney, basal ganglia, and cornea Pathologically, there are postnecrotic cirrhosi of the liver, degeneration of the renal tubula epithelial cells, spongy degeneration of th basal ganglia with large numbers of protoplas mic astrocytes, and granular clumping of coppe in the endothelial surface of Descemet's mem brane (cornea). On electron micrographs, cop per may be seen bound to hepatic mitochondri and sequestered in lysosomes; in the brain, thϵ copper is deposited primarily in astrocytes anϵ the pericapillary region (i.e., not neurons).

Although some patients present with a rapiϵ onset of hepatic failure in early childhood, thϵ typical neurological manifestations begiɪ around the age of 10 to 12 years and compris a slowly progressive dysarthria and dysphagia emotional lability sometimes merging with ϵ frank psychosis, a characteristic dystonic griɪ with a masklike facies, a flapping tremor of thϵ

Table 27-6. System Degenerations

Disorder	Defective enzyme	Inheritance pattern	Symptom onset	Clinical features	Laboratory features
GM$_1$ gangliosidosis	β-Galactosidase	AR	Childhood to adult	Progressive dystonia or ataxia, incoordination, dyarthria; no organomegaly	Findings as in Table 27-4, but less severe
GM$_2$ gangliosidosis	Hexosaminidase	AR	Childhood to adult	Spinocerebellar degeneration and motor neuron disease patterns; no visual loss; May have mild mental changes	Specific leukocyte enzyme assay required
Niemann-Pick disease (types C, D)	Sphingomyelinase, ?alleles	AR	2–4 yr	Ataxia, seizures, macular cherry-red spot, mild hepatosplenomegaly	As in Table 27-3; sea-blue histiocytes in bone marrow, spleen; liver: cholesterol accumulation (type D)
			6–14 yr	Progressive dystonia, dysarthria, ↓ upward gaze, hepatosplenomegaly, seizures	
Fabry's disease	α-Galactosidase A	XD	Late childhood to adult	Burning pain in feet, legs, fingers; punctate angiomatous papules on genitalia, abdomen; corneal opacities; renal failure	EKG: ↓ PR interval; skin biopsy: lipid inclusions; nerve biopsy: axonal swelling, inclusions in fibroblasts
Refsum disease	Phytanic acid oxidase	AR	4 yr to adult	Progressive polyneuropathy, ataxia, retinitis pigmentosa, hearing loss, ichthyosis	Slowed nerve conductions; ↑ CSF protein; EKG: widened QT, prolonged QRS

Table 27-6 (Continued).

Disorder	Defective enzyme	Inheritance pattern	Symptom onset	Clinical features	Laboratory features
Wilson's disease	Unknown	AR	Early childhood to adult	Acute hepatic failure in childhood; dysarthria, dysphagia, dystonia, tremor, rigidity, bradykinesia, Kayser-Fleischer rings	Blood: ↑ serum copper, ↓ ceruloplasmin; urine: aminoaciduria; CT scan/MRI: hypodensity or ↑ signal basal ganglia, thalamus
Lesch-Nyhan syndrome	Hypoxanthine-guanine phosphoribosyl transferase	XR	Infancy	Vomiting, choreoathetosis, self-mutilation, dystonia, seizures ± mental retardation, renal failure, gout	Blood: ↑ uric acid; urine: ↑ uric acid/creatinine ratio
Bassen-Kornzweig syndrome	Unknown	AR	Infancy	Malabsorption syndrome in infancy → progressive spinocerebellar ataxia; ± → visual acuity, night blindness, mental retardation	Blood: acanthocytosis, ↓ ↓ cholesterol, ↓ serum triglycerides, absent β-lipoproteins, → vitamin E levels, ERG abnormal
Cerebrotendinous xanthomatosis	Unknown	AR	Childhood to adult	Progressive tonsillar hypertrophy, retinitis pigmentosa, peripheral neuropathy (sensorimotor)	Blood: absent high-density lipoproteins, ↓ cholesterol; tonsils: storage of cholesterol esters; nerve biopsy: axonal loss, ↑ lipids in Schwann cells

AR = autosomal recessive; XD = X-linked dominant; XR = X-linked recessive; ERG = electroretinogram; ↓ = lowered; ↑ = raised.

mbs, generalized rigidity, and bradykinesia. The diagnosis is strongly supported by the findings of copper storage in the cornea on slit-lamp examination (the Kayser-Fleischer ring) nd generalized aminoaciduria, together with ow serum ceruloplasmin and high serum copper levels. Early diagnosis is crucial, as progresion of the hepatic and neurological features may be halted (with some attendant clinical recovery) by the use of copper-chelating drugs uch as penicillamine.

Diagnostic Tools

Even though the inherited metabolic neurological disorders are enormously complex and varied, accurate diagnosis can usually be made based on a characteristic clinical pattern and the results of a fairly small number of tests. Most of these tests are listed in the tables that summarize the various clinical patterns. As a cross-reference, the most useful blood, urine, CSF, radiological, and electrophysiological tests are summarized in Table 27-7. This table does not include specific enzymatic assays on cultured leukocytes or fibroblasts, however, as these investigations are not widely available and are only carried out when there is a high suspicion of a particular diagnosis.

Therapeutic Possibilities

A number of different treatment modalities for inherited metabolic defects have been mentioned in the tables summarizing the clinical patterns. The underlying strategies for these therapies fall into four main groups.

Reduce Intake of Substrate

By far the most widely used approach to the treatment of metabolic defects, dietary modifications that reduce the intake of the unmetabolized compound, or compounds, are particularly effective when the offending compound cannot be synthesized by body tissues. Examples of this method include the restriction of phenylalanine for phenylketonuria, branched-chain amino acids for maple-syrup urine disease (even for parenteral nutrition in comatose patients), and phytanic acid for Refsum disease. For other diseases, dietary approaches (e.g., decreased very-long-chain fatty acid intake and erucic acid supplementation for adrenoleukodystrophy) show promise, but further modifications of the treatment methods are probably required.

Enhance Elimination of Substrate

Enhancing the elimination of substrate is particularly useful when dietary restriction is impractical, or when the substrate can be synthesized within the body. Reference has already been made to augmenting copper excretion in Wilson's disease by administering chelating agents. Other examples, although less successful, include the use of sodium benzoate in the treatment of nonketotic hyperglycinemia, which converts excess glycine to hippurate, and alpha-ketoanalogues of branched-chain amino acids in the treatment of hyperammonemic disorders, which promotes inclusion of excess ammonia into excretable amino acids through the process of transamination.

Use of Cofactors to Help Push the Blocked Reaction to the Right

Pharmacological doses of reaction-specific cofactors (usually vitamins) may enhance the effective activity of remaining or defective enzymes such that the accumulation of substrate drops below the neurotoxic level. Examples of this approach include the use of cyanocobalamin (vitamin B_{12}) to enhance the activity of methylmalonyl-CoA mutase in patients with methylmalonic aciduria and the possible use of biotin to enhance the activity of propionyl-CoA carboxylase in some cases of propionic acidemia. For some disorders, the use of cofactors remains more of a theoretical possibility than a practical reality (e.g., the use of coenzyme Q in the treatment of mitochondrial encephalopathies).

Attempted Blockage of Brain Receptors to Neurotoxic Molecules

A very modest success has been achieved in cases of nonketotic hyperglycinemia through the use of strychnine to block spinal cord glycine receptors.

Enzyme Replacement

Although enzyme replacement would seem to be an obvious treatment modality on theoretical

Table 27-7. Screening Tests for Metabolic Disorders of the Nervous System

Diagnostic test	Disorder(s) in which test may be useful
Urine	
Ferric chloride	PKU, BCKAuria, propionic acidemia, methylmalonic aciduria
(Dinitrophenyl hydrazine)	PKU, BCKAuria, propionic acidemia, methylmalonic aciduria, glutaric aciduria
Benedict's	Galactosemia, hereditary fructose intolerance
Nitroprusside	Homocystinuria, glutathionuria, cystinuria
Acid albumin	GM₁ gangliosidosis, Hurler, Hunter, Sanfilippo, Sly, multiple sulfatase
Amino acid chromatography	Most disorders of amino acid metabolism, Hartnup, Wilson, Leigh
Organic acid chromatography	BCKAuria, isovaleric acidemia, propionic acidemia, methylmalonic acidemia, glutaric aciduria
Blood	
↓ Glucose, fasting	BCKAuria, propionic acidemia, methylmalonic aciduria, galactosemia, hereditary fructose intolerance, glycogen storage disorders
↑ Lactate	Leigh, MELAS syndrome
Venous gases (↓ pH)	BCKAuria, isovaleric acidemia, propionic acidemia, methylmalonic aciduria, carbamoyl phosphate synthetase deficiency, Leigh and MELAS syndromes
↑ Ammonia	Propionic acidemia, methylmalonic aciduria, CPS def., OTC def., citrullinemia, argininosuccinic aciduria
Amino acids	Most disorders of amino acid metabolism
CSF	
↑ protein	Krabbe, metachromatic leukodystrophy, Refsum
↑ glycine	Nonketotic hyperglycinemia
Skeletal survey	GM₁ gangliosidosis, Hurler, Hunter, Sanfilippo, Sly, I-cell disease, mannosidosis, fucosidosis, sialidosis type II, multiple sulfatase
Nerve conduction studies	Krabbe, metachromatic leukodystrophy, infantile neuroaxonal dystrophy, Refsum
Bone marrow aspirate	Niemann-Pick, Gaucher, GM₁ gangliosidosis
EEG	Santavuori-Haltia, Bielschowsky, Batten, Lafora, Rett
EKG	MELAS syndrome, Fabry, Refsum

PKU = phenylketonuria; BCKAuria = branched-chain ketoaciduria (maple-syrup urine disease); MELAS = mitochondrial encephalopathy with lactic acidosis and stroke; CPS def. = carbamoyl phosphate synthetase deficiency; OTC def. = ornithine transcarbamoylase deficiency; ↓ = lowered; ↑ = raised.

grounds, its practical applications are extremely limited, largely due to the problem of the immune reactions to parenterally administered enzyme and the difficulty of getting even purified human enzymes past the blood-brain barrier. Partial success has been achieved in some storage diseases (e.g., metachromatic leukodystrophy), with enzyme replacement accomplished through bone marrow transplant using tissue from a metabolically normal donor.

DEVELOPMENTAL DISORDERS OF THE NERVOUS SYSTEM

Basic Mechanisms

The normal process of brain and spinal cord development is extremely complex and poorly understood; we can only begin to guess at some of the fundamental mechanisms involved

Much of what is known of these mechanisms has been derived from the careful study of children with specific developmental disorders of the nervous system, and from the experimental manipulation of developmental processes in non-human animal species.

Human central nervous system development follows an ordered sequence, with a number of different processes occurring in series, and sometimes also in parallel. These developmental stages do not happen simultaneously everywhere in the nervous system; the cerebral cortex may have reached one stage in the rolandic area while the evolving frontal and occipital poles are still passing through an earlier phase. Thus a specifically timed teratogenic insult may lead to different patterns of malformation in different brain areas, depending on the developmental stage achieved in a given area. Acknowledging that there is considerable overlap temporally and spatially among them, the principal stages of nervous system development are as follows:

Dorsal Induction

The first stage of neural development, dorsal induction, takes place during the third and fourth weeks of embryonic life. After the dorsal thickening of the primitive neural plate, the ectodermal layer begins to infold to form the neural tube. Tube closure begins in the putative thoracic region and proceeds rostrally and caudally to form the brain and lumbosacral spinal cord, respectively.

Ventral Induction

At 5 to 6 weeks' gestation, the rostral pole of the neural tube divides into two telencephalic vesicles to become the embryonic cerebral hemispheres. Optic vesicles bud from the ventral aspect of the telencephalon to form the optic nerves and retina; these structures and the primitive olfactory apparatus participate in the induction of the eyes, nose, and related facial structures.

Neuronal Proliferation

From 2 to 4 months' gestation, primitive neural stem cells in the subependymal region differentiate into neuronal and glial lines, undergo rapid mitosis, and form dense germinal zones. Primitive glial cells establish footplates on the ependymal and pial surfaces, respectively, and begin to elongate into radial glia.

Neuronal Migration

In parallel with proliferation, primitive neurons attach themselves to radial glial processes and begin to migrate away from the subependymal area to the pial area to form the cortical plate. Successive waves of neurons migrate during the third to fifth month of gestation (and, to some extent, later) to form the cerebral cortex in an inside-out sequence. The same process also leads to the formation of the basal ganglia, thalami, and cerebellar nuclei, among other structures.

Neuronal Organization

Also in parallel with migration, neuronal organization includes the differentiation of neuronal and glial subtypes, axonal growth and the formation of tracts (including the cerebral commissures), dendritic proliferation, and synaptic bud maturation. This process continues throughout the rest of gestation and well into postnatal life.

Myelination

Beginning in the third trimester in the human, the process of oligodendroglial differentiation and axonal myelination starts in the spinal cord and proceeds rostrally in an orderly fashion to include brainstem tracts, internal capsules, optic nerves, the centrum semiovale, and subcortical U fibers. The velocity of intracortical myelination peaks around the ages of 2 to 5 years and continues (along with synaptic differentiation) into adult life.

Preprogrammed Cell Death and Axonal Pruning

Although the true significance of preprogrammed cell death and axonal pruning is just beginning to be appreciated, it is clear that a considerable amount of "remodeling" of the brain goes on throughout the other developmental stages already discussed. Many neuronal populations are generated in excess of what is ultimately required, then thinned out by selective "normal" cell death. Normal cortical volumetric asymmetries, such as the smaller area of the right planum temporale (in 65% of human brains), are a proposed example of such neuronal pruning. The failure to phase out pre-programmed cell death may explain the progressive loss of anterior horn cells seen in infantile spinal muscular atrophy.

Although most of the developmental mechanism involved in this sequence remain obscure, a number of quite disparate fundamental processes are beginning to emerge, disturbances of which can lead to an astonishingly varied array of developmental anomalies.

A cellular **biochemical milieu** appropriate for normal synthetic processes is obviously important for brain growth and development. As already noted in the first section of this chapter, enzymatic defects in normal amino acid, carbohydrate, and ammonia metabolism (to name a few) may severely disrupt neuronal organization and myelination. Excessive levels of enzyme may also interfere with brain development. For example, an extra copy of the superoxide dismutase gene in trisomy 21 (Down syndrome) appears to be responsible for the phenomenon of lipoperoxidation and altered membrane phospholipid content, with its various potential secondary effects on cell–cell interactions and on neuronal and glial maturation. The global absence of peroxisomal enzymes has already been linked with the neuronal migrational abnormalities seen in Zellweger syndrome.

In a related sphere, alterations in the normal **nutritional and environmental milieu** may result in abnormal nervous system development. A state of folate deficiency around the time of conception has been proposed on statistical grounds as a contributing factor in the production of spinal dysraphic states. So, too, has the maternal ingestion of valproic acid and ethanol.

Growth factors of various types (e.g., nerve growth factor) are being appreciated as vital to normal proliferative processes in brain development. The low production of growth factors may be at least partly responsible for the impaired development and maintenance of cholinergic neurons in Down syndrome. Excessive production of growth factors has been impli-

cated in disorders of neuronal and glial proliferation such as neurofibromatosis.

Cellular adhesion molecules are being increasingly identified as crucial to normal processes of brain differentiation such as neuronal migration. Various cellular and substrate adhesion molecules are expressed on neuronal and glial membranes at specific stages of brain maturation. What is intriguing about cell and substrate adhesion molecules is their close structural homology with antibody molecules, suggesting that circulating antibodies (e.g., maternally derived ones) might selectively interfere with specific adhesion molecules and, thus, with morphogenesis. Support for immune based causes of abnormal brain development comes from animal experiments; exposure of developing cerebellar cortical cultures to antibodies directed against the neural-glial cell–adhesion molecule impairs inward migration of cerebellar granule cells.

Finally, the integrity of the **vascular supply** is clearly important for normal brain maturation. Cerebrovascular occlusions in early pregnancy have been associated with areas of schizencephaly and porencephaly, malformations often containing regions of polymicrogyria, neuronal heterotopias, and other disturbances in neuronal migration.

Clinical Examples

Unlike the inherited metabolic defects, developmental disorders of the nervous system do not easily lend themselves to categorization according to their pattern of clinical presentation. The general lack of precise information about their respective pathogeneses also makes classification by metabolic pathway impractical. Instead, a descriptive approach will be used to present a few characteristic examples of developmental disorders that illustrate morphogenetic defects incurred at different stages of brain development.

Myelomeningocele. Along with anencephaly, myelomeningocele is one of the most common forms of a neurulation defect; in this disorder, the primary problem appears to be failed closure of the caudal end of the neural tube. The etiology is probably multifactorial with hereditary, nutritional, and possibly teratogenic factors playing a role. In this anomaly, the lower end of the spinal canal remains open, or is partially covered by skin and meninges; the lumbosacral spinal cord and associated nerve roots are often malformed and dysfunctional. Affected babies are almost invariably born with additional defects, the most important of which is a type II Arnold-Chiari malformation of the posterior fossa, consisting of the downward displacement of the cerebellar vermis and medulla, distortion of the fourth ventricle, hydrocephalus, and sometimes any or all of the following abnormalities: syringomyelia, syringobulbia, aqueductal stenosis, and polymicrogyria. Figure 27-7A shows a typical lumbosacral myelomeningocele prior to surgical repair; Figure 27-7B is an MRI portrayal of a type II Arnold-Chiari malformation.

The degree of the clinical disability obviously depends on the rostral extent of the neurulation defect. Meningeal sacs that are confined to the L3–L5 level permit considerable retention of motor and sensory function in the legs. Such patients are therefore incontinent of urine and have significant proximal and distal muscle weakness but are nevertheless able to walk independently. Patients with defects extending into the lower thoracic spine are profoundly paraplegic and suffer significant flexion spinal deformities.

Although neurosurgical, orthopedic, and urological interventions can prolong survival and promote some degree of independent living, the most effective treatment for this disorder remains prevention. Because of the leakage of the fetal glycoprotein, alpha-fetoprotein, from blood vessels within the open defect into the amniotic sac, early amniocentesis can be used to diagnose neural tube defects. The location and extent of the defect may then be confirmed by ultrasound examination. The possibility that gestational folate deficiency may play a pathogenetic role has prompted the use of folate supplementation prior to conception in at-risk women, but the effectiveness of such treatment is still unclear.

Down Syndrome (Trisomy 21). One of the best known and intensively studied disorders causing mental retardation, Down syndrome is still very imperfectly understood. The presence of an extra chromosome 21, either in whole or in part, implies excessive activity of a large number of (triplicated) genes, but the connection between this distortion of the nuclear genome and the array of neural and nonneural anomalies that characterize Down syndrome remains almost entirely conjectural. Some progress in deciphering the pathogenesis of this disorder may come from the intensive study of the trisomy-16 mouse, an animal model that shares many features with human trisomy 21. The mouse chromosome 16 contains, for example, the same superoxide dismutase gene that possibly plays a key role in causing certain types of aberrant nervous system development.

The characteristic facial and limb features of patients with Down syndrome are well known, and consist of almond-shaped, slanted palpebral fissures, a round face, Brushfield's spots on the iris, a fissured tongue, brachycephaly, transverse palmar creases, and short stubby digits. The other most characteristic nonneurological anomalies include duodenal atresia, an atrioventricular septal defect, and congenital hypothyroidism. From the neurological perspective, the most obvious problem is the impaired mental function that can vary from a profound retardation to near normal. Other neurological features include a characteristic oral-facial-lingual dyskinesia, severe hypotonia, a high incidence of sensorineural hearing loss, autistic features, seizures including infantile spasms, and the almost inevitable eventual appearance of Alzheimer's dementia.

A number of neuropathological findings are encountered in patients with Down syndrome, although few are really specific to the disorder. The brain, particularly the superior temporal gyrus, is characteristically small, possibly reflecting an impairment in neuronal or glial proliferation, or both. At a more basic, neurobiological level, Golgi staining of brain tissue from Down syndrome patients has disclosed a relative lack of production of aspiny neurons. There is also recent evidence that suggests progressive dendritic atrophy takes place in early childhood. The brains from older patients also show many Alzheimer-type plaques and neuro-

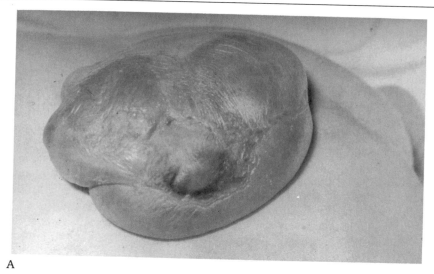

A

B

Fig. 27-7. *(A) Dorsal view of the lumbosacral area of a neonate with a large meningomyelocele with a closed membranous sac. The infant's head is to the left. (B)* T_1-*weighted MRI scan of an infant with a meningomyelocele (not shown) and associated Arnold-Chiari malformation (parasagittal section). Note the downward hernation of the cerebellum through the foramen magnum* (white arrow) *and the compression and distortion of the fourth ventricle* (black arrowhead). *Although not well-demonstrated in this section, the MRI scan also showed agenesis of the posterior portion of the corpus callosum and associated gyral abnormalities* (star).

fibrillary tangles. Current evidence suggests, therefore, that brain maturation in Down syndrome is disturbed at several different stages, the most important of which are neuronal proliferation, differentiation, and organization.

There is usually little difficulty in clinically

diagnosing trisomy 21 at birth, although diagnosis in mosaic patients with cellular mixtures of 46 and 47 chromosomes may prove more difficult. Many cases are diagnosed in utero by amniocentesis in women known to be at risk. Unfortunately, the persistent lack of precise information about the pathogenesis of the clinical features means that rational forms of treatment do not yet exist.

Tuberous Sclerosis and Neurofibromatosis.

We now turn to two classic examples of what are often referred to as the *phakomatoses*—developmental brain disorders that are accompanied by parallel disturbances in the differentiation of other tissues of ectodermal and mesodermal origin (e.g., heart, blood vessels, liver, kidney, and bones). The actual term *phakomatosis* (*phakos*, meaning "birthmark") was inspired by the presence of retinal hamartomas of various types that are frequently noted in this group of disorders. Although the pathogenesis of the phakomatoses is unknown, one must presume (for each type) the existence of a specific aberration of normal tissue growth and differentiation, which produces ostensibly different pathological changes in different tissues. The most common phakomatoses are neurofibromatosis, the Sturge-Weber syndrome, (Fig. 27-8), von Hippel–Lindau disease, and tuberous sclerosis. Tuberous sclerosis causes the most widespread and severe neurological manifestations.

Tuberous Sclerosis.

An autosomal dominant condition with a high mutation rate and variable expressivity, tuberous sclerosis has protean manifestations. In the most characteristic clinical presentation, infantile spasms and hypomelanotic skin macules start to appear around 6 months of age, with the patient going on to suffer severe mental retardation. Other clinical features that may appear include multiple round retinal hamartomas, adenoma sebaceum (angiofibromas) in the malar area, periungual fibromas, cardiac rhabdomyomas, shagreen patches (raised skin lesions with the texture of an orange peel), renal angiomyolipomas, and hamartomas of the liver and lung. In some patients, seizures do not appear early in life; instead these patients develop normally and only later present with the typical facial and skin lesions (Fig. 27-9), or even with an isolated cerebral giant-cell astrocytoma. When seizures do develop after infancy, they are usually the generalized tonic-clonic type.

Because tuberous sclerosis is so common, the unexplained development of seizures in a young child, particularly infantile spasms, should always prompt a search for hypomelanotic skin macules, or the so-called ash-leaf spots.

Hamartomatous lesions or tubers scattered throughout the cerebral cortex with intervening normal areas constitute the characteristic neuropathological finding in tuberous sclerosis. The cortical neuronal architecture is grossly disturbed within the tubers. Loose clusters of neurons and glia may be intermixed with groups of giant cells that are shown to contain eosinophilic cytoplasm on standard hematoxylin-eosin–stained preparations. These giant cells are the microscopic signature of tuberous sclerosis, and their features are encountered in cells of both neuronal and glial origin. They stain positively using immunoperoxidase methods that employ antiserum to neuronal-specific enolase. On electronmicrographs, the giant cells are found to possess giant multipolar processes containing glial filaments, glycogen, and membrane-bound dense bodies—all suggestive of partial differentiation inclining in the glial direction. These same cells, on the other hand, may develop atypical synaptic structures at some cell–cell contact points. Those cells within tubers that seem to be more typically neuronal are actually found to possess fairly primitive differentiation on Golgi-stained preparations.

The giant cells of tuberous sclerosis are also the predominant cell type contained in the subependymal nodules also characteristic of this disease. Unlike the cortical lesions, the subependymal hamartomas have a tendency to calcify; some may also enlarge and create giant-cell "astrocytic" tumors that then occlude the foramen of Monro, with resulting unilateral hydrocephalus.

Available evidence suggests, therefore, that the tuberous sclerosis gene causes a multifocal disturbance in neuronal–glial cell differentiation and an arrest in neuronal maturation.

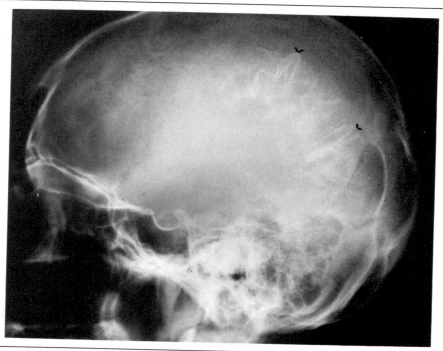

Fig. 27-8. *An 18-year-old man with Sturge-Weber syndrome (portwine stain in the trigeminal distribution, epilepsy, and leptomeningeal vascular malformation). (A) Skull x-ray study showing characteristic "tram-track" calcifications* (arrowheads) *in the cortical gyri underlying the vascular anomaly.*

There is also an abnormal proliferation of an intermediate neuronal–glial cell type, presumably related to the abnormal proliferation of mesodermal cell types in the angiofibromas, subungual fibromas, and angiomyolipomas.

The diagnosis of tuberous sclerosis is prompted largely by a strong clinical suspicion arising from the finding of hypomelanotic skin macules in an infant or child with epileptic seizures. It may then be confirmed by CT or MRI scans of the head. Figure 27-10 shows the typical CT finding of multiple small calcified nodules scattered throughout the cerebral hemispheres, particularly in the subependymal region.

Although the precise neurobiological defect responsible for tuberous sclerosis is unknown, and no specific treatment is possible, some of the manifestations of the disease can be treated. Infantile spasms, with their associated hypsarrhythmic EEG pattern, may respond well to treatment with ACTH, prednisone, or various benzodiazepines. Cardiac and renal tumors can sometimes be surgically removed when the space-occupying effect of the tumor compromises function of the organ involved. Finally, hydrocephalus resulting from the occlusion of the CSF pathways by subependymal tumors may be treated either by CSF shunting or by removal of the tumor.

Neurofibromatosis. Neurofibromatosis is one of the most common genetic diseases, with an incidence of about 1 per 4000. The two major forms of neurofibromatosis now recognized are NF-1 and NF-2, with some authors distinguishing up to eight clinical variants. NF-1, which is an autosomal dominant trait, shows 100 percent penetrance but a markedly variable expressivity. There is a high mutation rate, with about half the cases appearing sporadically. There is a possibility of genetic heterogeneity among

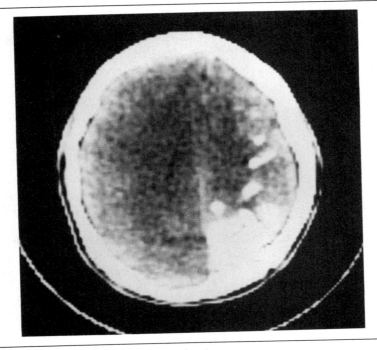

Fig. 27-8. *(B) CT scan showing the abnormal calcifications.*

Fig. 27-9. *Close-up photograph of a depigmented skin lesion in the right posterior thoracolumbar region of a school-aged child with tuberous sclerosis. Note the two small depigmented macules below and to the right of the large lesion.*

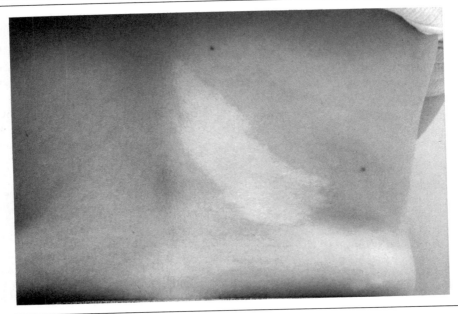

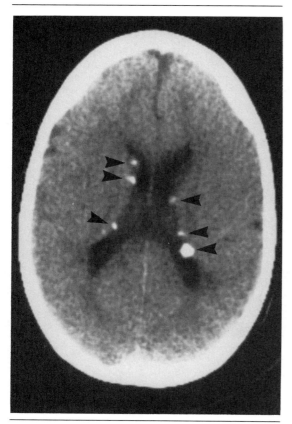

Fig. 27-10. *Unenhanced axial CT scan from a 3-year-old boy with tuberous sclerosis who had presented in infancy with infantile spasms, cardiac rhabdomyoma, and multiple renal cysts. Note the multiple hyperdense periventricular lesions* (arrowheads) *typical of the disease.*

families. The abnormal gene has now been localized to chromosome 17.

The diagnostic criteria for NF-1 have recently been formulated by an NIH consensus conference, and consist of:

1. Six or more café-au-lait macules greater than 5 mm in diameter in prepubertal individuals, or greater than 15 mm in diameter in postpubertal individuals (Fig. 27-11)
2. Two or more neurofibromas of any type or one plexiform neurofibroma
3. Axillary or inguinal freckling
4. Optic glioma
5. Two or more iris hamartomas (Lisch nodules)
6. A distinctive osseous lesion, such as sphenoid dysplasia or thinning of long-bone cortex, with or without pseudoarthrosis
7. A first-degree relative with NF-1 according to the preceding criteria

The diagnosis is based on the presence of two or more of these criteria. The disease is progressive and manifestations may become more apparent with age. Café-au-lait spots are usually present before age 2. Lisch nodules may be apparent only on slit-lamp examination. The cutaneous neurofibromata are widely variable in size and extent. A giant plexiform neurofibroma may cause considerable disfigurement, and the sarcomatous transformation of tumors can occur rarely. Neurofibromas or schwannomas may be found on cranial nerve V (intracranially or extracranially), the extracranial vagus nerve, spinal roots or ganglia, major plexuses, peripheral nerves of variable size, autonomic nerves, and visceral nerves and plexuses. Optic gliomas (pilocytic astrocytomas), which can be an associated finding, may cause visual loss in children and are best detected by MRI. Occasionally the optic foramina may be enlarged but without an optic glioma. Astrocytomas may develop in deep cerebral structures or in the posterior fossa. Pheochromocytomas form with increased frequency. Excessive norepinephrine production may also result from the formation of large cervical neurofibromata.

Kyphoscoliosis is a common problem. Secondary deficits may stem from the compression of various structures such as the spinal cord by adjacent neurofibromata. A concurrent aqueductal stenosis may occasionally lead to hydrocephalus in early life. Patients may often have a large head (macrocephaly) as an associated developmental abnormality. Dysplasia of the sphenoid wing can produce a pulsating exophthalmos.

Functional deficits in this disorder arise from the direct effects of neurofibromata such as pain, disfigurement, and segmental weakness; from the attendant cerebral developmental abnormalities (mental retardation in 8%, learning disabilities in 40%, and seizures in 5%); as the result of neoplasms of the central nervous system and internal organs; and from the psychosocial con-

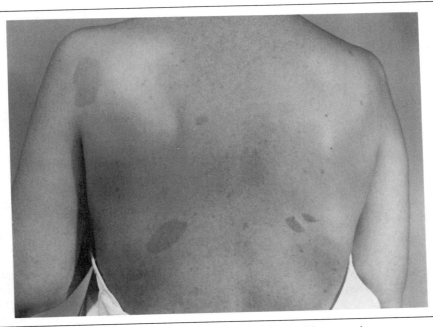

Fig. 27-11. *Typical café-au-lait spots on the back of a patient with neurofibromatosis type 1.*

sequences of what is often a disfiguring illness. Management is based on surgical treatment, when necessary, for cosmetic or other reasons, the symptomatic treatment of headaches and seizures, and other such problems, and screening for neoplasms by MRI. The Neurofibromatosis Foundation and its local chapters can furnish information and psychological support.

NF-2, or the "central" form of the disease, is genetically distinct from NF-1 and arises from a defective gene on chromosome 22. This form of the disease is much rarer than NF-1. In it, the skin lesions tend to be insignificant and it usually presents in the third or fourth decade. The hallmark of the condition in at least 90 percent of the cases is bilateral acoustic neuromas (see Fig. 20-13). The finding of posterior subcapsular cataracts, wedge-shaped cataracts in young patients, or epiretinal membranes should alert the opthalmologist to the possibility of this condition. Spinal and intracranial meningiomas and ependymomas are also seen in affected patients. Various methods of detection, such as MRI scanning, auditory evoked potentials, and vestibular testing, have been used to screen individuals at risk, since early surgical removal of an acoustic

neuroma offers a much better chance for the preservation of hearing.

BIBLIOGRAPHY

Adams, R. D., and Lyon, G. *Neurology of Hereditary Metabolic Diseases in Children.* New York: McGraw-Hill, 1982, Pp. 6–8.

Ampola, M. G., et al. Prenatal therapy of a patient with vitamin B_{12} responsive methylmalonic acidemia. *N. Engl. J. Med.* 293:313–317, 1975.

Balazs, R., and Brookbank, B. W. L. Certain Neurochemical Aspects of the Pathogenesis of Down Syndrome. In C.J. Epstein (editor). *The Neurobiology of Down Syndrome.* New York: Raven, 1986, Pp. 59–72.

Batshaw, M. L., Brusilow, S., and Walser, M. Long-term management of a case of carbamyl phosphate synthetase deficiency using ketoanalogues and hydroxyanalogues of essential amino acids. *Pediatrics* 58:227–235, 1976.

Becker, L. E., Armstrong, D.L., and Chan,

F. Dendritic atrophy in children with Down's syndrome. *Ann. Neurol.* 20:520–526, 1986.

Brown, E. W., et al. MR imaging of optic pathways in patients with neurofibromatosis. *AJNR* 8:1031–1036, 1987.

Centers for Disease Control. Valpoic acid in pregnancy—association with spina bifida: a preliminary report. *Clin. Pediatr.* 22:336–337, 1983.

Chatel, P. Dévelopement de l'isocortex du cerveau humain pendant les périodes embryonnaires et foetales jusqua'à la 24ième semaine de gestation. *J. Hirnforsch.* 17:189–212, 1976.

Dekaban, A. Large defects in cerebral hemispheres associated with cortical dysgenesis. *J. Neuropathol. Exp. Neurol.* 24:512–530, 1965.

Dimauro, S., et al. Cytochrome c oxidase deficiency in Leigh syndrome. *Ann. Neurol.* 22:498–506, 1987.

Dimauro, S., et al. Mitochondrial encephalomyopathies. *Neurol. Clin.* 8:483–506, 1990.

Dyken, P. R. The neuronal ceroid lipofuscinoses. *J. Child. Neurol.* 4:165–174, 1989.

Edelman, G. Topobiology. *Sci. Am.* 260:76–88, 1989.

Evrard, P., et al. The mechanism of arrest of neuronal migration in the Zellweger malformation: an hypothesis based upon cytoarchitectonic analysis. *Acta Neuropathol.* (Berl.) 41:109–117, 1982.

Fisher, D. A. Thyroid Function in the Fetus. In D. A. Fischer and G.N. Burrow (editors). *Perinatal Thyroid Physiology and Disease.* New York: Raven, 1978, P. 21.

Galaburda, A. Clinical Studies of Developmental and Acquired Neurobehavioral Disorders and Their Possible Immunologic Bases. In C. W. Cotman, et al. (editors). *The Neuro-Immune-Endocrine Connection.* New York: Raven, 1987, Pp. 117–144.

Goldstein, H. R., and Arulanantham, K. Neural tube defect and renal anomalies in a child with fetal alcohol syndrome. *J. Pediatr.* 93:636–637, 1978.

Harker, L. A., et al. Homocystinemia. Vascular injury and arterial thrombosis. *N. Engl. J. Med.* 291:537–543, 1974.

Huson, S., Jones, D., and Beck, L. Ophthalmic manifestations of neurofibromatosis. *Br. J. Opthalmol.* 71:235–238, 1987.

Huttenlocher, P. R. Tuberous sclerosis. *Recent Adv. Clin. Neurol.* 4:281–298, 1984.

Huttenlocher, P. R., and Heydemann, P.T. Fine structure of cortical tubers in tuberous sclerosis: a Golgi study. *Ann. Neurol.* 16:595–602, 1984.

Kissel, J. T., et al. Magnetic resonance imaging in a case of autopsy-proven adult subacute necrotizing encephalomyelopathy (Leigh's disease). *Arch. Neurol.* 44:563–566, 1987.

Kretzschmar, H. A., et al. Pyruvate dehydrogenase complex deficiency as a cause of subacute necrotizing encephalopathy (Leigh disease). *Pediatrics* 79:370–373, 1987.

Krieger, I., Winbaum, E. S., and Eisenbrey, A. B. Cerebrospinal fluid glycine in non-ketotic hyperglycinemia: effect of treatment with sodium benzoate and a ventricular shunt metabolism. *Metabolism* 26:517–524, 1977.

Krivit, W., et al. Treatment of late infantile metachromatic leukodystrophy by bone marrow transplantation. *N. Engl. J. Med.* 322:28–32, 1990.

Lindner, J., et al. Experimental modification of postnatal cerebellar granule cell migration in vitro. *Brain Res.* 377:298–304, 1986.

Liptak, G. S., et al. The management of children with spinal dysraphism. *J. Child Neurol.* 3:3–20, 1988.

Lott, I. T. The Neurology of Down Syndrome. In C. J. Epstein (editor). *The Neurology of Down Syndrome.* New York: Raven, 1986, Pp. 17–28.

MacDermot, K. D. et al. Attempts at use of strychnine sulfate in the treatment of nonketotic hyperglycinemia. *Pediatrics* 65:61–64, 1980.

McManaman, J. L., et al. Cholinergic Neurotrophic Factors. In C. J. Epstein (editor). *The Neurobiology of Down Syndrome.* New York: Raven, 1986, Pp. 179–193.

Mulvihill, J. J. Neurofibromatosis 1 (Recklinghausen disease) and neurofibromatosis 2 (bilateral acoustic neuromatosis). An update. *Ann. Intern. Med.* 113:39–52, 1990.

Naidu, S., and Moser, H. W. Peroxisomal disorder. *Neurol. Clin.* 8:507–528, 1990.

Nakano, T., et al. A new point mutation within exons of β-hexosaminidase α gene in a Japanese infant with Tay-Sachs disease. *Ann. Neurol.* 27:465–473, 1990.

NIH Consensus Development Conference. Neurofibromatosis. Conference statement. *Arch. Neurol.* 45:575–578, 1988.

Nishikawa, Y., et al. Long-term coenzyme Q_{10} therapy for a mitochondrial encephalomyopathy with cytochrome c oxidase deficiency: A^{31}P NMR study. *Neurology* 39:399–403, 1989.

Parnes, S., et al. Hexosaminidase deficiency presenting as atypical juvenile-onset spinal muscular atrophy. *Arch. Neurol.* 42:1176–1180, 1985.

Polten, A., et al. Molecular basis of different forms of metachromatic leuokodystrophy. *N. Engl. J. Med.* 324:18–22, 1991.

Poser, C. M. Dysmyelination revisited. *Arch. Neurol.* 35:401–408, 1978.

Rapin, I., et al. Adult (chronic) GM$_2$-gangliosidosis—atypical spinocerebellar degeneration in a Jewish sibling. *Arch. Neurol.* 33:120–130, 1976.

Riccardi, V. M. Neurofibromatosis. *Neurol. Clin.* 5:337–349, 1987.

Riopelle, R. J., and Riccardi, V. M. Neuronal growth factors from tumors of Von Recklinghausen neurofibromatosis. *Can. J. Neurol. Sci.* 14:141–144, 1987.

Rizzo, W. B., et al. Dietary erucic acid therapy for X-linked adrenoleukodystrophy. *Neurology* 39:1415–1422, 1989.

Rosen, G. D., Galaburda, A. M., and Sherman, G.F. Mechanisms of Brain Asymmetry: New Evidence and Hypotheses. In D. Ottoson (editor). *Duality and Unity of the Brain, Unified Functioning and Specialization of the Hemispheres.* New York: Macmillan, 1987, Pp. 29–36.

Ross, M. H., Galaburda, A. M., and Kemper, T. L. Down's syndrome: is there a decreased population of neurons? *Neurology* 34:909–916, 1984.

Scriver, C. R., et al. *The Metabolic Basis of Inherited Disease.* New York: McGraw-Hill, 1989.

Scriver, C. R., and Clow, C. L. Phenylketonuria: epitome of human biochemical genetics. *N. Engl. J. Med.* 303:1336–1342; 1394–1400, 1980.

Seashore, M. R., et al. Loss of intellectual function in children with phenylketonuria after relaxation of dietary phenylalanine restriction. *Pediatrics* 75:226–232, 1985.

Shah, S., Peterson, N., and McKean, C. Lipid composition of human cerebral white matter and myelin in phenylketonuria. *J. Neurochem.* 19:2369–2376, 1972.

Smithells, R. W., et al. Further experience of vitamin supplementation for prevention of neural tube defect recurrences. *Lancet* 1:1027–1031, 1983.

Sorensen, S. A., Mulvihill, J. J., and Nielsen, A. Long-term follow-up of Von Recklinghausen neurofibromatosis. Survival and malignant neoplasms. *N. Engl. J. Med.* 314:1010–1015, 1986.

Stefansson, K., and Wollmann, R. Distribution of the neuronal specific protein, 14-3-2, in the central nervous system lesions of tuberous sclerosis. *Acta Neuropathol.* (Berl.) 53:113–117, 1981.

Steinberg, D. Refsum Disease. In C. R. Scriver, et al. (editors). *The Metabolic Basis of Inherited Disease.* New York: McGraw-Hill, 1989, Pp. 1533–1550.

Tahmoush, A. J. et al. Hartnup disease. *Arch. Neurol.* 33:787–807, 1976.

Taubinan, B., Hale, D. E., and Kelley, R. I. Familial Reye-like syndrome: a presentation of medium chain acyl-coenzyme A dehydrogenase deficiency. *Pediatrics* 78:382–385, 1987.

Trombley, I. K., and Mirra, S. S. Ultrastructure of tuberous sclerosis: cortical tuber and subependymal tumor. *Ann. Neurol.* 9:174–181, 1981.

Wertelecki, W., et al. Neurofibromatosis 2: clinical and DNA linkage studies of a large kindred. *N. Engl. J. Med.* 319:278–283, 1988.

Wolf, B. Reassessment of biotin-responsiveness in "unresponsive" propionyl CoA carboxylase deficiency. *J. Pediatr.* 97:964–966, 1980.

Woods, S. E., and Colon, V. F. Wilson's disease. *Am. Fam. Phys.* 40:171–178, 1989.

Central Nervous System Trauma

HEAD INJURY

Despite concerted efforts at prevention such as the enforcement of stricter seat belt laws, the manufacture of safer vehicles and sporting equipment, and the mandatory requirement for motorcycle helmets, head trauma remains a major public health problem worldwide. Trauma is the leading cause of death in men under age 35 and head injury is a major factor in at least 50 percent of these trauma-related deaths. In the United States, the incidence of significant head trauma is approximately 250/100,000 annually, with a yearly mortality rate of approximately 9/100,000. The annual incidence in children is about 200/100,000. Men are the victims twice as frequently as women, and motor vehicle accidents account for about half of these cases. Other common civil causes are assaults, falls, sports injuries, and industrial accidents. Many survivors are left with significant neurological and psychological sequelae. Because of the massive overall problems posed by such injuries, a major effort is under way to improve prevention measures as well as the approaches to acute management and rehabilitation.

Head injuries can present a spectrum of severity, ranging from minor scalp lacerations through blunt closed-head trauma to high-velocity penetrating missile injuries of the brain. Rational management is predicated on an understanding of the pathophysiological mechanisms that underlie the various forms of head injury.

Pathophysiology

There are two main effects of head injury: primary damage arising as a direct consequence of the physical forces exerted by the impact on brain tissue and secondary delayed effects arising from mechanisms such as the release of neurotransmitters and vasoactive substances, brain ischemia, delayed hemorrhages, cerebral edema, and brain shifts. Cerebral compromise may also result from the combination of hypoxia and ischemia secondary to apnea, hypotension, or seizures.

When the skull is struck by a moving object, abruptly hits a fixed object, or suddenly decelerates, various impact forces come into play. The most important determinants of the degree of injury are the area and site involved as well as the velocity and the duration of impact; whether the skull is fixed or mobile; and the shape of the impacting object. Compressive forces arise when the fixed skull is crushed by a slow-moving object. This frequently causes a linear fracture with compaction of brain tissue. The brain, being a relatively incompressible structure, responds to sudden acceleration and deceleration by gliding or rotating within the cranial cavity. However, these rotational or angular forces are a major factor in brain injury and create shearing forces that not only physically disrupt axons at particular locations but also damage vessels.

Bony and dural protuberances (e.g., the floor of the middle and anterior fossae, the sphenoid wings, and the falx) restrict brain movement and thereby enhance shear stresses. The anatomical features of the various skull compartments surrounding the brain determine, in part, the distribution of lesions, as observed in pathological specimens or neuroimaging studies obtained after head injury.

Skull Fractures

Fractures of the skull are associated with 80 percent of the fatal head injuries. Although often inconsequential in themselves, their presence indicates a powerful blow has been delivered to the head and also a substantial risk of consequent epidural or subdural hematoma. Linear fractures result from high-magnitude forces acting over an area of at least 13 cm² and tend to extend from the point of impact toward the base of the skull. In children, a "greenstick" fracture with inward bending of the bone may be produced. Linear fractures crossing branches of the middle meningeal artery put the patient at particular risk for epidural hematoma.

Depressed skull fractures result from forces that are imposed over a smaller surface area and are often asymptomatic. If there are focal contusions, the risk of epilepsy as a long-term sequela is increased. Most such fractures are accompanied by scalp laceration, and this can provide a communication between the surface, sinuses, or middle ear canal and the intracranial compartment (i.e., compound fracture). However, the laceration may not be over the site of the fracture, which the examiner may best detect by carefully probing the area with a sterile gloved finger. The dura mater may be lacerated and bone chips may have been driven into the cerebral cortex.

Compound fractures that include a dural tear provide a route for infection and may lead to bacterial meningitis (particularly if a CSF leak occurs), brain abscess, or osteomyelitis of the skull. Fractures in which the bone is depressed greater than the thickness of the skull (approximately 5 mm) are usually elevated surgically, although the ultimate neurological outcome is not influenced by doing so. Such fractures, when located in frontal areas or when particularly deep, may also be elevated for cosmetic reasons.

Basilar skull fractures may either be contiguous with convexity fractures or constitute independent injuries. They are often difficult to detect radiologically. The most common type parallels the petrous bone in the middle fossa or involves the sphenoid bone, running toward the sella turcica. Transverse fractures that cross the petrous bone are less common and are particularly likely to damage the facial nerve. **Rhinorrhea** (discharge of CSF from the nose) may stem from tears of the dura mater that allow leakage of CSF through the cribriform plate or paranasal sinuses. **Otorrhea** (leakage of CSF from the ear), a carotid-cavernous fistula, or pneumocephalus (intracranial air resulting from a fracture that creates a communication with a paranasal sinus) are other potential consequences. Damage to the eighth nerve at the base of the skull can precipitate hearing loss and severe vertigo with petrous fractures. The less common transverse petrous fractures may cause seventh nerve damage, but this is usually a reversible injury.

Other cranial nerves may be damaged by head injury even without a skull fracture. Anosmia due to the tearing of olfactory fibers in the anterior fossa and vertical diplopia due to a fourth nerve palsy are relatively common.

Concussion, Contusion, and Brain Laceration

Concussion, contusion, and brain laceration refer respectively to brain injuries of increasing severity. A **concussion** is a transient arrest of brain activity due to a blow to the head or sudden acceleration and deceleration of the skull ("whiplash") without a detectable pathological change. The underlying pathophysiology is poorly understood but likely relates to the transient disruption of neuronal activity within the ascending reticular activating system. In experimental models of concussion, animals are found to undergo brief apnea, hypotension, bradycardia, a sudden rise in intracranial pressure, EEG slowing, and in some cases neurogenic pulmonary edema at the time of concussion.

The degree of amnesia exhibited by a head trauma victim is a rough indication of the severity of concussion. Normally there is both an anterograde and retrograde amnesia after a concussion is sustained. The retrograde amnesia, pertaining to events occurring prior to the head injury, shrinks gradually and disappears. The so-called posttraumatic amnesia, regarding events following the head injury, is the best indicator of the severity of injury. Posttraumatic amnesia lasting less than one hour is arbitrarily considered to indicate mild injury. In some cases, the concussion may not be severe enough to produce unconsciousness but may nevertheless cause posttraumatic amnesia lasting hours. This phenomenon has been recognized in football players ("the ding").

A **contusion** produces hemorrhage and necrosis of brain tissue but leaves the overlying pial membrane intact. The lesion penetrates right to the cortical surface, in contrast to primary hemorrhages which are usually deeper. A **laceration** is the physical disruption or an actual tear of the cortical surface. Damage to major vessels can lead to significant associated hemorrhage or ischemia. These lesions are associated with penetrating injuries.

Pathological studies performed in patients who died from severe closed-head trauma have disclosed the existence of multiple areas of hemorrhage (large and small) and tissue necrosis that tend to involve the tips of the gyri, the subpial areas, the lateral brainstem, and the corpus callosum. The undersurface of the frontal lobes, the tips of the temporal and frontal lobes, and lips of the sylvian fissure are particularly vulnerable sites because of their contact with sharp and bony prominences such as the floor of the anterior fossa and sphenoid wings. The "coup" injury refers to damage incurred directly beneath the site of impact. The "contrecoup" injury, which is often more extensive, applies to damage involving brain sites directly opposite the area of impact and stems from movement of the brain within the cranial cavity.

Cerebral Edema

Of the secondary consequences of severe head injury, cerebral edema is an almost universal problem and can lead to serious morbidity. Cerebral edema of the vasogenic type is caused by disruption of the blood-brain barrier at the capillary level and is worsened when cerebral autoregulation is impaired. Respiratory compromise with its attendant hypoxia and carbon dioxide retention may accentuate the overall brain congestion. Brain swelling, congestion, and rostral-caudal deterioration (see Chapters 5 and 20) can appear suddenly, particularly in cases of pediatric head trauma in which an abrupt rise in cerebral blood flow appears to be the major underlying factor. A vicious cycle of raised intracranial pressure (ICP) with worsening edema, brain herniation, cerebral ischemia, and brainstem compromise leading to hypotension and apnea often contributes to a precipitous decline in neurological status. It is possible that the endogenous opioid peptides released during head trauma may participate in the production of secondary injury by adversely affecting the microcirculation.

Expanding intracranial hematomas within the subdural or epidural spaces or within the brain parenchyma frequently contribute to rapid rostral-caudal deterioration and a poor outcome in many patients with severe head injury.

Extracerebral Hematoma

An **acute epidural hematoma,** which consists of a collection of blood that forms between the dura mater and inner table of the skull, is a frequent component of skull fractures, and occurs in about 10 percent of the cases of severe head injury. About 85 percent are due to arterial tears involving branches of the middle meningeal artery. These tears are most commonly in the temporal and frontal areas and assume a lenticular biconvex shape. The rest are due to trauma inflicted on venous structures such as the meningeal vein, or the transverse, lateral, or sagittal sinuses. The severity of the initial injury may be mild and the impairment of consciousness insignificant. A lucid interval ensues in about half the patients before their level of consciousness steadily deteriorates. Ipsilateral or occasional contralateral pupillary dilatation and hemiparesis are common. Such a picture should arouse a high index of suspicion, and a linear fracture crossing a vascular skull marking on a skull x-ray study should be an alerting sign.

An **acute subdural hematoma,** appearing within the first week of injury, is due to shearing forces that cause tearing of the veins bridging the subdural space. Impact of the skull is not essential, provided the rotational forces are sufficiently strong. About 50 percent of the cases are associated with skull fracture. Low-velocity injuries such as those caused when the head strikes a broad flat object (e.g., the pavement) most often give rise to subdural hematomas. Commonly there are underlying brain contusions in these patients and they are often a more important determinant of the clinical picture and long-term outcome. They are usually located over the frontoparietal convexities and rarely involve the posterior fossa. The clinical picture is often identical to that seen in patients with epidural hematomas. However, subdural hematomas are often far more extensive than epidural hematomas and frequently have a crescent shape. Bilateral hematomas are found in about 15 to 20 percent of cases with hematoma.

Chronic subdural hematomas appear several weeks after the initial injury, which in itself may be trivial. They are particularly common in the elderly, alcoholics, and other patients with brain atrophy, as well as in patients on hemodialysis or with coagulation disorders. A berry aneurysm or arteriovenous malformation

may occasionally rupture into the subdural space and give rise to a chronic subdural hematoma. The hematoma is often encased in a thick fibrotic membrane that is rich in capillaries and contains a thick yellowish fluid high in protein and blood breakdown products. The hematoma may gradually expand; at times it may also resolve spontaneously or even undergo calcification.

Chronic subdural hematomas are associated with a wide variety of clinical pictures and can be easily missed by the unwary clinician. Headaches, seizures, personality change, dementia, slowly progressing hemiparesis or stupor, and symptoms that resemble transient ischemic attacks are among the more common presentations. Contrast-enhanced CT scanning or MRI studies are very helpful for establishing the diagnosis. Occasionally isodense subdural hematomas, especially if they are bilateral and do not produce much midline shift, can be missed on CT scanning. Lumbar puncture yields little information that can aid in diagnosis and may be dangerous in the presence of an expanding hematoma. An EEG often shows widespread slowing with attenuation of activity over the area of the hematoma. Cerebral angiography clearly demonstrates the hematoma by showing an avascular area between the inner skull table and the terminal branches of the major cortical arteries.

Intracerebral Hemorrhage
Intracerebral hemorrhages occur when deeper vessels within the brain are physically disrupted, and ependymal tears can lead to intraventricular hemorrhage. Small upper brainstem hemorrhages may also occasionally account for cases involving prolonged coma plus pupillary and gaze abnormalities. The use of serial CT scanning has made possible the increased detection of **delayed intracerebral hemorrhages** that appear several days following the initial head trauma. These hemorrhages, which can be responsible for late deterioration in the patient's state, are thought to result from damage to deep vessels, possibly in conjunction with elevated blood pressure.

Subarachnoid hemorrhage may also be a consequence of head trauma, particularly after blows to the occiput. Its clinical consequences are usually minimal but it can lead to the development of vasospasm and focal ischemia as well as normal-pressure hydrocephalus.

Subdural hygromas (collections of CSF within the subdural space) can form as the result of tears in the arachnoid membrane that create a valvelike effect. They are particularly common in children and may have to be drained if they become symptomatic (e.g., headaches or raised ICP).

Initial Assessment of the Patient

The initial management of the patient who has sustained a head injury depends on the severity of the injury and whether the patient has incurred multiple trauma. In comatose patients, resuscitative measures, neurological and physical assessments, and preparation for radiological or surgical procedures may all have to be carried out virtually simultaneously.

Various measures that can grade the severity of brain injury have been proposed. In a concussion victim, the duration of posttraumatic amnesia correlates with severity: <5 minutes, very mild; <1 hour, mild; 1–24 hours, moderate; 1–7 days, severe; and >7 days, very severe. In more severe cases, in which diffuse axonal injury is likely, the duration of loss of consciousness (which is not always easy to determine) provides an indication of severity: mild, 6–24 hours; moderate, over 24 hours; and severe, days to weeks. The widely used Glasgow coma scale provides a quantitative measure of the depth of coma, and can be applied by nursing staff in a consistent manner to monitor a patient's progress. Three easily observable indicators are measured: eye opening, verbal response, and motor response (see Table 5-4). A score of 13 to 15 implies mild injury; 9 to 12, moderate injury; and 8 or less, more severe injury and a comatose state.

In patients whose head injury is mild without a skull fracture and who are alert and oriented without focal neurological signs, a few hours of observation in the emergency room usually suffices. Such patients can usually be sent home to be watched by family or friends for any deterioration in the level of consciousness. These people are instructed to try to rouse the patient every few hours throughout the night. Patients with more severe injury are admitted for observation and, if necessary, intensive care. Vomiting, dizziness, headache, photophobia, irritability, and fluctuating drowsiness are common even following a mild concussion. A syndrome of agitated delirium with unaccustomed combativeness and swearing is encountered in younger patients, often those with temporal lobe contusions, and constitutes a need for hospital admission. Patients with fractures, focal neurological signs, persistent stupor, severe memory loss, confusion, or intractable vomiting should undergo CT scanning and be admitted to the hospital for observation.

The initial efforts of emergency room personnel in the care of a head trauma patient are focused on making certain the airway is patent, respiration is adequate, blood pressure is maintained, and cardiac rate and rhythm are not compromised. Rapid assessment is carried out to determine whether there is ongoing thoracoabdominal hemorrhage (e.g., from a ruptured spleen) or hemorrhage related to longbone fractures. The cause of severe hypotension is rarely head injury alone, and other sources such as hemorrhagic shock or spinal injury should be suspected. Because of the possibility of cervical spine injury in all patients with significant head injury, the patient's head and neck should always be immobilized with sandbags until a cervical injury is ruled out. Scalp wounds should be carefully inspected to determine whether a compound fracture exists. Exploration with a gloved finger is often necessary because small depressed skull fractures may not be readily evident even on a skull x-ray study.

The most important neurological feature to note initially is the patient's level of consciousness. When patients are alert, this permits a fairly full rapid neurological examination to be performed. In comatose patients, the examination is tailored to localize the sites and level of CNS involvement and to determine whether rostral-caudal deterioration is in progress. However, an impaired level of consciousness following head injury may also result from concomitant intoxication with alcohol or drugs or a postictal state rather than from the head injury itself, and this must be recognized. Neurological signs following head injury may be due to an underlying acute neurological event such as subarachnoid hemorrhage, which preceded and actually provoked the accident responsible for the head injury.

Evidence for basal skull fracture should be sought. Battle's sign (ecchymoses over the mastoid), "raccoon eyes" (periorbital ecchymoses), otorrhea, hemotympanum, rhinorrhea, and frank blood draining from the ear or nose, all point to the existence of a basilar skull fracture. Involvement of cranial nerves I, VII, or VIII is also a suggestive finding.

Certain aspects of the neurological examination yield important information concerning whether rostral-caudal deterioration is occurring. Papilledema is an unusual early sign in a patient with head injury, even in the presence of raised ICP. Assessment of pupillary size and reaction to light may reveal unilateral pupillary dilatation, which is an early sign of transtentorial uncal herniation. A transient phase of pupillary constriction may precede pupillary dilatation, however. With progression, ophthalmoparesis appears, with the eye assuming a down-and-out position. Third nerve palsy or pupillary dilatation resulting from direct orbital trauma, possibly with an orbital blowout fracture, must be distinguished from the pupillary dilatation due to herniation. A Horner's syndrome with miosis and ptosis can signify injury to the cervicothoracic spinal cord, brachial plexus, or internal carotid artery (e.g., dissection). Bilateral constricted pupils suggest pontine injury or drug intoxication. A Marcus Gunn pupil (afferent pupillary defect), which dilates rather than constricts when the light is swung from the opposite eye onto it, implies underlying optic nerve or retinal damage.

Examination of eye movements provides important localizing clues. In the alert patient, eye movements can be tested by having the patient gaze in various directions. A sixth nerve palsy can be seen with fractures involving the petrous tip but may also constitute a nonlocalizing sign of elevated ICP, particularly in a stuporous or comatose patient. A fourth nerve palsy or the equivalent may be seen with

involvement of the superior oblique tubercle in the orbit or damage to the nerve intracranially. Vertical diplopia, which can be corrected by tilting the head to the contralateral side, is the result. The third nerve may also be damaged intracranially.

In the comatose patient, the oculocephalic (doll's eye) or oculovestibular (cold water caloric testing) reflex eye movements are examined. The latter is preferable, unless a cervical fracture has been absolutely ruled out. Cold water caloric testing should not be performed if there is blood or CSF draining from the ear or the eardrum has been pierced. Conjugate eye deviation or a gaze weakness to one side usually indicates a frontal lesion, but is also seen with involvement of one pontine gaze center. Fifth nerve function is tested by examining the corneal reflex and pinprick sensation over the face. An internuclear ophthalmoplegia or absent oculocephalic eye movements point to the existence of a pontine lesion, either intrinsic or secondary to rostral-caudal deterioration. Absent oculovestibular movements indicate medullary impairment. The symmetry of the resting facial expression, blinking, the cheeks during expiration, and grimace in response to noxious stimuli can be used to assess seventh nerve function. Eighth nerve function is tested by observing whether blinking or an arousal response occurs in reaction to a loud noise such as hand clap.

Asymmetries of spontaneous movements or withdrawal responses to noxious stimuli may reveal a hemiparesis. A Babinski's sign may also be present. Hemiparesis represents an important sign of a contralateral expanding intracranial hematoma, but may occasionally be ipsilateral to the lesion. Decorticate or decerebrate responses are seen when the rostral-caudal deterioration involves diencephalic or upper brainstem structures or intraaxial lesions at these locations.

Neuroradiological Procedures

X-ray Studies. Skull x-ray studies may furnish important information and should be obtained in all patients with severe injuries. Whether this is necessary in patients with mild head injury who have not lost consciousness is somewhat controversial. A linear fracture, which is often not readily detectable clinically, markedly increases the chances of a hematoma developing later, and serves as one good reason for obtaining such studies. Depressed skull fractures are also easily missed clinically and may be associated with subsequent neurological deficits. On the other hand, fractures are extremely rare in head-injured patients who have not lost consciousness. Medicolegal considerations also frequently sway the assessing physician to order skull x-ray studies.

Besides fractures, foreign intracranial bodies, air-fluid levels in the sinuses or the existence of intracranial air pointing to basilar fractures, and a displaced pineal gland resulting from an intracranial mass lesion are examples of findings that can be disclosed by these studies. Special views such as tangential views to demonstrate depressed fractures, Towne's views to visualize the occipital area, or basilar views may be indicated.

Cervical spine films should also be obtained in all patients except those with very mild injuries, but are particularly important in the elderly. These can reveal the existence of unexpected fractures and subluxations. Swimmer's views or downward traction on the patients' arms may be necessary for demonstrating the C7–T1 junction.

Computed Tomography.   CT scanning has proved invaluable in evaluating patients with moderate or severe head injury. Comatose or moderately severely injured patients should be transported to a center where CT scanning is available, once their condition is stabilized. CT scanning should not be delayed for other tests such as skull x-ray studies when an intracranial hematoma is suspected (e.g., comatose patients). In agitated or uncooperative patients, sedation or general anesthesia may be required in order to obtain an adequate scan. Fractures can be demonstrated using a "bone window."

The scan may show various combinations of intracranial hematomas, contusions, brain swelling, or shifts (Figs. 28-1 to 28-3). Hydrocephalus may be present with clots impinging on the ventricular system. Small hemorrhages

in the corpus callosum or upper brainstem signify diffuse axonal injury. Primary intraparenchymal lesions are seen principally in patients with deep and long-lasting coma. The CT scan has not been especially useful for determining the nature and extent of injury because of its low sensitivity in defining nonhemorrhagic lesions, the difficulties in obtaining multiplanar views, and artifacts.

Magnetic Resonance Imaging.   Although a much more sensitive imaging technique, MRI scanning is generally less practical in the acute stages of head injury because of the greater degree of patient cooperation required and the difficulties of scanning a patient who is receiving assisted ventilation. Once the patient's condition has stabilized, however, the MRI scan may be very useful to detect areas of contusion or hemorrhage that are not revealed by CT. Widespread white matter lesions are frequently detected, even in patients who have sustained a relatively mild injury. These are most commonly seen in frontotemporal areas. Multiple cortical contusions are also readily demonstrable in the early phases.

Cerebral Angiography.   Cerebral angiography may occasionally be necessary to aid in the diagnosis of an isodense extracerebral hematoma, carotid-cavernous fistula, and the dissection or laceration of vessels in the neck or at the base of the brain.

Management

The most important principle to adhere to for reducing the mortality and morbidity that attend head injury is the early diagnosis and surgical treatment of intracranial hematomas. The features of subdural and extradural hematoma have already been discussed. Early CT scanning to detect these lesions is mandatory in patients with linear skull fracture, focal neurological signs, or a depressed level of consciousness. In comatose patients or those showing rapid deterioration, some neurosurgeons have recommended the routine placement of bilateral burrholes in the skull even before diagnostic studies are undertaken.

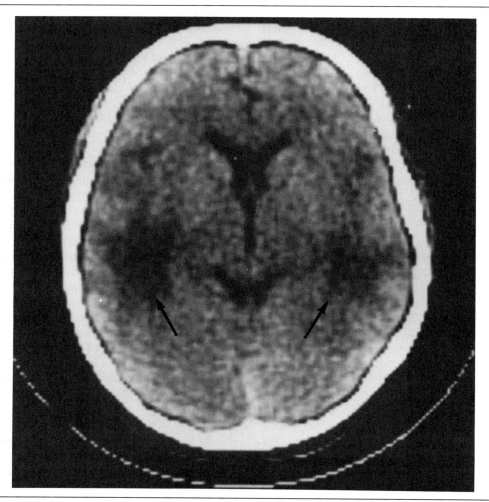

Fig. 28-1. *Unenhanced CT scan showing bilateral temporal lobe contusions* (arrows) *following acute head injury.*

Prevention of hypoxia and hypotension is extremely important if the maximum preservation of brain tissue is to be achieved. Arterial blood gases are obtained early and oxygen given by endotracheal tube and mechanical ventilation if necessary. Hypovolemic shock is treated with blood replacement or colloid instillation. Undue hypotension is particularly dangerous in these patients because cerebral autoregulation may already be compromised and elevated ICP is a further factor in reducing cerebral blood flow.

Management of elevated ICP is a major challenge in many head-injuried patients. Initially hyperventilation by mechanical ventilator is employed, keeping the arterial P_{CO_2} between 25 and 30 mm Hg. This brings about cerebral arteriolar constriction and reduces brain congestion and swelling. However, cerebral blood flow may be further reduced by this method, and thus it is at best only a temporary solution.

When raised ICP is suspected or anticipated, continuous ICP monitoring is often carried out. An extradural transducer is often used for this purpose but an intraventricular catheter can also be employed (in patients whose ventricles are not compressed), which additionally allows the drainage of CSF as a means of lowering

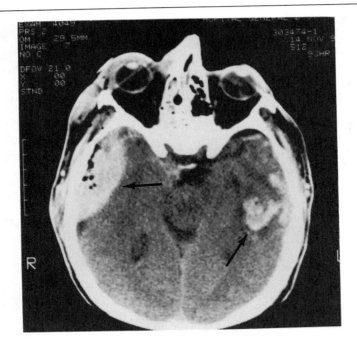

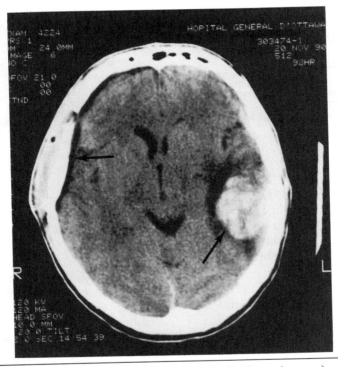

Fig. 28-2. *CT scans showing a right temporal epidural hematoma* (horizontal arrows) *underlying a temporoparietal fracture and a left temporal intracerebral hematoma* (oblique arrows) *resulting from a contrecoup injury. The patient was a 64-year-old man who had sustained a 12-foot (3.5-meter) fall.*

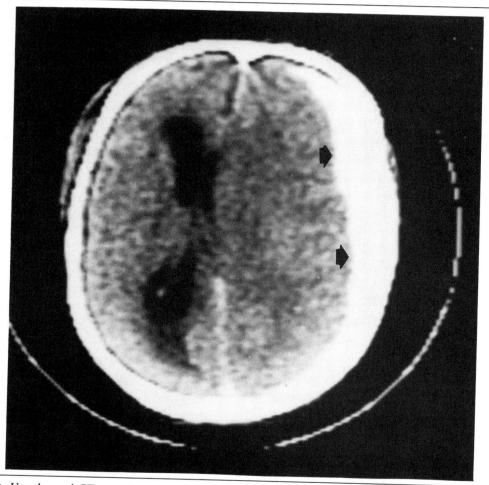

Fig. 28-3. *Unenhanced CT scan showing a subacute right subdural hematoma* (arrows). *Note the marked midline shift and compression of the right lateral ventricle.*

the ICP. Keeping levels of ICP at 25 mm Hg in the first 48 hours or 30 mm Hg thereafter requires vigorous treatment. Elevated ICP may result from intracranial hematoma, increased cerebral blood flow, diffuse cerebral edema, or ventricular dilatation (obstructive hydrocephalus), either alone or in combination (Table 28-1). It is seen more commonly in patients with intracranial hematomas and contusions than in those with diffuse axonal injury.

Cerebral edema, which is vasogenic in origin, usually peaks 24 hours or more following the injury. It may respond to mannitol therapy, often given in combination with a diuretic such as furosemide. The other causes have specific

therapies. Resectable intracranial hematomas or areas of severe cerebral contusion with hemorrhage are surgically evacuated; hyperventilation and a modest reduction in severe hypertension are measures that can reduce cerebral congestion; and ventricular drainage or shunt placement is performed to reduce ventricular size with hydrocephalus. Attention must also be paid to nonspecific measures that further elevate ICP. Patients should be nursed with their heads elevated (30 degrees) if possible, and undue neck flexion and airway suctioning avoided. Many advocate prophylactic therapy to prevent seizures (consisting of a phenytoin loading dose of 18 mg/kg delivered slowly intra-

Table 28-1. Treatable Factors Contributing to Elevated ICP

Hypoxia/hypercapnia
Straining against the ventilator
Use of positive end-expiratory pressure
Frequent airway suctioning
Jugular venous obstruction
Seizures
Fever
Arterial hypertension
Fluid overload
Hyponatremia
Hypoproteinemia

venously) because seizures can provoke marked elevations in ICP.

Hypothermia (33°C) combined with anesthesia (barbiturates) is a measure that has been advocated by some practitioners, particularly in pediatric cases of severe head injury. However, at this time, the use of barbiturates has largely been abandoned.

The intensive care management of the head-injuried patient ideally includes hemodynamic cardiac and cerebral monitoring through central venous pressure lines, indwelling arterial pressure lines, pulmonary venous pressure lines Swan-Ganz catheters), arterial blood gas sampling, continuous electrocardiographic monitoring, frequent EEG sampling, and regular determinations of Glasgow coma scale scores. Once intracranial hematomas, raised ICP, and seizures have been optimally treated, the next primary goal becomes the maintenance of adequate cerebral oxygenation and the prevention of infection and other systemic complications inherent to a prolonged comatose state. Atelectasis, aspiration, and pulmonary infection should be prevented or adequately managed if they occur. Rarely neurogenic pulmonary edema is a consequence of head injury. Fat embolism may occur in patients with long-bone fractures. Fluid and electrolyte balance should be carefully maintained using mainly colloid fluids or normal saline. Dehydration should be prevented and serum osmolarity monitored. The head trauma may precipitate a degree of syndrome of inappropriate antidiuretic hormone secretion (SIADH) in some patients, and this may necessitate water restriction. Diabetes insipidus occurs in a small percentage of patients and is usually a temporary consequence of injury to the pituitary stalk. Fluid replacement of the previous hour's urinary loss is carried out until the problem subsides. Vasopressin is occasionally required to reverse the diabetes.

The resting energy requirements are increased by a mean value of 40% following head injury and there is also an increased catabolism of protein resulting in excessive nitrogen excretion. Replacement of the calories expended should be attempted, usually by enteral feeding via a nasogastric tube, which can later be replaced by a smaller feeding tube. A gastrostomy tube is used in patients needing prolonged support.

Gastric ulcers or erosions, which may bleed or perforate, are well-known complications of head injury, most commonly within the first week after injury. Prophylactic treatment with cimetidine or frequent antacid administration is carried out routinely.

A low-grade disseminated intravascular coagulation may occasionally arise as a result of thromboplastic material that is released into the systemic circulation from damaged brain tissue.

Adequate eye, bladder, bowel, and skin care and the prevention of contractures are an important part of the long-term management of these patients.

Prognosis and Long-Term Sequelae

Severe Head Injury

The outcome in patients who have sustained head trauma depends on the severity of the injury, the patient's age, the patient's premorbid personality, and the availability of rehabilitation services. Seventy percent of head injury–related deaths occur in the first 24 hours. The prognosis for recovery is almost always evident within the first 3 to 6 months after trauma. In one series of patients admitted in coma after head injury and receiving aggressive medical and surgical care, the mortality was 32 percent and 11 percent suffered eventual severe disability. In some series, survival following severe head injury (prolonged coma or intracranial hematoma, or both) is less than 50 percent. The Glasgow coma scale correlates well with the ultimate outcome (Table 28-2). The following features carry a poor prognosis: presence of intracranial hematoma; severe disturbance of brainstem function (apnea, absent pupillary responses, absent oculovestibular responses, and decerebrate posturing); and an ICP exceeding 25 mm Hg.

Those patients who survive the acute phases but remain in a permanent state of complete dependence with no meaningful interaction with the environment are deemed to be in a **chronic vegetative state,** which occurs in 1 to 5 percent of cases of severe head injury. These patients exhibit preservation of eye opening, rudimentary brainstem and other reflexes, and sleep-wake cycles. The cerebral cortex is diffusely damaged in these patients and many die within the first year.

Difficult ethical issues come into play when considering support for long-term survivors. However, some patients with severe head injury and poor initial prognostic signs may eventually experience recovery of useful function. In one series of patients who were comatose for less than 2 weeks, up to one third had made a satisfactory recovery one year later. Younger patients, particularly children, may eventually make a surprisingly good recovery despite poor initial indicators. Aggressive management, at least until prognosis can be firmly determined, is therefore indicated in all patients. Somatosensory or multimodality evoked potential measurements have shown promise both for identifying the site of major pathology and for determining prognosis.

Posttraumatic Syndrome Following Concussion

It is now known that, when a mild head injury is associated with even a brief loss of consciousness, this is likely to inflict some degree of permanent white matter axonal damage. The consequences of this damage, which is usually localized to frontotemporal regions, is somewhat variable (Table 28-3). Many patients with minor behavioral and personality changes following mild head injury were once thought to be suffering from purely psychiatric consequences of their injury or exaggerating their deficits to qualify for compensation. With the increasing ability to detect mild structural damage using MRI scanning and to define neuropsychological deficits more precisely, plus the recognition of relatively stereotyped symptoms in these patients, it is now accepted that the so-called posttraumatic or postconcussive syndrome likely has an organic basis. The common features seen in these patients are listed in Table 28-3.

Certain problems experienced by these patients may result from anxiety and depression consequent to their reduced abilities. Specific rehabilitative measures should be implemented to help patients learn to recognize and compensate for their deficits and patients can also benefit from psychological counseling. Although there is a tendency toward gradual improvement, many patients are left with permanent deficits of learning, information processing, communication, and emotional control.

There is a small group of patients who present with an obvious picture of malingering and exaggeration of their deficits following head injury so that they might qualify for compensation. These patients are often easy to identify on the basis of histrionic behavior, deficits that are grossly disproportionate to the degree of injury, and a nonanatomical pattern of deficits.

Posttraumatic Epilepsy

The overall risk for epilepsy developing in patients who are hospitalized for their head injuries is approximately 5 percent. The results of population-based studies have shown an overall incidence of only 2 percent in all head-injured patients. Jennet has delineated the factors that predict an increased risk of late epilepsy developing (after the first week) following head injury. Early seizures (within the first week) are seen in 5 percent of patients and are more com-

Table 28-2. Correlation of Glasgow Coma Scale Score with Outcome

Glasgow coma score	Death or severe disability
3 or 4	80%
5–7	54%
8–10	27%
11–15	6%

Table 28-3. Long-Term Behavioral Consequences in Head-Injured Patients

Severity of symptoms	Moderate	Mild
Behavioral symptoms	Irritability Impulsivity Emotional lability Impaired judgment Anxiety Depression Altered libido Childish behavior Aggressivity Apathy Disinhibition	Irritability Anxiety Depression
Cognitive symptoms	Memory impairment Slowed information processing Poor concentration Slowed reaction time Deficits in processing and sequencing of information Poor planning Language deficits	Memory impairment Poor concentration Slowed information processing
Other symptoms	Headache Dizziness Vertigo	Headache Dizziness Vertigo Fatigability Insomnia
Pathology	Subcortical white matter lesions	? Mild subcortical white matter lesions

mon in children. Once they occur, the risk for the development of late epilepsy is increased. Late epilepsy is more commonly associated with more severe head injury and with factors that are known to cause brain scarring. It is extremely rare for a brief uncomplicated concussion to cause posttraumatic epilepsy.

Posttraumatic amnesia lasting more than 24 hours, depressed skull fracture, intracranial hematoma, tearing of the dura mater or brain laceration, and missile injuries are all factors that are linked to an increased incidence of late epilepsy. Surprisingly, the EEG recording is a relatively poor tool for predicting the risk of subsequent epilepsy. Most patients developing posttraumatic epilepsy do so within the first year, although up to 25 percent of the patients suffer the onset 4 or more years after the injury. Seizures are usually complex partial with secondary generalization, an indication of the susceptibility of the frontal and temporal lobes to traumatic damage.

Patients who face an elevated risk are often put on prophylactic antiepileptic drugs following injury, but the results from a recent randomized, controlled study have shown that phenytoin given for the first year following injury does not appear to prevent late posttraumatic epilepsy from occurring.

SPINAL CORD INJURY

The annual incidence of acute spinal cord injury in the United States is about 5/100,000. Half of the cases are the result of motor vehicle accidents, with motorcycle accidents accounting for increasing numbers. Other causes include bicycle accidents, sports injuries (especially diving, gymnastics, rugby, hockey, and horseback riding), industrial accidents, penetrating knife or missile wounds, and falls. These patients frequently incur multiple trauma, with associated systemic and head injuries in about 15 percent. Brachial plexus lesions often accompany mid-thoracic fractures.

Young men are the most likely victims of spinal cord trauma. Although the mortality has now been reduced to under 10 percent in most centers as the result of advances in acute medical and surgical care and improved rehabilitation measures, many patients are left with permanent paraplegia or quadriplegia, which has devastating physical, psychological, and socioeconomic consequences. The high cost to society of such injuries, which remove large numbers of young adults from enjoying a productive life and generate significant long-term medical care needs, is evident. The management of spinal cord injury, which is still a controversial matter, is centered on early efforts to reverse the pathophysiological mechanisms responsible for the progression of neural damage; to detect and reverse spinal compression caused by an unstable vertebral column or bony fragments, discs, or hematoma in the spinal canal; and to provide early specialized rehabilitation to prevent long-term complications and foster independence and social reintegration.

Pathophysiology

The most mobile segments of the vertebral column, the cervical spine (C5–C7) and thoracolumbar spine (T10–L2), are those most susceptible to injury. The less mobile thoracic spine, which is also stabilized by attachment to the ribs, is less frequently affected. Whether the spinal cord undergoes compression within the spinal canal partially depends on the space available, which is maximal at C1 and in the lumbosacral spine. A congenitally narrow canal or a preexisting disease such as cervical spondylosis (which may cause a reduction in the space surrounding the spinal cord) or ankylosing spondylitis (which reduces the mobility of the vertebral column) predisposes to a less favorable outcome following spinal injury.

The various spinal elements—the bony vertebral column and supporting soft tissues, spinal cord, roots (including the cauda equina), and blood vessels—may be injured alone or in combination. Although spinal cord injury may occur without vertebral fractures or dislocations, the two more commonly occur in tandem (Table 28-4).

The forces involved in spinal cord injury are dictated by the mechanism of injury, and include hyperflexion, hyperextension (e.g., whiplash or a fall on the chin), lateral flexion, rotation, compression (e.g., blow to the top of the head), or distraction. Hyperextension injuries account for the largest number of lower cervical injuries. In extreme cases, the anterior ligament may rupture, leading to temporary vertebral subluxation. The inward bulging of the ligamentum flavum during hyperextension may also impinge on the spinal cord. With subluxation, articular facets may become locked, and this creates a persistent spinal compression. If the laminal arch separates from the body in a vertebral fracture/dislocation, the spinal cord may escape serious injury. Posteriorly displaced bony fragments may also produce direct spinal cord compression following a vertebral fracture, traumatic intervertebral disc herniation, or epidural hematoma.

Experimental studies as well as clinical observations have revealed that, following the primary cord injury, a series of events take place including the release of vasoactive substances, impaired microcirculation, expanding intramedullary gray matter hemorrhages, and progressive edema in the white matter. These events compound the neurological deficits and may be responsible for converting a partial lesion into a complete transverse myelopathy within 4 to 8 hours of injury. The resulting hemorrhagic necrosis, which is always maximal within the central cord area where microcirculation is most tenuous, can theoretically be prevented or minimized if this cascade of events can be interrupted. Many of the same cellular and biochemical mechanisms responsible for neuronal damage following the onset of focal brain ischemia are also active in spinal cord injury. Most of the attempts to reverse the secondary consequences of injury on spinal cord microcirculation have shown little benefit to date.

Clinical Picture

Complete lesions above C4 cause diaphragmatic paralysis and rapid death. Quadriplegia and respiratory impairment requiring a ventila-

Table 28-4. Vertebral Fractures and Dislocations

Fracture and/or dislocation	Typical mechanism of injury
Atlantooccipital dislocation	Twisting force to head
Base of odontoid	Blow to back or front of head, extreme flexion
Burst fracture of ring of atlas (Jefferson's)	Blow to top of head — *land on head*.
C2–C3 fracture/dislocation ("hangman's")	Hyperextension/distraction
Fracture/dislocation of cervical spine (upper cervical vertebrae dislocated anteriorly)	Sudden arrest of forward motion while patient sitting (hyperflexion; e.g., motor vehicle accident)
Compression fracture of cervical vertebra (fragments may project backward into spinal canal)	Blow to top of head plus flexion
Thoracic	Severe direct trauma
Lumbar compression fracture (T12, L1)	Fall on back or epileptic seizure (possibly preexisting osteoporosis)
Fracture/dislocation of lumbar spine	Weight falling on back while bending forward; seat-belt injury

tor are the consequences of a transverse lesion at C4–C5. Injuries at C5–C6 cause biceps weakness, while those one segment lower produce weakness in the triceps, wrist extensors, and forearm pronators. Injuries at T1 and below may result in paraplegia. Injuries to the thoracolumbar area can bring about complex neurological findings stemming from the involvement of the conus medullaris as well as cauda equina. Cauda equina injuries result from lesions below L1–L2, and are often asymmetrical and incomplete.

Spinal shock represents a transient state of flaccidity, areflexia and hyporeflexia, and absence of function below the level of a complete lesion, which is replaced within weeks by spasticity and hyperreflexia. Autonomic hyperreflexia can be a consequence of complete lesions above the midthoracic level, and is due to disinhibition of spinal autonomic reflexes. Paroxysmal severe hypertension, sweating, piloerection, penile erection, bradycardia, anxiety, and headache are often precipitated by a full bladder or when the lower body is exposed to noxious stimuli. The provoking stimulus must be eliminated and antihypertensive therapy instituted acutely in extreme cases.

The **central cord syndrome** is produced by transient cervical cord compression that causes edema or impairs the microcirculation of the central gray matter. Affected patients suffer weakness and sensory loss over the arms with the lower extremities spared because the lower extremity fibers are located more superficially in the ascending spinothalamic and descending corticospinal tracts. The **anterior cord syndrome,** which stems from compromise of the anterior spinal artery, produces paralysis and loss of pain and temperature sensation below the lesion, with sparing of posterior column sensation. Patients who suffer a direct penetrating injury may exhibit a **Brown-Séquard syndrome** (hemicord syndrome) (see Fig. 19-2). This consists of weakness and posterior column sensory loss ipsilaterally combined with contralateral loss of pain and temperature sensation.

A **whiplash injury,** which is due to sudden neck extension such as occurs when riding in an automobile which is struck from behind, is a soft tissue injury that spares the neural elements. There are stretching and tearing of the cervical muscle fibers and the anterior fibers of the intervertebral disc and anterior longitudinal ligament may be lacerated. Persistent neck, upper back and upper arm pain, especially with neck extension, may be a sequela of this sort of injury. Some patients may sustain a concurrent concussion without an actual blow to the head.

Radiological Assessment

Radiological investigation of the cervical spine following trauma is indicated for all patients who (1) complain of neck pain or tenderness;

(2) show stupor, coma, or confusion following a head injury; (3) have had a significant high-risk injury; and (4) exhibit neurological deficits. It is important to bear in mind that spinal cord injury may occur without bony injury, and vice versa.

In the cervical spine, most of the vertebral injuries involve the vertebral arch, with the C2 and C6 vertebrae most commonly involved. The first study that should be obtained is a cross-table lateral cervical x-ray film, which can disclose evidence of subluxation, vertebral body fractures, narrowing of disc spaces, and alterations of the normal lordotic curvature (Figs. 28-4 and 28-5).

Subluxation, and particularly unilaterally dislocated articular facets, may be easily missed on a single lateral view. Studies that employ anteroposterior and special views such as oblique or pillar views and open-mouth odontoid views should be obtained when cervical injury is suspected. It is extremely important to visualize the C7–T1 vertebral area, which is often obscured by the shoulders. This can be accomplished by exerting gentle downward traction on the arms or by placing the patient in a "swimmer's position" with one arm extended above the head. Once evidence of instability has been thoroughly ruled out, views obtained with the patient gently placed in flexion and extension can be obtained, if indicated, provided the patient has no neurological deficits.

High-resolution, thin-section CT scanning can add useful information to that furnished by plain x-ray studies and may visualize fractures that were not apparent (see Fig. 28-5). Fractures and soft tissue injury can be more clearly delineated and multiple injuries may become apparent. This technique is particularly valuable for visualizing the craniocervical junction. Tomographic x-ray evaluation may supply additional information when CT is not available.

Myelography, with or without CT, allows the rapid review of the whole spinal cord and it can rule out significant compression or complete block. A C1–C2 lateral puncture can be utilized to minimize the amount of patient movement required.

If patients can cooperate and are not on ventilator support, they can undergo MRI scanning,

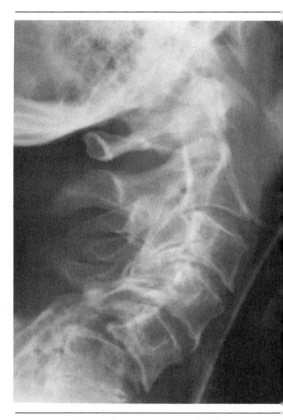

Fig. 28-4. *Cervical spine x-ray study showing sever subluxation of C5 onto C6. The patient was a 74-year-old man who had sustained a whiplash injury when the car he was sitting in the backseat of was struck from behind. The patient was not wearing a seat belt at the time. When this film was taken, he wa ambulatory and complaining of some pain and tingling in his hands. There was weakness affecting most muscle groups of the right arm and reduced sensation over the right hand and left fingertips. Th cervical spine x-ray study obtained immediately afte the accident had been normal.*

which furnishes a direct view of the spinal cor and vertebral column in the longitudinal axi and can detect disc herniations, vertebral mis alignment, extrinsic impingement on the spina cord, spinal cord swelling, or intramedullar hemorrhage.

Management

Acute Stages

Because many patients with spinal cord injur have sustained multiple injuries, and high spina

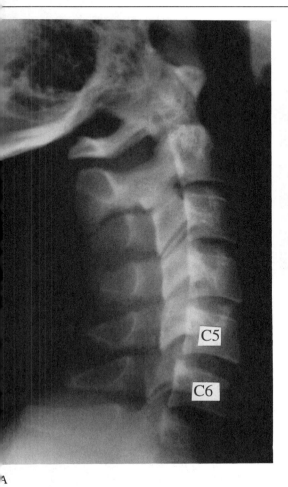

A

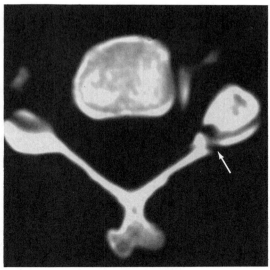

B

Fig. 28-5. *This 18-year-old man was involved in a motor vehicle accident in which his car turned over completely into a ditch. Initially in the emergency room, he complained only of minimal neck pain and a plain cervical spine x-ray study (A) was considered normal, despite the mild subluxation of C5 onto C6. He returned 12 hours later because of the acute onset of total right hemibody numbness and reduced sensation. (B) An axial CT scan revealed a fracture through the lamina of C5 (arrow).*

injuries (above C6) entail respiratory compromise, attention is first directed to the airway and ensuring adequate ventilation. Patients with lesions above C4 usually die from respiratory paralysis within minutes of injury. If intubation is necessary, it can usually be accomplished by the blind insertion of a nasotracheal tube. Other vital signs are stabilized as necessary, hemorrhage controlled, and long-bone fractures splinted. Because hypotension can compound spinal cord damage, measures should be instituted to prevent it. The neck must not be moved until cervical vertebral stability has been established. This is particularly important in comatose head-injured patients who cannot report symptoms and lack protective neck muscle reflexes. Extrication of the patient (e.g., from a damaged motor vehicle) must be done cautiously with a minimum of neck movement. The patient's head is supported by sandbags and further immobilized by a cervical collar with the patient's head taped to a special neck board. A conscious patient may be able to indicate the presence of spinal

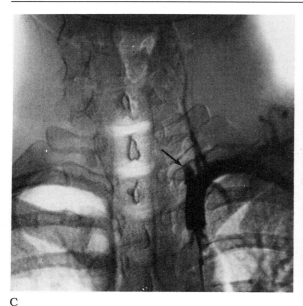

C

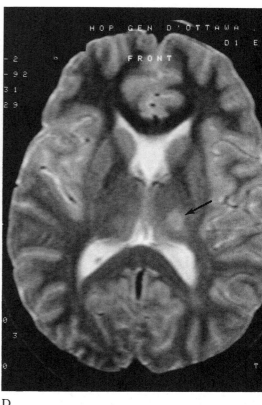

D

Fig. 28-5 *(Continued). (C) An angiogram showed that the left vertebral artery was sharply occluded just after it branched off from the aortic arch (arrow). (D) An MRI scan showed a small left thalamic infarct (arrow) that was causing the right-sided sensory symptoms. There was presumably an embolus to the thalamogeniculate artery from the vertebral dissection at the site of the fracture close to the vertebral canal. The patient underwent anticoagulation treatment and experienced a full recovery within 3 weeks.*

injury by reporting localized neck or back pain, especially with attempts to move. The patient may also describe numbness or weakness if there is spinal cord damage. The patient must be carefully and rapidly transported to a center that is adequately equipped to deal with the assessment of spinal cord injury, plus its management and, ideally, rehabilitation. Comprehensive neuroradiological assessment should be carried out as soon as possible.

Early management is directed toward preventing secondary spinal injury through the diagnosis and treatment of spinal instability or compression caused by bone fragments, a dislocated disc, or hematoma. Palpation of the cervi-

cal spine may reveal the existence of a step deformity, which signifies a dislocation. Many patients need to be placed in cervical traction with tongs and applied weights in order to stabilize the cervical spine or correct a subluxation. Halo traction is the preferred method for more long-term stabilization, but certain patients require surgical fusion. Perhaps the most difficult aspect of managing cervical spinal cord injuries is to decide whether surgical intervention is indicated. If paraplegia appears at some point after the injury, the patient's neurological status deteriorates, or foreign bodies are suspected in the spinal canal, these all constitute reasons for surgical intervention.

The findings from a full and careful neurological examination must be recorded initially, which can then serve as a baseline for the subsequent determination of neurological deterioration. It is important to determine whether the spinal cord lesion is complete or incomplete, as even minimal evidence of voluntary movement or preserved sensation below the level of involvement indicates that a complete or good functional recovery may be possible.

The early intravenous administration of very high doses of methylprednisolone can improve the ultimate neurological outcome, probably by stabilizing the spinal cord microcirculation.

Whether the severely injured patient survives the early phases depends largely on the prevention and management of complications that can arise from spinal cord injury. Patients with lesions above T6 may exhibit **autonomic instability,** with either hypotension or hypertension. This is due to a "functional sympathectomy." Attention to bladder care is important in the early phases to prevent infection and minimize hypertensive episodes. An indwelling catheter is required for this purpose.

Patients must not be given excessive amounts of intravenous fluids, as this may precipitate pulmonary edema. Gastric paralysis, ileus, and air swallowing can cause abdominal distention and worsen the respiratory compromise. Insertion of a nasogastric tube is normally necessary for the emptying of gastric contents. Adequate skin care is essential, both in the acute and chronic phases, to prevent bed sores and sepsis from occurring. The patient should be "log-rolled" every 2 hours to prevent both skin breakdown and atelectasis. Gastrointestinal bleeding from stress ulcers is not uncommon and the prophylactic administration of antacids or histamine H_2 blockers is required. A possible pulmonary embolus from deep vein thrombosis poses a serious danger and patients should generally receive low doses of heparin administered subcutaneously. When there are functional transverse sections above T8, temperature regulation poses a problem and measures must be instituted to prevent undue overheating or cooling. Early attention to the psychological management of both the patient and family must be undertaken in what often represents a catastrophic situation for all.

Long-term rehabilitation is best carried out at specialized spinal cord injury centers and should begin as early as possible. The aim is to gain maximum use, through various aids and devices, of muscles that are still functioning. In addition, long-term care must include careful attention to pulmonary and bladder function and skin care as well as the detection and prevention of heterotopic ossification around joints, hypercalcemia, deep vein thrombosis, and autonomic hyperreflexia. Spasticity and painful spasms can be ameliorated by agents such as baclofen.

Patients with a lesion at C6 can generally feed themselves using mechanical aids; those with lesions at C7 can generally be taught to grip. Patients with C8 lesions will have a claw-hand deformity, but maintain a prehensile grasp. In some cases, a progressing neurological deficit due to posttraumatic syringomyelia may arise years after the initial injury.

The ultimate success of rehabilitation and the eventual reintegration of the patient into society depend not only on the status of his or her neurological function but also on psychological adaptation. With the advent of modern-day technological devices, including computerized and voice-driven aids, more and more neurologically impaired patients are now able to function independently and even accomplish productive work.

BIBLIOGRAPHY

Head Injury

Adams, J. H., et al. Diffuse axonal injury in non-missile head injury. *J. Neurol. Neurosurg. Psychiatry* 54:481–483, 1991.

Annegers, J. F., et al. Seizures after head trauma: a population study. *Neurology* 30:683–689, 1980.

Becker, D. P., and Gudeman, S. K. (editors). *Textbook of Head Injury.* Philadelphia: Saunders, 1989.

Becker, D. P., and Povlischock, J. T. (editors). *Central Nervous System Trauma Status Report—1985.* Bethesda: National Institute of

Neurological and Communicative Disorders and Stroke, 1985.

Caveness, W. F., et al. The nature of posttraumatic epilepsy. *J. Neurosurg.* 50:545–553, 1979.

Coxe, W. S., and Grubb, R. L. Trauma to the Central Nervous System. In S.G. Eliasson, A. L. Prensky, and W. B. Hardin, Jr. (editors). *Neurological Pathophysiology,* 2nd ed. New York: Oxford University Press, 1978, Pp. 321–347.

Desai, B. T., et al. Seizures and civilian head injuries. *Epilepsia* 24:289–296, 1983.

Dikmen, S., McLean, A., and Temkin N. Neuropsychological and psychosocial consequences of minor head injury. *J. Neurol. Neurosurg. Psychiatry* 49:1227–1232, 1986.

Dornan, J. The long-term sequelae of head injury: I. *Mod. Med. Can.* 40:244–258, 1985.

Dornan, J. The long-term sequelae of severe head injury: II. *Mod. Med. Can.* 40:484–500, 1985.

Dublin, A. B., French, B. N., and Rennick, J.M. Computed tomography in head trauma. *Radiology* 122:365–369, 1977.

Frazee, J. G. Head trauma. *Emerg. Med. Clin. North Am.* 4:859–874, 1986.

Friedman, W. A. Head injuries. *CIBA Clin. Symp.* 36:1–32, 1984.

Gentry, L. R., Godersky, J.C., and Thompson, B. MR imaging of head trauma: review of the distribution and radiopathologic features of traumatic lesions. *AJNR* 9:101–110, 1988.

Jenkins, A., et al. Brain lesions detected by magnetic resonance imaging in mild and severe head injuries. *Lancet* 2:445–446, 1986.

Jennett, B. Assessment of the severity of head injury. *J. Neurol. Neurosurg. Psychiatry* 39:647–655, 1976.

Jennett, B. *Epilepsy After Non-Missile Head Injury.* Chicago: Year Book, 1975.

Jennett, B., and Teasdale, G. *Management of Head Injuries.* Philadelphia: Davis, 1981.

Kingston, W. J. (editor). Head injury. *Semin Neurol.* 5:195–264, 1985.

Kingston, W. J. Treatable neurologic complications encountered during rehabilitation of the head-injured adult. *Semin. Neurol.* 5:260–264 1985.

Langfitt, T. W., and Gennarelli, T. A. Can the outcome from head injury be improved? *J Neurosurg.* 56:19–25, 1982.

Levin, H. S., et al. Magnetic resonance imaging after "diffuse" nonmissile head injury: a neurobehavioral study. *Arch. Neurol.* 42:963–968 1985.

Majkowski, J. Post-traumatic Epilepsy. In M Dam and L. Gram (editors). *Comprehensive Epileptology.* New York: Raven, 1991, Pp 281–288.

Mendelow, A. D. The early management of head injury. *Curr. Opin. Neurol. Neurosurg* 4:5–11, 1991.

Salazar, A. M. Traumatic brain injury: the continuing epidemic. In V. Hachinski (editor). *Challenges in Neurology.* Philadelphia: Davis 1992, Pp. 55–67.

Schaffer, L., Kranzler, L. I., and Siqueira, E B. Aspects of evaluation and treatment of head injury. *Neurol. Clin.* 3:259–274, 1985.

Sosin, D. M., Sacks, J.J., and Smith, S. M Head injury–associated deaths in the United States from 1979 to 1986. *JAMA* 262:2251–2255, 1989.

Swann, K. W. Management of Severe Head Injury. In A.H. Ropper, S.K. Kennedy, and N. T. Zervas (editors). *Neurological and Neurosurgical Intensive Care.* Baltimore: University Park Press, 1983, Pp. 207–230.

Temkin, N. R., et al. A randomized, double-blind study of phenytoin for the prevention of post-traumatic seizures. *N. Engl. J. Med.* 323:497–502, 1990.

Van Dellen, J. R., and Becker, D. P. Craniocerebral Trauma. In W. G. Bradley, et al. (editors). *Neurology in Clinical Practice.* Boston: Butterworth-Heinemann, 1991, Pp. 861–892.

Vollmer, D. G., Dacey, R. G., and Jane, J. A. Craniocerebral Trauma. In R. J. Joynt (editor). *Clinical Neurology.* Philadelphia: Lippincott, 1991, Vol. 3, Pp. 1–80.

Weiderholt, W. C., et al. Short-term outcomes of skull fracture: a population-based study of survival and neurologic complications. *Neurology* 39:96–102, 1989.

Spinal Cord Injury

Albin, M. S. Acute cervical spinal injury. *Crit. Care Clin.* 1:267–284, 1985.

Becker, D. P., and Povlischock, J. T. (editors). *Central Nervous System Trauma Status Report—1985.* Bethesda, MD: National Institute of Neurological and Communicative Disorders and Stroke, 1985.

Bracken, M. B., et al. A randomized, controlled trial of methylprednisolone or naloxone in the treatment of acute spinal-cord injury. Results of the second national acute spinal cord injury study. *N. Engl. J. Med.* 332:1407–1411, 1990.

Cloward, R. B. Acute cervical spine injuries. *CIBA Symp.* 32:1–32, 1980.

Collins, W. F., and Chehrazi, B. Concepts of the Acute Management of Spinal Cord Injury. In W. B. Matthews and G. H. Glaser (editors). *Recent Advances in Clinical Neurology—3.* Edinburgh: Churchill Livingstone, 1982, Pp. 67–82.

Coxe, W. S., and Grubb, R. L. Trauma to the Central Nervous System. In S.G. Eliasson, A. L. Prensky, and W. B. Hardin, Jr. (editors). *Neurological Pathophysiology,* 2nd ed. New York: Oxford University Press, 1978, Pp. 321–347.

Faden, A. I. Neuropeptides and central nervous system injury. Clinical implications. *Arch. Neurol.* 43:501–504, 1986.

Janssen, L., and Hansebout, R. R. Pathogenesis of spinal cord injury and newer treatments: a review. *Spine* 14:23–32, 1989.

Karbi, O. A., Caspari, D. A., and Tator, C. H. Extrication, immobilization and radiologic investigation of patients with cervical spine injuries. *Can. Med. Assoc. J.* 139:617–621, 1988.

Meyer, P. R., Jr., et al. Spinal cord injury. *Neurol. Clin.* 9:625–661, 1991.

Murphy, K. P., et al. Cervical fractures and spinal cord injury: outcome of surgical and nonsurgical management. *Mayo Clin. Proc.* 65:949–959, 1990.

Penny, D., et al. Radiologic clues to cervical spine injuries. *Can. J. Diagn.,* Sept. 1990, Pp. 81–94.

Teasell, R. W. The Whiplash Patient: A Sympathetic Approach. In V. Hachinski (editor). *Challenges in Neurology.* Philadelphia: Davis, 1992, Pp. 29–52.

Van Dellen, J. R., and Becker, D. P. Spinal Cord Trauma. In W. G. Bradley, et al. (editors). *Neurology in Clinical Practice.* Boston: Butterworth-Heinemann, 1991, Pp. 893–902.

Complications of Pregnancy, Medical Illness, Alcohol and Substance Abuse, Toxins, and Vitamin Deficiencies

PREGNANCY

Pregnancy represents an altered physiological state that changes as gestation advances. The following adaptations take place in normal pregnancy: increased heart rate and cardiac output, increased plasma volume, increased extracellular fluid volume, decreased glucose tolerance, decreased serum albumin concentration, increased minute ventilation (compensated respiratory alkalosis), hypercoagulability (increased levels of fibrinogen and factors VII, VIII, IX, and XII), and a decreased serum magnesium content. The neurological aspects of pregnancy can be categorized into those conditions that occur coincidentally, those that are not specific to pregnancy but appear to be more common during pregnancy, those that are preexistent and may be exacerbated by pregnancy, and those that are specific complications of pregnancy or delivery. There are also other conditions that do not strictly represent complications of pregnancy but re-

quire special management or consideration of the fetal effects (Table 29-1).

Eclampsia

Eclampsia and preeclampsia constitute a form of hypertensive encephalopathy that is probably immunologically mediated. It tends to appear mainly in primigravidas late in pregnancy and even postpartum. Eclampsia, which occurs in about 1 out of 1,000 deliveries, is the most notable cause of maternal mortality in Western countries. It is a multisystem disease that stems from fibrin deposition in small vessels and resultant tissue necrosis and hemorrhages.

The principal features of eclampsia are hypertension (or a significant increase in blood pressure from earlier levels), proteinuria, renal impairment, and a coagulopathy that resembles disseminated intravascular coagulation (DIC). Laboratory tests may reveal elevated uric acid and liver enzyme levels as well as thrombocytopenia. Headache, vomiting, and hyperreflexia are common. Convulsions,

Table 29-1. Neurological Aspects of Pregnancy

Eclampsia
Epilepsy
  Differential diagnosis of seizures beginning in
    pregnancy
  Management of epilepsy in pregnancy
Cerebrovascular disease
  Cortical venous and sagittal sinus thrombosis
  Ruptured aneurysms and arteriovenous
    malformations
  Emboli (e.g., fat, air, amniotic fluid)
  Anticardiolipin antibody
  Disseminated intravascular coagulation,
    thrombotic or idiopathic thrombocytopenic
    purpura
Headaches
  Preexisting headaches worsening in pregnancy
    (e.g., migraine, common and classic)
  Headaches appearing in pregnancy
Brain tumors
  Meningiomas
  Choriocarcinoma metastatic to brain
  Pituitary tumors
Effects of pregnancy on chronic neurological
    conditions and special management problems
  Multiple sclerosis
  Myasthenia gravis
  Myotonic dystrophy
  Paraplegia
  Chronic vegetative state
  Wilson's disease
Entrapment and other neuropathies
  Acroparesthesias and carpal tunnel syndrome
  Guillain-Barré syndrome
  Bell's palsy
  Lumbosacral disc disease
  Abdominal cutaneous nerve entrapment
Complications of delivery
  Obstetrical palsies: brachial plexus, common
    peroneal, obturator, sciatic, femoral
  Complications of epidural anesthesia
Miscellaneous
  Meningitis (tuberculous, *Listeria*)
  Hyperemesis gravidarum (hyponatremia,
    Wernicke-Korsakoff)
  Chorea gravidarum
  Syncope

cortical blindness, retinal arteriolar constriction, cerebral edema (often seen on CT scans), and intracranial hemorrhage are major neurological complications. In uncontrolled cases, one of the most common causes of death is intracerebral hemorrhage.

Therapy consists of keeping the patient as relaxed and quiet as possible, controlling blood pressure with antihypertensive agents, treating convulsions with phenytoin or diazepam, or both, the administration of magnesium sulfate, which is a smooth muscle relaxant, and inducing early delivery.

Headache in Pregnancy

Hormonal changes, stress, and sleep disturbances may cause preexisting migraine or muscle contraction headache to worsen in pregnancy. However, some migraine patients remain remarkably free of headaches during pregnancy. Sinus headaches may be aggravated because of increased congestion in the nasal mucosa. A not uncommon event in migraineurs is the new appearance of classic migraine. The accompanying signs of hemianopia, hemianesthesia, aphasia, or hemiparesis are often mistaken for transient ischemic attacks (TIAs) or stroke.

The treatment options are somewhat limited in such instances because all medication should be avoided during the first trimester. Later in pregnancy, acetaminophen, codeine, and beta-blockers appear to be relatively safe for the fetus. Newly appearing headache in pregnancy may also herald serious intracranial or systemic disease such as eclampsia, intracranial hemorrhage, cortical venous thrombosis, or an expanding tumor. CT scanning that includes adequate fetal shielding or MRI scanning may be required in this situation.

Epilepsy in Pregnancy

Endocrine changes, fluid retention, stress, and sleep disturbances may exacerbate seizures during pregnancy in from a third to half of epileptic women. In addition, antiepileptic drug levels may fall, particularly during the later phases of pregnancy, due to poor absorption, increased metabolic rate, and reduced patient compliance. The actual adverse effects of seizures on the fetus or the outcome of pregnancy have been poorly studied, but status epilepticus, a rare complication during pregnancy, frequently provokes spontaneous abortion. It is therefore important to watch the patient closely and measure serum antiepileptic drug levels (ideally free levels) frequently during pregnancy. Doses of antiepileptic drugs often have to be increased as pregnancy advances.

An important consideration in all epileptics who are or who wish to become pregnant is the potential teratogenic effects of virtually all of the antiepileptic drugs. There appears to be a two- to threefold (about 5–10%) risk of malformations, such as digital dysplasia, cleft lip and palate, and heart defects, in the offspring of patients on phenytoin or barbiturates. Valproic acid use may cause spina bifida in 1 to 2 percent of exposed fetuses and recently carbamazepine has also been implicated. Rarely, a full-blown fetal anticonvulsant syndrome has been described that comprises growth retardation, multiple congenital anomalies, and mental retardation. The teratogenicity of benzodiazepines is less well established and ethosuximide appears to be safe.

Recommendations in pregnant epileptics include eliminating any unnecessary antiepileptic drugs and optimizing serum levels before conception, as well as monitoring patients on valproic acid and carbamazepine at approximately 19 weeks' gestation. At this time the serum alpha-fetoprotein level should be checked and fetal ultrasound carried out to detect possible spina bifida. Further measures consist of folate supplementation, monitoring of the serum antiepileptic drug levels as pregnancy advances to determine whether doses need to be increased, and administering vitamin K prepartum and to the fetus postpartum to prevent hemorrhagic disease in the newborn.

The new onset of seizures in pregnancy may reflect a variety of underlying conditions, some potentially serious (Table 29-2).

Cerebrovascular Disease in Pregnancy

Hemorrhagic Disorders

Subarachnoid or intracerebral hemorrhages resulting from ruptured aneurysms or arteriovenous malformations increase in incidence during pregnancy, the former tending to occur in the last trimester and the latter, in the second trimester. Rerupture, and at times initial rup-

ture, may also take place during delivery due to the inherent cardiovascular stresses and the use of the Valsalva maneuver. The management adopted is generally similar to that in the nonpregnant woman, with definitive surgical treatment performed when possible. If the rupture occurs in the last weeks of pregnancy or definitive treatment is not possible, then cesarean section is generally recommended followed by surgical treatment.

Ischemic Disease

There is an increased risk of cerebral infarction during pregnancy arising from various causes. The mild hypercoagulable state of pregnancy may predispose to infarction. Certain hematological disorders such as thrombotic thrombocytopenic purpura (TTP) tend to be exacerbated during pregnancy. Patients with systemic lupus erythematosus (SLE) can suffer a worsening cerebral vasculitis during pregnancy that then leads to cerebral infarction, encephalopathy, and seizures. A cerebral embolism is probably the most common cause of ischemic stroke in pregnancy, and potential sources include rheumatic valvular disease, mural thrombus complicating the cardiomyopathy of pregnancy, subacute bacterial endocarditis, paradoxical embolus arising from pelvic thrombophlebitis and a patent foramen ovale, a prolapsed mitral valve, and air or amniotic fluid embolism that occurs during delivery. The **anticardiolipin antibody syndrome** is being increasingly recognized in pregnant women and may be responsible for causing cerebral infarction and increased fetal wastage.

Cortical venous and sagittal sinus thrombosis is a well-known and feared complication of pregnancy that tends to occur peri- and postpartum. Rarely it can happen as early as 6 weeks in the first trimester. The usual presenting symptoms are headache and focal signs that may progress to an encephalopathy, seizures, elevated intracranial pressure, and coma. CT scanning (Fig. 29-1), MRI, and digital intravenous subtraction angiography have facilitated diagnosis. Heparin should be administered unless large hemorrhagic brain infarcts are identified. Patients who survive the initial phases often recover completely.

Table 29-2. Differential Diagnosis of Seizures Appearing in Pregnancy

Etiology	Usual time of appearance
Eclampsia	Late
Idiopathic epilepsy	Variable
Cerebrovascular disease	
Arteriovenous malformation	Late
Subarachnoid hemorrhage	Late
Cortical venous thrombosis	Peripartum
Embolus (e.g., amniotic fluid, air)	Peripartum
Tumor	Mid-late
Hyponatremia (oxytocin)	Peripartum
Intravenous lidocaine with epidural anesthesia	Peripartum
Vasodepressor syncope	Variable
Psychogenic pseudoseizure	Peripartum

Peripheral Nerve Involvement

Acroparesthesias and **carpal tunnel syndrome of pregnancy** are fairly frequent problems in pregnancy and are likely due to swelling of the tissues in the carpal tunnel that involves the median nerve. This is a transient phenomenon that is best treated using conservative measures such as cock-up wrist splints.

Bell's palsy is probably a more common affliction in pregnancy, especially in the later phases, but carries a good prognosis for recovery.

Abdominal cutaneous nerve entrapment is a relatively rare condition that produces upper abdominal paresthesias, dysesthesias, and bothersome pain late in pregnancy. Symptoms resolve postpartum.

Meralgia paresthetica (entrapment of the lateral femoral cutaneous nerve of the thigh under the inguinal ligament) occasionally occurs in pregnancy and likely stems from the attendant postural changes. Symptoms resolve postpartum.

Lumbosacral degenerative disc disease and low back pain worsen because of the hyperlordotic posture produced by pregnancy.

The obturator, femoral, sciatic, and saphenous nerves may sometimes be compressed due to the fetal head position or to pressure or stretching during delivery (especially in the lithotomy position). Although rapid resolution is the rule, if axonal damage is incurred, recovery may take several months.

The administration of **epidural anesthesia** carries its own risks of neurological complications and sequelae, including paralysis with escape of the anesthetic agent into the CSF pathways and post–lumbar puncture headache if the subarachnoid space is entered.

Other Conditions

Chorea gravidarum is a form of acute chorea during pregnancy that likely represents basal ganglia involvement from SLE or some other vasculitic process.

Brain tumors such as meningiomas or pituitary adenomas may undergo rapid growth and become symptomatic during pregnancy.

About 10 percent of the cases of **pseudotumor cerebri** commence in pregnancy and symptoms often begin in the first trimester. The disorder may recur in subsequent pregnancies. Management generally consists of performing repeated lumbar punctures, with preservation of vision the principal goal.

The incidence of **tuberculous meningitis** is increased during pregnancy and is especially common in the women of developing countries such as India.

Myasthenia gravis is encountered mainly in women of childbearing age and neonatal myasthenia appears in up to a third of the offspring of affected mothers. Symptomatic treatment with pyridostigmine is safe. Plasmapheresis has been used to treat myasthenia gravis success-

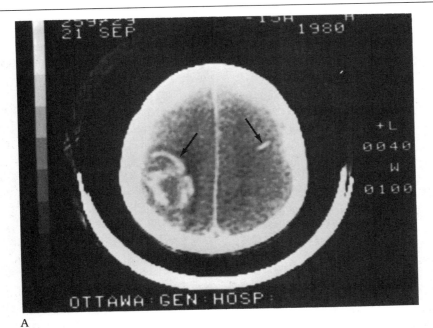

A

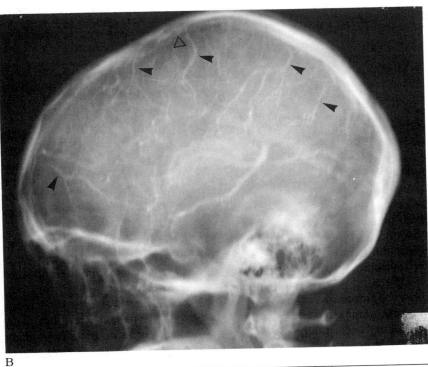

B

Fig. 29-1. *Cortical venous and sagittal sinus thrombosis in early pregnancy. This 22-year-old woman's last menstrual period had occurred 6 weeks previously and she was not known to be pregnant. She presented with a 2-week history of headache, low-grade fever, and Wernicke's aphasia. (A) A CT scan obtained a few days later showed left parietal and small right frontal hemorrhagic lesions (arrows). (B) An initial angiogram showed several cortical veins (solid arrowheads) and opacification of part of the sagittal sinus (open arrowhead). The patient's condition deteriorated over the subsequent week, with coma, seizures, and decerebration, and repeat CT scans showed extensive bilateral edema and new hemorrhagic lesions.*

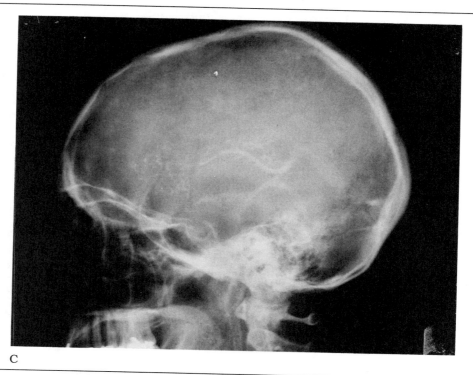

C

Fig. 29-1 *(Continued). (C) A repeat angiogram revealed filling only of the deep venous system due to occlusion of the sagittal sinus. The patient eventually died as the result of severe brain swelling, and pregnancy was confirmed. The unusual feature of this case is its occurrence in the early phase of pregnancy, as most cases tend to occur postpartum.*

fully during pregnancy, but steroids and immunosuppressants should be avoided.

Patients with **myotonic dystrophy** are at increased risk of complications such as polyhydramnios, spontaneous abortion, and dysfunctional uterine contraction during labor.

Exacerbations of **multiple sclerosis** may arise more commonly in pregnancy, especially during the postpartum period, but the long-term course of the disease is unaltered.

HEPATIC DISEASE

Hepatic encephalopathy is a common cause of metabolic encephalopathy and coma in hospitalized patients. One variety occurs in the context of **acute fulminant hepatic failure** and is due to exposure to toxins, or drugs, or to viral illness. In such cases, often in younger patients,

severe encephalopathy often leads to coma accompanied by decerebration and intracranial pressure is significantly elevated.

More commonly, patients with hepatic encephalopathy present a picture of chronic gradual deterioration of cerebral function that is punctuated by acute reversible episodes of a precoma state or of coma. Alcoholic liver disease with portosystemic shunts, and viral or immunologically mediated hepatitis are among the most common causes. Acute episodes of neurological deterioration can be provoked by the use of sedative or hypnotic drugs, excessive protein intake, gastrointestinal bleeding, intercurrent infection, or excessive diuresis that precipitates hypokalemia and metabolic alkalosis.

The neuropsychiatric and neurological manifestations of hepatic encephalopathy are highly variable but can usually be categorized according to their severity. Many of the signs point to frontal involvement. In stage 1, the patient exhibits insomnia with reversal of sleep patterns, mild confusion, agitation, attention deficits, postural tremor, and incoordination. In stage 2, the encephalopathy worsens and is accompanied by disorientation, memory deficits, and stupor. Asterixis, dysarthria, and ataxia are prominent symptoms and primitive reflexes emerge. Stage 3 includes worsening delirium and deepening stupor. Corticospinal tract involvement, hyperventilation, seizures, and myoclonus may be seen. In stage 4, the patient is comatose and may manifest oral or facial dyskinesias, brisk oculocephalic responses, and decerebrate movements.

The diagnosis is based on the clinical picture in the context of clear-cut liver disease, often with jaundice, elevated liver enzyme levels, and other telltale laboratory findings. Asterixis, although a frequent component of hepatic encephalopathy, is a nonspecific finding and may also occur in conjunction with uremic encephalopathy, carbon dioxide narcosis, and certain drug intoxications. The EEG shows progressive slowing and commonly triphasic delta waves in the intermediate stages (see Fig. 4-1). Although the serum ammonia level is often elevated, the levels do not always correlate with the severity of the encephalopathy. The CSF glutamine level is also elevated and correlates well with the clinical state, but this substance is not routinely measured.

The neurological features of hepatic encephalopathy may be compounded and even overshadowed by other factors that produce independent symptoms and signs. The likelihood of intracerebral hemorrhages is increased because of the coagulation deficits involved. Electrolyte and acid/base disturbances that include hyponatremia, the effects of alcohol and nutritional deficiencies, concurrent renal failure, hypoxia, and hypoglycemia may all add to the overall clinical picture. **Central pontine myelinolysis** is also occasionally seen in these patients.

The pathogenesis of hepatic encephalopathy is still not completely understood, although it is likely related to the CNS effects of various toxic substances that are normally metabolized by the liver. Both experimental and clinical evidence point strongly to a primary role for am-

monia in this process. However, because ammonia levels are not always elevated and in some cases correlate poorly with the clinical state, this suggests the involvement of additional factors. One hypothesis purports that substances such as octopamine may serve as false transmitters at dopaminergic and noradrenergic synapses when their levels are elevated in the brain. Because of this theory, attempts to improve the neurological picture through the administration of L-dopa and bromocriptine have been mounted, with some success. Interest is now focused on excessive GABAergic activity as the possible source of the CNS depression observed in hepatic encephalopathy. This may be related to abnormally elevated levels of benzodiazepine-like substances, either stemming from endogenous production or from ingestion. The neuropathological changes in the brain are unimpressive and consist mainly of an increase in the number of type II Alzheimer astrocytes.

The strategy in the treatment of hepatic encephalopathy is directed toward lowering the serum ammonia level. Standard measures are reducing the dietary protein intake, administering tap water enemas to remove blood from the gastrointestinal tract, administering neomycin, which depopulates the gut of ammonia-producing bacteria, and lactulose, which changes the pH of the gut. Other more radical measures include exchange transfusions and liver transplantation in selected cases.

A rare manifestation of chronic liver failure is nonwilsonian hepatocerebral degeneration. These patients exhibit both cortical and basal ganglia involvement.

A **myelopathy** with spastic paraparesis is an unusual complication of liver failure and is seen in patients with spontaneous or surgically produced portosystemic shunts.

Reye's syndrome is a rare form of acute fulminant fatty degeneration of the liver that appears mainly in children or adolescents following a viral infection and at times are triggered by aspirin ingestion. There appears to be a hepatic mitochondrial dysfunction in this disorder. The illness is often heralded by severe vomiting, which is followed rapidly by a severe encephalopathy with coma, raised intracranial pressure, and decerebration. Liver enzyme levels are markedly elevated, and there are hepatic necrosis, a coagulopathy, and hypoglycemia. The mortality associated with the syndrome has now diminished because such patients receive meticulous intensive care and attention is devoted to lowering the intracranial pressure, correcting the coagulopathy and electrolyte imbalances, and reversing the hypoglycemia.

RENAL FAILURE

Uremic Encephalopathy

Acute renal failure can provoke an encephalopathy that is not distinct from other metabolic encephalopathies. In the early phases, personality changes, inattention, and lethargy alternating with restlessness may be seen. Later, decreased cognitive function, sleep disturbance, and emotional lability progress to a frank confusional state together with dysarthria, cranial nerve abnormalities, asymmetrical deep tendon reflexes, asterixis, multifocal myoclonus, seizures, and finally coma. A similar pattern with a slower and fluctuating course is seen in patients suffering from chronic renal failure. The EEG is slowed, but more so in acute renal failure. Several metabolic imbalances are likely responsible for this state, including an increase in the concentration of osmotically active particles in the brain (idiogenic osmoles), increased ammonia, calcium, and parathyroid hormone levels in the brain, and imbalances in neurotransmitter function.

This encephalopathy can be reversed by dialysis or renal transplantation. Phenytoin is the best treatment for the seizures, which may be part of the encephalopathy or secondary to focal brain ischemic or hemorrhagic lesions. Because of the decreased protein binding of phenytoin, it is the free levels that should ideally be monitored.

Dialysis Encephalopathy (Dementia)

Dialysis encephalopathy is a rare, fatal progressive syndrome that sometimes appears in patients who have been on hemodialysis for over 2 to 3 years. The clinical picture consists of dysar-

thria, asterixis, myoclonus, dementia, focal seizures, and multifocal sharp- and slow-wave EEG abnormalities. The accumulation of aluminum in the cerebral cortex, which is derived from aluminum-containing antacids or dialysate fluid, is blamed for this disorder, and its incidence has decreased with greater emphasis on the preparation of ionic-free dialysate fluids.

Dialysis Dysequilibrium

Over-rapid dialysis may precipitate brain swelling, the major cause of dialysis dysequilibrium. Affected patients typically experience headache, nausea, restlessness, muscle cramps, and tremulousness during or after dialysis. Improved scheduling of dialysis and greater attention to maintaining optimal fluid balance have reduced the incidence of this syndrome.

Uremic Neuropathy

Peripheral neuropathy is an almost universal feature of severe end-stage renal disease. Typically the patient initially has symptoms of restless legs and then a distal sensorimotor symmetrical polyneuropathy affecting the lower extremities later develops. Burning feet, uncomfortable dysesthesias, and autonomic symptoms such as orthostatic hypotension and impotence may occur. Nerve conduction velocities may be mildly impaired, but, because the pathology mainly consists of axonal degeneration, F- and H-wave measurements are the most sensitive tests. The neuropathy often abates considerably following the institution of dialysis, and especially following transplantation. In addition, uremic patients may be subject to polyneuropathies or mononeuropathies because of such underlying conditions as diabetes mellitus, polyarteritis nodosa, or SLE.

Other Neurological Complications of Renal Failure

Hypertension as well as other conditions such as diabetes mellitus and collagen disease predispose the patient with renal failure to ischemic vascular disease, and **cerebral infarction** is a relatively common complication. Cerebral emboli may also originate from clotted arterial shunts. A **subdural hematoma** can be a complication of dialysis. Uremic patients manifest a bleeding diathesis with impaired platelet function and are given anticoagulants to preserve shunt patency.

Renal Transplantation

Renal transplantation, with its attendant long-term use of immunosuppressants such as cyclosporine, can make recipients susceptible to neurological complications such as CNS infection with opportunistic pathogens (e.g., herpes zoster, cytomegalovirus, *Cryptococcus*, and progressive multifocal leukoencephalopathy) as well as CNS lymphoma or glioma. In addition, cyclosporine itself can be responsible for causing epileptic seizures, tremors, burning dysesthesias of the palms and soles, ataxia, and weakness of the extremities.

SYSTEMIC CANCER

The neurological effects of cancer and its treatment are numerous and varied (Table 29-3). Direct effects due to metastatic or invasive tumors are common and must always be sought first in any patient with cancer who exhibits neurological, particularly focal, signs (see Chapter 20). Cancer metastasizes to the brain in 20 to 40 percent of affected patients. Such neoplasms most commonly involve the cerebral hemispheres and are multiple in 50 percent of the cases. They are usually associated with primary cancers of the lung, breast, kidney, gastrointestinal tract, cervix and uterus, choriocarcinoma, and melanoma. Carcinomatous or lymphomatous meningitis is being seen more commonly as an aftermath of the otherwise successful treatment of systemic malignancy. It occurs particularly in the presence of adenocarcinomas, melanomas, lymphomas, and leukemia. The clinical picture may consist of acute or subacute syndrome with headache, raised intracranial pressure, fever, signs of meningeal irritation, cranial nerve palsies, and radicular sensory or motor signs, or both. However, it may also be more

Table 29-3. Neurological Complications of Cancer and its Treatment

Direct
  Metastases to brain or spinal cord
  Epidural spinal cord compression
  Carcinomatous meningitis
  Metastases to base of skull with cranial nerve
    involvement
  Peripheral nerve plexus and root invasion
Secondary effects
  Cachexia and muscle weakness
  Nutritional neuropathies and encephalopathies
    (e.g., Wernicke's)
  Cerebral venoocclusive disease
    (hypercoagulability)
  Cerebral vasculitis
  Marantic endocarditis embolizing to CNS
  Other causes of stroke (e.g., disseminated
    intravascular coagulation, thrombocytosis)
  Metabolic encephalopathies (e.g., hypercalcemia)
Paraneoplastic syndromes (remote effects
    presumably immunologically mediated)
  Eaton-Lambert myasthenic syndrome
  Polymyositis/dermatomyositis
  Subacute sensory neuronopathy
  Subacute motor neuronopathy
  Syndrome resembling amyotrophic lateral
    sclerosis
  Peripheral sensorimotor neuropathy
  Myelopathy
  Subacute cerebellar degeneration
  Ataxia/myoclonus/opsoclonus
  Limbic encephalitis
Complications of treatment
  Neurotoxicity of chemotherapeutic agents (e.g.,
    cisplatin or vincristine neuropathy, cerebellar
    syndrome with 5-fluorouracil)
  Steroid encephalopathy or myopathy
  CNS infections with opportunistic agents
  CNS hemorrhage due to low platelet counts
  Early and late neurotoxic effects of radiotherapy

indolent and comprise headache, nausea, vomiting, mild confusion with seizures, and possibly cranial nerve palsies. Several lumbar punctures may be necessary before the abnormal cytology can be discovered. CT or MRI scanning with contrast enhancement may show diffuse meningeal or more localized tumor deposits, or both (Fig. 29-2). Treatment consists of radiotherapy and intrathecal chemotherapy. Patients with lymphoma or leukemia may do well.

Other neurological complications of cancer

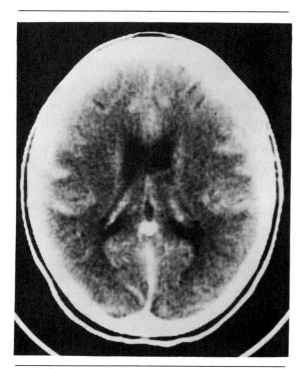

Fig. 29-2. *Enhanced CT scan in a 29-year-old woman with carcinomatous meningitis stemming from metastatic breast cancer. She presented with headache, stupor, nuchal rigidity, and vomiting. CSF was xanthochromic with a markedly elevated protein level (580 gm/dl), 52 WBCs (60% neutrophils), 5 malignant cells, and negative Gram's staining. Note the diffuse enhancement of the meninges over the surface of the brain. She responded well to intrathecal methotrexate.*

are termed *remote* or *paraneoplastic* because they occur a certain distance from the primary tumor, are not due to direct tumor cell involvement of the tissues or organs affected, and, for the most part, their pathogenesis is unknown. Some of these syndromes are specific to the underlying cancer, or at least highly associated with a primary neoplasm, and therefore, when encountered, should prompt a search for an occult malignancy. This is especially important because frequently these remote nervous system symptoms antedate the appearance of other signs of the cancer by months and sometimes by as much as 5 years. These syndromes assume additional importance because they are often associated with severe neurological symptoms, which can

occasionally be somewhat ameliorated by th successful treatment of the primary cancer In addition, understanding the pathogenesi of these syndromes may give some insigh into the pathophysiology of cancer and it immunological effects.

Although the pathogenesis of most of thes syndromes is poorly understood, an autoim mune mechanism has recently been invoke to explain several of them. Three strikin; clinical features of these syndromes are tha they tend to run a course that is independen of the underlying cancer, occur in combinatio or as "overlap" syndromes, and have a hig association with certain cancers such as smal cell carcinoma of the lung, gynecological an breast cancers, neuroblastoma in children, an lymphomas or Hodgkin's disease. Recognitio of these syndromes is not only important from the standpoint of early diagnosis of an occul malignancy, but also for differentiating thes syndromes from other neurological problem related to cancer, some of which may b treatable.

The immunosuppression in cancer patient also makes them susceptible to a host o opportunistic infections, especially viral an fungal, which can affect the nervous system Herpes zoster radiculitis, progressive multifo cal leukoencephalopathy, and cryptococca meningitis are examples of such infections The malnutrition that accompanies advanced and gastrointestinal cancer may foster vitamin deficiency neuropathies and rarely Wernicke's encephalopathy. Cachexia with loss of muscle and subcutaneous tissue in a bedridden patient may predispose to the development of compression palsies of peripheral nerves, such as the common peroneal. Certain metabolic effects of cancer can produce neurological symptoms. Small-cell lung cancers can secrete antidiuretic hormone, which in turn can cause hyponatremia and its neurological consequences of confusion and seizures. Hypoglycemia can be a complication of pancreatic islet cell tumors. The hypercalcemia that can occur with metastatic breast and other cancers, or as a paraneoplastic effect, can spawn behavioral changes, confusion, and stupor. Through the operation of various mechanisms, stroke is a elatively frequent problem in cancer patients. A hypercoagulable state may be associated with several types of cancer. Cortical venous thrombosis is occasionally the presenting symptom of an underlying pancreatic cancer. Marantic endocarditis, which may embolize to the brain, is especially common with thoracic cancers.

The medications used for pain control and sedation may themselves precipitate an encephalopathy and the antiemetic agents commonly prescribed to control the nausea and vomiting provoked by chemotherapy can precipitate extrapyramidal symptoms. Corticosteroids, used particularly in treating the reticuloses, occasionally cause neurological complications such as psychosis and myopathy. A number of the chemotherapeutic agents used to treat cancer, either given intravenously or intrathecally, are very neurotoxic.

Radiotherapy, when administered in high doses and delivered to central or peripheral nervous structures, either deliberately or inadvertently, can have both acute and chronic effects on nervous tissues. Neurons are generally more impervious to these effects than are glial cells or the vascular endothelium, and many of the effects are likely mediated by the slowly progressive occlusion of small vessels that then leads to tissue ischemia with resultant myelin breakdown or necrosis. Radiation plexopathies, which may appear in the brachial plexus years after cobalt treatment for breast cancer or in the lumbosacral plexus years after cobalt treatment for uterine and cervical cancer, must be distinguished from metastatic plexus invasion by the primary tumor. Unlike a radiation plexopathy, the latter is usually a painful condition and, in the brachial plexus, involves the distal arm and hand muscles rather than the proximal ones. MRI or CT scanning of the plexus areas may help discriminate between the two conditions. The internal carotid artery may undergo accelerated atherosclerotic narrowing or thrombotic occlusion years following irradiation for head or neck cancer and is due to endothelial vascular damage.

Some of the more important paraneoplastic syndromes are discussed in the following sections.

Limbic Encephalitis

Patients with cancer (usually small-cell lung carcinoma or Hodgkin's disease) often manifest the signs and symptoms of limbic encephalitis by as much as several years before their cancer is diagnosed. The subacute onset of memory loss, behavioral change, psychiatric disturbances, and generalized or complex partial seizures are common features of the syndrome. Neuronal loss, perivascular inflammatory cell infiltrates, gliosis, and microglial nodules are found in the hippocampus, amygdala, and other limbic structures. Similar structures may also be scattered throughout other areas of the nervous system, including the brainstem, cerebellum, spinal cord, and dorsal root ganglion, but may or may not cause symptoms. Diagnosis is mainly based on the clinical findings because the results of special tests are relatively nonspecific. The CSF protein level may be mildly elevated with a mild pleocytosis. CT and MRI scans may show mild atrophy, particularly in conjunction with enlargement of the temporal horns.

The pathogenesis of the syndrome is unclear, although a viral or autoimmune etiology, or both, is likely. The anti-Ho antineuronal antibody, which is highly linked to various paraneoplastic neurological syndromes in patients with small-cell carcinoma of the lung, has been detected in several patients with limbic encephalitis. In some cases, partial regression is achieved once the underlying neoplasm has been treated.

Subacute Cerebellar Degeneration

Subacute cerebellar degeneration is the most common paraneoplastic syndrome affecting the brain and is strongly associated with cancer of the ovary, breast, and uterus, although it may also occur in patients with Hodgkin's disease or small-cell lung carcinoma. The signs and symptoms indicate diffuse dysfunction of the cerebellum and consist of gait ataxia, dysarthria, nystagmus, and limb dysmetria or ataxia. A more diffuse encephalomyelitis, including cognitive deterioration and Babinski's signs as well as peripheral neuropathy, is not uncommon. Deficits are usually moderately severe but often plateau after several months. As with several other paraneoplastic syndromes, the CSF findings often only consist of a mildly elevated protein level, pleocytosis, and oligoclonal bands. CT scanning may reveal the existence of cerebellar atrophy and an enlarged fourth ventricle.

The course of the cerebellar syndrome is usually independent of that of the underlying cancer. Pathological examination discloses a striking loss of Purkinje cells throughout the cerebellum with proliferation of astrocytes as well as mild inflammatory changes, which may also be seen scattered throughout areas outside the cerebellum. High titers of anti–Purkinje cell antibodies ("anti-Yo") are typically found in the serum and CSF of patients with subacute cerebellar degeneration and underlying gynecological cancers. These antibodies likely participate in the pathogenesis of the condition and are directed at a tumor antigen, which shares features with Purkinje cells and other neurons.

Opsoclonus-Myoclonus-Ataxia Syndrome

The opsoclonus-myoclonus-ataxia syndrome, with its striking, nearly continuous spontaneous conjugate saccadic eye movements, is associated with an underlying neuroblastoma in children in about 50 percent of cases (see Chapter 18). It may occur in adults with underlying lung carcinoma as well. However, it can also constitute a viral or postviral complication and be a part of certain toxic reactions. Symptoms pursue an unpredictable course but often abate with treatment of the underlying neuroblastoma.

Myelopathies

The rare syndrome of necrotizing myelopathy presents as a painless acute transverse myelopathy consisting of paraplegia, together with sensory level and sphincter disturbances. Extensive transverse segmental spinal cord destruction is seen pathologically. A vasculitic pathogenesis has been hypothesized. Clinically this syndrome must be distinguished from spinal cord compression due to epidural metastases or abscess.

A less severe, often patchy and asymmetric myelitis forms a part of the diffuse encephalomyelitis that affects various levels of the nervous system in patients with an underlying malignancy.

Motor Neuron Disorders

Rarely, otherwise typical cases of amyotrophic lateral sclerosis (ALS) may be associated with an underlying cancer. There have been a few reports in which treatment of the cancer effected remission of the ALS. A characteristic syndrome, possibly caused by a poliolike virus and affecting anterior horn cells, is termed *subacute motor neuronopathy*. It is strongly linked to underlying Hodgkin's disease or lymphoma and may regress with treatment of the lymphoma. Although patients often suffer a significant paraparesis, this frequently abates. Other varieties of motor neuron disorders that can resemble ALS have been associated with paraproteinemias, particularly IgM. Treatment of the monoclonal gammopathy with immunosuppressive agents may occasionally ameliorate the neurological syndrome.

Peripheral Neuropathies

A nonspecific distal, often mild, sensorimotor peripheral neuropathy is relatively common in cancer patients with advanced disease. It can constitute a remote effect of the underlying cancer but also can stem from other factors such as malnutrition with consequential vitamin deficiency. The most characteristic neuropathy seen with cancer is a **subacute sensory neuronopathy** that stems from inflammatory involvement of the dorsal root ganglion cells. Burning dysesthesias and severe pain involving the feet are the hallmark of this syndrome, but profound large-fiber sensory loss later produces ataxia and pseudoathetosis. This severely incapacitating syndrome is strongly associated with small-cell carcinoma of the lung. It is regarded as part of the spectrum of autoimmune disorders that are associated with carcinoma because there is a high incidence of neuronal antinuclear antibodies (anti-Hu), which, as already mentioned, also exist in ome patients with other neurological paraeoplastic syndromes.

A similar sensory ganglionitis has been observed in the context of Sjögren's syndrome, yridoxine toxicity, cisplatin toxicity, and "idiopathic ataxic neuropathy." A predominantly **utonomic neuropathy** is a rare component f a paraneoplastic syndrome. An otherwise ypical **Guillain-Barré syndrome** or **chronic nflammatory demyelinating polyneuropathy** ay occur in conjunction with underlying carinoma or Hodgkin's disease. However, these emyelinating neuropathies in cancer patients ay represent little more than coincidental vents. There have been reports of patchy nononeuropathies in cancer patients that are ue to **microvasculitis.** Multiple myeloma is articularly associated with peripheral neuropthy, especially the osteosclerotic type. Amyiidosis in patients with multiple myeloma ends to produce a painful small-fiber neuropthy that exhibits autonomic features. In cerain cases of multiple myeloma, an antibody as been identified that is directed against nyelin-associated glycoprotein. Waldentrom's macroglobulinemia is also associated /ith a peripheral neuropathy.

In any cancer patient who exhibits a neuropthy, even a diffuse symmetrical neuropathy, lirect tumor invasion must be ruled out before paraneoplastic etiology is postulated. ymphomas, myelomas, and rarely carcinoas can extensively and relatively selectively nvade peripheral and cranial nerves, even /ithout systemic metastases. These invasive europathies are exquisitely painful.

Eaton-Lambert Myasthenic Syndrome

A neuromuscular junction disorder, the Eaton-Lambert myasthenic syndrome is particularly common in middle-aged men suffering from small-cell carcinoma of the lung. Its pathogenesis has been fairly well worked out. Autoantibodies are produced to presynaptic voltage-dependent calcium channels, which then malfunction and this interferes with the release of acetylcholine. Patients exhibit proximal weakness with sparing of the cranial musculature, except for occasional ptosis and dysphagia. Increasing strength with sustained muscular effort is a hallmark of the syndrome and can be demonstrated clinically as well as electrically. The motor action potential has a low amplitude and shows a decremental response at low-frequency stimulation rates but increases to supramaximal levels at higher-frequency rates. Other telltale features are dry mouth and areflexia, suggesting an associated neuropathy. The syndrome subsides with treatment of the underlying cancer. Drugs such as 3,4-diaminopyridine, which enhance acetylcholine release, improve the patient's strength. There may also be a partial response to anticholinesterase drugs such as pyridostigmine.

Muscle Disease

Polymyositis and particularly dermatomyositis are associated with cancer in approximately 10 to 50 percent of cases, which represents about a twofold increased risk compared to the general population. A rare necrotizing myopathy can constitute a remote effect of cancer. Proximal weakness is common in patients with carcinoid tumors. Cachexia produces generalized weakness and possibly a specific myopathy.

COLLAGEN VASCULAR DISEASES

Systemic Lupus Erythematosus

SLE is a multisystem disease with an autoimmune pathogenesis that largely affects young to middle-aged women. Among the organs most commonly involved are the skin (photosensitive butterfly rash over the face), the joints (arthritis and arthralgias), the kidneys (glomerulonephritis), the heart (pericarditis and endocarditis), and the blood (thrombocytopenia). Serological findings include antinuclear antibodies, anti–double-stranded DNA antibodies, and a positive VDRL. There is central or peripheral nervous system involvement in approximately 50 percent of the patients.

The pathogenesis of the CNS involvement is variable. Autoantibodies to neurons, serum lymphocytotoxic antibodies, and antiribosomal P protein antibodies have been detected and their presence correlated with neurological deficits in some studies. Immune complex deposition has been noted in the choroid plexus and may be responsible for causing alterations in the blood-brain barrier. Small arteries and arterioles within the brain may undergo hyaline degeneration and inflammation, but a true vasculitis is not observed. Some patients have circulating antiphospholipid antibodies (lupus anticoagulant). This sets up a condition that predisposes to the occurrence of TIAs and cerebrovascular thromboocclusive disease. The complete antiphospholipid antibody syndrome also includes recurrent deep vein thromboses, spontaneous abortions, thrombocytopenia, and a prolonged partial thromboplastin time.

The most common CNS manifestations of SLE are seizures, psychosis (organic delirium), or personality changes, but often without clear-cut structural correlates depicted by neuroimaging studies. The EEG is often a sensitive indicator of brain involvement. These symptoms may be due to microvascular involvement or to the existence of specific antibodies directed against neurons or cellular components. A migraine-like syndrome can occur in patients with lupus and heralds its onset. As already mentioned, cerebral infarcts and TIAs may be seen, especially in the context of antiphospholipid antibodies. Libman-Sacks endocarditis, which most commonly affects the mitral valve, may rarely embolize to the brain and also predisposes the patient to infective endocarditis.

Chorea can occur, possibly due to the involvement of small vessels in the basal ganglia. Rarely a picture resembling multiple sclerosis with optic neuritis or transverse myelitis, or both, may occur, even without signs of systemic involvement. To further confuse the picture, oligoclonal bands are found in the CSF in up to 50 percent of cases and the MRI scan may show multifocal subcortical and periventricular white matter lesions that are indistinguishable from those typical of multiple sclerosis. The deficits may be relapsing and remitting and responsive to steroids; these are other characteristics of multiple sclerosis. Recurrent aseptic

meningitis, pseudotumor cerebri, and progressive multifocal leukoencephalopathy are also seen in some patients.

The peripheral nervous system is less commonly involved, but a symmetrical sensorimotor distal polyneuropathy and occasionally multiple mononeuropathy (also affecting the cranial nerves) can occur.

Besides the direct effects of SLE on the nervous system, neurological complications stemming from renal failure, hypertension, and steroid and immunosuppressant treatment can arise. Thrombotic thrombocytopenic purpura may afflict patients in the preterminal phase and cause multifocal CNS involvement.

Progressive Systemic Sclerosis (Scleroderma)

A trigeminal sensory neuropathy, which is often bilateral and potentially painful, is the most well recognized neurological complication of progressive systemic sclerosis (PSS). In addition, the seventh and eighth cranial nerves may be involved. Vasculitic involvement of the CNS is rare.

Necrotizing Vasculitis

Necrotizing vasculitis represents a group of disorders, of which **polyarteritis nodosa** (PAN) is the best example. These disorders are characterized by inflammation and fibrinoid necrosis of small and medium-sized arteries in various organs, especially the skin, gut (mesenteric artery), heart, and kidney, and likely result from immune complex deposition and complement activation in the vessel walls.

Features of PAN, which tends to affect older men, include renal failure, hypertension, intestinal ischemia, and eosinophilia. Mesenteric or cerebral arteries may show nodular beading on angiograms. CNS involvement in PAN occurs in about 11 percent of cases and is a late phenomenon. Diffuse and multifocal brain involvement is a rare feature and produces an encephalopathy that consists of seizures or focal signs. More commonly a multiple mononeuropathy afflicts the peripheral nervous system and, more rarely, a symmetrical distal polyneuopathy resulting from vasculitic involvement of the vasa nervorum.

Churg-Strauss Syndrome

Churg-Strauss syndrome (allergic angiitis and granulomatosis) that affects the CNS occurs in the context of systemic disease, typically asthma, allergic rhinitis, and eosinophilia. In the advanced phases, fever, weight loss, arthralgias and arthritis, skin rash, myositis, and cardiac involvement affect up to three fourths of the patients.

Wegener's Granulomatosis

Wegener's granulomatosis is a type of systemic necrotizing vasculitis that affects the lower and upper respiratory tracts, including the paranasal sinuses. Nasal pain and ulcerations are common ailments, as are skin lesions, kidney involvement, and arthralgias. Granulomas originating from the paranasal sinuses or middle ear may invade the orbit or intracranial structures such as the cavernous sinus. Rarely, isolated granulomas may form in the CNS or cranial nerves. Vasculitis may also occur in the CNS but much more commonly in the peripheral nervous system, where it can produce a multiple mononeuropathy.

Rheumatoid Arthritis

CNS vasculitis is a rare component of systemic rheumatoid vasculitis. When the CNS is affected, symptoms can include seizures, dementia, strokelike manifestations, cranial nerve palsies, and blindness.

Rheumatoid involvement of the transverse ligament of the atlas can cause atlantoaxial subluxation in up to 25 percent of the cases, which is usually asymptomatic. However, patients may experience occipital headache, ataxia, vertigo, weakness, and paresthesias, particularly with neck flexion, and a severe, acute myelopathy that is possibly due to vertebral artery compression is a constant danger in these cases.

There are a variety of compression neuropathies that are due to nerve entrapment and result from rheumatoid synovitis and joint de-

formity. Carpal tunnel syndrome is the most common abnormality, but entrapment of the ulnar nerve at the elbow or wrist, the posterior tibial, or common peroneal nerves also occurs. A digital neuropathy causing discomfort and sensory loss on one side of a finger can result from joint deformity and rheumatoid inflammation. A painful distal sensory neuropathy characterized by burning dysesthesias in the feet is relatively common. A more severe distal sensorimotor neuropathy can accompany rheumatoid vasculitis. Gold, which is used to treat rheumatoid arthritis, can precipitate a neuropathy.

Ankylosing Spondylitis

Ankylosing spondylitis is an inflammatory disease that affects the sacroiliac and posterior intervertebral joints. It is highly associated with the HLA27 antigen. Cervical myelopathy due to atlantoaxial subluxation can produce quadriparesis, but it may also be a clinically silent defect. A cauda equina syndrome that includes bladder impairment, sacral anesthesia, and motor involvement has been described as a late complication of this disorder.

Sjögren's Syndrome

Sjögren's syndrome (keratoconjunctivitis sicca), with or without arthritis, has been increasingly recognized to encompass neurological complications that may be the presenting feature. Psychiatric and cognitive dysfunction, trigeminal sensory neuropathy, facial weakness, recurrent aseptic meningoencephalitis, and a relapsing and remitting multifocal CNS or spinal disease that resembles multiple sclerosis have all been observed. MRI scans may disclose the existence of multifocal cerebral white matter disease. A peripheral sensory or sensorimotor neuropathy occurs in 10 to 20 percent of the affected patients.

Mixed Connective Tissue Disease

Mixed connective tissue disease includes features of SLE and polymyositis. The neurological features comprise the CNS manifestations seen in SLE (particularly aseptic meningitis) and trigeminal sensory neuropathy.

Other Vasculitides

Other conditions causing or related to vasculitis, including giant-cell arteritis, sarcoidosis, Behçet's disease, and granulomatosis angiitis of the nervous system, have been discussed in previous chapters.

DISTURBANCES OF ELECTROLYTE BALANCE

Electrolyte disturbances accompany a wide variety of systemic illnesses and iatrogenic disorders, are commonly encountered in clinical practice, and are apt to give rise to neurological or neuromuscular symptoms. The most important derangements likely to cause neurological and neuromuscular dysfunction are listed in Table 29-4. When sodium balance is disturbed in conjunction with osmolality derangements, this is particularly likely to lead to permanent neurological sequelae if either severe or improperly managed. In patients with hyponatremia, the absolute value of the serum sodium concentration may be less important in the production of symptoms than the rate of fall. Many patients, however, exhibit a definite encephalopathy with seizures when levels are less than 110 mEq/L. Acute severe hyponatremia, often due to water intoxication or the syndrome of inappropriate ADH secretion, can produce brain swelling and also interfere with neurotransmitter release.

There is controversy over the maximum rate at which hyponatremia should be corrected. Rapid correction (i.e., >0.5 mEq/L/hr) has been implicated in the development of central pontine and extrapontine myelinolysis, but it appears that a more relevant factor is correction to normal or hypernatremic levels within the first 48 hours. The absolute amount of correction (i.e., >25mEq/L in 48 hours) may be a more important determinant than the rate of correction.

The osmotic demyelination syndrome is also more common in malnourished alcoholic pa-

tients who suffer from potassium deficiency. Patients with serum sodium levels below 12 mEq/L who are asymptomatic generally d well when treatment consists of water restric tion or intravenously administered sodiu chloride (154 mEq/L). Patients with level below 120 mEq/L who are symptomatic ar candidates for receiving 3% hypertonic salin and furosemide. The mortality and morbidit are high in patients with severe hyponatremi resulting from cerebral edema, brain hernia tion, and possible respiratory arrest. This i especially true for previously healthy wome whose hyponatremia is induced postopera tively. A prudent guideline for the manage ment of symptomatic hyponatremia that is o unknown duration but likely acute is a fairl prompt 10 percent increase in the serum so dium level, and then slower correction accom plished by water restriction at a rate of les than 2.5 mEq/L/hr or 20 mEq/L/day.

Hypernatremia due to dehydration brough about by gastroenteritis, diuretic use, wate deprivation, or diabetes insipidus causes wate to be lost from the brain, leading to shrinkag and focal hemorrhages. Focal signs, seizures and coma may result and permanent brain dam age is relatively common in severe cases. Re bound cerebral edema may occur if rehydratio is too rapid.

Disturbances in potassium balance produc mainly neuromuscular and not CNS symptoms. However, both hyper- and hypocalcemia ar associated with a variety of CNS disturbance (see Table 29-4).

ENDOCRINE DISEASE

Diabetes Mellitus

Both juvenile (type 1) and adult-onset (type 2) diabetes are associated with a host of central and peripheral neurological complications whose pathogenesis is frequently not well understood.

Diabetic Ketoacidosis
Diabetic ketoacidosis constitutes a medical emergency in insulin-dependent diabetics. Pa-

Table 29-4. Electrolyte Derangements Commonly Associated with Neurological and Neuromuscular Complications

Electrolyte derangement	CNS effects	Neuromuscular effects	Other/comments	Causes
Hyponatremia	Confusion, seizures, coma	—	Neurological symptoms correlate with rapidity of fall of sodium concentration, central pontine myelinolysis (osmotic demyelination can occur with over-rapid correction of hyponatremia)	SIADH, dehydration (vomiting, diarrhea, sweating), water intoxication, liver failure, congestive heart failure, nephrotic syndrome, excessive renal sodium loss
Hypernatremia	Coma, focal cerebral damage, seizures	—	—	Failure to drink, diarrhea/vomiting, diabetes insipidus, osmotic diuresis, burns, excessive sweating
Hypokalemia	—	Weakness (vacuolar myopathy), myalgia, periodic paralysis	—	Diarrhea/vomiting, glucocorticoid excess, diuretics, hyperaldosteronism

Table 29-4 (Continued).

Electrolyte derangement	CNS effects	Neuromuscular effects	Other/comments	Causes
Hypocalcemia	Seizures, neuropsychiatric	Tetany	Pseudotumor, extrapyramidal (chorea, rigidity)	Vitamin D deficiency, malabsorption, hypoparathyroidism, pseudohypoparathyroidism, acute pancreatitis, renal tubular acidosis
Hypercalcemia	Behavioral change, psychosis, coma	Myopathy in hyperparathyroidism	—	Remote effect of cancer, hyperparathyroidism, excessive intake
Hypomagnesemia	Seizures, delirium, myoclonus	Weakness, hyperreflexia, tetany	—	Starvation, alcohol, malabsorption, diuretics, cisplatin
Hypermagnesemia	Confusion, stupor	Paralysis, depressed deep tendon reflexes	—	Renal failure and excessive intake
Hypophosphatemia	Seizures, myoclonus, paresthesias, tremor, stupor	—	—	Alcohol withdrawal, diabetic ketoacidosis, phosphate-binding antacids, extensive burns, refeeding after starvation, hyperalimentation, severe respiratory acidosis

nts may be comatose or more often stuporous
t rarely exhibit seizures or focal neurological
gns. The pathogenesis of the neurological
mptoms is obscure and they do not appear to
em from the acidosis, although the pH of CSF
es correlate somewhat with the level of con-
iousness. Over-rapid correction of the hyper-
ycemia and hyperosmolality can precipitate
rebral edema, which is often fatal.

yperosmolar Nonketotic Coma

yperosmolar nonketotic coma afflicts older
tients with mild or new diabetes, often with
underlying infection. Blood glucose levels
d osmolality are exceedingly high and pa-
nts are markedly dehydrated. This syndrome
also rarely encountered in burn and heat
roke victims, patients with thyrotoxicosis, and
tients undergoing corticosteroid therapy or
nal dialysis. Affected patients frequently
esent with strokelike symptoms such as hemi-
resis, aphasia, or visual field deficits. Sei-
res, including generalized tonic-clonic and
cal motor seizures (including epilepsy par-
lis continua), are common. These patients
rmally recover well with the cautious admin-
tration of insulin, fluid, and potassium, al-
ough occasionally cerebral edema may
evelop.

ypoglycemia

ypoglycemia, which is due to an excessive
nount of circulating insulin, exhibits a variety
f symptoms. In its mildest form, there may be
btle changes in personality accompanied by
ritability or aggressive behavior. Patients may
xperience hunger and symptoms of sympa-
etic hyperactivity such as sweating and tachy-
ardia, unless there is an underlying autonomic
europathy. Symptoms depend not only on the
bsolute serum glucose level but also on the
egree and rate of the reduction. Patients may
lso suffer seizures, and hypoglycemia must al-
ays be suspected when nocturnal seizures
ccur in a diabetic.

More profound hypoglycemia may produce
eversible focal neurological deficits such as
emiparesis and deep coma. Repeated bouts of
ypoglycemia can lead to cognitive impairment,
erebellar signs, and possibly motor neuron

damage. The pathological changes brought
about by severe hypoglycemia resemble those
following anoxia, and mainly involve the deep
cortical layers. Hippocampal, striatal, and cerebellar cell damage may result from excessive
calcium influx, phospholipase activation, and
free radical formation. However, the brain appears to be able to tolerate hypoglycemia better
than it does hypoxia, and full recovery is the
rule, even when profound hypoglycemia lasts
for periods of up to an hour or more. Other
causes of hypoglycemia include hepatic diseases, myxedema, insulinoma, and severe
starvation.

Cerebrovascular Disease
The risk of stroke is increased two to three
times in diabetics, and this is largely attributed
to the higher incidence of concurrent atherosclerosis and hypertension in these patients, but
diabetes-related small-vessel degenerative disease is also an important contributing factor.
In addition, alterations in platelet aggregability
and blood clotting factors tend to produce a
hypercoagulable state. The outcome is
worsened if hyperglycemia ensues after the cerebral infarction.

Peripheral Neuropathy
Peripheral nervous system complications of diabetes are exceedingly common and often contribute significantly to the discomfort and
morbidity seen in advanced disease (Table 29-
5). Although the currently available treatment
of most diabetic neuropathies is less than satis-

Table 29-5. Diabetic Neuropathies

Symmetrical neuropathies
  Distal sensorimotor neuropathy
    Mainly large-fiber
    Mainly small-fiber
  Truncal neuropathy
  Autonomic neuropathy
Mononeuropathies
  Cranial
    Third nerve
    Sixth nerve
  Peripheral
  Plexopathy (diabetic amyotrophy)
  Radiculopathy

---

factory, it is important to recognize typical patterns so that patients can be spared investigations aimed at uncovering other etiologies; this also aids in the formulation of a prognosis. The pathogenesis of the symmetrical distal polyneuropathies is likely dependent on vascular and metabolic factors. The cranial and peripheral mononeuropathies, radiculopathies, and plexopathies are likely the outcome of ischemia resulting from a diabetic vasculopathy that affects the vasa nervorum. In addition, such patients are more susceptible to various compression neuropathies.

Symmetrical Sensorimotor Neuropathy. Symmetrical sensorimotor neuropathy is the most common neuropathy in diabetics and its prevalence increases as the illness advances, although occasionally it may be severe within a few years of the diagnosis of diabetes. There is often electrophysiological evidence of neuropathy even in asymptomatic individuals. It bears an uncertain relationship to the degree of diabetic control, although many believe careful regulation of the blood glucose level to be the mainstay of management. Retinopathy and nephropathy are more likely to afflict patients with neuropathy.

The neuropathy is deemed a length-related neuropathy of the dying-back type. Multiple accumulating ischemic lesions that occur at random throughout the length of the nerves could also account for the histological and clinical deficits observed. Another hypothesis, which has been supported by experimental findings, is founded on the effects of hyperglycemia on the intracellular metabolism of sorbitol and *myo*-inositol. Because nerves do not require insulin for glucose uptake, high levels of glucose can accumulate intracellularly. The *myo*-inositol store is depleted, which then causes interference with Na-K-ATPase, disruption of sodium channels, and disjunction at the nodes of Ranvier. This leads to impaired nerve conduction. Both Schwann cells and axons are likely affected by these mechanisms, although the neuropathy is mainly axonal. Axonal regeneration, demyelination, and onion bulb formation are also seen. When large fibers are mainly affected, findings include distal loss of vibration

and proprioception, ataxia in severe cases ("diabetic pseudotabes"), and loss of deep tendon reflexes. Uncomfortable distal burning dysesthesias and a stocking-and-glove loss of pain sensation arise in the presence of small-fiber involvement. This loss of pain sensation partly responsible for the formation of painless foot ulcers and, in some cases, for painless joint destruction in the lower extremities (Charcot joints). There may be a truncal neuropathy with loss of sensation over the central portions of the thoracolumbar areas, but this is often asymptomatic. The hand and foot muscles become wasted, but weakness is usually minimal. A fairly acute distal painful neuropathy following marked weight loss has also been described.

Autonomic Neuropathy. The autonomic neuropathy of diabetes often accompanies the distal sensorimotor neuropathy and, when present, indicates a poorer prognosis for survival. Orthostatic hypotension (with or without syncope), sweating abnormalities, nocturnal diarrhea or gastroparesis, impotence in males, atonic bladder, and pupillary abnormalities (rarely Argyll Robertson pupils) are the most common manifestations.

Cranial Neuropathy. The sudden onset of a painful third, or less commonly sixth, cranial nerve palsy is the common mode of presentation of a cranial neuropathy. Pupillary light reaction is characteristically preserved because the ischemic lesion probably affects the central part of the nerve and not the more circumferentially located pupilloconstrictor fibers. Recovery within 3 to 6 months is the rule.

Peripheral Mononeuropathy. Various nerves such as the ulnar, median, or common peroneal nerves can be involved in patients with a peripheral mononeuropathy. Ischemia is the likely triggering event, although compression plays a role in some cases. Recovery within several months can be expected. The wrists can be splinted in patients with carpal tunnel syndrome and patients are told to avoid leaning on their elbows or crossing their legs, depending on the nerves involved. These are helpful interventions.

lexopathy. The syndrome of "diabetic myotrophy" is seen predominantly in middle-aged men with mild diabetes. Patients suffer severe proximal thigh pain as well as wasting and weakness of their quadriceps, often accompanied by weight loss. An ischemic plexopathy/radiculopathy or femoral neuropathy, both, are blamed for the disorder. It may be necessary to institute pain management with tricyclic antidepressants, carbamazepine, narcotic analgesics. Improvement often takes several months and coincides with weight gain.

adiculopathy. An acutely painful thoracic or abdominal radiculopathy may be mistaken for ischemic cardiac or serious intraabdominal disease. It must also be distinguished from root compression stemming from disc protrusion.

ther Complications

lucormycosis (phycomycosis) is a fungal infection encountered mainly in diabetics. It causes invasive destruction of the nose and paranasal sinuses and may extend into the orbit and intracranially. Invasion of the blood vessels brings about arterial and venous occlusion and brain infarction. The condition is often fatal. **Malignant otitis externa** is a *Pseudomonas* infection that is seen mainly in diabetics; it produces multiple cranial nerve palsies and may be life-threatening.

Thyroid Disease

The thyroid gland is important to the development of the nervous system as well as to normal neurological and neuromuscular functioning. There are numerous neurological and neuromuscular complications of thyroid excess or deficiency, some occurring as the presenting symptom of an underlying thyroid disorder.

Hyperthyroidism

Graves' disease is frequently associated with unilateral or bilateral **thyroid orbitopathy** and is due to an inflammatory infiltration of the extraocular muscles and orbital tissues (see Fig. 11-4). Secondary vascular compromise compounds the edema and congestion of the globe as well as produces varying degrees of ophthalmoplegia. Diplopia with or without mild proptosis, which does not correlate well with the degree of thyrotoxicosis, may be the presenting symptom of this illness. The condition may abate with management of the hyperthyroid state, but optic nerve compromise can occur. Steroid treatment, administered locally or systemically, and, in severe cases, orbital decompression have been tried to reverse the consequences of the disorder.

The neuropsychiatric and neuromuscular signs of thyrotoxicosis are well known and consist of irritability, hypomanic behavior or possibly delirium, decreased attention and concentration, fine tremor (exaggerated physiological tremor), hyperreflexia, muscle irritability, weakness, and fatigability. In the apathetic form of hyperthyroidism, which typically occurs in older patients, the usual signs of thyroid excess may not be obvious, but the patient may exhibit depression and slowed mentation. In thyroid storm, the neurological signs become exaggerated, there is sympathetic overactivity, and the patient may become comatose. Seizures occur for unknown reasons in a small percentage of patients with thyrotoxicosis. The EEG may show diffuse slow or fast activity. Chorea is also rarely encountered in patients with hyperthyroidism.

A proximal myopathy with hip- and shoulder-girdle weakness and wasting is relatively common. Occasionally, bulbar weakness can appear. **Thyrotoxic periodic paralysis** is a rare complication that gives rise to attacks of extremity weakness without bulbar involvement; these can last as long as several hours. This complication is seen most commonly in Asian males and resembles familial hypokalemic periodic paralysis. Attacks can be provoked by exercise or carbohydrate intake, and serum potassium levels are often found to be low. These neuromuscular consequences of excess thyroid hormone levels resolve gradually once a euthyroid state is restored. The incidence of myasthenia gravis is also increased in patients with hyperthyroidism of autoimmune origin.

Hypothyroidism

A rare manifestation nowadays of congenital hypothyroidism, which attests to the importance of thyroid hormone for brain development, is **cretinism.** Affected children are mentally retarded and underdeveloped physically, and may show deafness and seizures.

In its milder forms, hypothyroidism produces mental slowing, a dull apathetic mental state, and depression. If prolonged, more pronounced thyroid deficiency can lead to dementia, which is reversible with thyroid replacement. The EEG shows slowing of the background rhythms, which increase in frequency in parallel with improved mentation. **Myxedema madness** refers to the more florid psychotic delirium with hallucinations that can appear in patients with profound deficits. With more advanced myxedema, **coma** can supervene and this represents a medical emergency that carries a relatively high mortality. Manifestations of myxedema coma include marked hypothermia, hypoglycemia, coagulopathy, and cardiac arrhythmias. Treatment includes the cautious administration of thyroid and adrenal steroid hormones plus the management of the medical complications.

Cerebellar ataxia is an uncommon problem that may be the presenting symptom of hypothyroidism. Sensorineural deafness and tinnitus are also well-described aspects of hypothyroidism.

Delayed or "hung-up" deep tendon reflexes, especially at the ankle, are common in patients with hypothyroidism. Muscle weakness and a mild myopathy may be seen but are less common than they are in hyperthyroidism. However, the serum level of creatine kinase is frequently elevated, even in the absence of overt weakness. A rare manifestation is enlarged muscles and tongue, and this constitutes the Kocher-Debré-Sémélaigne syndrome in children. On the other hand, a peripheral sensorimotor neuropathy is more common in hypothyroidism than it is in hyperthyroidism, although it is not usually too severe. Myxedema is one of the more common causes of carpal tunnel syndrome, and is due to entrapment of the median nerve through the deposition of mucopolysaccharide-like material.

Other Endocrine Disorders

Hyperparathyroidism

Symptoms from primary or secondary (wi renal failure) hyperparathyroidism result fro hypercalcemia and hypophosphatemia as we as possibly from the direct effects of parathyro hormone on brain and muscle tissue. Beha ioral disturbances, psychosis, and other neur psychiatric symptoms are exhibited by significant proportion of the patients and m be incipient signs of the disorder. A proxim myopathy likely resulting from an excess parathyroid hormone is also seen in patien suffering from osteomalacia and is due to eith a decreased intake or absorption of calcium.

Hypoparathyroidism

Primary or secondary (due to parathyroide tomy) hypoparathyroidism or pseudohypopar thyroidism may produce marked hypocalcemi which has an impact on central and peripher neuronal excitability. Epilepsy, either genera ized or partial, is a frequent component of t clinical picture and correlates with multifocal ar generalized paroxysmal EEG disturbances, ofte with photosensitivity. CT scans reveal the pre ence of cerebral calcification bilaterally in t basal ganglia, frontal areas, and, at times, t cerebellum. This finding may serve as the initi clue to the diagnosis. Rarely parkinsonian or e trapyramidal signs occur. Cognitive symptom dementia, and a variety of psychiatric sympton are relatively common. Pseudotumor cerebri a rare finding. Tetany manifested by paresthesi and carpopedal spasm provoked by exercise c hyperventilation are symptoms of peripher nerve hyperexcitability. A Chvostek sign (faci twitch elicited when the facial nerve over th parotid area is tapped) or Trousseau's sign (carp spasm provoked by the inflation of a blood pre sure cuff around the upper arm) can indicat latent tetany.

Cushing's Disease

Neurological and neuromuscular symptoms c endogenous or exogenous corticosteroid exces are common in patients with Cushing's disease Behavioral disturbances, including frank psy chosis, are frequent aspects of the disorder, an eudomotor cerebri can occur either in the presence of glucocorticosteroid excess or as the result of withdrawal. A proximal myopathy that mainly affects the legs and a selective type II fiber atrophy seen on histological specimens are encountered in most cases.

HEMATOLOGICAL DISORDERS

Several hematological disorders that predispose to stroke by creating a hypercoagulable state or hemorrhagic tendency have already been mentioned (see Chapter 23). Other selected hematological disorders with a high incidence of neurological complications are discussed here.

Sickle-Cell Anemia

Sickle-cell disease is a hemoglobinopathy that is due to genetically determined alterations in the beta-globin chain of the hemoglobin A molecule. Under conditions of low oxygen tension, the abnormal hemoglobin molecule causes the red blood cell to assume a sicklelike shape, which eventually becomes permanent. Stroke occurs in at least 10 percent of patients with sickle-cell disease. Although small-vessel occlusions do occur in these patients, possibly due to impaired microcirculation, the principal site of the pathology is situated at the terminal portion of the internal carotid artery and in the proximal middle and anterior cerebral arteries. Intimal proliferation and disruption with thrombotic stenosis and occlusion take place in the first two decades and may ultimately lead to the acute onset of hemiplegia in childhood. Watershed infarcts also occur, and recurrent strokes are the rule. Intracranial, and often intracerebral, hemorrhages constitute about one third of the strokes in patients with sickle-cell anemia and tend to afflict adults. They may occur in the context of a previous ischemic stroke and could possibly be related to the rupture of fragile collateral vessels. Screening patients with sickle-cell disease for the existence of large-vessel occlusive disease has been attempted using transcranial Doppler studies and MRI angiography. The prevention of stroke consists of exchange transfusions, which keep hemoglobin S levels below approximately 30 percent.

Polycythemia

Polycythemia rubra vera is a myeloproliferative disorder and secondary polycythemia is a component of a number of conditions that cause oxygen desaturation, such as chronic pulmonary disease, smoking, and prolonged exposure to high altitudes. In both forms of the disorder, hyperviscosity and accelerated atheroma formation accentuate the risk of TIA and cerebral infarction, often with a subcortical distribution. Patients often suffer multiple thromboembolic events and sometimes venous sinus or cortical venous thrombosis. The incidence of intracerebral and subdural hemorrhages is also increased. In addition, a number of nonspecific symptoms such as headache, dizziness, visual disturbances, weakness, and paresthesias are prevalent among patients with polycythemia. A painful distal sensory neuropathy that is characterized by burning dysesthesias in the feet may actually precede the diagnosis of polycythemia rubra vera. Disturbances in the microcirculation of peripheral nerves may be the triggering event, or it may be a remote effect of what is essentially a neoplastic process. Repeated phlebotomies to reduce the hematocrit below 45 percent are the mainstay of treatment.

Hemophilia

Intracranial hemorrhage that can present as a massive intracerebral or subdural hematoma, especially following head trauma, poses a serious risk in patients with either type of hemophilia and is a leading cause of death in these patients. Focal compressive mononeuropathies may result from hematomas that form at other locations (e.g., hematoma compressing the femoral nerve).

Platelet Disorders

Thrombotic Thrombocytopenic Purpura
Patients with TTP commonly manifest a diffuse and multifocal encephalopathy that includes prominent neurological symptoms. Headache, alterations in mental status, seizures, and focal

signs such as aphasia are all typical findings. A microangiopathic hemolytic anemia, thrombocytopenia, fever, and renal impairment also form part of the clinical picture. Despite widespread involvement of the cerebral small vessels by thrombi, patients often experience complete recovery. Treatment consists of corticosteroids and plasmapheresis.

Thrombocytosis

Essential thrombocythemia is a myeloproliferative disorder in which a marked elevation in the number of platelets produces a hypercoagulable state, which then increases the risk of TIA or cerebral infarction. Secondary thrombocytosis, such as can occur in association with malignancy, also increases the risk of stroke.

Disseminated Intravascular Coagulation

Although a low platelet count is a feature of disseminated intravascular coagulation (DIC), it is not strictly a platelet disorder but is rather characterized by the release of thromboplastic substances into the circulation and the subsequent fibrin deposition and formation of thrombi in small vessels throughout the body, which then causes ischemic and hemorrhagic lesions. The disorder occurs secondary to several conditions, such as sepsis, malignancy, heat stroke, obstetrical complications, burns, trauma, surgery, allograft rejection, and even brain injury, that precipitate the release of thromboplastins. A low platelet count and increased fibrin split products are hallmarks of the condition. The brain is frequently involved and affected patients manifest a picture of diffuse encephalopathy with alterations in mental status, coma, seizures, and multifocal signs. Signs frequently fluctuate, and complete recovery may ensue even in comatose patients.

Multiple Myeloma and Paraproteinemias

Multiple myeloma is associated with a host of neurological and neuromuscular complications. It can cause discrete "punched out" skull lesions and may invade the dura mater or the brain beneath. A solitary plasmacytoma of the brain is rare, but spinal cord or cauda equina compression resulting

from vertebral involvement is relatively commo[n] and may be the presenting symptom. Hypercalc[e]mia with accompanying neurological manifest[a]tions is a late complication. With high levels [of] circulating immunoglobulin (especially IgA), h[y]perviscosity syndromes can eventuate that predi[s]pose to stroke. Compression or local infiltratio[n] is responsible for causing neuropathies and r[a]diculopathies. Very rarely, a myeloma can inf[il]trate peripheral or cranial nerves in a diffuse a[nd] relatively selective fashion, thereby producing [a] painful multiple mononeuropathy that eventua[lly] becomes symmetrical. Secondary amyloidosis c[an] arise and causes an ischemic neuropathy that is d[ue] to either infiltration of the vasa nervorum or di[f]fuse infiltration of nerves. A paraneoplastic sens[o]rimotor neuropathy is also seen.

In the POEMS syndrome (*p*lasma cell dyscr[a]sia with polyneuropathy, *o*rganomegaly, end[o]crinopathy, *M* protein, and *s*kin changes), the[re] is a progressive sensorimotor neuropathy th[at] usually includes osteosclerotic bone lesions an[d] circulating light chains.

The neuropathies that have excited the mo[st] interest are immune-mediated demyelinatin[g] neuropathies caused by the formation of ant[i]body to myelin-associated glycoprotein. Thes[e] entities may be associated with monoclonal gam[-] mopathies of unknown significance that afflic[t] 30 percent of the population over the age of 7[0] and progress to become multiple myeloma o[r] other lymphoproliferative disorders about 1[0] percent of the time. These neuropathies may b[e] associated with IgG, IgA, and especially IgM monoclonal proteins and produce a clinic[al] picture that resembles that of idiopathic chron[ic] inflammatory demyelinating polyradiculopa[thy]. In come cases, immunohistochemical tech[-] niques have been used to demonstrate th[e] binding of antibody to myelin-associated glyco[]protein. Intensive immunosuppressive therap[y] with prednisone plus cyclophosphamide therap[y] and plasmapheresis have been used to revers[e] the disease process.

Idiopathic Hypereosinophilic Syndrome

Persistent eosinophilia (>1500 cells/mm³) tha[t] lasts for more than 6 months may occur for n[o] own cause and provoke damage to the heart, ngs and upper airway, spleen, kidney, skin, es, muscles, and nervous system. Neurological and neuromuscular complications appear in o thirds of the cases and consist of an early bacute encephalopathy with memory deficits, asticity, ataxia, and seizures. Patients also stain stroke due to cardiac emboli, which are lated to endomyocardial fibrosis, and a peoheral sensory neuropathy.

orphyrias

he hepatic porphyrias represent disorders that volve autosomal dominant, partial enzyme dects in heme biosynthesis and consist of acute termittent porphyria (AIP), variegate poriyria, and hereditary coproporphyria. In AIP, orphobilinogen deaminase activity is reduced, sulting in the accumulation of the porphyrin ecursors delta-aminolevulinic acid and poriobilinogen, both of which are likely neuroxic. Delta-aminolevulinic acid may inhibit imma-aminobutyric acid (GABA)–receptor nding in the CNS. Drugs that induce porphy1 synthesis, such as the sulfonamides, barbitutes, and most antiepileptic agents, may ovoke acute crises in patients with porphyria. eurological features of the disorders include izures, psychosis, and a neuropathy resem)ing Guillain-Barré syndrome with prominent itonomic features. Other manifestations are ine-colored urine and photosensitivity. Treatent consists of high carbohydrate intake and travenous hematin.

ernicious Anemia

he neurological effects of pernicious anemia em from B_{12} deficiency. These are discussed Chapter 19 under the topic of subacute comned degeneration of the spinal cord.

IISCELLANEOUS MEDICAL ONDITIONS

aget's Disease

iget's disease represents a chronic progresve disease of bone in which patients suffer from skeletal deformities related to accelerated bone resorption and unregulated bone repair and remodeling. Skull enlargement (manifested by an increased hat size), vertebral column deformity (gibbus formation), and hypercalcemia may be features of the disease. The cranial nerves may be affected by bony overgrowth at their exit foramina at the base of the skull, particularly the eighth cranial nerve, which causes deafness.

Basilar impression can produce stretching, distortion, and compression of the cranial nerves as well as the brainstem. A syndrome of tic douloureux and hemifacial spasm has been described, and spinal nerve roots may also be compromised. Most importantly, spinal cord compression can occur. Treatment has been attempted with antineoplastic agents as well as calcitonin.

Acute Pancreatitis

Pancreatic encephalopathy is a rare disorder seen in conjunction with acute pancreatitis that produces a toxic encephalopathy with seizures and focal signs. The pathogenesis is unclear but may stem partially from the direct effects of released pancreatic enzymes on the brain as well as from hypocalcemia.

Lymphomatoid Granulomatosis

Lymphomatoid granulomatosis fits into the spectrum of T-cell lymphomas, although it also includes elements of vasculitis. The disorder mainly affects middle-aged men and often presents with clinical or radiological signs of pulmonary lesions. A skin rash occurs in 40 percent of the cases. About 20 to 30 percent of the patients exhibit CNS involvement that affects the cerebral hemispheres, cranial nerves, and, less commonly, the cerebellum. A peripheral neuropathy appears in about a fourth of the cases. CT and MRI reveal fairly discrete enhancing lesions and, at times, multiple or periventricular involvement. The mortality is high despite the use of steroids, antineoplastic agents, or radiotherapy.

ALCOHOL ABUSE

The consumption of ethanol-containing drinks is an extremely prevalent custom in our society. Approximately 10 to 15 percent of the population over the age of 12 drink alcohol excessively on a regular basis and 10 percent of men and up to 5 percent of women develop true alcoholism—a dependence on ethanol with predictable behavioral, physical, and social consequences. These figures vary from country to country, depending on cultural and socioeconomic factors.

The mechanisms of alcohol's effects on the nervous system are multiple and include a reduction of depolarization-induced calcium entry into cells and increase in the number of calcium channels with chronic use, direct disruption of brain lipid levels in neuronal membranes, raised concentrations of excitatory neurotransmitters such as glutamate and glutamate-receptor binding sites in the brain, enhancement of GABA inhibitory effects on neuronal firing and reduced GABA effects during withdrawal, and impaired adenosine-stimulated cyclic AMP levels in the brain leading to hyperexcitability. Low-dose effects, higher-dose effects, and withdrawal effects must all be distinguished. The manifold neurological complications related to excessive alcohol consumption are listed in Table 29-6.

Acute Intoxication

The individual's acute response to alcohol ingestion depends on the degree of chronic alcohol use, amount and rate of ingestion, genetic variations in the rate of metabolism, and the concurrent use of sedative or excitant substances.

Alcohol is normally absorbed rapidly from the gastrointestinal tract, then widely distributed throughout the body and metabolized by alcohol dehydrogenase in the liver to form acetaldehyde. Acetaldehyde is then converted to acetate by aldehyde dehydrogenase. In a nonalcoholic, a blood concentration of 30 to 65 mg/dl (approximately 7–15 mmol/L) causes a measurable impairment in motor coordination, sensory perception, and cognition. The early signs of intoxication, due to disinhibition of cerebral function, consist of euphoria, loss of social inhibitions (garrulousness, hilarity, and so on), and emotional lability. Ataxia, nystagmus, dysarthria, and sympathetic stimulation (sweating, tachycardia, mydriasis) appear when blood levels exceed 100 mg/dl (22 mmol/L). At even higher levels, depressant effects supervene and consist of stupor or coma (level over 300 mg/dl or 65 mmol/L), hyporeflexia, hypotension, and respiratory depression.

Alcoholics characteristically complain of periodic "blackouts" or memory lapses for events related to episodic heavy drinking. These symptoms are likely due to direct effects on hippocampal memory circuits and may also be observed in nonalcoholic drinkers.

Table 29-6. Neurological Complications of Alcoholism

ACUTE

Acute alcohol intoxication
  Drunkenness
  Pathological intoxication
Withdrawal syndromes
  Tremulousness, confusion
  Seizures
  Alcoholic hallucinosis
  Delirium tremens
  Movement disorders

CHRONIC

Due to direct or secondary effects on nervous system
  Wernicke's encephalopathy
  Korsakoff's syndrome
  Alcoholic dementia and brain atrophy
  Alcoholic cerebellar degeneration
  Alcoholic neuropathy
  Pellagra
  Alcoholic amblyopia
  Central pontine myelinolysis
  Marchiafava-Bignami disease
  Acute and chronic myopathy
Due to effects on other organs
  Hepatic encephalopathy and myelopathy
  Acquired hepatocerebral degeneration
Due to other secondary effects
  Predisposition to head trauma, subdural hematoma
  Predisposition to cerebral infarction
  Associated intoxication (e.g., methanol, ethylene glycol)

Pathological intoxication is the idiosyncratic rapid development of aggressive and violent behavior following the ingestion of even small amounts of alcohol.

Withdrawal States

Minor withdrawal states can appear in alcohol-dependent individuals as early as 6 to 8 hours after the cessation or reduction of alcohol intake. **Alcoholic tremulousness** is accompanied by mild confusion, anxiety, irritability, and sympathetic overactivity. This condition is often apparent upon awakening in the morning following a night of heavy drinking, and may prompt alcohol ingestion soon thereafter to "calm the nerves." More pronounced symptoms may occur around 24 hours after withdrawal and include worsening confusion, agitation, perceptual distortions, and visual or auditory hallucinations.

Withdrawal seizures ("rum fits") occur in a small proportion of alcoholics, most commonly between 18 and 24 hours following either the cessation of drinking or a dramatic reduction in intake. Typically, these individuals suffer one to six generalized tonic-clonic seizures within a space of 6 hours. Status epilepticus is rare. It is a self-limited condition that does not normally require antiepileptic drugs, although benzodiazepines (e.g., diazepam 5–10 mg delivered intravenously) are often used if two or more seizures occur and may also reduce other withdrawal symptoms such as tremulousness.

Full-blown **delirium tremens (DTs)** most commonly occurs 72 hours following withdrawal and usually lasts for less than 3 days. Occasionally it may appear as late as 3 weeks after the cessation of drinking. This major withdrawal state still carries a mortality rate of approximately 5 percent, despite advances in medical management, and must be treated as a medical emergency. Withdrawal seizures precede DTs in a significant percentage of cases but generally occur independently. These patients are usually in an extreme state of agitation, disorientation, and global confusion with perceptual illusions, marked attention deficits, sleeplessness, and visual and tactile hallucina-

tions (e.g., bugs crawling on the wall or on the skin). Autonomic hyperactivity is manifested by tachycardia and hypertension and may lead to dehydration, cardiac arrhythmias, and cardiovascular collapse. A superimposed infection such as pneumonia is not uncommon in these patients because they are generally nutritionally deprived and immunologically deficient.

Management consists of intensive medical and nursing care, reassurance and reality orientation, avoidance of excessive sensory stimuli, rehydration, vitamin replacement including thiamine (see later discussion), and sedation. Benzodiazepines, which share a cross-tolerance with alcohol and are relatively free of hypotensive and respiratory depressant effects, have been the preferred sedative drugs. An initial loading dose of diazepam 60 mg orally followed by 20 mg/hr until mild sedation is achieved has been recommended. Chlordiazepoxide (100 mg/hr), sublingual lorazepam, or oxazepam has also been recommended. Because of their hypotensive and seizure-exacerbating effects, the phenothiazines are best avoided but haloperidol given intravenously has been used safely.

Chronic Effects of Heavy Alcohol Intake

Wernicke-Korsakoff Syndrome

Wernicke's encephalopathy is a specific neuropathological entity that is due to thiamine deficiency. It is seen not only in chronic undernourished alcoholics but also in other states of malnutrition such as hyperemesis gravidarum, gastric carcinoma, or prolonged starvation, as well as in dialysis patients. Thiamine (vitamin B_1) is a cofactor for the enzymes pyruvate dehydrogenase, transketolase, alpha-ketoglutarate dehydrogenase, and branched-chain alpha-keto acid dehydrogenase. Because thiamine is necessary for the proper functioning of the glycolytic and pentose phosphate pathways, the administration of a glucose load to a thiamine-deficient patient may precipitate Wernicke's encephalopathy. The pathological finding in these patients consists of symmetrical bilateral necrotic, hemorrhagic lesions that are located in the diencephalon, around the third ventricle, the aqueduct, and the fourth ventricles, and especially affecting the mammillary bodies (Fig. 29-3). MRI scans may show atrophy of the mammillary bodies in alcoholics.

The classic clinical triad includes a global confusional state, oculomotor disorders, and ataxia. The most common eye findings are nystagmus, unilateral or bilateral sixth nerve palsy, gaze palsies, or a third nerve palsy (usually with pupillary sparing). There is often a concurrent peripheral neuropathy, which, in addition to a cerebellar deficit, contributes to the ataxia. A rare presentation of Wernicke's encephalopathy is hypothermic coma. Autopsy studies have shown that the neuropathological findings of Wernicke's encephalopathy in alcoholics are far more common than would be expected judging from their clinical histories and that many patients do not have documented classic symptoms. Although most cases present acutely, a subacute or even chronic condition may occur.

Prompt treatment with parenteral thiamine (at least 100 mg intravenously and 50 mg intramuscularly) is essential in alcoholics who exhibit neurological symptoms or patients with undiagnosed coma. Nystagmus and ocular signs usually remit within 6 hours; the ataxia and confusion abate over several days.

Korsakoff's psychosis is a prototypical amnestic syndrome that ensues in 80 percent of the patients with acute Wernicke's encephalopathy. However, some patients do not have a clear-cut history of preceding Wernicke's encephalopathy. Lesions in the dorsal median nuclei of the thalamus as well as possibly the mammillary bodies are likely responsible for the severe short-term (anterograde) memory deficits. Additional symptoms include a retrograde memory deficit, general apathy and decreased spontaneity, and a tendency toward confabulation (possibly due to a combination of retrograde memory deficit and an inability to distinguish the time order of past events). As much as 50 to 75 percent of these patients show significant improvement over the course of several months, but most continue to have at least some memory deficits. In the more severe cases, the amnestic deficit is extremely disabling.

Alcoholic Dementia

Whether an alcohol-induced dementia exists separately from Korsakoff's psychosis, and not attributable to repeated seizures with hypoxia or head injuries, is controversial. Chronic alcoholics often show a general decline in their cognitive function, frequently in addition to a more pronounced memory deficit. Neuroimaging studies have repeatedly shown evidence of brain atrophy with predominant involvement of the white matter. This atrophy appears to be partially reversible after a month or more of abstinence. The neuropathological substrate for the atrophy and dementia has not been well defined. **Marchiafava-Bignami disease** is a rare disorder encountered in heavy drinkers which may appear subacutely or chronically. It involves dementia, dysarthria, spasticity, and ataxia and may lead to coma. Neuropathological and imaging studies show a characteristic necrosis of the corpus callosum and adjacent white matter.

Epilepsy and Alcoholism

The findings from recent studies imply that there is an increased incidence of epilepsy in heavy alcohol users independent of withdrawal seizures. Alcohol use in general tends to lower the seizure threshold and may provoke seizures in patients with epilepsy arising from other causes and due to a variety of mechanisms. Disturbance of sleep patterns, poor compliance, as well as poor absorption and accelerated metabolism of antiepileptic drugs all tend to foster seizures in these patients. A syndrome of subacute encephalopathy with generalized tonic-clonic and simple partial seizures, confusion, focal neurological signs and periodic lateralized epileptiform EEG discharges that resolves over several days has been described in alcoholics.

Cerebellar Degeneration

Loss of Purkinje cells and atrophy of midline cerebellar structures, particularly the anterior and superior vermis, are common after years of heavy alcohol intake and are possibly the consequence of thiamine deficiency (see Fig. 29-3). Men are more frequently affected than women. Symptoms include a wide-based unsteady gait, lower limb ataxia, tremor, and dys-

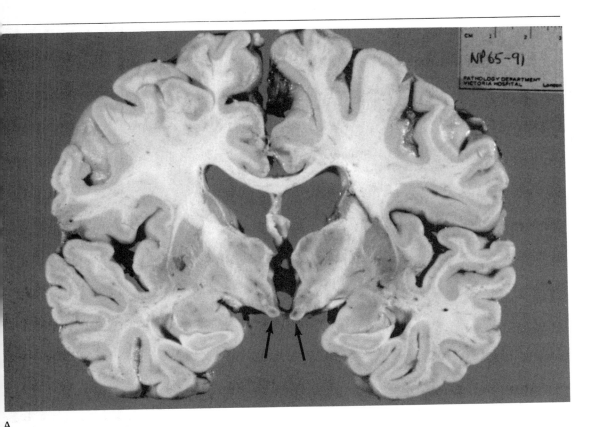

A

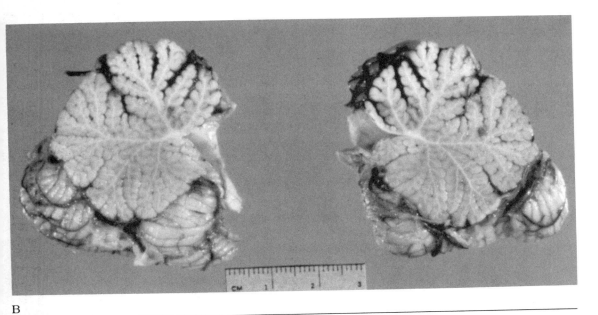

B

Fig. 29-3. *Brain appearance seen at autopsy in a severe alcoholic. (A) Coronal section showing diffuse cortical atrophy and enlarged lateral ventricles. The mammillary bodies* (arrows) *are shrunken and necrotic, typical of Wernicke-Korsakoff syndrome. (B) Marked cerebellar atrophy affecting mainly the superior vermis.*

arthria. Symptoms may appear or worsen quite abruptly, perhaps because a threshold level of compensation is suddenly exceeded or a second cerebellar insult occurs. Abstinence and thiamine replacement can bring about improvement in these patients.

Central Pontine Myelinolysis

Central pontine myelinolysis is a rare condition and is more common in alcoholics, but appears to be related to the over-rapid correction of hyponatremia resulting from any cause. Demyelination occurs in central pontine regions as well as in symmetrical subcortical sites. Affected patients may present in a lock-in syndrome or coma with a spastic quadriparesis. The pontine lesions can usually be visualized by CT or MRI scanning.

Neuropathy

A peripheral sensorimotor neuropathy is commonly found in alcoholics and is thought to be due to a deficiency of thiamine and other B vitamins. Painful burning dysesthesias of the feet, distal weakness, wasting, and ataxia are the symptoms. Pathologically the nerves show a wallerian degeneration. Alcoholics are also susceptible to various compression mononeuropathies. The so-called Saturday night palsy results from the prolonged compression of the radial nerve in the upper arm after the patient falls asleep in an alcoholic stupor with the arm abducted and pressing against a hard surface such as the back of a chair. A more acute generalized severe neuropathy resembling the Guillain-Barré syndrome has also been noted. Unlike acute inflammatory polyradiculoneuropathy, the nerves in this disorder show axonal degeneration and the CSF protein level is not elevated. An **optic neuropathy** may also occur in the syndrome of tobacco-alcohol amblyopia.

Myopathy

Chronic proximal muscle weakness and wasting are seen in a high proportion of alcoholics and may be analogous to the cardiomyopathy caused by alcohol consumption. In addition, a severe acute necrotizing painful myopathy with myoglobinuria can occur following a bout of heavy drinking.

Miscellaneous

Many other neurological complications encountered in alcoholics are the result of concurrent processes to which the alcoholic is particularly susceptible.

There is an increased risk of both hemorrhagic and, for unknown reasons, ischemic strokes in alcoholics. Head injuries and subdural hematomas are a natural consequence of repeated episodes of ataxia and stupor. Hepatic encephalopathy subsequent to alcoholic liver disease leads to various neurological manifestations that have already been discussed. There is also an increased incidence of movement disorders related to alcohol withdrawal, including parkinsonism, chorea, and especially tremor. Finally, ethanol abusers may at times ingest other toxic alcohols that give rise to an encephalopathy and other neurological signs such as optic neuritis (methanol use) or facial nerve palsies (ethylene glycol intake). Permanent basal ganglia damage can occur following ingestion of large amounts of methanol (Fig. 29-4).

DRUG AND SUBSTANCE ABUSE

Drug abuse has become a major social and medical problem, particularly in the major cities of North America and Western Europe. In many cases, more than one drug is used in conjunction with alcohol.

Cocaine

Cocaine is a psychostimulant alkaloid prepared from the leaves of the coca plant that fosters strong psychological dependence without the physical dependence characteristic of the narcotics. Recently, freebase or "crack" cocaine, a nearly pure and very potent form of the drug, has become readily available. It can be administered in a variety of ways, including intranasally, intramuscularly, or intravenously, or by smoking it. Recreational use of the drug has now reached epidemic proportions. Besides the dependency and all that that entails, a number of serious cardiovascular and neurologic complications can result from its use.

Cocaine is a local anesthetic but acts centrally

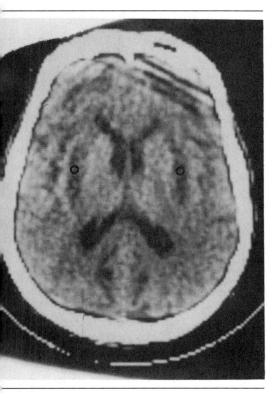

ig. 29-4. *CT scan showing destruction of the globus allidus bilaterally* (circles) *in a 59-year-old man after large overdose of methanol.*

decrease the presynaptic uptake of norepinephrine and dopamine. It is strongly ympathomimetic and induces tachycardia, hypertension, mydriasis, and euphoria. The euphoric effects last for 20 to 90 minutes, epending on the form and route of administraon. This is followed by a sudden depletion of nergy, or the "crash," and a dysphoric mood nat lasts for days, during which there is an ntense craving for another dose. Long-term se may bring about a number of psychiatric isturbances, including a paranoid psychotic allucinatory state.

Reports of ischemic strokes (including spinal) s well as subarachnoid or intracerebral hemorhages have multiplied with the more widepread use of the drug. Some users are found have underlying berry aneurysms or arteriovenous malformations that rupture, likely beause of the acute hypertension induced by the rug. Ischemic strokes may be due to vaso-

spasm or cardiac emboli subsequent to arrhythmias and possibly cardiomyopathies. Acute convulsive seizures are a well-described complication of cocaine use. Fungal cerebritis can result from intravenous use. Overdose precipitates CNS depression with coma and respiratory depression. Treatment of overdose includes the intravenous administration of diazepam to control the seizures and beta-blockers to reduce sympathetic overactivity.

Narcotics

Narcotics are alkaloid derivatives of the opium plant and their synthetic analogues, including heroin, morphine, codeine, oxycodone, propoxyphene, methadone, pentazocine, and the narcotic antagonist naloxone. They act at specific opiate receptors within the CNS that are confined mainly to the limbic system (amygdala), periaqueductal gray matter, nucleus solitarius, and substantia gelatinosa. Naturally occurring endogenous peptides, known as *enkephalins* and *endorphins,* serve as ligands for these receptors and play a neuromodulatory role. The central regulation of pain and emotional behavior is one of the main functions of this system. There are also extensive effects on other neurotransmitters, including acetylcholine, the monoamines, and GABA.

Narcotic abuse constitutes an ancient and worldwide problem that reached major proportions in the United States in the 1960s. Narcotics such as heroin produce physical dependence plus a marked rapidly developing tolerance, with users requiring ever higher doses. Narcotic effects include euphoria, analgesia, respiratory depression, miosis, nausea and vomiting, constipation, cough suppression, reduced body temperature, and orthostatic hypotension. Symptoms of overdose include coma, cardiorespiratory depression, pinpoint reactive pupils, and occasionally hypothermia. Addicts, who misjudge their own tolerance and are often unaware of the true potency of the preparation they acquire, are subject to fatal overdoses. To treat an overdose, a small dose (to prevent withdrawal symptoms and respiratory depression) of the narcotic antagonist naloxone (e.g., 0.4 mg intravenously) is given, and this is sometimes repeated.

The major withdrawal syndrome from narcotics begins with a craving for the drug starting 6 hours after the previous dose. During the next 24 to 72 hours, addicts exhibit anxiety, restlessness, irritability, weakness, lacrimation, rhinorrhea, sneezing, yawning, sweating, dilated pupils, gooseflesh that rapidly appears and disappears, tachycardia, hypertension, vomiting, diarrhea, muscle and bone pain, abdominal cramps, and shivering. These symptoms subside over several days and are usually not life-threatening. To treat withdrawal, either the "cold-turkey" method can be adopted or methadone can be given and gradually withdrawn. Clonidine has been used to reduce the effects of excessive sympathetic activity.

The neurological consequences of heroin addiction include strokes (often embolic due to the embolization of injected impurities or from endocarditis), rarely cerebral vasculitis, AIDS and its vast array of neurological complications, rarely seizures, and peripheral nerve palsies caused by direct damage or pressure.

Amphetamines

Amphetamines are stimulant sympathomimetic agents that are also appetite suppressants. Their mechanism of action is related to the release of norepinephrine from presynaptic terminals and subsequent interference with re-uptake. The acute hypertension induced by amphetamine intake can precipitate intracerebral hemorrhage. Cerebral arteritis can also occur with methamphetamine use and this can be responsible for causing ischemic strokes. The cerebral embolization of talc or cornstarch granules is a risk posed by intravenous injections. Chronic users commonly suffer a schizophreniform psychosis with market paranoid features.

Marijuana (Cannabis)

Marijuana and hashish are usually smoked for their euphoria-producing and relaxant qualities. Hallucinations and seizures may be provoked by high doses but, in general, the neurological effects are few with moderate consumption.

Phencyclidine

Phencyclidine (PCP), an uncompetitiv NMDA-receptor antagonist, has become i creasingly popular because of its hallucinogen properties. In low doses, it produces a sta resembling alcohol intoxication with vertig nystagmus, and illusions. At higher doses, fra psychosis with hallucinations and bizarre b havior ensue and this is accompanied by musc rigidity, analgesia, anesthesia, and then com PCP is also a sympathomimetic that precipitat tachycardia and hypertension. Phenothiazin are best avoided in the treatment of overdose

Aromatic Hydrocarbons and Inhalants

The inhalation of various substances to achiev a "high" is fairly prevalent among children an adolescents. The substances commonly abuse include airplane glue, cleaning fluids, pai thinners, lacquers, and gasoline. The offendir chemicals include toluene, chlorinated hydr carbons, various ketones, esters, and alcohol The immediate effects of inhalation are euph ria, ataxia, diplopia, dysarthria, and, at highe doses, vivid visual hallucinations, seizures, an loss of consciousness. Chronic behavioral e fects as well as cerebellar ataxia may be seen long-term users. Peripheral neuropathy, whic may be severe, can occur from glue-sniffin possibly due to the *n*-hexane in the glue.

ENVIRONMENTAL AND OTHER TOXINS

With the increasing public awareness of enviror mental and occupational safety, neurotoxico ogy has been given greater emphasis in recer years. The identification of toxins such as MPTI which can produce a parkinsonian syndrom (see Chapter 12), or substances in the cycad plar that may be responsible for causing the Guamar ian ALS-parkinsonian-dementia complex (se Chapter 12) has given new impetus to the searc for toxic substances that might play a role in th pathogenesis of certain "degenerative" neurc logical disorders of unknown etiology. In add

...on, the proliferation of chemical substances and drugs has increased the likelihood of exposure to potentially neurotoxic substances. The mechanisms by which neurotoxins inflict their damage are largely unknown. In many cases, a direct toxic effect on the cell is likely, but other mechanisms such as interference with intracellular energy supplies leading to unblockage of NMDA receptors and excessive excitotoxic effects are theoretically possible.

Establishing a definite relationship between a potential neurotoxin and a particular neurological syndrome or disease is not always a simple task. Few toxic substances produce specific syndromes, substances can precipitate widely varying manifestations depending on the level and chronicity of exposure, and, in some cases, neurological effects may persist as the result of exposure to substances that took place months or years before. When a miniepidemic of neurotoxicity cases occurs, it is usually relatively easy to identify the cause, but this is the exception. In many cases, toxins do their damage without producing any specific laboratory-detected abnormalities or neuroimaging changes, or there is no means for measuring their presence in tissues. In such cases, when a toxic etiology is suspected, history-taking is by far the most important tool for identifying the cause (Table 29-7). In some cases, episodic symptoms may occur as the result of repeated acute exposure to a specific substance at a particular location.

To establish a likely etiological role for a potential neurotoxin, it is necessary to determine

Table 29-7. Points in History-Taking in Patients with Suspected Neurotoxic Illness

Occupational details
  Exposure to chemicals, vapors, and the like
  Wearing of protective devices such as gloves, masks, clothing
  Abatement of symptoms on weekends and holidays
  Eating in the workplace
  Ventilation, heating, and so on
Home environment
  Surrounding pollution, factories, and so on
  Ventilation and heating
  Cleaning fluids, solvents, chemicals
  Pesticides, herbicides
  Drugs
  Water source
  Health of family members
  Animal exposure, pets
Habits
  Dietary
  Hobbies
  Travels

that (1) there has been exposure; (2) the neurological symptoms are compatible with the known effects of the substances; (3) there is no better explanation for the symptoms; and (4) the cessation of exposure to the toxin results in improvement or at least stabilization of the condition. In some cases, the demonstration of elevated tissue levels of the offending substance or distinctive biochemical or neuroanatomical changes are helpful. Only some of the more distinctive, well-recognized, and common neurotoxins and their characteristics are listed in Table 29-8.

Table 29-8. Neurotoxic Substances

Substance	Syndrome/symptoms	Source of exposure	Special features
HEAVY METALS			
Lead			
Inorganic lead salts	Encephalopathy: cognitive slowing; severe cases: elevated intracranial pressure, seizures	Chewing chips of lead-based paint in older houses, lead pipes, home-distilled whisky in old car batttery cases, lead vapor inhalation from stained-glass making, eating off china painted with lead-based paint	Seen in children, blue line in the gums, lead line in long bones on x-ray studies, paint chips seen in abdominal x-ray studies, abdominal pain, basophilic stippling

Table 29-8 (Continued).

Substance	Syndrome/symptoms	Source of exposure	Special features
	Polyneuropathy (subacute, symmetrical, proximal, predominantly motor)	Lead mining and smelting, automobile radiator mechanics, construction work, plastic production, ceramics	Myelin breakdown, low-dose effects with blood level <100 μg/dl
Organic lead	Irritability, insomnia, emotional instability	Industrial, inhalation of gasoline	—
Mercury			
Methylmercury	Minamata disease: sensory neuropathy, visual field constriction, hearing loss, tremor, mild confusion	Industrial (electrical apparatus, chloralkali, paints, pulp and paper, drug and pesticides), eating fish contaminated with mercury, mining	—
Inorganic mercurous salts	Pink disease in infants: irritability, pink appearance, sweating, peripheral neuropathy	Calomel teething powder	—
Inorganic mercuric salts	Shyness, confusion, insomnia, tremor	Industrial	—
Arsenic			
Pentavalent	Hemorrhagic encephalopathy, polyneuropathy (mainly motor), exfoliative dermatitis, optic neuritis, myelitis, vestibulopathy	Insecticides, therapeutic	—
Trivalent	Polyneuropathy (symmetrical, distal, painful, mainly motor)	Food or beer contaminant, arsine, balloonists and submariners	Hair loss, anemia, gastroenteritis, hyperpigmentation, Mees' lines in nails, wallerian degeneration of nerves
Thallium	Acute: vomiting, diarrhea; subacute: sensorimotor neuropathy resembling Guillain-Barré syndrome, hair loss, exfoliative dermatitis, Mees' lines	Industrial, fungicide, ant killer, rodenticide	—
Manganese	Parkinsonian syndrome, muscle twitching, cramps, "manganese madness"	Manganese mining (dust inhalation), production of alloys, dry batteries, paints, varnishes, enamel, linoleum, matches, fireworks	—
Triethyltin/diethyltin	Elevated ICP, psychiatric symptoms	Industrial, fungicides, molluscacides	Intramyelinic edema
Gold	Peripheral neuropathy	Therapy of rheumatoid arthritis	—

Table 29-8 (Continued).

Substance	Syndrome/symptoms	Source of exposure	Special features
INDUSTRIAL CHEMICALS, SOLVENTS, INSECTICIDES, ETC.			
Acrylamide	Psychiatric symptoms, distal sensory neuropathy, dysarthria, nystagmus, ataxia, sphincter disturbances	Industrial	Neuropathy preceded by contact dermatitis of hands, wallerian degeneration with giant axonal swellings
Carbon disulfide	Psychiatric symptoms, delirium, peripheral neuropathy (mainly sensory)	Industrial (solvent in various insecticides, rubber industry, preparation of rayon viscose fibers)	—
Carbon tetrachloride	Headaches, vertigo, ataxia, optic atrophy, neuropathy	Solvent, cleaning fluid	Renal and hepatotoxic
Cyanide (chronic)	Peripheral neuropathy, encephalopathy	Consumption of apricot, peach, or wild cherry seeds	Extremely rare in Western countries
DDT, lindane	Hyperirritability, ataxia, tremor, seizures	Insecticide	—
n-Hexane	Peripheral sensorimotor neuropathy, optic neuritis	Industrial, glue-sniffing	—
Methyl *n*-butyl ketone	Similar to *n*-hexane	Industrial, glue-sniffing	—
Methyl bromide	Behavioral disturbances, psychosis, seizures, diplopia, ataxia, tremor, peripheral neuropathy (chronic)	Fumigant, insecticide, refrigerant	—
Toluene	Mental changes, cerebellar ataxia	Industrial, glue- and solvent-sniffing	—
Trichloroethylene	Multiple cranial mononeuropathy (e.g., V, VI, VII), upper cervical radiculopathy	Degreasing solvent	Circumoral herpex simplex
Organophosphates Aryl compounds (e.g., triorthocresyl phosphate)	"Ginger Jake paralysis"; severe peripheral neuropathy (mainly motor): paralysis, ataxia, excessive sweating, mild corticospinal tract involvement, laryngeal paralysis	Contaminant of salad or cooking oil	Axonal degeneration
Alkyl compounds (e.g., pesticides: parathion, carbaryl, dimethoate, methamidophos)	Subacute peripheral neuropathy and myelopathy (corticospinal tracts); also "intermediate" syndrome of proximal	Suicide attempts, spraying	Early GI upset, cramps, bradycardia, pupilloconstriction

Table 29-8 (Continued).

Substance	Syndrome/symptoms	Source of exposure	Special features
Alkyl compounds (cont.)	muscle and respiratory weakness with certain agents		
Methanol (see Fig. 29-4)	Optic neuritis, retinal edema, photophobia, blindness, headache, vomiting, coma, seizures	"Rubbing alcohol," contaminant of alcoholic beverages	Treatment with ethanol to prevent oxidation to formaldehyde
Ethylene glycol	Seizures, coma, bilateral seventh nerve palsy	Antifreeze, substitute for alcohol	Renal failure
CARBON MONOXIDE	Symptoms: headache, dizziness, weakness, nausea, trouble thinking, visual symptoms, unconsciousness Examination: cortical blindness, field defects, red retinal veins, retinal hemorrhages, hearing loss, vestibular dysfunction Pathology: cerebral edema, leukoencephalopathy, globus pallidus lesions	Incomplete combustion of organic fuels (e.g., vehicle exhaust, fire, heaters, charcoal), air pollution	CO binds to cytochrome a_3, >10% carboxyhemoglobin in blood Treatment: hyperbaric oxygenation
FISH, MARINE, AND FOOD TOXINS			
Ciguatera poisoning	GI upset, acute or subacute sensory disturbances (especially oral), vertigo, hypersalivation, blurred vision, tremor, ataxia, coma	Eating contaminated fish in coastal or tropical areas (especially barracuda, grouper, snapper, sea bass)	Affects calcium regulation of sodium channels, neurological symptoms may persist for months
Scombroid poisoning	Acute flushing, headache, dizziness, oral burning sensation, palpitations	Fish, including tuna, mackerel, jacks, dolphin, bluefish	Probable histamine-like toxin, recovery the rule
Paralytic shellfish poisoning (e.g., saxitoxin)	Acute oral and limb paresthesias, headache, vertigo, ataxia, cranial nerve dysfunction, paralysis, GI upset	Ingestion of contaminated bivalve mollusks (mussels, clams, oysters, scallops)	9% mortality, inhibition of sodium channels
Tetrodotoxin	Lethargy, paresthesias, vomiting, salivation, ataxia, weakness, dysphagia, respiratory paralysis	Puffer fish ingestion (Japan)	Blockade of voltage-dependent sodium channels

Table 29-8 (Continued).

Substance	Syndrome/symptoms	Source of exposure	Special features
Domoic acid	Seizures, confusion, delirium, amnesia	Contaminated mussels (epidemic in Prince Edward Island, Canada)	Glutamate analogue—excitotoxin
Lathyrus toxin (beta-*N*-oxalylamino-L-alanine)	Lathyrism: spastic paraparesis, pain, paresthesias	Chickpeas	Glutamate analogue—excitotoxin
Cyanide	Konzo: an acute spastic paraparesis found in Zaire	Improperly soaked cassava flour	—
BMAA (2-amino-3[methylamino]-propanoic acid)	Possibly responsible for ALS-parkinsonian-dementia complex of Guam	Cycad flour (*Cycas circinalis* seeds)	—
PHARMACOTHERAPEUTIC AGENTS			
Antiepileptics	Acute dose-related neurotoxicity: ataxia, blurred vision, diplopia, drowsiness, encephalopathy	All antiepileptics	—
	Diplopia, myoclonus	Carbamazepine	
	Choreoathetosis	Phenytoin	
	Chronic neurotoxicity		
	Peripheral neuropathy	Phenytoin	
	Cerebellar degeneration	Phenytoin	
	Encephalopathy	Phenytoin, valproic acid	
	Worsening seizures	Phenytoin, carbamazepine, clobazam	
	Tremor	Valproic acid, carbamazepine	
	Cognitive impairment	All agents	
Antimicrobials, antiviral agents	Seizures, encephalopathy	Penicillin (high-dose, especially with renal failure or cardiac bypass), ciprofloxacin, acyclovir	—
	Ototoxicity, vestibular toxicity, weakness	Aminoglycosides (e.g., streptomycin, gentamicin)	
	Peripheral neuropathy	Metronidazole, nitrofurantoin, INH (pyridoxine deficiency), sulfonamides	
	Optic neuropathy	Ethambutol	
	Retinal degeneration	Chloroquine	
	Pseudotumor cerebri	Tetracycline	
Antineoplastics	Peripheral neuropathy	Vincristine, vinblastine	—
	Ototoxicity, peripheral neuropathy	Cisplatin	

Table 29-8 (Continued).

Substance	Syndrome/symptoms	Source of exposure	Special features
	Encephalopathy, cerebellar syndrome	Cytarabine	
	Cerebellar syndrome	5-Fluorouracil	
	Encephalopathy, delayed leukoencephalopathy, chemical meningitis	Methotrexate given into CSF	
Immunosuppressants	Psychosis, euphoria, insomnia, myopathy	Corticosteroids	—
	Hallucinations, seizures, tremor, paresthesias	Cyclosporine	
Nonsteroidal antiinflammatory agents, etc.	Aseptic meningitis	Ibuprofen	—
	Confusion, headache, dizziness, encephalopathy	Indomethacin	
	Myopathy, neuropathy	Colchicine	
Antihypertensives	Headache, depression, nervousness	Calcium channel blockers	
	Neuropathy	Hydralazine	Due to pyridoxine deficiency
	Orthostatic hypotension	Several	
	Dizziness, confusion	Beta-blockers	
	Taste impairment, dizziness, headache, paresthesias	Captopril	
Antiparkinsonian agents	Acute confusion	Anticholinergics	—
	Hallucinations, confusion, orthostatic hypotension, involuntary movements	L-Dopa, bromocriptine, pergolide, amantadine	
Antipsychotics	Seizures	All phenothiazines and butyrophenones lower threshold	Clozapine particularly
	Extrapyramidal syndromes: akathisia, parkinsonism, acute dystonia, tardive dyskinesia	Most agents	
	Orthostatic hypotension	Phenothiazines	
Tricyclic and other antidepressants, lithium	Seizures, myoclonus	Especially tricyclics	—
	Peripheral neuropathy	Tricyclics	
	Encephalopathy, seizures, myoclonus, tremor, cerebellar syndrome	Lithium	
Miscellaneous	Optic neuropathy	Amiodarone	—

Table 29-8 (Continued).

Substance	Syndrome/symptoms	Source of exposure	Special features
	Loss of taste, polymyositis, myasthenic reaction, optic neuritis	Penicillamine	
	Confusion, dizziness, hallucinations with sudden withdrawal	Baclofen	

ICP = intracranial pressure; GI = gastrointestinal; ALS = amyotrophic lateral sclerosis.

Several categories of drugs produce prominent central or peripheral neurotoxic effects, and these are discussed in appropriate places throughout the text. The drugs most frequently implicated in the production of neurotoxic effects include the chemotherapeutic agents, antiepileptics, antiparkinsonian agents, antimicrobials, nonsteroidal antiinflammatory agents, antidepressants, and major and minor tranquilizers.

VITAMIN DEFICIENCIES

Vitamins are organic substances contained in natural foodstuffs and serve as important cofactors for various enzyme systems. Neurological disorders may arise as the result of both deficiencies and excesses of certain vitamins. Individual variability in the impact of vitamin deficiencies may be governed by genetic factors

Table 29-9. Neurological Complications Related to Vitamins

Vitamin	Neurological symptom/syndrome	Mechanism
DEFICIENCY		
B_1	Wernicke-Korsakoff, peripheral neuropathy, beriberi	Alcoholism, excessive vomiting (e.g., hyperemesis gravidarum), gastric plication, renal dialysis
B_6	Peripheral neuropathy, neonatal seizures	Starvation, INH, hereditary
Niacin	Pellagra: dementia, psychiatric syndromes, extrapyramidal or cerebellar deficits	Starvation, alcoholism
B_{12} (cobalamin)	Subacute combined degeneration of the spinal cord, peripheral sensory neuropathy, optic neuropathy (tobacco-alcohol amblyopia), dementia, ? neuropsychiatric symptoms	Pernicious anemia, strict vegetarianism, gastrectomy, gastric cancer, intestinal disorders
A	Night blindness, pseudotumor cerebri	Malabsorption
E	Peripheral neuropathy; spinocerebellar degeneration: weakness, ataxia, proprioceptive loss; ophthalmoplegia; impaired vision; myopathy	Malabsorption, Bassen-Kornzweig syndrome (vitamin E deficiency, retinitis pigmentosa, acanthocytosis, abetalipoproteinemia)
EXCESS		
B_6	Sensory neuronopathy: paresthesias, ataxia	Megavitamin self-medication
A	Pseudotumor cerebri	Self-administration, eating polar bear liver

as well as concurrent nutritional or toxic factors such as alcohol use. Early recognition of these syndromes is essential because generally early vitamin replacement therapy can reverse the effects. The main neurological and neuromuscular syndromes related to vitamins are summarized in Table 29-9.

BIBLIOGRAPHY

Pregnancy

General

Donaldson, J. O. (editor). Neurologic problems of pregnancy. *Semin. Neurol.* 8:181–246, 1988.

Donaldson, J. O. *Neurology of Pregnancy,* 2nd ed. London: Baillière Tindall, 1989.

Goldstein, P. J. (editor). *Neurological Disorders of Pregnancy.* Mount Kisco, NY: Futura, 1986.

Epilepsy

Dansky, L., et al. Anticonvulsants, folate levels and pregnancy outcome: a prospective study. *Ann. Neurol.* 21:176–182, 1987.

Delgado-Escueta, A. V., Janz, D., and Beck-Mannagetta, G. (editors). Pregnancy and teratogenesis in epilepsy. *Neurology* 42(suppl. 5):7–160, 1992.

Janz, D., et al (editors). *Epilepsy, Pregnancy and the Child.* New York: Raven, 1982.

Knight, A. H., and Rhind, E. G. Epilepsy and pregnancy: a study of 153 pregnancies in 59 patients. *Epilepsia* 16:99–110, 1975.

Ramsay, R. E., and Sanchez, R.M. Antiepileptic drugs, pregnancy and breast-feeding. *Merritt Putnam Q* 1:3–13, 1988.

Yerby, M. S. Problems and management of the pregnant woman with epilepsy. *Epilepsia* 28(suppl. 3):529–536, 1987.

Vascular Disease and Headaches

Digre, K. B., Varner, M. W., and Corbett, J. J. Pseudotumor cerebri and pregnancy. *Neurology* 34:721–729, 1984.

Guberman, A. Headache in pregnancy. *Med Clin. North Am.* 38:6842–6848, 1989.

Robinson, J. L., Christopherson, S. H., and Sedzimir, C. B. Arteriovenous malformations aneurysms and pregnancy. *J. Neurosurg.* 41:63–70, 1974.

Sommerville, B. W. A study of migraine in pregnancy. *Neurology* 22:824–828, 1972.

Stein, G. S. Headaches in the first postpartum week and their relationship to migraine. *Headache* 21:201–205, 1981.

Wiebers, D. O. Ischemic cerebrovascular complications of pregnancy. *Arch. Neurol.* 42:1106–1113, 1985.

Eclampsia/Toxemia

Beck, D. W., and Menezes, A. H. Intracerebral hemorrhage in a patient with eclampsia. *JAMA* 246:1442–1443, 1981.

Beeson, J. H., and Duda, E. E. Computed axial tomography scan demonstration of cerebral edema in eclampsia preceded by blindness. *Obstet. Gynecol.* 60:524–532, 1982.

Sheehan, H. L., and Lynch, J. B. *Pathology of Toxemia of Pregnancy.* Baltimore: Williams & Wilkins, 1973.

Will, A. D., et al. Cerebral vasoconstriction in toxemia. *Neurology* 37:1555–1557, 1987.

Peripheral and Cranial Neuropathies in Pregnancy and Postpartum

Gonzales, R. C., Gonzales-Cantu, N., and Rizzi-Hernandez, H. Recurrent polyneuropathy with pregnancy and oral contraceptives. *N. Engl. J. Med.* 282:1307–1308, 1970.

McCombe, P. A., et al. Chronic inflammatory demyelinating polyradiculoneuropathy associated with pregnancy. *Ann. Neurol.* 21:102–104, 1987.

McGregor, J. A., et al. Idiopathic facial nerve paralysis (Bell's palsy) in late pregnancy and he early puerperium. *Obstet. Gynecol.* 9:435–438, 1987.

chachter, S. C., and Ronthal, M. Intrapartum rachial plexus injury. *Arch. Neurol.* 9:673–674, 1982.

Chronic Neurological Diseases

Birk, K., and Rudick, R. Pregnancy and multiple sclerosis. *Arch. Neurol.* 43:719–726, 1986.

Jaffe, R., et al. Myotonic dystrophy and pregnancy: a review. *Obstet. Gynecol. Surv.* 41:272–278, 1986.

Levine, S. E., and Keesey, J. C. Successful plasmapheresis for fulminant myasthenia gravis during pregnancy. *Arch. Neurol.* 43:197–198, 1986.

Scheinberg, I. H., and Sternlieb, I. Pregnancy in penicillamine-treated patients with Wilson's disease. *N. Engl. J. Med.* 293:1300–1302, 1975.

Brain Tumors, Other Neurological Considerations, and Chronic Vegetative States

Fisher, R. G., et al. Metastatic cerebral choriocarcinoma without pelvic or pulmonary metastases. *Surg. Neurol.* 11:57–59, 1979.

Hill, L. M., Parker, D. P., and O'Neill, B. P. Management of maternal vegetative state during pregnancy. *Mayo Clin. Proc.* 60:469–472, 1985.

Roelvink, N. C. A., et al. Pregnancy-related primary brain and spinal tumors. *Arch. Neurol.* 44:209–215, 1987.

Hepatic Disease

Basile, A. S., et al. Elevated brain concentrations of 1,4 benzodiazepines in fulminant hepatic failure. *N. Engl. J. Med.* 325:473–478, 1991.

De Vivo, D. C. Reye syndrome. *Neurol. Clin.* 3:95–115, 1985.

Fraser, C. L., and Arieff, I. Hepatic encephalopathy. *N. Engl. J. Med.* 313:865–872, 1985.

Lockwood, A. H. Hepatic Encephalopathy and

Other Neurological Disorders Associated with Gastrointestinal Disease. In M. J. Aminoff (editor). *Neurology and General Medicine.* New York: Churchill Livingstone, 1989, Pp. 211–230.

Misra, P. Hepatic encephalopathy. *Med. Clin. North Am.* 65:209–226, 1981.

Rothstein, J. D., and Herlong, H.F. Neurologic manifestations of hepatic disease. *Neurol. Clin.* 7:563–578, 1989.

Renal Failure

Alfrey, A. C., LeGendre, G. R., and Kaehny, W. D. The dialysis encephalopathy syndrome. Possible aluminum intoxication. *N. Engl. J. Med.* 294:184–188, 1976.

Bruno, A., and Adams, H.P. Neurologic problems in renal transplant recipients. *Neurol. Clin.* 6:305–325, 1988.

Fraser, C. L., and Arieff, A. I. Nervous system complications in uremia. *Ann. Intern. Med.* 109:143–153, 1988.

Lockwood, A. H. Neurologic complications of renal disease. *Neurol. Clin.* 7:617–628, 1989.

Raskin, N. H., and Fishman, R. A. Neurologic disorders in renal failure. *N. Engl. J. Med.* 294:143–147, 204–210, 1976.

Raskin, N. H., and Fishman, R. A. Neurologic Aspects of Renal Failure. In M. J. Aminoff (editor). *Neurology and General Medicine.* New York: Churchill Livingstone, 1989, Pp. 231–246.

Systemic Cancer

Anderson, N. E., et al. Autoantibodies in paraneoplastic syndromes associated with small-cell lung cancer. *Neurology* 38:1391–1398, 1988.

Brennan, L. V., and Craddock, P. R. Limbic encephalopathy as a nonmetastatic complication of oat cell cancer: its reversal after treatment of the primary lung lesion. *Am. J. Med.* 75:518–520, 1983.

Chad, D. A., and Recht, L. D. Neuromuscular

complications of systemic cancer. *Neurol. Clin.* 9:901–918, 1991.

Dropcho, E. J. The remote effects of cancer on the nervous system. *Neurol. Clin.* 7:579–604, 1989.

Newsom-Davis, J., and Murray, N. M. F. Plasma exchange and immunosuppressive drug treatment in the Lambert-Eaton myasthenic syndrome. *Neurology* 34:480–485, 1984.

O'Neill, J. H., Murray, N.M.F., and Newsom-Davis, J. The Lambert-Eaton myasthenic syndrome. A review of 50 cases. *Brain* 111:577–596, 1988.

Posner, J. B. Paraneoplastic syndromes. *Neurol. Clin.* 9:919–936, 1991.

Rodriguez, M., et al. Autoimmune paraneoplastic cerebellar degeneration. Ultrastructural localization of antibody-binding sites in Purkinje cells. *Neurology* 38:1380–1386, 1988.

Sigurgeyirsson, B., et al. Risk of cancer in patients with dermatomyositis or polymyositis. A population-based study. *N. Engl. J. Med.* 326:363–367, 1992.

Steck, A. J., and Schluep, M. Neuromuscular Manifestations of Plasma Cell Dyscrasias. In S. H. Appel (editor). *Current Neurology.* Chicago: Mosby–Year Book, 1989, Vol. 9, Pp. 219–244.

Collagen Vascular Diseases and Vasculitis

Alexander, E. L., et al. Magnetic resonance imaging of cerebral lesions in patients with the Sjögren syndrome. *Ann. Intern. Med.* 108:815–823, 1988.

Bonfa, E., et al. Association between lupus psychosis and anti-ribosomal P protein antibodies. *N. Engl. J. Med.* 317:265–271, 1987.

Brick, J. E., and Brick, J. F. Neurologic manifestations of rheumatologic disease. *Neurol. Clin.* 7:629–640, 1989.

Davidson, R. C. Brainstem compression in rheumatoid arthritis. *JAMA* 238:2633–2634, 1977.

Devinsky, O., Petito, C. K., and Alonso, D. R. Clinical and neuropathological findings in systemic lupus erythematosus: the role of vasculitis, heart emboli and thrombotic thrombocytopenic purpura. *Ann. Neurol.* 23:380–384, 1988.

Harris, E. N., et al. Cerebral infarction in systemic lupus erythematosus: association with anticardiolipin antibodies. *Clin. Exp. Rheumatol.* 2:47–51, 1984.

Johnson, R. T., and Richardson, E. P. The neurological manifestations of systemic lupus erythematosus: a clinical-pathological study of 24 cases and review of the literature. *Medicine* 47:337–369, 1968.

Jongen, P. J. H., et al. Diffuse CNS involvement in systemic lupus erythematosus: intrathecal synthesis of the 4th component of complement. *Neurology* 40:1593–1596, 1990.

Kissel, J. T. Neurologic manifestations of vasculitis. *Neurol. Clin.* 7:655–674, 1989.

Malinow, K. L. Neuropsychiatric dysfunction in primary Sjögren's syndrome. *Ann. Intern. Med.* 103:344–349, 1985.

Moore, P. M., and Cupps, T. R. Neurological complications of vasculitis. *Ann. Neurol.* 14:155–167, 1983.

O'Connor, P. Diagnosis of central nervous system lupus. *Can. J. Neurol. Sci.* 15:257–260, 1988.

Shannon, K. M., and Goetz, C. G. Connective Tissue Diseases and the Nervous System. In M. J. Aminoff (editor). *Neurology and General Medicine.* New York: Churchill Livingstone, 1989, Pp. 389–412.

Sigal, L. H. The neurologic presentation of vasculitic and rheumatologic syndromes. A review. *Medicine* 66:157–180, 1987.

Steck, A. J. Antibodies in the neurologic clinic. *Neurology* 40:1489–1492, 1990.

Tsokos, G. C., et al. A clinical and pathologic study of cerebrovascular disease in patients with systemic lupus erythematosus. *Semin. Arthritis Rheumatol.* 16:70–78, 1986.

ndocrine Disease

abetes Mellitus

own, M. J., and Asbury, A. K. Diabetic neu-
pathy. *Ann. Neurol.* 15:2–12, 1984.

eene, D. A., Lattimer, S. A., and Sima, A.
F. Sorbitol, phosphoinositides and sodium-
tassium-ATPase in the pathogenesis of dia-
tic complications. *N. Engl. J. Med.*
6:599–605, 1987.

arati, Y. Diabetic Peripheral Neuropathies.
S. H. Appel (editor). *Current Neurology.*
icago: Mosby–Year Book, 1987, Vol. 7, Pp.
30.

alouf, R., and Brust, J. C. M. Hypoglycemia:
uses, neurological manifestations and out-
me. *Ann. Neurol.* 17:421–430, 1985.

izisin, A. P., and Powell, H. C. Diabetes and
urologic complications. *Curr. Opin. Neurol.
eurosurg.* 3:418–424, 1990.

aff, M. C., Sangalang, W., and Asbury, A. K.
chemic mononeuropathy multiplex associated
ith diabetes mellitus. *Arch. Neurol.*
:487–499, 1968.

aid, G., et al. Severe early-onset polyneurop-
hy in insulin-dependent diabetes mellitus. A
inical and pathological study. *N. Engl. J. Med.*
26:1257–1263, 1992.

/indebank, A. J., and McEvoy, K. M. Diabe-
es and the Nervous System. In M. J. Aminoff
editor). *Neurology and General Medicine.*
lew York: Churchill Livingstone, 1989, Pp.
73–304.

hyroid Disease

bend, W. K., and Tyler, H. R. Thyroid Dis-
ase and the Nervous System. In M. J. Aminoff
editor). *Neurology and General Medicine.*
lew York: Churchill Livingstone, 1989, Pp.
57–272.

Dresner, S. C., and Kennerdell, J. S. Dysthy-
oid orbitopathy. *Neurology* 35:1628–1634,
985.

Glaser, G. H. Neurological aspects of Thyroid
Disease. In W. B. Matthews and G. H. Glaser

(editors). *Recent Advances in Clinical Neurology—4.* Edinburgh: Churchill Livingstone,
1984, Pp. 141–158.

Kaminski, H. J., and Ruff, R. L. Neurologic
complications of endocrine diseases. *Neurol.
Clin.* 7:489–508, 1989.

Royce, P. C. Severely impaired consciousness
in myxedema—a review. *Am. J. Med. Sci.*
261:46–49, 1971.

Swanson, J. W., Kelly, J. J., Jr., and McCona-
hey, M. Neurologic aspects of thyroid dysfunction. *Mayo Clin. Proc.* 56:504–512, 1981.

Parathyroid Disease

Cogan, M. G., et al. Central nervous system
manifestations of hyperparathyroidism. *Am. J.
Med.* 65:963–970, 1978.

Guberman, A., and Jaworski, Z. F. G. Pseudo-
parathyroidism and epilepsy: diagnostic value
of computerized cranial tomography. *Epilepsia*
20:541–553, 1979.

Electrolyte Disorders

Arieff, A. I. Hyponatremia, convulsions, respiratory arrest and permanent brain damage after
elective surgery in healthy women. *N. Engl. J.
Med.* 314:1529–1535, 1986.

Berl, T. Treating hyponatremia: what is all the
controversy about? *Ann. Intern. Med.*
113:417–419, 1990.

Fraser, C. L., and Arieff, A. I. Symptomatic
hyponatremia: management and relation to
central pontine myelinolysis. *Semin. Neurol.*
4:445–452, 1984.

Howsky, B. P., and Laureno, R. Encephalopathy and myelinolysis after rapid correction of
hyponatremia. *Brain* 110:855–867, 1987.

Knochel, J. P. Neuromuscular manifestations
of electrolyte disorders. *Am. J. Med.*
72:521–535, 1982.

Layzer, R. B. *Neuromuscular Manifestations of
Systemic Disease.* Philadelphia: Davis, 1985.

Miller, G. M., et al. Central pontine myelinolysis and its imitators—MR findings. *Radiology* 168:795–802, 1988.

Riggs, J. Neurologic manifestations of fluid and electrolyte disturbances. *Neurol. Clin.* 7:509–524, 1989.

Sterns, R. H. Severe symptomatic hyponatremia: treatment and outcome—a study of 64 cases. *Ann. Intern. Med.* 107:656–664, 1987.

Hematological Disorders

Becker, D. M., and Kramer, S. The neurological manifestations of porphyria: a review. *Medicine* 56:411–423, 1977.

Brott, T. (editor). Neurologic complications of clotting disorders. *Semin. Neurol.* 11:305–418, 1991.

Davies-Jones, G. A. B. Neurological Manifestations of Hematological Disorders. In M. J. Aminoff (editor). *Neurology and General Medicine.* New York: Churchill Livingstone, 1989, Pp. 187–210.

Massey, E. W., and Riggs, J. E. Neurologic manifestations of hematologic disease. *Neurol. Clin.* 7:544–562, 1989.

Samuels, M. A. Neurologic Aspects of Hematologic Disease. In S. H. Appel (editor). *Current Neurology.* St Louis: Mosby–Year Book, 1992, Vol. 12, Pp. 215–240.

Miscellaneous Medical Conditions

Chen, J. R., et al. Neurologic disturbances in Paget disease of bone: response to calcitonin. *Neurology* 29:448–457, 1979.

Jones, H. R., Jr., and Siekert, R. G. Neurological manifestations of infective endocarditis. *Brain* 112:1295–1315, 1989.

Moore, P. M., Harley, J. B., and Fauci, A. S. Neurologic dysfunction in the idiopathic hypereosinophilic syndrome. *Ann. Intern. Med.* 102:109–114, 1985.

Alcohol Abuse

Carlen, P. L. Alcoholic brain disease and the Wernicke-Korsakoff syndrome. *Curr. Opinion Neurol. Neurosurg.* 1:372–376, 1988.

Carlen, P. L., Wartzman, G., and Holgate, C. Reversible cerebral atrophy in recently abstinent chronic alcoholics measured by CT scan. *Science* 200:1076–1078, 1978.

Chan, A. W. K. Alcoholism and epilepsy. *Epilepsia* 26:323–333, 1985.

Charness, M. E., and Diamond, I. Alcohol and the Nervous System. In S. H. Appel (editor) *Current Neurology.* New York: Wiley, 198 Vol. 5, Pp. 383–422.

Charness, M. E., Simon, R. P., and Greenberg, D. A. Ethanol and the nervous system. *N. Engl. J. Med.* 321:442–454, 1989.

Gorelick, P. V. Alcohol and stroke. *Stroke* 18:268–271, 1987.

Lang, A. E., et al. Alcohol and Parkinson disease. *Ann. Neurol.* 12:254–256, 1982.

Messing, R. O., and Greenberg, D. A. Alcohol and the Nervous System. In M. J. Aminoff (editor). *Neurology and General Medicine* New York: Churchill Livingstone, 1989, Pp 533–548.

Neiman, J., et al. Movement disorders in alcoholism: a review. *Neurology* 40:741–746, 1990.

Reuler, J. B., Girard, D. E., and Cooney, T. G. Wernicke's encephalopathy. *N. Engl. J. Med.* 312:1035–1039, 1985.

Sellers, E. M. Alcohol, barbiturate and benzodiazepine withdrawal syndromes: clinical management. *Can. Med. Assoc. J.* 139:113–118 1988.

Victor, M., Adams, R. D., and Collins, G. H. *The Wernicke-Korsakoff Syndrome and Related Neurologic Disorders due to Alcoholism and Malnutrition* (Contemporary Neurology series Vol. 3). Philadelphia: Davis, 1989.

Drug and Substance Abuse

Cregler, L. L., and Mark, H. Medical complications of cocaine abuse. *N. Engl. J. Med.* 315:1495–1500, 1986.

Korobkin, R., et al. Glue-sniffing neuropathy. *Arch. Neurol.* 32:158–162, 1975.

vine, S. R., et al. Cerebrovascular complications of the use of the "crack" form of alkaloidal cocaine. *N. Engl. J. Med.* 323:699–704, 1990.

ody, C. K., et al. Neurologic complications of cocaine abuse. *Neurology* 38:1189–1193, 1988.

icaurte, G. A., and Langston, J. W. Neurological complications of substance abuse. In M.J. Aminoff (editor). *Neurology and General Medicine.* New York: Churchill Livingstone, 1989, Pp. 549–558.

Roth, D. R., et al. Acute rhabdomyolysis associated with cocaine intoxication. *N. Engl. J. Med.* 319:673–677, 1988.

Environmental and Other Toxins

Burkhart, K. K., and Kulig, K. W. The other alcohols: methanol, ethylene glycol and isopropanolol. *Emerg. Med. Clin. North Am.* 8:913–928, 1990.

Eastaugh, J., and Shepherd, S. Infectious and toxic syndrome from fish and shellfish consumption. *Arch. Intern. Med.* 149:1735–1740, 1989.

Feldman, R. G. Effects of Toxins and Physical Agents on the Nervous System. In W.G. Bradley, et al. (editors). *Neurology in Clinical Practice.* Boston: Butterworth-Heinemann, 1991, Pp. 1185–1209.

Macdonald, D. R. Neurologic complications of chemotherapy. *Neurol. Clin.* 9:955–968, 1991.

Mallya, K. B., Mendis, T., and Guberman, A. Bilateral facial paralysis following ethylene glycol ingestion. *Can. J. Neurol. Sci.* 13:340–341, 1986.

Moen, B. E. Environmental and occupational toxins. *Curr. Opinion Neurol. Neurosurg.* 4:442–446, 1991.

Perl, T. M., et al. An outbreak of toxic encephalopathy caused by eating mussels contaminated with domoic acid. *N. Engl. J. Med.* 322:1775–1787, 1990.

Richter, R. W., and Corder, C. N. Neurotoxic Syndromes. In R.R. Rosenberg (editor). *Comprehensive Neurology.* New York: Raven, 1991, Pp. 845–885.

Schaumburg, H. H., and Spencer, P. S. Recognizing neurotoxic disease. *Neurology* 37:276–278, 1987.

Spencer, P. S., and Schaumburg, H. H. An expanded classification of neurotoxic responses based on cellular targets of chemical agents. *Acta Neurol. Scand.* 100(suppl.):9–19, 1984.

Teitelbaum, J. S., et al. Neurologic sequelae of domoic acid intoxication due to the ingestion of contaminated mussels. *N. Engl. J. Med.* 322:1781–1787, 1990.

Vitamin Deficiencies

Lindenbaum, J., et al. Neuropsychiatric disorders caused by cobalamin deficiency in the absence of anemia or macrocytosis. *N. Engl. J. Med.* 318:1720–1728, 1988.

Mancall, E. Nutritional Disorders of the Nervous System. In M. J. Aminoff (editor). *Neurology and General Medicine.* New York: Churchill Livingstone, 1989, Pp. 323–340.

Satya-Murti, S., et al. The spectrum of neurologic disorders from vitamin E deficiency. *Neurology* 36:917–921, 1986.

Schaumburg, H. H., et al. Sensory neuropathy from pyridoxine abuse. *N. Engl. J. Med.* 309:445–448, 1983.

So, Y. T., and Simon, R. P. Deficiency Diseases of the Nervous System. In W. G. Bradley, et al. (editors). *Neurology in Clinical Practice.* Boston: Butterworth-Heinemann, 1991, Pp. 1167–1184.

ndex

Note: Page numbers in italics indicate illustrations; those followed by *t* indicate tables.